# Hospitalist Neurology

Blue Books of Practical Neurology
*(Volumes 1–14 published as BIMR Neurology)*

# Hospitalist Neurology

Edited by

**Martin A. Samuels, M.D.**
Professor of Neurology, Harvard Medical School, Boston;
Neurologist-in-Chief, Brigham and Women's Hospital, Boston

with 40 Contributors

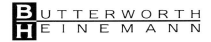

Boston    Oxford    Auckland    Johannesburg    Melbourne    New Delhi

**Library of Congress Cataloging-in-Publication Data**
Hospitalist neurology / edited by Martin A. Samuels.
        p.   cm. -- (Blue books of practical neurology  ;  20)
     Includes bibliographical references and index.
     ISBN 0-7506-9779-2
     1. Nervous system--Diseases--Diagnosis.  2. Medical consultation.
  3. Nervous system--Diseases--Hospitals.  I. Samuels, Martin A.
  II. Series.
     [DNLM: 1. Diagnostic Techniques, Neurological.  2. Nervous System
  Diseases--therapy.  3. Neurologic Examination.  WL 141 H828 1999 /
  W1 BU9749 v.20 1999]
  RC348.H62    1999
  616.8--DC21
  DNLM/DLC
  for Library of Congress                                          98-46555
                                                                        CIP


**British Library Cataloguing-in-Publication Data**
A catalogue record for this book is available from the British Library.

The publisher offers special discounts on bulk orders of this book.
For information, please contact:
Manager of Special Sales
Butterworth–Heinemann
225 Wildwood Avenue
Woburn, MA 01801-2041
Tel: 781-904-2500
Fax: 781-904-2620

For information on all Butterworth–Heinemann publications available,
contact our World Wide Web home page at: http://www.bh.com

10 9 8 7 6 5 4 3 2 1

Printed in the United States of America

# Contents

# Contributing Authors

*Peter R. Bergethon, M.D.*
Director, Symmetry Research, Sherborn, Massachusetts

*James L. Bernat, M.D.*
Professor of Medicine (Neurology), Dartmouth Medical School, Hanover, New Hampshire; Attending Neurologist, Dartmouth-Hitchcock Medical Center, Lebanon, New Hampshire

*Charles F. Bolton, M.D., F.R.C.P.C.*
Professor Emeritus of Neurology, University of Western Ontario Faculty of Medicine, London, Ontario; Consultant Neurologist, London Health Sciences Centre, London, Ontario

*Jon Brillman, M.D., F.R.C.P.I.*
Professor of Neurology, Allegheny University of the Health Sciences, Pittsburgh; Chairman of Neurology, Allegheny General Hospital, Pittsburgh

*Edward B. Bromfield, M.D.*
Assistant Professor of Neurology, Harvard Medical School, Boston; Director of Electroencephalography and Epilepsy, Brigham and Women's Hospital, Boston

*John C.M. Brust, M.D.*
Professor of Clinical Neurology, Columbia University College of Physicians and Surgeons, New York; Director of Neurology, Harlem Hospital Center, New York

*John J. Caronna, M.D.*
Professor and Vice-Chairman of Clinical Neurology, Weill Medical College of Cornell University, New York; Attending Neurologist, The New York Hospital–Cornell Medical Center, New York

*Michael B. Chancellor, M.D.*
Associate Professor of Urologic Surgery, University of Pittsburgh School of Medicine

*Raymond Tak Fai Cheung, M.B., B.S., Ph.D.*
Associate Professor of Medicine, The University of Hong Kong; Consultant Neurologist, Tung Wah Hospital and Queen Mary Hospital, Hong Kong

*Lisa M. DeAngelis, M.D.*
Professor of Neurology, Weill Medical College of Cornell University, New York; Chairman of Neurology, Memorial Sloan-Kettering Cancer Center, New York

*Adré J. du Plessis, M.B.Ch.B., M.P.H.*
Assistant Professor of Neurology, Harvard Medical School, Boston; Assistant in Neurology, Children's Hospital, Boston

*John Edmeads, M.D.*
Professor of Medicine (Neurology), University of Toronto Faculty of Medicine; Physician-in-Chief, Sunnybrook Health Science Centre, Toronto

*Mustapha Ezzeddine, M.D.*
Fellow, Neurointensive Care and Stroke, Department of Neurology, Massachusetts General Hospital, Boston

*Edward Feldmann, M.D.*
Associate Professor of Neurology, Brown University School of Medicine, Providence, Rhode Island

*Steven K. Feske, M.D.*
Assistant Professor of Neurology, Harvard Medical School, Boston; Director, Stroke Division, Brigham and Women's Hospital, Boston

*Vladimir Hachinski, M.D., F.R.C.P.C., M.Sc.(D.M.E.), D.Sc.(Med)*
Richard and Beryl Ivey Professor and Chair, Department of Clinical Neurological Sciences, University of Western Ontario Faculty of Medicine, London, Ontario; Chief of Clinical Neurological Sciences, London Health Sciences Centre, London, Ontario

*Frances Jensen, M.D.*
Associate Professor of Neurology, Harvard Medical School, Boston; Neurologist, Brigham and Women's Hospital and Children's Hospital, Boston

*Igor J. Koralnik, M.D.*
Assistant Professor of Neurology, Harvard Medical School, Boston; Director, Human Immunodeficiency Virus/Neurology Center, Beth Israel Deaconess Medical Center, Boston

*Walter J. Koroshetz, M.D.*
Associate Professor of Neurology, Harvard Medical School, Boston; Medical Director, Neurointensive Care, Neurology Service, Massachusetts General Hospital, Boston

*Kalpathy S. Krishnamoorthy, M.D.*
Assistant Professor of Pediatrics and Neurology, Harvard Medical School, Boston; Associate Neurologist and Associate Pediatrician, Massachusetts General Hospital, Boston

*Jerome E. Kurent, M.D., M.P.H.*
Associate Professor of Neurology and Medicine, Medical University of South Carolina, Charleston; Acting Director of the Center for the Study of Aging and Interim Medical Director for Quality, Medical University of South Carolina Medical Center, Charleston

*Robert Laureno, M.D.*
Professor of Neurology, George Washington University School of Medicine and Health Sciences, Washington, D.C.; Chairman of Neurology, Washington Hospital Center, Washington, D.C.

*Steven Mandel, M.D.*
Clinical Professor of Neurology, Jefferson Medical College of Thomas Jefferson University, Philadelphia

*Ramon Mañon-Espaillat, M.D.*
Clinical Professor of Neurology, Jefferson Medical College of Thomas Jefferson University, Philadelphia

*Patricia M. Moore, M.D.*
Professor of Neurology, University of Pittsburgh School of Medicine

*Kenneth K. Nakano, M.D., M.P.H., S.M., F.R.C.P.C.*
Neurologist, Straub Clinic and Hospital, Honolulu

*Roy A. Patchell, M.D.*
Associate Professor of Neurosurgery, University of Kentucky College of Medicine, Lexington; Chief of Neuro-Oncology, University of Kentucky A.B. Chandler Medical Center, Lexington

*Dawn M. Pearson, M.D.*
Fellow in Neurology, Division of Behavioral Neurology, Beth Israel Deaconess Medical Center, and Harvard Medical School, Boston

*Jonathan H. Pincus, M.D.*
Professor of Neurology and Chairman Emeritus, Georgetown University School of Medicine, Washington, D.C.; Attending Neurologist, Georgetown University Hospital, Washington, D.C.

*Misha Pless, M.D.*
Assistant Professor of Ophthalmology and Neurology, University of Pittsburgh School of Medicine; Director of Neuro-Ophthalmology, University of Pittsburgh Medical Center

*Bruce H. Price, M.D.*
Assistant Professor of Neurology, Harvard Medical School, Boston; Chief of Neurology, McLean Hospital, Belmont, Massachusetts; Assistant in Neurology, Massachusetts General Hospital, Boston

*David A. Rivas, M.D.*
Assistant Professor of Urology, Jefferson Medical College of Thomas Jefferson University, Philadelphia; Attending Physician, Department of Urology, Thomas Jefferson University Hospital, Philadelphia

*Lawrence Rodichok, M.D.*
Chief of Neurology, Central Pennsylvania NeuroCenter, Lancaster General Hospital, Lancaster

*Garfield B. Russell, M.D.*
Professor of Anesthesia, Pennsylvania State University College of Medicine, Hershey; Director, Neuroanesthesia and Intraoperative Neurophysiological Monitoring, Milton S. Hershey Medical Center, Pennsylvania State Geisinger Health System, Hershey

*Thomas D. Sabin, M.D.*
Clinical Professor and Vice-Chairman, Department of Neurology, Tufts University School of Medicine, Boston; Lecturer on Neurology, Harvard Medical School, Boston

*Nasrollah Samiy, M.D.*
Vitreo-Retinal Services, Carolina Eye Associates, Charlotte, North Carolina

*Martin A. Samuels, M.D.*
Professor of Neurology, Harvard Medical School, Boston; Neurologist-in-Chief, Brigham and Women's Hospital, Boston

*S. Clifford Schold, Jr., M.D.*
Professor and Chair of Neurology, University of Texas Southwestern Medical Center at Dallas

*Albert Pall Sigurdsson, M.D.*
Stroke Fellow, Department of Neurology, Brown University School of Medicine and Rhode Island Hospital, Providence

*Joerg-Patrick Stübgen, M.D., F.R.C.P.C.*
Assistant Professor of Neurology and Neuroscience, Weill Medical College of Cornell University, New York; Assistant Attending Neurologist and Neurologist for Intensive Care Unit, The New York Hospital–Cornell Medical Center and Hospital for Special Surgery, New York

*G. Bryan Young, M.D., F.R.C.P.C.*
Professor of Clinical Neurological Sciences, University of Western Ontario Faculty of Medicine, London, Ontario; Director of Electroencephalography Laboratory, London Health Sciences Centre, London, Ontario

# Series Preface

The *Blue Books of Practical Neurology* series is the new name for the *BIMR Neurology* series, which was itself the successor of the *Modern Trends in Neurology* series. As before, the volumes are intended for use by physicians who grapple with the problems of neurological disorders on a daily basis, be they neurologists, neurologists in training, or those in related fields such as neurosurgery, internal medicine, psychiatry, and rehabilitation medicine.

Our purpose is to produce monographs on topics in clinical neurology in which progress through research has brought about new concepts of patient management. The subject of each monograph is selected by the Series Editors using two criteria: first, that there has been significant advance in knowledge in that area and, second, that such advances have been incorporated into new ways of managing patients with the disorders in question. This has been the guiding spirit behind each volume, and we expect it to continue. In effect we emphasize research, both in the clinic and in the experimental laboratory, but principally to the extent that it changes our collective attitudes and practices in caring for those who are neurologically afflicted.

C. David Marsden
Arthur K. Asbury
*Series Editors*

# Preface

Medical care is undoubtedly changing. Although the rate of penetration of managed care into the health care marketplace is somewhat slower than predicted by many pundits, the forces of cost-effectiveness nonetheless continue to alter the way in which physicians practice. As the economic cycle inevitably turns down, the rate of change will probably increase as large companies feel more financial pressure to offer less expensive health care insurance to their employees.

To avoid the perception of rationing care, a concept that is anathema to Americans, society has chosen an approach based on enhancing the number and status of so-called gate-keepers who are primary care physicians consisting mainly of internists, family physicians, pediatricians, and some gynecologists. These busy practitioners are given strong incentives to reduce the number and length of hospitalizations by emphasizing ambulatory evaluation and procedures. Driven by these forces, many traditional hospitals have merged and developed networks of affiliated primary care providers to offer the consumer a full-service, soup-to-nuts, cradle-to-grave system of health care. At the core of these networks still lie more or less recognizable hospitals filled to overflowing with more acutely ill patients requiring a pace of evaluation unprecedented anywhere in the world.

Paradoxically in this era of the primary care physician, circumstances have spawned a new specialist known as the *hospitalist*. These physicians and surgeons spend all of their time in the hospital, where they are capable of meeting current demands for speed and efficiency that the army of gate-keepers can no longer provide given their heavy load and emphasis on less acute ambulatory medicine.

In this context, the hospitalist is frequently faced with a dizzying array of neurologic problems in patients who are not under the primary care of a neurologist. In 20 years of experience working in a general hospital as a neurologist and internist, I have been struck by the difference between these patients and those with traditional neurologic problems who are hospitalized on a standard neurology service. The hospitalist, whether he or she be a neurologist, internist, emergency physician, or surgeon, has an urgent need to recognize, diagnose, and treat neurologic problems that arise in his or her patients. It was out of this practical need that this book arose.

The text is organized to reflect the organizational scheme of a modern hospital. When asked to consult on a patient in the hospital, the consultant faces problems that are more or less specific to the service where the patient resides. By thinking about the problems in this way, the consulting physician can reduce the enormous number of possible diagnoses to a manageable few commonly encountered in each clinical context. The book is meant to provide consulting hospitalists a rational approach to evaluating neurologic problems in a busy general hospital.

I am indebted to Susan Pioli, Director of Medical Publishing at Butterworth–Heinemann, for crystallizing the idea for this project and for her patience and wisdom during its preparation. Leslie Kramer, also of Butterworth–Heinemann, provided invaluable editorial and organizational skills, without which this project could never have been completed. I also thank Carole Warkel for her tireless, cheerful, and skilled efforts in assembling the manuscript and Kim Langford, of Silverchair Science + Communications, who produced the final product painlessly and in record time.

*MAS*

# Hospitalist Neurology

# ONE

## MAJOR NEUROLOGIC ISSUES FACED BY THE CONSULTING NEUROLOGIST

# I
# SYMPTOMS

# 1
# Headache

John Edmeads

Headaches occur in the hospitalized patient in three general contexts:

1. The disease that has led the patient to hospitalization has produced headache as one of its symptoms.
2. A diagnostic or therapeutic intervention in the hospital has caused headache.
3. The patient may bring benign dysfunctional headaches, such as migraine or tension-type headaches into hospital or, much less commonly, develop them for the first time in the hospital.

An obvious example of headache occurrence within the first context is a patient in the respiratory service who has chronic obstructive pulmonary disease (COPD) with carbon dioxide retention and hypoxia, with headaches due to cerebral vasodilatation. Less obvious is the patient in the oncology ward with multiple myeloma, whose headache may be the result of hypercalcemia or hyperviscosity, or both. Typically, as in the case of the respirologist caring for the patient with COPD, the attending physician is well aware that the headache is a result of the lung disease and requires the help of the neurologic consultant simply to confirm this, to exclude other causes, and to collaborate in the management of the headache. Sometimes, the relationship between the headache and the admitting disease is far from evident to the attending physician; the neurologist, by raising the possibility that headache in the myeloma patient may be due to unrecognized hyperviscosity, may expedite the diagnosis and treatment of this complication.

Examples within the second context are headache after lumbar puncture, carotid endarterectomy, and antibiotic treatment. Some of these headaches, such as postpuncture headache, are immediately obvious to the attending physician; the consultant's usefulness is again simply to confirm the diagnosis, exclude other causes, and assist with the treatment of the headache. Often, however, the attending staff can be puzzled by the headache. Not all gastroenterologists know, for example, that ranitidine and some other $H_2$ blockers can be potent causes of headache in some patients, and not all rheumatologists are aware that some nonsteroidal anti-inflammatory drugs (NSAIDs) can produce intracranial hypertension with

5

intractable headache. The neurologist's consultation in the gastrointestinal (GI) service can promptly relieve headache and, in the rheumatology service, may prevent serious, permanent neurologic disability such as blindness.

Within the third context, diagnosis is seldom a problem. The difficult task of the consulting neurologist here is to treat the benign headache within the context of the considerable limitations imposed by the disease that has hospitalized the patient. How does one treat an acute attack of severe migraine in a depressed patient being withdrawn from narcotics in the psychiatry service, for example, in which the antidepressant medications militate against serotonergic agents and the situation renders narcotic analgesics illogical? What treatment can be offered safely to the patient with cluster headaches who has just been admitted to the coronary unit with an acute myocardial infarct?

In this chapter, we proceed on neurology consultation rounds through the inpatient services of a general hospital. For each service we discuss the following:

- Those diseases likely to be found on that service that can cause headache as a symptom severe enough to call for a neurologic consultation; and the management of that headache in the context of the causative disease
- The diagnostic and therapeutic procedures (including medications) usually performed on that service that may result in headaches; and the management of those headaches
- The management of benign dysfunctional headaches that the patient has either "imported" into the hospital or, much less commonly, developed for the first time in the hospital

## ONCOLOGY SERVICE

### Headache Caused by Oncologic Diseases or Their Complications

In one major cancer center, headache was the third most common reason for referring patients with systemic cancer to a neurologist [1]: 18% had back pain, 17% had alteration of mental status, and 15% had headaches. Of these patients with headache, 30% of their headaches were related to brain or skull base tumor metastases, and 60% had such "nonstructural" causes as tension-type headache, migraine, or headaches associated with fever and sepsis. Just as only a minority of headaches in cancer patients are due to brain tumors, so it is that only a minority of brain tumor patients present with headaches [2]. Children are more likely than adults to develop headaches from brain tumors because these headaches tend to be located in the posterior fossa, where mass lesions can readily produce increased intracranial pressure. In adults, in whom most brain tumors are located in the cerebral hemispheres, seizures, weakness, and altered mental state are more common early manifestations. When headaches do occur in these adult patients, they tend not to exhibit the textbook characteristics: more prevalent in the early morning, worse with straining or the head-low position, and accompanied by vomiting [3]. These headaches are, in fact, nondescript. Their relationship to brain metastases is suggested by their recent onset in patients who (usually) are middle-aged or older, by their failure to conform to diagnostic criteria (such as those of the International Headache Society [4]) for benign dysfunctional headaches and by their association (usually) with abnormalities of the neurologic examination. Contrast-enhanced computed tomographic (CT) scans or magnetic resonance imaging (MRI) remove any doubt. Treatment of headaches of brain metastases is, of course, that of the metastases themselves (e.g., radiation or surgery), but short-term relief can be obtained from systemic corticosteroids such as dexamethasone, 4 mg q6h intramuscularly, to relieve perilesional edema and increased intracranial pressure, and from analgesics.

The headache of *meningeal carcinomatosis* occurs in about one-half of patients as the first manifestation of systemic cancer. These cases are more likely to present to primary care physicians than to oncologists. In the other half of patients with meningeal carcinomatosis, the systemic cancer (typically breast, bronchus, gut, or melanoma) is known to be present, sometimes for months to years. The headache typically runs a course of several weeks (if the condition is untreated). It is most often diffuse, progressive, and severe, and is often accompanied by other symptoms. Associated features of this headache may include decreasing consciousness, cranial nerve palsies, papilledema, diabetes insipidus, meningeal irritation, vomiting, and back pain. The diagnosis is made suspect by clinical findings and by the appearance of enhancing meninges on MRI; it is confirmed by cytologic examination of the cerebrospinal fluid (CSF). Treatment of the headache is that of the meningeal carcinomatosis—irradiation and chemotherapy—and the prognosis is bad.

Although not usually described as headache, pain in the angle of the jaw or in the ear may occur as a manifestation of a mediastinal tumor, usually lung carcinoma, that irritates pain fibers in the ipsilateral vagus nerve. Treatment of the pain is that of the tumor.

Cancer patients are prone to develop hypercoagulable states that may cause headaches should they result in *intracranial venous thrombosis*. There may not be associated symptoms or signs, particularly early in the course. A new headache, progressively worsening in a cancer patient, should indicate an MRI of the intracranial venous channels; if this is unavailable, cerebral angiography with venous phase studies can make the diagnosis. Later in its course, with the advent of increased intracranial pressure with papilledema and of venous cortical infarcts with seizures and neurologic deficits, the diagnosis is more apparent.

Partial or complete *obstruction of the superior vena cava*, usually by extrinsic compression from a mediastinal tumor but sometimes by thrombosis from a subclavian line being used to deliver chemotherapy, can produce progressive venous engorgement of the head, neck, arms, and upper trunk. Symptoms include worsening headache, cough, dyspnea, and hoarseness; the physical signs are those of congestion. Death can occur from airway obstruction, increased intracranial pressure, or cerebral hemorrhage. The extent of the obstruction can be assessed by contrast-enhanced CT scan or MRI of the thorax, neck, and head and by transbrachial venography. Treatment is usually directed by the oncology service and may include thrombolysis, anticoagulation, irradiation, chemotherapy, and corticosteroids for brain and laryngeal edema.

*Hyperviscosity* states, such as may occur in myeloma, and *polycythemia* and *thrombocytosis* occurring in hematologic malignancies may present with headaches due either vascular congestion or frank venous occlusion. *Thrombocytopenia*, which may result from marrow invasion by cancer cells or from chemotherapy, can produce headaches from intracranial bleeding, which is usually not difficult to diagnose. Occasionally, the thrombocytopenia of idiopathic thrombocytopenic purpura (ITP) or systemic lupus erythematosus (SLE) may produce recurrent headaches that resemble migraine [5] but this has not been reported in the thrombocytopenia of malignancy.

Infections of the brain and meninges are not a frequent complication of malignancy, but can be seen especially in patients with leukemia and lymphoma. Often, in these very ill patients, the symptoms and signs of meningitis and cerebritis are subtle; headache is not severe, meningeal irritation is not marked and fever is low-grade or absent [6]. A high index of suspicion is often a prerequisite to diagnosis.

## Headache Caused by Oncologic Diagnostic and Therapeutic Measures

Radiotherapy to the brain (for tumors) may produce symptoms in three time frames: (1) acute reactions that occur during the course of treatment (and thus are most likely to be seen by the hospital neurologic consultant), (2) early delayed reactions that occur a few weeks to a few months after radiotherapy, and (3) late delayed reactions that occur several months to a few years after treatment. Only in the acute reactions are headaches a symptom. These acute reactions are quite uncommon with dose-fractionation protocols that employ small doses (e.g., 200 cGy per day) given frequently (e.g., 5 days per week, for a total of 6,000 cGy). With larger doses over a shorter period (e.g., 750 cGy per day for 2 days), acute reactions are much more frequent, occurring in up to 50% of cases. The symptoms are likely caused by radiation-induced vasogenic edema, and include headache, nausea, and vomiting. Such symptoms respond well to systemic corticosteroids [7].

*Chemotherapeutic agents*, like any other medication, may cause headaches as a nonspecific adverse event, but this is seldom a problem. In some circumstances, however, chemotherapy may bring about severe headaches.

Methotrexate, given intrathecally either for prophylaxis in acute leukemia or for the treatment of meningeal metastases, can produce acute aseptic meningitis that presents as headache, stiff neck, nausea, vomiting, fever, and CSF pleocytosis; treatment is symptomatic and may involve the administration of systemic corticosteroid. Methotrexate given intrathecally in tandem with craniospinal irradiation for the treatment of acute leukemia may, after some months, produce a severe encephalopathy characterized by stupor, focal signs, and seizures, often ending in death. Milder cases, especially in children, may present with headache, nausea, and lethargy, sometimes culminating in intellectual deficit. These milder cases may present earlier, sometimes shortly after receiving combined therapy.

## Benign Dysfunctional Headaches in Cancer Patients

Patients with cancer may continue to have the same migraine they experienced before developing their malignancy, but sometimes the cancer, or the treatment for it, may appear to change the migraine pattern. In one study [8] of migraine in cancer, fully 63% did not have their first attack until receiving chemotherapy or radiotherapy; 26% had their first attack before chemotherapy or radiotherapy; and 11% never had chemotherapy or radiotherapy. Those migraineurs who had received chemotherapy had a high incidence (31%, or approximately 10 times normal) of recurrent migraine auras without accompanying headaches.

Treatment of migraine in the cancer patient may raise special problems in terms of associated liver disease, cachexia, and other conditions that indicate special precautions when using some antimigraine medications.


## NEPHROLOGY SERVICE

### Headache Caused by Kidney Diseases or Their Complications

Headache is not a common or prominent symptom of acute or chronic renal failure, possibly because the main neurologic feature of uremic encephalopathy, drowsiness, inhibits complaining. It is more likely, however, because it is truly uncommon. Rarely, people with *uremia* complain of diffuse and sometimes throbbing headaches that ease after dialysis or transplantation.

When *hyponatremia* complicates renal disease, it may, in its early stages, produce headache, likely through the agency of cerebral edema and increased intracranial pressure. As the hyponatremic encephalopathy worsens, such other features as impaired cognition and diminishing consciousness emerge, obscuring the headache.


### Headache Caused by the Treatment of Kidney Disease

In some institutions, about half the patients undergoing *hemodialysis* have recurrent headaches associated with the procedure. Typically, the headache appears in isolation, but rarely may present as part of a full-blown "dialysis dysequilibrium syndrome" with nausea, vomiting, irritability, confusion, obtundation, and even seizures. During dialysis, water may shift into the brain, causing cerebral edema, especially if the dialysis is overly vigorous. Thus, headaches tend to occur toward the end of a dialysis or even after its completion, and persist for several hours until osmotic equilibrium between the brain and the systemic compartment is reestablished. Headaches are more likely to occur in headache-prone individuals, especially migraineurs, and may loosely mimic the migraine. Almost always, they can be prevented by using shorter dialysis times at more frequent intervals.

Renal transplantation itself is not associated with headaches, but late complications, such as the *CNS infections* or *lymphomas* that arise from prolonged immunosuppression, may present with head pain.


### Benign Dysfunctional Headaches in Renal Patients

Many of the medications used for the treatment of headaches, such as NSAIDs, beta blockers, ergotamine, and sumatriptan, are either metabolized or excreted by the kidney. Their use in patients with renal failure is thus decidedly problematic.

The reverse problem can occur when easily dialyzable drugs such as the salicylates are prematurely flushed from the pained person's plasma during dialysis. Sometimes, only consultation among the neurologist, nephrologist, and pharmacologist can resolve these situations.

## HEMATOLOGY SERVICE

### Headache Caused by Hematologic Diseases or Their Complications

Severe *anemia* from any cause may produce headache through cerebral vasodilatation, which, by increasing cerebral blood flow, attempts to compensate for the diminished oxygen-carrying capacity of the blood. The degree of anemia necessary to produce headache is variable, though, as a rule, hemoglobin levels lower than 8 g/dl are necessary. The headache tends to be diffuse, throbbing, and aggravated by exertion. It may be associated with other neurologic symptoms of severe anemia, including faintness, postural giddiness, and tinnitus. Certain types of anemia may rarely produce special types of headache. Iron deficiency anemia has been found in a few cases to be associated with the syndrome of benign intracranial hypertension (BIH) [9], and a syndrome of frontal headache, proptosis, and lid edema due to infarction of the orbital bones has been described in sickle cell disease [10].

*Polycythemia*, whether primary or secondary, may paradoxically produce the same kind of diffuse throbbing headaches as severe anemia, probably because of the passive cerebral vasodilatation resulting from increased blood volume and viscosity. As with anemia, the headaches of polycythemia may be accompanied by faintness, postural giddiness, and tinnitus. If intravascular stasis results in brain infarction, then a more lateralized headache may supervene, in association with a neurologic deficit or with signs of increased intracranial pressure. Cerebellar hemangioblastomas, by secreting erythropoietin, can produce polycythemia and sometimes an etiologic variety of headaches—a diffuse headache from polycythemia, another diffuse headache from hydrocephalus, and possibly a posterior headache from the tumor—plus focal signs such as nystagmus and ataxia.

*Thrombocytopenia* may be associated with two types of headache. Migrainous headaches may accompany sudden falls in platelet count in patients with ITP (5), and in the much more ominous syndrome of thrombotic thrombocytopenic purpura, focal or diffuse headaches may herald or accompany brain hemorrhage or infarction. Paradoxically, headaches have also been described as developing in tandem with essential *thrombocytosis* [11].

*Leukemias and lymphomas*, through studding the cranial meninges, may cause headaches that are usually diffuse, progressively severe, and may be associated with cranial nerve signs, meningeal irritation, papilledema, or hydrocephalus. Rarely, *myeloma* may do the same. Infections complicating these hematologic malignancies may produce headaches by involving brain or meninges. *Hyperviscosity* syndromes resulting from marked increases in white blood cell counts or from paraproteinemias can cause headaches and transient or persisting multifocal neurologic disturbances.

*Bleeding disorders,* such as hemophilia and Christmas disease, frequently cause cerebral hemorrhage, with headaches and focal neurologic signs and symptoms. Disseminated intravascular coagulation causes both brain hemorrhage and infarction, again with headaches associated with multifocal neurologic signs.

## Headache Caused by the Treatment of Hematologic Disorders

The headaches that may result from the treatment of hematologic malignancies with radiation or chemotherapy have already been described. Most of the other treatments for hematologic disorders, such as iron, vitamins, and so on, are not likely to result in headaches. An exception is *intravenous immune globulin* (IV Ig) [12], which may produce a nondescript mild to moderate headache that responds to NSAIDs. IV Ig may trigger a migraine attack in patients known to have migraine; propranolol prophylaxis for subsequent infusions has been recommended. In up to 10% of patients, IV Ig may produce aseptic meningitis that settles in 24–48 hours and is managed with analgesics.

## Benign Dysfunctional Headaches in Hematology Patients

Migraine can be unmasked or precipitated, as noted, by severe fluctuations in platelet count, and by the administration of IV Ig. Anemia is not a contraindication to the use of conventional antimigraine drugs, but because anemia can produce worsening in migraine, it is preferable to make treatment of the anemia an early part of the treatment of migraine. Because some drugs used for migraine, such as valproate and methysergide, can produce thrombocytopenia or neutropenia, it is prudent not to use them in patients with low white blood cell or platelet counts.

## CARDIOVASCULAR SERVICE

### Headaches Caused by Cardiovascular Diseases or Their Complications

*High blood pressure*, as a cause of headache, is part of medical folklore. Only three situations exist in which high blood pressure causes headaches: (1) early *morning headaches* produced by long-standing, severe (diastolic >120 mm Hg) hypertension; (2) *acute hypertensive crisis*, as may occur when sympathomimetic substances are taken with monoamine oxidase (MAO) inhibitors or in pheochromocytoma; and (3) *hypertensive encephalopathy*, in which patchy edema, hemorrhages and infarcts of the brain produce headaches accompanied by obtundation, seizures, or multifocal deficits. Some medications prescribed for the treatment of high blood pressure (e.g., hydralazine, diltiazem) may produce headaches de novo, and others (e.g., reserpine) may trigger pre-existent migraine. Aside from these four considerations, it is clear that the great majority of hypertensive cases with headaches have the same migraine or tension-type headaches as normotensive cases.

Heart disease seldom causes headache. Children with congenital cyanotic heart disease may develop secondary *polycythemia* that can sometimes cause chronic headache, and right-to-left shunting may lead to brain abscesses that can produce progressively worsening headaches. In both of these situations, it is rare for the headache to be the only symptom; other features are present, which give the diagnosis. Atrial myxoma, valvular heart disease, atrial fibrillation, and postinfarction mural thrombus may all, through *cerebral embolization*, cause single or recurrent headaches, but again these headaches seldom occur without other neurologic symptoms or signs. Leakage of blood from a mycotic aneurysm caused by septic cerebral embolism in bacterial endocarditis may cause fulminating severe headache. The association between *mitral valve prolapse and migraine* is well documented [13], but it is not known whether the relationship is causal.

## Headaches Caused by the Treatment of Cardiovascular Disease

Cardiovascular medications are a prominent cause of iatrogenic headache. The nitrates (nitroglycerine, isosorbide dinitrate, etc.) used to treat ischemic heart disease regularly produce diffuse throbbing headaches that tend to attenuate with continued intake. In treating hypertension, adrenergic inhibitors that work through vasodilatation may produce headaches; these include hydralazine, minoxidil, and reserpine. Some of the calcium channel blockers, such as diltiazem and the dihydropyridines, frequently cause headaches.

The surgical treatment of cardiovascular disease may provoke headache. *Cardioembolism to the brain* during or after cardiac or great vessel surgery may cause headache; as noted above, this is nearly always accompanied by, and overshadowed by, prominent focal neurologic deficits.

Headache alone may follow carotid endarterectomy, particularly when the stenosis has been tight. This is a moderate to severe throbbing headache, sometimes diffuse and sometimes ipsilateral to the previous stenosis, lasting hours to days and occasionally weeks, eventually clearing spontaneously. We have seen these same headaches after internal carotid angioplasty and stenting. Ergotamine, dihydroergotamine, or sumatriptan transiently relieves these *postendarterectomy headaches*, although the cardiovascular disease that accompanies the carotid stenosis contraindicates their use. Corticosteroids are said to be helpful [14]. The pathophysiology of these headaches is believed to be as follows: As the carotid stenosis increased, vasodilatation distal to the stenosis occurred in an attempt to maintain cerebral perfusion by decreasing peripheral resistance. Endarterectomy, by removing the stenosis, allows unimpeded flow of blood into the dilated cerebral vessels, distending them further to the point of causing vascular headache. Ultimately, autoregulation reasserts itself, the cerebral vessels return to their normal diameter and the headache disappears.

Severe intractable headaches may rarely follow surgery for *carotid body tumor* [15]. In the one case in which details are given, the headaches were migraine-like, ipsilateral to the side of surgery, and resistant to all therapy (KL Moore, personal communication, 1997).

## Benign Dysfunctional Headaches in Cardiovascular Patients

Migraine tends to attenuate with age, and thus its concurrence with severe cardio-vascular disease is fortunately uncommon. Ergotamine, dihydroergotamine, and sumatriptan are contraindicated in most instances of cardiovascular disease. The intravenous administration of neuroleptics (e.g., chlorpromazine, 15–25 mg, or haloperidol, 5 mg), very useful in treating severe attacks of migraine in otherwise healthy people, is dangerous in cardiac patients due to its tendency to produce hypotension. Analgesics are usually safe, although there may be interactions among some of them (e.g., those containing acetylsalicylic acid) and some cardiovascular medications (e.g., anticoagulants). Attacks of severe headaches in inpatients with heart or peripheral vascular disease are probably best managed with careful admin-istration of narcotics and antinauseants. Some migraine prophylactic medications, such as tricyclic antidepressants and methysergide, are contraindicated in most or all instances of cardiovascular disease. Others are contraindicated in some instances of heart disease and helpful in others; beta blockers, for example, are contraindi-cated in congestive heart failure, but may be especially useful in the patient with concurrent migraine and hypertension or arrhythmia.

## ENDOCRINOLOGY SERVICE

## Headaches Caused by Endocrine Diseases or Their Complications

A number of endocrine or metabolic disorders may cause chronic, recurring dif-fuse headaches by producing BIH (or pseudotumor cerebri). These disorders include obesity, various menstrual disorders, hypoparathyroidism, hypothy-roidism, hyperthyroidism, and adrenocortical insufficiency due either to disease or to corticosteroid withdrawal. Paradoxically, the corticosteroid triamcinolone, often prescribed for arthritis, has been associated with the development of BIH. The neurologic consultant will, of course, be familiar with the clinical picture of BIH and with the fact that papilledema may be absent in this syndrome.

   Some of these same conditions, and others, may present with or be accompa-nied by recurrent headaches that are not mediated through the mechanism of BIH, but rather appear to be produced by cranial *vasodilatation*. These include hypothyroidism, hyperthyroidism, hyperparathyroidism, hyperaldosteronism, mineralocorticoid excess of various causes, cortisol withdrawal, and hypo-glycemia. Some disorders of the urea cycle, notably ornithine transcarbamylase deficiency in females (in males this condition produces other symptoms so severe that headache is masked), can present as migrainous headaches triggered by eat-ing meat. Acquired partial lipodystrophy may be associated with headaches. In all of these conditions, the headaches are usually recurrent, holocephalic, or hemicranial; of variable intensity and duration; and sometimes associated with nausea or vomiting. These headaches can mimic migraine. Diagnosis is aided by the presence of other features of the underlying endocrinopathy. The treatment is that of the primary condition, plus symptomatic analgesics.

*Tumors* of the hypophyseal-pituitary axis may cause various endocrinopathies and headaches. Larger tumors are more likely to be associated with headaches. The *empty sella syndrome* is said to be associated with chronic headaches, but the 10% prevalence of headaches in those with this condition is no greater than in the general population.

## Headaches Caused by the Treatment of Endocrinologic Diseases

Iatrogenic headaches are seldom a problem on the endocrine service. *Corticosteroid withdrawal* may trigger pre-existent migraine or evoke headaches de novo. The treatment of Bartter's syndrome (increased plasma renin, hyperaldosteronism, and hypokalemic alkalosis, occurring in the absence of edema or hypertension) with *indomethacin* has led to BIH with headaches [16].

## Benign Dysfunctional Headaches in Endocrine Patients

The presence of an underlying endocrinopathy such as hyperthyroidism may provoke or exacerbate migraine and make it resistant to conventional treatment until the endocrine condition has been corrected.

There are relatively few adverse interactions between migraine and endocrine medications. Corticosteroids may enhance the renal excretion of salicylates [17], causing decreased blood salicylate levels, and reduction of the dose of corticosteroids may cause salicylism. Propranolol and other beta blockers are contraindicated in diabetics on insulin and oral hypoglycemic agents. The beta blockers also may reduce triiodothyronine concentrations in patients who take thyroxine.

## GASTROENTEROLOGY SERVICE

## Headaches Caused by Gastrointestinal Diseases or Their Complications

Although *encephalopathy* due to liver disease is common in the gastroenterology service, headache is not. This is, perhaps, because as in all the other progressive encephalopathies, the emergence of impaired cognition and altered consciousness overshadow any headache that might occur as an early encephalopathic symptom.

Headache may be more common in patients with *inflammatory bowel diseases* (IBDs) such as Crohn's disease and ulcerative colitis. Sometimes diffuse, sometimes hemicranial, these recurrent headaches may be associated with the "toxicity" of IBD, they may be intercurrent or concurrent migraine [18], or they may be related to the treatment of the disease.

Any of the *infective enteritides*, whether bacterial, viral, or parasitic, may be accompanied by a so-called toxic vascular headache; this fades as the underlying disease resolves spontaneously or responds to treatment.

## Headaches Caused by the Treatment of Gastrointestinal Diseases

Some $H_2$ blockers, such as ranitidine and famotidine, widely used for the treatment of peptic ulcer disease, are well known to produce headache; cimetidine is less so. Proton inhibitors such as omeprazole, prostaglandin analogues such as misoprostol, and cytoprotectives such as sucralfate all have a lower incidence of headache. In the treatment of IBD, older agents such as sulfasalazine have a significant incidence of headache, whereas newer drugs such as mesalamine and olsalazine appear not to.

## Benign Dysfunctional Headaches in Gastrointestinal Patients

Salicylate analgesics and NSAIDs are contraindicated in the management of headache in people with peptic ulcer disease and IBD. Acetaminophen is not, but it should not be given to patients with liver disease. Patients taking metoclopramide on a maintenance basis may have accelerated absorption of acetaminophen, which can produce toxicity. The primary antimigraine drugs ergotamine, dihydroergotamine, and sumatriptan should not be given to those with liver disease but are not contraindicated in peptic ulcer or IBD. Narcotic analgesics are safe for most people with GI disease but should be given cautiously to those with liver dysfunction; administration to those taking cimetidine has been reported to enhance depressive and sedative side effects [19].

Similarly, for migraine prophylaxis, those on cimetidine who are given amitriptyline or propranolol may have increased side effects from these medications, likely due to interference with their hepatic metabolism produced by cimetidine. People with diseased livers should not be given these medications.

## RESPIRATORY SERVICE

## Headaches Caused by Respiratory Diseases or Their Complications

Most lung diseases, when severe, can produce *hypoxia* and *carbon dioxide ($CO_2$)* *retention*. These, in turn, can produce headache through the agency of cerebral vasodilatation. *Secondary polycythemia* resulting from chronic hypoxia may increase this vasodistention. These headaches tend to be diffuse, recurrent or constant, of variable severity, and worse with the coughing that may accompany respiratory disease. These headaches also tend to be worse in the morning due to impaired respiratory efficiency during sleep and may increase hypoxia and $CO_2$ retention, which summates with the head-low position to increase the cephalic congestion. The treatment of these headaches is treatment of the underlying respiratory disease.

Even in the absence of hypoxia or $CO_2$ retention, some respiratory diseases, notably the pneumonias, can be accompanied by severe headaches. Although any infection anywhere in the body can produce a *toxic vascular headache*, some are more likely to do so. *Mycoplasma pneumoniae*, notorious for producing, and not infrequently presenting with, an intense generalized throbbing headache that is much exacerbated by coughing, is a good example. Sometimes, the headache is based on the concurrent meningitis caused by the spread of *M. pneumoniae* from lung to meninges, but much more often, is not. Nevertheless, it is a good rule to always perform a lumbar puncture when significant headache occurs in the context of a systemic infection.

Malignancies of the respiratory system frequently metastasize to the brain, and these *metastases* may cause headaches (see the section on Oncology). Posterior fossa metastases may present with a cough headache that, clinically, is indistinguishable from that suffered by many people with chronic chest disease.

Bronchiectasis and empyema may "seed" infection to the nervous system, causing *brain abscesses*, which, in turn, cause headaches indistinguishable from those of metastases; rarely, these abscesses may rupture, causing meningitis and an acute, severe diffuse headache. Pulmonary tuberculosis may produce the same sequence of events, though in a slower tempo.

## Headaches Caused by the Treatment of Respiratory Diseases

Bronchodilators, used in the treatment of asthma and COPD, can cause headache in some people; these drugs include theophylline, aminophylline, salbutamol, and terbutaline. Cromolyn (cromoglycate sodium) and inhaled corticosteroids are not associated with headaches. One antibiotic often prescribed for respiratory infections, trimethoprim-sulfamethoxazole, is well known to cause headaches; other antibiotics appear not to.

## Benign Dysfunctional Headaches in Respiratory Patients

Aspirin and other NSAIDs are contraindicated in some asthmatics who show hypersensitivity reactions to these analgesics; acetaminophen is safe. The primary antimigraine drugs ergotamine, dihydroergotamine, and sumatriptan are generally safe in people with respiratory disease, but dihydroergotamine may cause severe peripheral vasoconstriction in a patient on erythromycin (a commonly used antibiotic for respiratory infections) [20].

For migraine prophylaxis, beta blockers are contraindicated in people with asthma and other forms of bronchospasm. Methysergide should be avoided in people who already have either pulmonary fibrosis or a disease likely to produce pulmonary fibrosis.

## MUSCULOSKELETAL SERVICE

## Headaches Caused by Musculoskeletal Diseases or Their Complications

Many rheumatologic conditions have headache as a major or minor symptom. *Rheumatoid arthritis* of the upper cervical spine may cause neck stiffness and occipital headaches, and when it produces atlantoaxial subluxation, it may cause cervical cord compression with weak legs, extensor plantar responses, ataxia, and other symptoms. Debate exists about whether *cervical spondylosis* causes headache [21]; this is probably a rare event because spondylosis affects chiefly the lower cervical spine, which does not refer pain to the head. Controversial in a different sense is *fibromyalgia*, in which there is argument about its nosologic status and its pathogenesis, but certainly there are many patients on a rheumatology service with a symptom concatenation of chronic multifocal muscle aching, particularly in the region of the trunk and neck, typically with multiple tender pressure points in muscles and tendons, sometimes with some peripheral joint symptoms, and very frequently with prominent headaches indistinguishable from tension-type headaches.

SLE may be associated with a wide variety of neurologic features, including headaches. Typical migraine, sometimes with visual aura, may occur coincident with flare-ups of SLE [22]. More continuous headaches may occur when SLE has a cranial vasculitic component (this is believed to be uncommon), or when it produces pseudotumor cerebri or aseptic meningitis. Aseptic meningitis may also occur in *Sjögren's syndrome*, as may episodic migraine-like headaches [23].

*Vasculitis* usually produces headache when it involves cranial vessels; examples include polyarteritis nodosa, giant cell arteritis, Takayasu's disease, Wegener's granulomatosis, lymphomatoid granulomatosis, and Cogan's syndrome. Multifocal neurologic deficits caused by brain infarcts typically punctuate the chronic course of the headache. The clinical diagnosis of cranial arteritis rests on three aspects: (1) the demonstration of an underlying disease that can cause cranial arteritis; (2) the presence of multiple infarcts on MRI; and (3) the uncovering of changes of vasculitis on cerebral angiography, though not infrequently such angiography fails to uncover it. Sometimes, drastic treatment with corticosteroids and other powerful immunosuppressant drugs may be used, based on a suggestive history, abnormal results from blood tests, and results from the MRI. Diagnostic biopsy of a cranial vessel, however, provides the means for a definitive diagnosis.

Some of these collagen-vascular diseases can produce headache through the mechanism of *meningeal infiltration with granulomata*; examples include Wegener's granulomatosis, lymphomatoid granulomatosis, and sarcoidosis. Others, such as Behçet's disease, Vogt-Koyanagi-Harada syndrome, Cogan's syndrome, and Sjögren's syndrome, can be associated with *aseptic meningitis*, which can declare itself as headache. Some of these conditions with meningeal involvement have multiple cranial nerve deficits occurring with their headaches—a potent diagnostic clue that impels the consultant to consider MRI and CSF examination.

## Headaches Caused by the Treatment of Musculoskeletal Disorders

The tendency for NSAIDs, such as indomethacin, to produce headache either by a direct vascular effect or through causing a syndrome of BIH is well known. The consultant should recall that benign intracranial hypertension may exist without papilledema, and should therefore not hesitate to measure CSF pressure by lumbar puncture (after CT scan or MRI) in a patient who develops a new persistent diffuse headache while taking an NSAID, even if the fundi are normal.

*Antimalarial drugs*, used sometimes for the treatment of rheumatoid arthritis, SLE, and other rheumatologic conditions, may occasionally, produce headache; switching to another antimalarial sometimes allows treatment to continue without headaches. Some rheumatologists use *sulfasalazine* for the treatment of rheumatoid arthritis, and this may produce headaches as an adverse effect (see section on Gastroenterology, inflammatory bowel disease). Corticosteroids by themselves seldom cause headaches, but *withdrawal from corticosteroids* can, either through a presumed direct vasodilatation effect or by producing pseudotumor cerebri.

## Benign Dysfunctional Headaches in Musculoskeletal Patients

The increased incidence of migraine in SLE and in Sjögren's syndrome has been noted; it has also been described in Behçet's disease. There is controversy about whether migraine-like headaches are more common in people with SLE who have antiphospholipid antibodies in their blood. The treatment of migraine in these and other patients with rheumatologic disease differs very little from that of people without such diseases. It is worthwhile trying to minimize or discontinue their NSAIDs, particularly indomethacin.

In cluster-headache patients who need to be on NSAIDs for rheumatologic disease, care should be taken when prescribing lithium; NSAIDs reduce renal lithium clearance and may tip the patient into serious lithium toxicity.

Patients with the fibromyalgia syndrome frequently complain of chronic headaches indistinguishable from tension-type headaches; prescription of a tricyclic antidepressant sometimes helps not only the headaches but the musculoskeletal complaints.

## INFECTIOUS DISEASES SERVICE

## Headaches Caused by Infectious Diseases or Their Complications

So common are headaches in the infectious diseases service that merely listing the entities associated with this symptom would fill several pages. Instead, following is an account of how infectious diseases may cause headaches and a description of what these headaches may be like.

Toxic Vascular Headaches

Toxic vascular headaches are poorly defined but extremely common headaches that may complicate any infection. It is theorized that various inflammatory mediators or by-products gain access to the systemic circulation and act on the pain-sensitive cranial vasculature, distending and perhaps inflaming it to produce bilateral moderate to intense throbbing headaches that, like all vascular headaches, are increased by exertion, straining, and the head-down position. Although they are more likely to occur with fever, fever is not necessary for their production. Although any infection can cause these headaches, some, such as *M. pneumoniae*, are notorious for doing so. Aspirin or other NSAIDs are useful in treating mild to moderate toxic vascular headaches; for more severe ones, narcotic analgesics may have to be added temporarily.

Infections may trigger an attack of migraine in someone who already has this condition, and these migraine headaches may be difficult to disentangle, diagnostically, from a toxic vascular headache, especially if the migraine is bilateral and not accompanied by conspicuous nausea or vomiting, or by aura. Recall that treatment of migraine by ergot in the presence of an infection may, even with normal doses, result in ergotism.

## Meningitis

Meningitis, like toxic vascular headache, can result from any systemic infection—viral, bacterial, fungal, or protozoal—and cause a diffuse severe headache. Meningeal irritation can be inconspicuous, particularly in very early meningitis, or in the very young, the very old, or the very sick, and thus, on occasion, meningitis may mimic a toxic vascular headache. When vomiting is present in meningitis, particularly in a patient known to have a history of headaches, considerations of migraine may obscure the diagnosis. Conversely, a patient with toxic vascular headache or migraine who also has tender cervical adenopathy or neck muscle soreness may appear to manifest "a stiff neck" on neurologic examination and thus mimic meningitis. The consultant who resorts freely to lumbar punctures is most likely to establish a proper diagnosis.

## Encephalitis

Headache is usually not as prominent in encephalitis as it is in meningitis for a number of reasons: the meninges may not be sufficiently involved by the organism to become inflamed and painful; other symptoms, such as seizures or paralysis, may overwhelm a relatively minor headache complaint; or altered consciousness may prevent the patient from communicating the presence of a headache.

## Brain Abscess

The headache of brain abscess is produced by a combination of mass effect (usually considered to be the main mechanism) and meningeal irritation (if the abscess is abutting on the pain-sensitive meninges). Headache may be absent with small abscesses unless they are multiple and, in aggregate, result in increased intracranial pressure. When present, the headache may be focal or diffuse, mild to severe, and intermittent or constant. Like the headache of brain tumor, the headache of brain abscess seldom exhibits the textbook behavior of early morning worsening and exacerbation by straining and the head-low position; more often, the headache of brain abscess is nondescript. Ready imaging (CT scan or MRI) of the infected patient with a new or worsening headache is a prudent policy.

## Headaches Caused by Diagnostic or Therapeutic Measures in Patients with Infections

Post–lumbar puncture headaches are not uncommon in the infectious disease service. They can be tricky, at times, to recognize, because they may be obscured by a toxic vascular headache or a meningitis headache and may thus present mainly as a worsening of the "usual" headache after the patient has been sitting up for a while. Management of this headache should be conservative, consisting mainly of the head-down position and analgesics and perhaps caffeine as a vasoconstrictor; in particular, there are good theoretical reasons for forbidding the performance of an epidural blood patch in a patient known or suspected to have an infection.

Trimethoprim-sulfamethoxazole may cause headache either by a direct presumably vascular effect or, rarely, by producing an aseptic meningitis syndrome. Tetracyclines, nitrofurantoin, and nalidixic acid can produce a pseudotumor cerebri syndrome with headache. Zidovudine (AZT) may cause headaches, especially in the first few weeks of treatment; the mechanism is unknown. Interferon-alpha commonly causes headaches, again by an unknown mechanism. Aside from these instances, antibiotics rarely cause headaches.

## Benign Dysfunctional Headaches in Patients with Infections

Migraine sufferers may have their attacks precipitated by an infection. Usually, these headaches are straightforward in their presentation, but if the patient already has a toxic vascular headache or a postpuncture headache, it may be difficult to discern the migraine. Doing so is important, however, because the treatment of these multiple headache syndromes varies. Recall that the vasoconstrictor effects of ergotamine (and perhaps dihydroergotamine) may be potentiated in the presence of infection to the point of causing ergotism. The literature to date does not indicate that this may occur with sumatriptan, but it may be that some of the newer triptans, with longer durations of action, could be problematic in the context of infection. As noted, dihydroergotamine may interact with erythromycin to produce severe peripheral vasoconstriction [20]. Acetaminophen may interact with zidovudine azidothymidine to produce a higher incidence of hematologic toxicity [24] and may enhance chloramphenicol-induced agranulocytosis [25]. Meperidine can interact with isoniazid to produce hypotension [26].

## OBSTETRIC SERVICE

### Headache Caused by Pregnancy or its Complications

Pregnancy is a normal state and not a disease, but it may, nonetheless, be associated with headaches. Pregnancy may precipitate BIH in some women, producing a chronic diffuse headache and usually (but not always) papilledema. This syndrome needs to be distinguished from *intracranial venous thrombosis*, which also may complicate pregnancy or the postpartum period. When additional neurologic features such as focal deficits, altered awareness, or seizures are present, this differentiation is not difficult; when these features are not present, MRI may be required to make the distinction. Pregnancy is complicated by *pre-eclampsia* in about 5% of cases; this last trimester triad of hypertension, proteinuria, and edema may have headache as a symptom, especially if the pre-eclampsia is severe. The syndrome, and the headaches, usually clear after delivery; if delivery must be delayed (because of fetal immaturity), then bed rest and treatment of the hypertension with a drug reasonably safe for the fetus (e.g., beta blocker) should help the headache. Rarely, intracranial tumors such as *meningiomas* may expand very rapidly in pregnancy, producing headaches and sometimes other symptoms of increased intracranial pressure. Subarachnoid hemorrhage from *aneurysm* can occur in pregnancy, especially during the third trimester, with greatest risk for rebleeding in the postpartum period, whereas *arteriovenous malformations* (AVMs) are more likely to bleed in the second trimester and to rebleed during delivery or in subsequent pregnancies.

## Headaches Produced in Obstetric Delivery

Occasionally, a lumbar epidural puncture, performed for the purpose of administering an epidural block for analgesia during delivery, inadvertently becomes a true spinal tap, as the needle breaches the arachnoid; in such instances, a *postpuncture headache* may develop. The anesthesiologist generally knows when an epidural has "gone spinal," but sometimes this accident is unrecognized, and the subsequent headache may remain mysterious until the neurologic consultant, by eliciting a history of a diffuse headache that appears and worsens with the head up and resolves with the head down, makes the diagnosis. The treatment is conscientious bed rest for a few days but, not infrequently, the new mother, with too much to do to remain in bed for very long, opts for an early epidural blood patch.

Rarely, the straining of labor and delivery will cause an AVM or, even more rarely, an *aneurysm*, to rupture; the diagnosis of the suddenly appearing severe headache is usually obvious.

## Benign Dysfunctional Headaches in Pregnancy and the Puerperium

Typically, *migraine* tends to continue at its usual frequency during the first trimester and then, as estrogen levels (from the placenta) rise, improve, or disappear [27]. This is most likely to occur in women with a history of menstrual migraine. The migraine may recur with great suddenness once the placenta is delivered, raising alarms of some intracranial catastrophe, particularly if the obstetrician is unaware of, or has forgotten, the history of migraine.

Migraine does not always improve during pregnancy, and indeed may come on for the first time during pregnancy. When it does, the presentation may be somewhat atypical, with auras that may be predominantly sensory rather than visual. In such cases, cortical venous thrombosis or a tumor may need to be excluded (preferably by MRI, which does not involve radiation).

The treatment of migraine or other benign dysfunctional headaches during pregnancy is made difficult by the potential teratogenic and other adverse effects of some of the drugs normally used. Ideally, all drugs should be avoided, but if pain relief is essential, then acetaminophen, codeine, or meperidine (Demerol) is least likely to affect the fetus. Ergotamine and dihydroergotamine are contraindicated, and there is insufficient evidence of the safety of sumatriptan, in terms of the fetus, to permit its use in pregnancy. For those rare patients in whom migraine prophylaxis is necessary in pregnancy, beta blockers are least dangerous to the fetus.

## SURGICAL SERVICES

### Headaches Produced by Surgical Diseases or Their Complications

The neurologic consultant seldom encounters headaches in surgical patients. Typically, these patients are hospitalized for only the briefest possible time, and during much of their admission, they are under the influence of postoperative analgesics or have other more serious and painful problems to distract them. Some surgical services do have their share of headache patients, and most of these are dealt with in this chapter under the appropriate medical service (e.g., headaches in cardiac surgery patients are described in the section on Cardiovascular Service).

### Headaches Produced by Surgical Therapy

Headaches after *carotid endarterectomy, carotid angioplasty,* and *carotid body surgery* are described under Cardiovascular Service.

Postoperative headache after *surgery for acoustic neuroma* is a common problem [28]: Approximately 70% of women and 25% of men develop a dull headache in the region of the incision. In most people (75%), the headache clears in 3 days to 10 weeks (median, 3 weeks), but in some it lasts much longer, and often takes the form of recurrent jabs in the incisional area. These headaches likely result from damage to regional nerves necessarily incurred during surgery. Treatment with analgesics, NSAIDs, and possibly carbamazepine may be helpful.

*Post–gamma knife headache* [29] has resulted from stereotactic surgery of cerebral AVMs using this radiosurgical technique. Such headaches are believed to be rare. They may come on as de novo headaches postoperatively (sometimes long postoperatively) or as exacerbations of the preoperative headaches that were ascribed to the AVM. They may resemble migraine in their severity and pulsatility. Their etiology is uncertain: They may be related to the cerebral edema that is sometimes seen on MRI or to intracranial hypertension produced by radiation-induced venous changes. These headaches usually resolve gradually, and until they do, treatment is symptomatic.

### Benign Dysfunctional Headaches in Surgical Patients

The practice of keeping patients NPO (nil per os, or fasting) before surgery may precipitate headache, particularly in known migraine sufferers. Not as frequent are postoperative headaches induced by the NPO regimen, probably because these patients usually have some postoperative analgesic extant. Fasting headaches may respond to intravenous glucose, to intramuscular or intravenous dihydroergotamine (after premedication with a parenteral antinauseant to prevent vomiting), or to subcutaneous sumatriptan. A patient with a severe attack of migraine should likely have anything except emergency surgery deferred until the migraine is under control and full rehydration has been achieved.

## PSYCHIATRIC SERVICE

### Headaches Produced by Psychiatric Disease

It is natural for the neurologic consultant assessing the headache of a patient on the psychiatry service to consider the possibility that it is a symptom of the psychiatric disease that hospitalized the patient. Sometimes, especially in the *anxious* or *depressed* patient or in the patient with a *somatoform disorder*, this is correct. In these conditions, the headaches may resemble migraine or tension-type headaches or appear quite nondescript. When appearing as a part of a psychiatric disease, these headaches typically require treatment of that disease and do not respond (at least, not significantly) to symptomatic treatment alone. The difficulty here is that anxiety, depression, and somatoform disorders confer no immunity against lesions such as brain tumors or subdural hematomas (which not infrequently mimic and are misdiagnosed as psychiatric disorders), nor do they protect against migraine or other benign dysfunctional headaches. Accordingly, special care should be taken when dealing with headache in these patients so as not to miss neurologic disease or benign dysfunctional headaches, which respond only to specific therapy.

Many people find themselves in a psychiatric facility because of drug or substance abuse; either the toxic or the withdrawal state may produce prominent headache. The headache associated with *withdrawal from alcohol or opiates* is well known. *Cocaine* commonly causes severe headache in the intoxicated state, likely produced by hypertension and often associated with other signs of sympathetic overactivity. Headache occurring in the cocaine addict can also result from cocaine-induced migraine (perhaps precipitated by serotonin release and depletion) or a cocaine-induced subarachnoid or intracranial hemorrhage. Because these patients may not be able to cooperate well in terms of history and examination, it is prudent to resort quickly to imaging and to lumbar puncture.

### Headaches Associated with the Treatment of Psychiatric Disease

Severe hypertension, with or without intracranial hemorrhage, can also result from the unwitting consumption of sympathomimetic drugs such as bronchodilators and nose sprays by people taking *MAO inhibitors*. A much less dramatic headache—dull, low grade, and rather nondescript—may occur in patients started on *benzodiazepines* for anxiety or restlessness. This headache may be more or less constant through the day or may appear first thing in the morning when the patient wakes up in need of his or her first benzodiazepine "fix" for the day. In such patients, a tricyclic antidepressant with mild sedative side effects (e.g., amitriptyline) is often better for settling anxiety; neuroleptics are more effective but also considerably more likely to cause worrisome side effects such as extrapyramidal features.

## Benign Dysfunctional Headaches Occurring in Patients with Psychiatric Disease

In headaches occurring in patients with psychiatric disease, the challenge, largely, is to avoid interactions between the psychiatric drugs the patient is ingesting and the headache medications the neurologic consultant would like to prescribe.

MAO inhibitors contraindicate the following medications for the treatment of acute headache: demerol, sumatriptan, rizatriptan, zolmitriptan, isometheptene (Midrin), and metoclopramide. Aspirin, acetaminophen, naratriptan, ergotamine, and dihydroergotamine are safe. In terms of migraine prophylaxis, tricyclics and beta blockers are not recommended for patients on MAO inhibitors because hypertensive and hyperpyretic crises may occur, but other agents, including calcium channel blockers, valproic acid, and methysergide, appear to be safe.

*Specific serotonin-reuptake inhibitors* are said to contraindicate the use of sumatriptan due to the potential for the combination to cause a serotonin syndrome. This is a very rare occurrence, but it is probably prudent to use ergotamine, dihydroergotamine, and analgesics for the treatment of acute headaches in these patients.

## REFERENCES

1. Clouston PD, De Angelis LM, Posner JB. The spectrum of neurologic disease in patients with systemic cancer. Ann Neurol 1992;31:268–273.
2. Edmeads J. Brain Tumors and Other Space-Occupying Lesions. In PJ Goadsby, SD Silberstein (eds), Headache. Boston: Butterworth–Heinemann, 1997;313–326.
3. Forsyth PA, Posner JB. Headaches in patients with brain tumors. A study of 111 patients. Neurology 1993;43:1678–1683.
4. Headache Classification Committee of the International Headache Society. Classification and diagnostic criteria for headache disorders, cranial neuralgias and facial pain. Cephalalgia 1988;8(suppl 7):1–96.
5. Damasio H, Beck D. Migraine, thrombocytopenia, and serotonin metabolism. Lancet 1978;1:240–242.
6. Posner JB. Neurologic Complications of Cancer. Philadelphia: FA Davis, 1995;30.
7. Larson DA, Wora WM, Fike JR. Central Nervous System Manifestations of Radiotherapy. In AI Arieff, RC Griggs (eds), Metabolic Brain Dysfunction in Systemic Disorders. Boston: Little, Brown, 1992;389–398.
8. Kats S, Vecht CJ. Aura without headache in cancer. Neurology 1997;48(suppl 3):A342.
9. Parag KB, Omar MAK. Benign intracranial hypertension associated with iron deficiency anemia. S Afr Med J 1983;63:981–983.
10. Blank JP, Gill FM. Orbital infarction in sickle cell disease. Pediatrics 1981;67:879–883.
11. Hanington E. Platelet behaviour in migraine. Panminerva Med 1982;24:63–66.
12. Dalakos MC. Intravenous immune globulin therapy for neurologic diseases. Ann Intern Med 1997;126:721–730.
13. Gamberini G, D'Alessandro R, Labriola E, et al. Further evidence on the association of mitral valve prolapse and migraine. Headache 1984;24:39–40.
14. Fisher CM. Painful states: a neurologic commentary. Neurosurgery 1984;31:32–53.

15. Rabl H, Friehs I, Gutschi S, et al. Diagnosis and treatment of carotid body tumors. Thorac Cardiovasc Surg 1993;41:340–343.
16. Konomi H, Imai M, Nihei K, et al. Indomethacin causing pseudotumor in Bartter's syndrome. N Engl J Med 1978;298:855–858.
17. Koren G, Roifman C, Gelfard E, et al. Corticosteroids-salicylate interaction in a case of juvenile rheumatoid arthritis. Ther Drug Monit 1987;9:177–179.
18. Sacks O. Migraine. Berkeley, CA: University of California Press, 1992;48.
19. Guay DRP, Meatherall RC, Chalmers JL, Grahame GR. Cimetidine alters pethidine disposition in man. Br J Clin Pharmacol 1984;18:907–914.
20. Lefroy F, Asseman P, Pruvost P, et al. Dihydroergotamine-erythromycin induced ergotism. Ann Intern Med 1988;109:249.
21. Edmeads J. The cervical spine and headache. Neurology 1988;38:1874–1878.
22. Brandt KD, Lessell S. Migrainous phenomena in systemic lupus erythematosus. Arthritis Rheum 1978;21:7–16.
23. Pal B, Gibson C, Passmore J, et al. A study of headaches and migraine in Sjögren's syndrome and other rheumatic disorders. Ann Rheum Dis 1989;48:312–320.
24. Richman DD, Fischl MA, Grieco MH, et al. Toxicity of azidothymidine (AZT) in the treatment of patients with AIDS and AIDS-related complex: a double blind controlled trial. N Engl J Med 1987;317:192–197.
25. Buchanan N, Moodley GP. Interaction between chloramphenicol and paracetamol. BMJ 1979;2:307–308.
26. Gannon R, Pearsall W, Rowley R. Isoniazid, meperidine and hypotension. Ann Intern Med 1983;99:415.
27. Reik L. Headaches in pregnancy. Semin Neurol 1988;8:187–192.
28. Dodick DW, Mosek A, Ebersold MJ. Acoustic neuroma and postoperative pain. Neurology 1997;48(suppl 3):A259.
29. Rozen TD, Swanson JW. Post gamma knife headache: a new headache syndrome? Headache 1997;37:180–183.

# 2
# Altered Mental Status

Joerg-Patrick Stübgen and John J. Caronna

Few problems are more difficult to manage than those presented by the unconscious patient because the potential causes of an altered mental status are considerable and the time for diagnosis and effective intervention is relatively short. *Consciousness* may be defined as a state of awareness of self and the environment. The phenomenon of consciousness depends upon two intact and interdependent physiologic and anatomic components: (1) arousal (or wakefulness) and its underlying neural substrate, the ascending reticular activating system (ARAS) and diencephalon, and (2) awareness, which requires the functioning cerebral cortex of both hemispheres. Most disorders that acutely disturb consciousness are, in fact, impairments of arousal that create circumstances under which the brain's capacity for consciousness cannot be accurately assessed. Failure of the arousal system renders it impossible to test the awareness system.

Alterations in arousal level may be transient, lasting only several seconds or minutes (following seizure, syncope, and cardiac dysrhythmia), or sustained, lasting several hours or longer (the subject of this chapter).

Alterations in arousal do not actually form discrete levels but rather are made up of a continuum of subtly changing behavioral states that range from alert to comatose. These states are dynamic and may change with time. Four points on the continuum of arousal are often used in describing the clinical state of a patient: (1) *Alert* refers to a perfectly normal state of arousal. (2) *Stupor* is defined as unresponsiveness from which the patient can be transiently aroused only by vigorous and repeated stimuli. (3) *Coma* is unarousable unresponsiveness in which the patient lies with eyes closed, and, at best, only reflex responses can be elicited. (4) *Lethargy* lies between alertness and stupor. In practice, only the terms *alert* and *coma* have enough precision to be used without further qualification; possibly, coma has gradation in depth but this cannot be assessed accurately once the patient is no longer responsive to external stimuli. The terms *lethargy* and *stupor* cover a broad spectrum of behavioral states; definitions of these grades have not been fully standardized and are thus subject to misinterpretation and miscommunication when used without further qualification. It is best simply to describe observations and the patient's appearance in plain language.

## PATHOPHYSIOLOGY OF ALTERED CONSCIOUSNESS

Arousal and the state of wakefulness depend on an intact ARAS, a conceptual array of isodendritric nuclei and tracts extending from the medulla through the tegmentum of the pons and midbrain, which is continuous caudally with the reticular intermediate gray lamina of the spinal cord and rostrally with the subthalamus, the hypothalamus, and the thalamus. ARAS functions and interconnections are considerable, and its role is likely greater than only a cortical arousal system. Arousal was considered to depend on projections from the reticular formation via the midline thalamic nuclei to the thalamic reticular nucleus and the cortex. It now appears less certain that the thalamic reticular nucleus is the final relay, and the specific role of the various links from the reticular formation to the thalamus has yet to be identified. Furthermore, the cortex feeds back on the thalamic nuclei to contribute an important self-cycling loop to arousal mechanisms. The system contains cholinergic, monoaminergic, and other projecting fiber systems, none of which has been identified as the singular arousal neurotransmitter. It follows that acute structural damage to or metabolic-chemical derangement of either the ascending brain stem–thalamic activating system or the thalamo-corticothalamic loop is capable of producing an altered state of arousal.

Consciousness depends on the continuous interaction between the mechanisms that provide arousal and awareness. The brain stem and thalamus provide the activating mechanism, and the cerebrum provides for cognition and self-excitation. For the sake of this discussion, the content of consciousness can best be regarded as the amalgam and integration of all cognitive function that resides in the cerebral cortex of both hemispheres. Altered awareness arises from disruption of this cortical activity by diffuse pathology. Focal lesions can produce profound deficits, such as aphasia, alexia, amnesia, or hemianopsia, but only a diffuse bilateral process, sparing the ARAS and diencephalon, can lead to unawareness.

Thus, there are two kinds of altered mental states: (1) altered arousal due to dysfunction of the ARAS-diencephalon, and (2) altered awareness due to bilateral diffuse cerebral hemisphere dysfunction.

## COMA-LIKE BEHAVIORAL STATES

Several different behavioral states appear similar to, and can be confused with, coma. Differentiation of the states from true coma has important diagnostic, therapeutic, and prognostic implications. Moreover, coma is not a permanent state; patients who survive initial coma may evolve through and into these altered behavioral states.

### Locked-In Syndrome

In the locked-in syndrome, patients are alert and fully conscious but are de-efferented. Such patients suffer bilateral ventral pontine lesions with quadriplegia, horizontal gaze palsies, and lower cranial nerve palsies and are voluntarily capable only of vertical eye movements or blinking. Sleep may be abnormal with marked reduction in non–rapid eye movement (REM) and REM sleep phases. The most common etiology is pontine infarction due to basilar artery thrombosis, but also pontine hemorrhage, central pontine myelinolysis, and brain stem mass lesions. Neuromuscular causes include severe, acute inflammatory demyelinating or axonal polyradiculoneuropathies, myasthenia gravis, and neuromuscular blocking agents.

## Akinetic Mutism

*Akinetic mutism* describes a subacute or chronic state of altered behavior in which an alert-appearing patient is silent and immobile. External evidence of mental activity is unobtainable. The patient usually lies with eyes closed but retains cycles of self-sustained arousal, giving the appearance of vigilance. Skeletal muscle tone is flaccid, and movements are rudimentary even in response to unpleasant stimuli. Patients are doubly incontinent. Lesions that result in akinetic mutism have in common interruption of reticular-cortical or limbic-cortical integration with relative sparing of motor pathways. Responsible lesions involve bilateral, basal medial, frontal lobes, or incomplete lesions of the deep gray matter (paramedian reticular formation of the posterior diencephalon and adjacent midbrain) or diffuse cortical lesions. Electroencephalography (EEG) shows reactive alpha and theta rhythms in response to external stimuli.

## Catatonia

*Catatonia* is a symptom complex associated most often with psychiatric disease. This behavioral disturbance is characterized by stupor or excitement and variable mutism, posturing, rigidity, grimacing, and catalepsy. Catatonia can be caused by a variety of illnesses, both psychiatric (affective more than psychotic) disorders and structural or metabolic diseases (toxic and drug-induced psychoses, encephalitis, and alcoholic neurotoxicity). Psychiatric catatonia may be difficult to distinguish from organic disease because patients often appear lethargic to stuporous rather than totally unresponsive, and patients may have a variety of endocrine or autonomic abnormalities. Patients in catatonic stupor do not move spontaneously, and they appear unresponsive to the environment despite a normal level of consciousness and cognitive functions. This impression is supported by a normal neurologic examination and the patient's recall of most events that took place during the unresponsive period. Patients usually lie with eyes opened and may not blink to visual threat, but optokinetic responses are usually present. The pupils are dilated and reactive to light, oculocephalic reflexes are absent, and vestibulo-ocular testing evokes normal ocular nystagmus. Patients may hypersalivate and be doubly incontinent. Passive movement of the limbs meets with waxy flexibility, and catalepsy is seen in 30% of patients. Choreiform jerks of the extremities and facial grimaces are common. The EEG both of catatonic excitement and stupor most often shows a reactive, low-voltage fast normal record rather than the slow record of a comatose patient.

## Vegetative State

The *vegetative state* can be defined as wakefulness without awareness, and it is the consequence of various diffuse brain insults. It may be a transient phase through which patients in coma pass as the cerebral cortex recovers more slowly than the brain stem. Clinically, vegetative patients appear to be awake and to have cyclical sleep patterns; however, such individuals do not show evidence of cognitive function or learned behavioral responses to external stimuli. Vegetative patients may feature spontaneous eye opening and eye movements and stereotypic facial and limb movements; however, they are unable to demonstrate speech or comprehension, and they lack purposeful activity. Vegetative patients generate normal body temperature and usually have normally functioning cardiovascular, respiratory, and digestive systems, but are doubly incontinent. The persistent vegetative state is a condition lasting at least 1 month and requiring extended observation of the patient to assess behavioral responses to external stimulation and to demonstrate cognitive unawareness. EEG may be essentially isoelectric or may regain various patterns of rhythm and amplitude that are inconsistent from one case to the next. Normal EEG sleep-wake patterns are absent.

## APPROACH TO COMA

The initial approach to stupor and coma is based on the principle that all alterations in arousal are acute, life-threatening emergencies. The evaluation of a comatose patient demands a systematic approach with appropriate, directed diagnostic and therapeutic endeavors; time must not be wasted on irrelevant considerations. Urgent steps are required to prevent or minimize permanent brain damage from reversible causes. Patient evaluation and treatment must necessarily occur simultaneously. Serial examinations are needed with accurate documentation to determine a change in state of the patient. Accordingly, management decisions (diagnostic or therapeutic) must be made. The clinical approach to an unconscious patient logically entails the following steps:

1. Emergency management
2. History (from relatives, friends, and emergency medical personnel)
3. General physical examination
4. Neurologic profile (the key to categorizing the nature of coma)
5. Specific management
6. Prediction of outcome

## Emergency Management

The initial assessment must focus on the vital signs to determine the appropriate resuscitation measures; the diagnostic process begins later. Urgent, and sometimes empiric, therapy must be given to avoid additional brain insult.

## Oxygenation

Oxygenation must be assured by the establishment of an airway and ventilation of the lungs. The threshold for intubation should be low in the comatose patient, even if respiratory function is sufficient for proper ventilation and oxygenation: The level of consciousness may deteriorate, and respiration may decompensate suddenly and unexpectedly. An open airway must be assured and protected from aspiration of vomitus or blood. While preparing for intubation, maximal oxygenation can be assured by suction of the upper airway, gentle extension of the neck, elevation of the jaw, and manual ventilation with oxygen using a mask and bag. Maximal oxygenation ("bagging") and 1 mg atropine help prevent cardiac dysrhythmias. If severe neck injury is a possibility, intubation should be performed by the most skilled practitioner without extension of the patient's neck. A brief neurologic examination is mandatory before sedation required for intubation.

## Evaluate Respiratory Excursions

Arterial blood gas measurement is the only certain method to determine adequate ventilation and oxygenation. Pulse oximetry is useful because it provides immediate information regarding arterial oxygen saturation. The comatose patient ideally should maintain a $pO_2$ greater than 100 mm Hg and a $pCO_2$ between 34 and 37 mm Hg. Do not hyperventilate less than 35 mm Hg, as this constricts brain arteries. Positive end-expiratory pressure should be avoided if increased intracranial pressure (ICP) is suspected. Place a nasogastric tube to facilitate gastric lavage and to prevent regurgitation.

## Maintain Circulation to Assure Adequate Cerebral Perfusion

Appropriate resuscitation fluid is lactated Ringer's solution; normal saline is used when high ICP is suspected. A mean arterial pressure at about 100 mm Hg probably is adequate and safe for most patients. While obtaining venous access, collect blood samples for anticipated tests and others (Table 2.1). Treat hypotension by replacing any blood volume loss and the use of vasoactive agents (preferably dopamine). Judiciously manage elevated blood pressure with hypotensive agents that do not substantially raise ICP by their vasodilating effect (we use labetalol, hydralazine, or a titrated nitroprusside infusion for uncontrollable hypertension). For most situations, we feel comfortable with a systolic pressure of 150–160 mm Hg and a diastolic pressure of 90–100 mm Hg. Urine input should be maintained at least 0.5 ml/kg per hour; accurate measurement requires bladder catheterization.

## Glucose and Thiamine

Hypoglycemia is a frequent cause of altered consciousness; give glucose (25 g as a 50% solution) intravenously immediately and before the results of blood tests

*Table 2.1*   Emergency laboratory tests of metabolic coma

---

I. Immediate tests
   A. Venous blood
      1. Glucose
      2. Electrolytes (Na, K, Cl, $CO_2$, $PO_4$)
      3. Urea and creatinine
      4. Osmolality
   B. Arterial blood (check color)
      1. pH
      2. $pO_2$
      3. $pCO_2$
      4. $HCO_3$
      5. HbCO (if available)
   C. Cerebrospinal fluid
      1. Gram's stain
      2. Cell count
      3. Glucose
   D. Electrocardiogram
II. Deferred tests (initial blood sample, process later)
   A. Venous blood
      1. Sedative and toxic drugs
      2. Liver function tests
      3. Coagulation studies
      4. Thyroid and adrenal function
      5. Blood cultures
      6. Viral titers
   B. Urine
      1. Sedative and toxic drugs
      2. Culture
   C. Cerebrospinal fluid
      1. Protein
      2. Culture
      3. Viral and fungal titers

---

are available. Empiric glucose treatment prevents hypoglycemic brain damage and outweighs the theoretical risks of additional harm to the brain in hyperglycemic, hyperosmolar, or anoxic coma. Give thiamine (100 mg) with the glucose infusion to prevent precipitation of Wernicke's encephalopathy in a malnourished, thiamine-depleted patient. Rarely, an established thiamine deficiency can cause coma.

## Stop Repeated Generalized Seizures

Repeated generalized seizures damage the brain and must be stopped. Initial treatment should be intravenous benzodiazepines, lorazepam (2–4 mg) or diazepam (5–10 mg). Maintain seizure control with intravenous phenytoin (18 mg/kg at a rate of 25 mg per minute). Seizure breakthrough requires additional benzodiazepines.

## Sedation

Careful and mild sedation should be given to the agitated, restless patient to prevent self-injury. A quiet patient facilitates ventilator support and diagnostic procedures. Small doses of intravenous benzodiazepines, intramuscular haloperidol (1 mg as often as hourly until desired effect), or intravenous morphine (2–4 mg) are appropriate; in the supported patient, the effects set in quickly, can be reversed, and are short-lasting.

## Specific Antidotes

Drug overdose is the largest single cause (30%) of coma in the emergency room. Most drug overdose can be treated by supportive measures alone. However, certain antagonists specifically reverse the effects of coma-producing drugs. Intravenous naloxone (0.4–2.0 mg) is the antidote for opiate coma. The reversal of narcotic effect, however, may precipitate acute withdrawal in an opiate addict. Give the minimum amount necessary to establish the diagnosis by pupillary dilatation and to reverse depressed breathing and coma. Do not attempt to completely reverse all drug effects.

Intravenous flumazenil reverses benzodiazepine-induced coma. It follows that coma unresponsive to 5 mg flumazenil given over 5 minutes is not due to benzodiazepine overdose. Recurrent resedation can be prevented with 1 mg flumazenil every 20 minutes.

The sedative effects of drugs with anticholinergic properties, particularly tricyclic antidepressants, can be reversed with 1–2 mg physostigmine intravenously. Pretreatment with 0.5 mg atropine prevents bradycardia. Only full awakening is characteristic of an anticholinergic drug overdose, as physostigmine has nonspecific arousal properties. Physostigmine has a short duration of action (45–60 minutes), and repeated doses may be required to maintain a state of arousal.

## Body Temperature

Hyperthermia is dangerous because it increases brain metabolic demand and, at extreme levels, denatures brain proteins. Temperature above 40°C requires nonspecific cooling measures, even before the underlying etiology is determined and treated. Hyperthermia most often indicates infection but may also be due to intracranial hemorrhage, anticholinergic drug intoxication, or heat exposure. The neuroleptic malignant syndrome must be considered in a patient exposed to psychotropic drugs. A body temperature of less than 34°C should be slowly elevated to above 35°C to prevent cardiac dysrhythmia. Hypothermia accompanies profound sepsis, sedative-hypnotic drug overdose, near-drowning, hypoglycemia, or Wernicke's encephalopathy.

## History

Once vital functions have been protected and the patient's condition is stable, clues to the cause of coma must be sought by interviewing relatives, friends, bystanders, or medical personnel who may have observed the patient before or during the decline in consciousness. The history should include the following:

1. Witnessed events: head injury, seizure, details of a motor vehicle accident, circumstances under which the patient was found
2. Evolution of coma: abrupt or gradual, headache, progressive or recurrent weakness, vertigo, nausea and vomiting
3. Recent medical history: surgical procedures, infections, current medication
4. Past medical history: epilepsy, head injury, drug or alcohol abuse, stroke, hypertension, diabetes, heart disease, cancer, uremia
5. Previous psychiatric history: depression, suicide attempts, social stresses
6. Access to drugs: sedatives, psychotropic drugs, narcotics, illicit drugs, drug paraphernalia, empty medicine bottles

## General Physical Examination

A systematic, detailed examination is helpful and necessary in the approach to the comatose patient who obviously is in no condition to describe prior or current medical problems. This examination is an extension of the initial evaluation and includes the following:

1. Repeated assessment of vital signs to determine efficacy of resuscitation measures
2. External evidence of trauma
3. Evidence of acute or chronic medical illness
4. Evidence of ingestion or self-administration of drugs (needle marks, alcohol on breath)
5. Evaluation for nuchal rigidity; be careful if severe neck injury is possible, or has not been excluded

## Neurologic Profile

The establishment of the nature of coma is critical for appropriate management and requires the following:

1. The correct interpretation of neurologic signs that reflect the integrity or impairment of various functional levels of the brain
2. Determination of whether the pattern and evolution of these signs are best explained by a supratentorial or infratentorial structural lesion, a metabolic-toxic encephalopathy, or a psychiatric cause (Tables 2.2 and 2.3)

The clinical neurologic functions that provide the most useful information in making a categorical diagnosis are outlined in Table 2.4. These clinical indices are easily and quickly obtained, have a high degree of interexaminer consistency, and, when applied serially, accurately reflect the patient's clinical course. Once the cause of coma can be assigned to one of these categories, specific radiographic, electrophysiologic, or chemical laboratory studies are used to make a disease-specific diagnosis and to detect existing or potential complications.

*Table 2.2* Neurologic profile (a modified Glasgow Coma Scale)

Verbal responses
    Oriented speech
    Confused conversation
    Inappropriate speech
    Incomprehensible speech
    No speech
Eye opening
    Spontaneous
    Response to verbal stimuli
    Response to noxious stimuli
    None
Motor responses
    Obeys
    Localizes
    Withdraws (flexion)
    Abnormal flexion
    Abnormal extension
    None
Pupillary reactions
    Present
    Absent
Spontaneous eye movement
    Orienting
    Roving conjugate
    Roving dysconjugate
    Miscellaneous abnormal movements
    None
Oculocephalic responses
    Normal (unpredictable)
    Full
    Minimal
    None
Oculovestibular responses
    Normal (nystagmus)
    Tonic conjugate
    Minimal or dysconjugate
    None
Deep tendon reflexes
    Normal
    Increased
    Absent

## Specific Management

## Supratentorial Mass Lesion

If the cause of coma is a presumed supratentorial mass, determine the severity and rate of evolution of signs. A relatively stable patient next requires an emergent head computed tomographic (CT) scan or magnetic resonance imaging

*Table 2.3*    Correlation between levels of brain function and clinical signs

| Structure | Function | Clinical sign |
| --- | --- | --- |
| Cerebral cortex | Conscious behavior | Speech (including any sounds) Purposeful movement Spontaneous To command To pain |
| Brain stem sensory pathways (reticular activating system) | Sleep/wake cycle | Eye opening Spontaneous To command To pain |
| Brain stem motor pathways | Reflex limb movements | Flexor posturing (decorticate) Extensor posturing (decerebrate) |
| Midbrain (CN III) | Innervation of ciliary muscle and certain extraocular muscles | Pupillary reactivity |
| Upper pons CN V CN VII | Facial and corneal sensation Facial muscle innervation | Corneal reflex-sensory Corneal reflex-motor response Blink Grimace |
| Lower pons: CN VIII (vestibular portion) connects by brain stem pathways with CN III, IV, VI | Reflex eye movements | Doll's eyes Caloric responses |
| Medulla | Spontaneous breathing Maintained blood pressure | Breathing and blood pressure do not require mechanical or chemical support |
| Spinal cord | Primitive protective responses | Deep tendon reflexes Babinski's response |

(MRI). Carotid angiography is considerably less informative, and a skull radiograph is a waste of time.

The priority in deep coma or established/threatening transtentorial herniation is the empiric medical treatment of intracranial hypertension. Hyperventilation (to a pCO$_2$ between 25 and 30 mm Hg) is the most rapid technique to lower elevated ICP. This is achieved by adjusting the ventilation rate (10–16 per minute) and tidal volume (12–14 ml/kg). The vasoconstrictive effect is transient (lasting a few hours at most) so that an osmotic agent must be administered concurrently. The preferred agent is a 20% mannitol solution as a 1-g/kg intravenous bolus. Maximal ICP reduction occurs within 20–60 minutes, and the effect of a single bolus lasts about 6 hours. Corticosteroids probably are not indicated in the emergent, empiric management of elevated ICP because their full effects are observed only after a few hours. Furthermore, as steroids are effective only for certain lesions (e.g., edema around a tumor or abscess), their use can be delayed until after a diagnosis has been made by head CT.

*Table 2.4*  Characteristics of categories of coma

I. Supratentorial mass lesion affecting the diencephalon/brain stem
   Initial focal cerebral dysfunction
   Dysfunction progresses rostral to caudal
   Signs reflect dysfunction at one level
   Signs often asymmetric
II. Subtentorial structural lesion
   Symptoms of brain stem dysfunction or sudden-onset coma
   Brain stem signs precede or accompany coma
   Cranial nerve and oculovestibular dysfunction
   Early onset of abnormal respiratory patterns
III. Metabolic-toxic coma
   Confusion or stupor precede motor signs
   Motor signs usually symmetric
   Pupil responses generally preserved
   Myoclonus, asterixis, tremulousness, and generalized seizures common
   Acid-base imbalance common with compensatory ventilatory changes
IV. Psychogenic coma
   Eyelids squeezed shut
   Pupils reactive or dilated, unreactive (cycloplegics)
   Oculocephalic reflex unpredictable; nystagmus on caloric tests
   Motor tone normal or inconsistent
   No pathologic reflexes
   (Awake-pattern electroencephalogram)

After initial ICP management, a head CT scan or MRI is required. The scan demonstrates the nature of the supratentorial lesion and associated mass effect. Arrangements must be made to evacuate promptly an epidural or subdural hematoma. Intraparenchymal masses that acutely produce deep stupor or coma initially are best managed nonsurgically. If steroids are indicated, a dexamethasone bolus (up to 100 mg intravenously) should be given, followed by approximately 16 mg every 6 hours.

The patient's vital signs and neurologic condition require repeated examination. Keep the head slightly elevated. Mannitol may be repeated, if necessary, every 4–6 hours; serum electrolytes and fluid balance must be monitored.

When patients with presumed increased ICP do not respond clinically as expected to medical management, or when obstructive hydrocephalus complicates a supratentorial mass lesion, we favor placement of a ventriculostomy into the lateral ventricle. This allows accurate measurement of intraventricular ICP and provides a method for cerebrospinal fluid (CSF) drainage, if necessary. The placement of a ventriculostomy allows calculation of cerebral perfusion pressure (mean systemic arterial pressure minus ICP), a critical determinant of cerebral blood flow, and, therefore, oxygen and substrate delivery. Monitoring of ICP also allows adjustment of therapeutic intervention before clinical deterioration occurs in patients with diminished intracranial compliance. Drainage of CSF aims to relieve high ICP to maintain cerebral perfusion pressure (>80 mm Hg) and to improve intracranial compliance. The risk of ventricular infection (predominantly with *Staphylococcus epidermidis*) can be decreased by removing or changing the ventricular catheter every 5–7 days.

After increased ICP has responded to emergency management and the patient's condition has stabilized, definitive treatment of the mass lesion is required as deemed appropriate.

## Infratentorial Lesion

The evolution of neurologic symptoms and signs and the neurologic examination generally give sufficient information to localize a lesion to the posterior fossa; lesions may be intrinsic or extrinsic to the brain stem.

Rapid neurologic deterioration of a patient suspected of harboring an infratentorial lesion demands emergency treatment before a head CT scan is performed. Treatment of a presumed extrinsic compressive lesion of the brain stem entails measures that decrease ICP as outlined above. A cerebellar hemorrhage or infarction requires urgent evacuation if the patient is in stupor or coma, if the level of arousal is decreasing, or if signs of progressive brain stem compression develop. Intrinsic brain stem lesions are best treated conservatively; an incompleted stroke may benefit from heparin anticoagulation. Posterior fossa tumors are managed initially with osmotic agents and steroids; definitive treatment includes surgery or irradiation or both.

The placement of a ventricular catheter for acute hydrocephalus must be considered carefully in consultation with a neurosurgeon; the danger exists of potentially fatal upward transtentorial herniation.

## Metabolic-Toxic Coma

The task of the physician in first contact with the patient in metabolic coma is to preserve and protect the brain from permanent damage. Metabolic (see Table 2.3) and toxicologic studies must be performed on the first blood drawn. Treatable conditions that quickly and irreversibly damage the brain include the following:

1. Hypoglycemia: As noted above, glucose (50 ml of a 50% solution intravenously) should be administered during emergency treatment before blood results return. Prolonged hypoglycemic coma that has considerably damaged the brain will not be reversed by a glucose load; also, a glucose bolus may transiently worsen hyperglycemic, hyperosmolar coma. In contrast, the osmolar load of intravenous glucose may transiently decrease elevated ICP and lighten nonhypoglycemic coma. A glucose infusion is needed to prevent recurrent hypoglycemia.

2. Acid-base imbalance: For accurate assessment, an arterial blood gas is required. The hyperventilating comatose patient with acute, severe metabolic acidosis and threatening cardiovascular collapse requires emergency treatment. In this situation, an intravenous infusion of $NaHCO_3$ (1 mEq/kg body weight) can be life-saving; simultaneously, a search for, and specific treatment of, the cause must be initiated.

3. Hypoxia: Suspected or proven carbon monoxide poisoning requires hyperventilation with 100% oxygen to facilitate excretion of this toxin. Idiopathic and drug-induced methemoglobinemia is treated with methylene blue (1–2 mg/kg

intravenously over a few minutes; repeat dose after 1 hour if needed). Anemia alone does not cause coma but exacerbates other forms of hypoxia. Transfusion of packed red cells or whole blood is appropriate for severe anemia (hematocrit less than 25%). Cyanide poisoning causes histotoxic hypoxia of the brain. Treatment entails amyl nitrite (vapor of crushed ampule inhaled every minute), sodium nitrite (300 mg intravenously), followed by sodium thiosulfate (12.5 g intravenously).

4. Acute bacterial meningitis: A lumbar puncture must be considered on any unconscious patient with fever or signs of meningeal irritation. A high index of suspicion is appropriate, particularly as the elderly may not develop fever and meningismus may not be elicited in the comatose patient. A head CT scan should be performed before lumbar puncture on a comatose patient to rule out unexpected mass lesions. Increased ICP is present in all cases of bacterial meningitis, but a lumbar puncture is not contraindicated when this diagnosis is suspected. Cerebral herniation seldom occurs except in small children with *Haemophilus influenzae* meningitis. Clinica! correlates of impending herniation demand a more cautious approach to lumbar puncture: coma or rapidly deteriorating level of arousal, focal neurologic signs, and tonic or prolonged fits. (Papilledema is rare in bacterial meningitis.) Estimates of the risk of herniation vary from 1% to 12%. Should unexpected herniation occur after lumbar puncture, treatment with hyperventilation and intravenous mannitol is indicated. Appropriate antibiotic treatment can usually await the result of an urgent CSF Gram's stain. Empiric broad-spectrum antibiotic treatment with a third-generation cephalosporin (ceftriaxone) and vancomycin is necessary if the result of the Gram's stain is negative but a bacterial etiology is suspected.

5. Drug overdose: Certain general principles apply to all patients suspected of having ingested sedative drugs. Most drug overdoses are treated by emergency treatment (already discussed) and supportive measures. Once vital signs are stable, attempt to remove, neutralize, or reverse the effects of the drug. The patient in coma requires a gastric lavage after endotracheal intubation. Place a large, preferably double-lumen, gastric tube orally. The lavage is performed in the head-down position on the left side. Lavage is performed with 200- to 300-ml boluses of tap water or half-normal saline and continued until the return is clear. After lavage, pass 1–2 tbsp. of activated charcoal down the lavage tube. With meticulous supportive measures, patients with uncomplicated drug-induced coma should recover without neurologic deficit. The recovery from coma due to massive doses of phenobarbital or glutethimide can be hastened by hemodialysis.

Constant vigilance and attention to the patient's condition, with timely and appropriate diagnostic and therapeutic, and, if necessary, repeated evaluation ensure the best possible outcome of the unconscious patient. Effective care demands meticulous attention to the maintenance of tissue perfusion and oxygenation; the documentation and anticipation of acute neurologic events (particularly diminished cerebral perfusion, herniation, or seizures); aggressive, rapid treatment of initial or subsequent infections; and prevention of agitation. Deep venous thrombosis must be prevented with either subcutaneous heparin or full-length leg pneumatic compression boots. Enteral or parenteral feeding within 36–48 hours must satisfy nutritional needs. Corneal injury can be prevented by protecting the eyes with lubricants and taping the lids shut.

## Prediction of Outcome of Coma

A complete evaluation of the comatose patient must include an estimate of prognosis. The outcome in a given comatose patient cannot be predicted with absolute certainty. Available serial data are not sufficiently specific or selective to help in establishing the prognosis in an individual patient. Guidelines on the outcome of coma have been compiled based on serial examinations, and although the results are valuable in providing early, informed discussion with relatives of patients and medical colleagues, they should probably not be used to make decisions to withhold therapy. However, the early establishment of a highly probable outcome ideally should be made within 24 hours after hospital admission to ration intensive care services in futile cases. A logical and sensible approach to prognostication includes an etiologic subcategorization into medical, drug-induced, and traumatic coma.

Factors that are useful in determining the outcome of medical coma include the cause, the depth, and the duration of coma. Certain clinical signs, particularly brain stem responses (motor and verbal responses), are the most helpful and best validated predictors (confidence interval 0.95).

Overall, only 15% of patients in established *medical coma* for longer than 6 hours make a good or moderate recovery; others die (61%), remain vegetative (12%), or become permanently dependent on others for daily living (11%). Prognosis depends on the etiology of medical coma. Patients in coma due to a stroke or subarachnoid hemorrhage have a 9% chance of achieving independent function. Thirty-five percent of patients achieve moderate or good recovery if coma is due to metabolic causes, including infection, organ failure, and biochemical disturbances.

The depth of coma affects the individual prognosis. If patients open their eyes in response to painful stimuli after 6 hours of coma, they have a 20% chance of making a good recovery, versus 10% if eyes remain closed.

The longer the coma persists, the less likely is recovery; 15% of patients in coma for 6 hours make a good or moderate recovery compared with only 3% who remain unconscious at 1 week.

The severity of signs of brain stem dysfunction on admission inversely correlates with the chance of good recovery in medical coma. Absent pupillary responses at any time after onset and absent caloric reflexes 1 day after onset indicate a poor prognosis (<2% recovery). No patient with absent pupillary light reflexes, corneal reflexes, oculocephalic or caloric responses, or lack of a motor response to noxious stimulation at 3 days after onset is likely to ever regain independent function. Patients likely to recover speak words, open their eyes to noise, show nystagmus on caloric testing, or have spontaneous eye movements within 1–3 days.

Postanoxic convulsive status epilepticus (CSE) and myoclonic status epilepticus (MSE) imply a poor prognosis. Most patients die or become vegetative. Associated with clinical findings (e.g., loss of brain stem reflexes, eye opening at the onset of myoclonic jerks) and EEG patterns (e.g., suppression or burst suppression), CSE and MSE confirm a grim neurologic outcome for such patients. Autopsy studies show that cerebral and cerebellar damage can be ascribed to the initial ischemic-hypoxic event; there is no evidence that status epilepticus further contributes to this damage. We initially treat patients with an intravenous loading dose of a major anticonvulsant (phenytoin, 13–18 mg/kg at 25 mg per minute, and/or phenobarbital, 20 mg/kg at 50 mg per minute). MSE is generally resistant to therapy; we give intermittent doses of benzodiazepines (lorazepam, 2–4 mg, or clonazepam, 0.5 mg) intravenously as needed to suppress particularly severe myoclonus that interferes with ventilatory support. Anesthetic agents are rarely indicated and are unlikely to alter outcome.

The most accurate prediction of outcome in a patient in medical coma is obtained from the use of combinations of clinical signs. Within the first week, it is hard to justify the withdrawal of therapy for patients in medical coma unless they are already brain dead or lack all sings of brain stem function. There is little to be added by more sophisticated testing other than to identify the cause of the coma. Patients in medical coma who are in a vegetative state at 1 month have a 14% chance of recovery to independent life.

Patients in coma due to *exogenous agents* (except carbon monoxide poisoning) carry an overall good prognosis provided that circulation and respiration are protected by avoiding or correcting cardiac dysrhythmia, aspiration pneumonia, and respiratory arrest. Despite absent brain stem reflexes (and electrocerebral silence on EEG), patients with deep sedative drug intoxication have the potential for complete recovery. Therefore, in the emergent situation, patients in coma of uncertain etiology should be supported vigorously until the precise cause of coma has been fully established.

The outcome of *traumatic coma* is generally somewhat better than medical coma, and prognostic criteria are somewhat different because (1) many patients with head injury are young; (2) prolonged post-traumatic unconsciousness of up to several months does not preclude a satisfactory outcome; and (3) compared with the initial degree of neurologic abnormality, traumatic recover better than medical coma patients.

Patients in coma for longer than 6 hours after head injury have a 40% chance to recover to moderate disability or better at 6 months. The most reliable predictors of outcome at 6 months are (1) patient age (worse outcome especially over 60 years), (2) depth and duration of coma (an inverse correlation with the Glasgow Coma Scale), (3) pupil reaction and eye movements (absence at 24 hours predicts death or a vegetative state in 90% of such patients), and (4) motor response in the first week of injury. An independent poor prognostic indicator is sustained, uncontrollable increased ICP (>20 mm Hg). Factors that appear to have little influence on outcome are (1) the cause of head injury, (2) skull fracture, (3) lateralization of damage to one hemisphere, and (4) the extent of extracranial injury.

## ROLE OF SPECIAL INVESTIGATIONS

### Neurodiagnostic Imaging

Once the patient with an altered mental status is appropriately resuscitated and stabilized, more information is usually required to define a lesion because this determines specific therapy. CT scan and MRI provide morphologic information about intracranial contents and pathology that produces coma.

The CT scan is currently the most expedient imaging technique and gives the most rapid information about possible structural lesions with the least risk to the patient. The value of the CT scan to demonstrate mass lesions, hemorrhage, and hydrocephalus is well established. Axial cuts (10 mm for the cerebral hemispheres, 5 mm for the posterior fossa) are sufficient initially; intravenous iodinated dye highlights areas of blood-brain barrier breakdown such as tumor, abscess, and subacute strokes, and may be necessary to better define such lesions. The CT scan shows tissue shifts due to intracranial compartmental pressure gradients, but may somewhat underestimate resultant herniation syndromes compared to MRI. Certain lesions such as early (less than 12 hours) infarction, encephalitis, and isodense subdural hemorrhage may be difficult to visualize. Posterior fossa pathology may be somewhat obscured by bone artifact inherent in the CT technique. Raised ICP is suggested by a narrowed third ventricle and obliteration of the suprasellar or quadrigeminal cisterns but cannot otherwise be quantified.

MRI may be performed depending on the clinical setting and the stability of the patient's condition. The use of MRI is limited in the urgent setting of coma evaluation because of the length of time required to perform the imaging, image degradation by even a slight movement of the patient, and the relative inaccessibility of the patient for emergencies during the imaging process. However, MRI provides superb visualization of the posterior fossa and its contents, which is useful when intrinsic brain stem lesions are suspected as the cause of coma. Sagittal MRI views are particularly useful in the documentation of the degree of supratentorial or infratentorial herniations and may enable intervention before clinical deterioration.

## Electroencephalography

The EEG is a sensitive indicator of cerebral function and may give useful additional information in the evaluation of the unresponsive patient. With metabolic and toxic disorders, the EEG changes generally reflect the degree and severity of altered consciousness, characterized by a decreased frequency of the background rhythm, and the appearance of diffuse slow activity in the theta (4–7 Hz) or delta (1–3 Hz) range. Bilaterally synchronous and symmetric, medium- to high-amplitude, broad triphasic waves are seen in various metabolic encephalopathies, most often in hepatic coma. Rapid beta activity (>13 Hz) in a comatose patient suggests ingestion of sedative hypnotics, such as barbiturates and benzodiazepines. Acute, focally destructive lesions show focal slow activity, and when periodic lateralized epileptiform discharges are accentuated in one or both temporal lobes, herpes simplex encephalitis must be strongly considered. A nonreactive, diffuse alpha pattern in a comatose patient usually implies a poor prognosis and is most often seen after anoxic insults to the brain or acute, destructive pontine tegmental damage. Nonconvulsive generalized status epilepticus and repeated complex partial seizures may produce altered levels of arousal or awareness; the EEG is an indispensable tool in the diagnosis and management of both these disorders. Continuous EEG monitoring optimizes management of status epilepticus, as clinical assessment is insufficiently sensitive to detect continued electrographic seizures. Furthermore, continuous EEG monitoring in the intensive care unit setting has shown an unsuspected high incidence of electrographic seizure activity in critically ill neurologic patients. A normally reactive EEG in an unresponsive patient suggests psychiatric disease; however, relatively normal results from EEG are seen in the locked-in syndrome, akinetic mutism, and catatonia, which may all be caused by structural brain lesions.

Attempts have been made to correlate the pattern and frequency spectra of postresuscitation EEG with neurologic outcome. We do not use the EEG routinely for this purpose because the absolute predictive value of the EEG has not been established (at best, 88% accuracy). At present, the most useful information regarding patient prognosis is still obtained by the correct interpretation of physical signs.

## SUGGESTED READING

Ellenhorn MJ, Schonwald S, Ordog G, et al. Ellenhorn's Medical Toxicology: Diagnosis and Treatment of Human Poisoning (2nd ed). Baltimore: Williams & Wilkins, 1997.

Fisher CM. The neurological examination of the comatose patient. Acta Neurol Scand 1969; 45(suppl):5–56.

Hacke W, et al. (eds). Neurocritical Care. Berlin: Springer, 1994.

Jennett B, Teasdale G, Brackman R, et al. Prognosis of patients with severe head injury. Neurosurgery 1979;4:283–301.

Levy DE, Bates D, Caronna JJ, et al. Prognosis in non-traumatic coma. Ann Intern Med 1981;94:293–301.

Levy DE, Caronna JJ, Singer BH, et al. Predicting outcome from hypoxic-ischemic coma. JAMA 1985;253:1420–1426.

Plum F, Posner JB. The Diagnosis of Stupor and Coma (3rd ed). Philadelphia: Davis, 1980.

Reich JB, Sierra J, Camp W, et al. Magnetic resonance imaging measurements and clinical changes accompanying transtentorial and foramen magnum brain herniation. Arch Neurol 1993;33:159–170.

Ropper AH. Lateral displacement of the brain and the level of consciousness in patients with an acute hemispheral mass. N Engl J Med 1986;314:953–958.

Ropper AH (ed). Neurological and Neurosurgical Intensive Care (3rd ed). New York: Raven, 1993.

Salcman M (ed). Neurologic Emergencies (2nd ed). New York: Raven, 1990.

Schwartz GR: Poisonings, Emergency Toxicology, and General Principles of Medical Management of the Poisoned Patient. In GR Schwartz, P Safar, JH Stone (eds), Principles and Practice of Emergency Medicine. Philadelphia: Saunders, 1978;1316–1332.

Synek VM. EEG abnormality grades and subdivisions of prognostic importance in traumatic and anoxic coma in adults. Clin Electroencephalogr 1988;19:160–166.

Wijdicks EFM. Neurology of Critical Illness. Philadelphia: Davis, 1995.

Young GB, Gilbert JJ, Zochodne DW. The significance of myoclonic status epilepticus in postanoxic coma. Neurology 1990;40:1843–1848.

Young GB, Gordon KG, Doig GS. An assessment of nonconvulsive seizures in the intensive care unit using continuous EEG monitoring: an investigation of variables associated with mortality. Neurology 1996;47:83–89.

# 3
# Weakness

Thomas D. Sabin and Peter R. Bergethon

One of the greatest difficulties in neurologic evaluation is the lack of common language with which patients and non-neurologists can discuss weakness, one of the most frequent manifestations of neurologic disease. Although the most difficult assignment of language is probably associated with sensory disturbances, weakness is also very difficult to describe. Such language limitations may hamper the general physician who seeks to better understand the cause of the symptoms of weakness and consults a neurologic colleague. Perhaps it is for this reason that the experienced neurologic consultant suppresses a momentary roll of the eyes or other sign of impatience when consulted for evaluation of the weak patient. Inevitably, the first requirement of the consultant is a careful retaking of the patient's history to determine the precise nature of the complaint. No area of neurologic consultation demands a clearer formulation of a prime principle of neurology: Where is the lesion?

Patients most often use the term *weakness* when referring to a generalized lassitude. The term could refer to a loss of energy resulting from depression; systemic disease; or the poorly understood, diagnostically tenuous chronic fatigue and fibromyalgia syndromes. Such lassitude is not likely to represent a disorder in neurologic motor pathways but rather reflects the general medical or psychological status of the patient. Thus, a complaint of weakness must first be evaluated with respect to its general quality, duration, and focal nature. Patients with neurologically based weakness typically avoid the word *weakness* and complain instead of the difficulty in motor performance produced by the weakness.

Patients may also complain of "weakness" that is actually discomfort occasioned by robust contraction of a muscle, usually related to painful states in joints, tendons, or the muscles themselves. In such cases, the patient is referring to the limitation of muscle power engendered by pain. A variety of motor-system disorders without paralysis may cause the patient to think he or she is weak. This phenomenon includes, for example, spasticity, myotonia, "stiff man" syndrome, and rigidity, and is illustrated by the term selected by James Parkinson: *paralysis agitans*. Patients complain that they are weak when they sense a proprioceptive experience of increased resistance. Various sensory symptoms may also be erroneously described

45

*Table 3.1*   Examples of motor-performance difficulties associated
with dysfunction in specific nerves

| Lesion site | Complaint |
|---|---|
| Upper brachial plexus | Trouble lifting a glass to the lips |
| Suprascapular nerve | Difficulty in scratching the back of the head. Has to move the paper to left when writing a long line of words. Trouble turning a key or door knob clockwise with the arm outstretched. |
| Subscapular nerve | Cannot scratch the lower part of the back |
| Inferior gluteal nerve | Difficulty climbing stairs and rising from sitting |
| Anterior interosseous nerve | Difficulty pinching or using a needle for hand sewing |
| Ulnar nerve | Fingers slip laterally when tightly grasping the handle of a knife, paintbrush, or pencil. Little finger hands laterally. |
| Deep palmar branch of ulnar | Trouble holding pencil, buttoning clothes, and tying shoelaces |

as weakness. A patient who is losing proprioceptive sense in a severe sensory ataxia may conclude after falling to the side in the shower that his or her legs are weak.

The patient, if allowed to describe situations in which he or she is having difficulty, provides the consultant with the essential localizing information. A patient with proximal limb-girdle weakness complains of difficulty in rising from sitting to standing, especially from a low chair or a bathtub. Proximal weakness in the upper limbs results in difficulties doing his or her hair or performing tasks that require extension of the arms above the head, such as reaching up to high shelves. The complaint of "stiffness" of the muscles and difficulty in moving through the full range of motion may be the prime concern of patients with chronic spinal cord lesions or other conditions in which spasticity far outweighs upper motor-neuron weakness.

Patients suffering from a footdrop report focal weaknesses in terms of their liability to falling and tripping on stairs, curbings, or even at the edge of carpets. The patient with femoral nerve palsy usually reports that the affected knee may "buckle." Walking becomes impossible if femoral nerve palsy is bilateral. Many peripheral nerve syndromes are associated with motor performance failures that consultants are more likely to discover by allowing the patients to describe the details of their troubles using familiar language and everyday situations rather than immediately categorizing the complaint as a neurologic syndrome (Table 3.1).

The nature of a motor difficulty can be further sorted out by knowledge of the duration and penetration of the symptoms into daily life. For example, episodic weakness may be present with the syndromes of transient ischemic attack (TIA), migraines, periodic paralysis, and even the episodic ataxia and choreoathetotic syndromes. The consultant may also see a patient who is episodically weak in the postictal state. A patient may have an unseen or unrecognized occult seizure in the hospital bed, where the postictal hemiparesis or paralysis is noted by the staff. A physical examination is invaluable in identifying such cases because purely postictal weakness is never spastic or hyper-reflexic. Weakness affecting the bulbar innervated musculature may result in dysarthric speech that may be described as "tired" or "drunken" and there may be associated difficulty with swallowing. Such symptoms are seen secondary to myasthenia gravis, motor-neuron disease, or pseudobulbar palsy, but may be found in the direct bulbar peripheral palsies such as Guillain-Barré syndrome, sarcoidosis, Lyme disease, and human immunodeficiency virus infection.

On completion of the history, the consulting neurologist should suspect a localization that may be tested during the physical examination. In the evaluation of weakness, the mental status examination often provides important clues based on the ability and willingness of the patient to engage in tests that may suggest a psychological cause of weakness. The more directed issues of reflexes and power must include assessment of abnormal tone such as rigidity, spasticity, or gegenhalten, which are associated with abnormal motor performances and might be erroneously described as weakness.

Another form of "pseudoweakness" is apraxia. Here, a cooperative patient with no elementary neurologic deficits (i.e., adequate strength) has difficulty performing a learned motor task in response to a verbal command. Ordinarily a testing circumstance can be devised to normalize the performance; for example, the patient may be allowed to imitate the examiner or the actual rather than an imagined object is provided for the motor task. Examiners should, however, be alert for pseudoapraxia, illustrated by the following case. A physician called one of the authors urgently stating that she had a stroke in the middle of the night, manifested as an apraxia limited to the right hand. Her motor difficulty in performing fine manipulation was in fact a result of paralysis of the right adductor pollicis. She had damaged the deep palmar branch of the ulnar nerve during prolonged, vigorous use of a paint scraper on the previous night.

Once the possibility of erroneously described weakness is eliminated, the consultant should proceed to a detailed evaluation of each aspect of the power production system of the nervous system. These include the following:

1. The effector systems of the muscles and the neuromuscular junction
2. The command structures of the brain and spinal cord
3. The interlinked communication systems of the peripheral nerves

Neurologists know the details of operation of these aspects, and it is not our intention to review these familiar systems but rather to demonstrate some of the quirkier and more interesting anecdotal subtleties by which the bedside examination can determine the appropriate work-up and treatment of the hospitalized patient.

The experienced consultant's examination is directed toward localizing a diagnostically meaningful pattern of weakness and undergoes continuous modification as the findings accumulate. The pattern of weakness may be classified as bilateral, unilateral, or following a specific pattern. We focus on the more difficult area of bilateral weakness, because most unilateral and specific pattern weakness syndromes are readily recognizable as ischemic cerebral events and focal peripheral neuropathies. We include only a few interesting examples to illustrate the last two groups.

## BILATERAL WEAKNESS

The common in-house problem of widespread, often acute, bilateral weakness is useful in illustrating the approach of developing a useful pattern of weakness. We use the word *widespread* because the words *diffuse weakness* in a patient's chart nearly always reflect a failure to exploit the distinctive patterns of weakness associated with dysfunction at the various organizational levels of the neuraxis.

## Paresis Due to Myopathy

In primary muscle disease the most common pattern of weakness is a symmetric paresis of the proximal limb girdles and axial musculature. The patient's complaints usually involve respiratory function or difficulty in rising from a chair or bathtub, climbing stairs, rolling over in bed, or partaking in activities requiring elevation of the arms (e.g., shaving or grooming the hair).

Usually, the dystrophies and polymyositis do not constitute emergencies and thus allow time for thorough investigation. Occasionally, however, chronic muscular weakness can result in respiratory failure if sudden stress on the muscles of respiration occurs as a result of infection, asthma, or pulmonary disease with increased airway resistance.

## Myositis

Skeletal muscle may be affected by an inflammatory process associated with weakness and sometimes myalgias (i.e., tender, achy muscles). The examiner must differentiate between dermatomyositis, polymyositis, and inclusion-body myositis.

Dermatomyositis is often associated with carcinoma, though it has been reported in patients with infection (toxoplasmosis, hepatitis B), intoxication (ipecac abuse), hypothyroidism, and immune-mediated reactions (sarcoidosis, penicillamine reactions, and vaccination reactions). The skin and muscles are most likely both involved in an autoimmune attack of this kind. Skin rash and muscle weakness usually start together, but the rash may precede the achy, weak muscles by several weeks. The weakness pattern is proximal and the course of the disease rapid; it is usually a matter of weeks from onset to severe disability. Cranial muscles are usually spared, though neck muscles are affected. Diagnosis is clinical, based on the rash and myopathic pattern. Between 50% and 80% of patients respond to steroids, and often the malignancy has already been diagnosed.

Polymyositis is a subtler syndrome with diverse causes leading to the inflammatory myopathy. Usually a proximal pattern of weakness with dysphagia is present along with elevated creatine phosphokinase (CPK) levels and distinctive electromyographic changes. Despite the *-itis* suffix, the process may be entirely painless, and no neuropathic weakness is present. Polymyositis is associated with systemic disease about 50% of the time, and the etiologies are extensive (Table 3.2). The time course for disease progression is similar to dermatomyositis, but polymyositis is seen only after puberty, and the weakness in dermatomyositis is often more disabling. Treatment is aimed at the underlying disease when appropriate, and many cases of polymyositis respond to immunosuppressive treatment.

A differentiation between steroid-responsive polymyositis and the histologically distinct inclusion-body myositis can often be made clinically. Distinguishing features of inclusion-body cases are slow progression, low CPK levels, male sex, and a clinical pattern of knee-hip extensor weakness, asymmetric wrist and finger flexor–shoulder abduction weakness, and an associated peripheral neuropathy.

*Table 3.2*  Disorders associated with polymyositis

Systemic lupus erythematosus
Mixed connective-tissue syndrome
Sjögren's syndrome
Systemic sclerosis
Ulcerative colitis
Human lymphotrophic virus type I
Lupron therapy
Ranitidine therapy

## Periodic Paralysis

The rare hereditary condition known as *periodic paralysis* is characterized by acute widespread myopathic paralysis related to muscle membrane ion channel dysfunctions. Attacks of flaccid quadriplegia beginning during the second decade of life are seen in hypokalemic periodic paralysis. The individual attacks tend to occur after heavy meals or subsequent to resting that follows a burst of vigorous physical activity. Paralysis associated with hypokalemia lasts 6–48 hours. The diagnosis is suggested by a history of prior attacks and similarly affected relatives. Patients' genetic history reveals an autosomal dominant pattern with a male preponderance. The cranial nerves and the respiratory musculature are usually spared, and the attacks may be prevented or aborted by administration of oral potassium preparations.

The hyperkalemic form of periodic paralysis also follows an autosomal dominant pattern of inheritance. In contrast to the hypokalemic form, attacks are milder and occur during the first decade. Exposure to cold is the most consistent precipitant of the paralysis, though a heavy meal can also provoke an attack. The syndrome affects men and women equally. Myotonia, especially of the eyelids, is a characteristic finding. Treatment involves administering thiazide diuretics to lower serum potassium levels. Administration of oral potassium precipitates attacks.

Varieties of periodic paralysis without abnormal serum potassium have also been described. Paralyzed muscles demonstrate a loss of direct muscle excitability in all forms of periodic paralysis. A brisk tap of the reflex hammer on a normal muscle belly mechanically distorts muscle membrane and initiates depolarization with visible contraction. Observation of this phenomenon is useful in differentiating paralysis resulting from denervation from periodic paralysis because even when muscle is fully paralyzed because of denervation, direct muscle excitability is normal or enhanced, though tendon reflexes are absent.

## Paresis Caused by Medical Conditions

Metabolic derangements such as hyperthyroid storm can result in myopathic patterns of weakness. In very sick hospitalized patients, widespread muscle weakness may be associated with muscle necrosis. Reddish urine due to myoglobinuria results from disruption of muscle membranes and the release of myoglobin into the circulation. The myoglobin is rapidly cleared into the urine, which then becomes guaiac-

or benzidine-positive. Although the test for blood in the urine is strongly positive, few or no red blood cells are seen. The serum should be examined to distinguish this event from hemoglobinuria. Because hemoglobin is bound to proteins, the serum becomes pink, but myoglobin is unbound and excreted so rapidly that the serum remains clear.

At the Boston City Hospital, the most common cause of myoglobinuria was pressure necrosis of muscles resulting from the prolonged immobility associated with drug and alcohol overdose. Intense, repetitive exercise by formerly sedentary individuals is an occasional cause of myoglobinuria, usually reported at military training centers. The same etiology accounts for the myoglobinuria seen after a bout of status epilepticus. Crushing or thermal (e.g., "trench foot") injuries may be sufficient to cause disruption of muscle membranes. Alcohol, the glycyrrhizic acid found in licorice, carbon monoxide, and sea-snake venom have all been cited as toxic causes of myoglobinuria. In hereditary muscle phosphorylase deficiency (McArdle's disease), exertion causes painful, electrically silent cramps that are occasionally associated with myoglobinuria. Once myoglobinuria is recognized, the most urgent goal is to avert renal failure resulting from accumulation of myoglobin in the renal tubules.

Alcohol-induced, generalized muscle weakness may be caused by rhabdomyolysis associated with immobility or by other causes. A sometimes overlooked problem that can cause weakness is the low phosphate supply caused by dietary inadequacy in a patient with severe alcoholism. The inadequate dietary supply of phosphate can create clinical hypophosphatemia with widespread muscle weakness. Finally, hypokalemia may play a role in the patient with severe alcoholism. The patient may present to the hospital with combined electrolyte abnormalities that often include hyponatremia, hypokalemia, hypocalcemia, and hypophosphatemia. The metabolic causes of weakness in alcoholics are sometimes ignored because of the accompanying difficulties the patients may have with acute or chronic peripheral neuropathy, midline cerebellar dysfunction, and mental status alterations. In addition, the patient's hematologic picture, with high mean corpuscular volume, may lead the consultant to believe the patient is suffering from subacute combined degeneration, when in fact acute alcoholism is presented with either necrotizing myolysis or a form of induced hypokalemic periodic paralysis. Certainty of diagnosis of these alcohol-related diseases requires consideration of the differential, but may be assisted by the salutary response to repletion of the missing electrolytes and re-establishment of normal nutrition. The myopathies associated with the "failure to wean" problem are discussed later in this chapter, under Prolonged Neuromuscular Blockade in Hospitalized Patients.

## MYASTHENIA GRAVIS AND OTHER DISORDERS OF THE NEUROMUSCULAR JUNCTION

Except to the neurologic consultant, the neuromuscular junction (NMJ) may be one of the more enigmatic neurochemical devices in the body. In myasthenia gravis, the interaction of autoantibodies with the acetylcholine receptors on the postsynaptic membranes of the neuromuscular junction leads to blockade of neuromuscular transmission, resulting in weakness, abnormal fatigability, and delayed recovery from exercise-induced weakness. The weakness can be alleviated by increasing the effective concentration of acetylcholine either with anticholinesterase agents or by reducing the autoantibodies with suppression of the immune system. The disorder is rare (1 in 20,000) but may occur at any age, although onset in the second and third decades is usual, and women are more commonly affected than men. Myasthenia gravis is the most common NMJ disorder and remains a disease generally diagnosed and treated by the neurologist. The current tendency in practice when an NMJ disorder is suspected is to immediately order anti–acetylcholine receptor antibodies levels and to do a single fiber jitter study. This approach overlooks the more subtle clinical features of myasthenia, which can predict the usefulness of such tests.

The pattern of muscle involvement is a key feature of NMJ disorders. The characteristic initial symptoms are fluctuating weakness in the extraocular, facial, masticatory, or pharyngeal muscles. The patient notes intermittent diplopia, nasal voice, dysphagia, weakness in chewing, or nasal regurgitation. The flattening of the nasolabial folds with ptosis and a slightly slack jaw make the patient appear mentally dull. The relative preservation of the levator labii superioris and anguli oris when the zygomatics and buccinators are weak superimposes a slight snarl and results in a highly diagnostic facial appearance. The tongue may have two extra longitudinal furrows located midway between the normal central raphe and the lateral borders. Normal function may be present after sleep, but progressive weakness often develops during the day's activities. Paralysis does extend to limb and respiratory muscles, but severe paralysis below the neck without obvious weakness in the cranial musculature is extremely rare.

The examination of strength before and after muscular activity in such cases reveals the characteristic abnormal fatigability and delay in recovery of strength. For example, when the patient is asked to sustain an upward gaze, progressive ptosis or failure in maintaining the position of the eyes becomes apparent. When the limb muscles are affected, rapid repetitive tapping of a tendon may show a fatigue of the reflex as neuromuscular transmission fails. Having a patient repetitively squeeze an ergometer or a partially inflated blood pressure cuff may also be used for evaluation at the bedside, but using an electromyographer eliminates subjective factors by directly stimulating the nerve at a rapid rate and displaying the declining muscle potentials on the cathode ray tube.

Early symptoms of amyotrophic lateral sclerosis (ALS) may sometimes be difficult to distinguish from myasthenia gravis, particularly in the bulbar form of ALS in which dysphagia and dysphonia are presenting symptoms. The edrophonium (Tensilon) test can be useful in this differentiation, although, unless it is strongly positive, the diagnosis may remain unclear.

## Edrophonium (Tensilon) Test

A transient improvement in strength with intravenous administration of a short-acting anticholinesterase agent such as edrophonium (Tensilon) is diagnostic. A total of 10 mg is drawn into the syringe but only 2 mg is administered initially, and the patient is observed for changes in strength. If no clear change occurs after 1 minute, the remaining 8 mg is given. The dosage is staged in this manner to avoid cholinergic weakness in patients who are extremely sensitive to anticholinesterase agents. Increased weakness when Tensilon is administered is characteristic in a cholinergic crisis; a control test using intravenous saline is often very helpful. Electrocardiogram monitoring may be prudent in some patients.

## Myasthenic Crises

Patients with myasthenia are subject to sudden bouts of life-threatening profound weakness involving respiratory paralysis. Such crises are not a usual presenting feature of the disease, and most patients in crisis are known to have myasthenia and have been taking oral anticholinesterase medications. The patient may have tried to combat progressive weakness by increasing medications. In these cases, the physician must be aware that *the crisis may be due to either worsening of the myasthenia or to the neuromuscular blockade caused by excess anticholinesterase agents* (known as *cholinergic crisis*). Overdose of anticholinesterase drugs increases available acetylcholine to levels capable of causing continued depolarization of the muscle membrane and blocking neuromuscular transmission (depolarization blockage). *The distinction between myasthenic crisis and cholinergic crisis is of critical importance in the early management of these patients.* A Tensilon test worsens the weakness in cholinergic crisis and is apt to be accompanied by abdominal cramps and showers of fasciculations, especially around the eyelids. Patients with myasthenic crisis may show improved strength or no change with Tensilon. When no change occurs with Tensilon, the patient is in an anticholinesterase-resistant phase of the disease.

Confusion about the status of the patient's neuromuscular pharmacology should never delay prompt measures to secure an airway and adequate ventilation for the patient. The myasthenic patient is in jeopardy not only because of decreased tidal volume but also because the faulty swallowing mechanism allows aspiration of secretions. Tracheal intubation and frequent suctioning may be necessary. Search for the cause of the crisis should consider pneumonia, other systemic disease, or a harmful drug.

Medications that are potentially harmful to the myasthenic include opiates, barbiturates, muscle relaxants, quinine and quinidine, and some antibiotics (most of the aminoglycosides). Adrenocorticotropic hormone (ACTH) and steroids in large doses may precipitate or worsen myasthenic crises. These agents are sometimes very useful despite this problem because a remission may follow the steroid-induced exacerbation.

## Lambert-Eaton Myasthenic Syndrome

Lambert-Eaton myasthenic syndrome (LEMS) results when IgG autoantibodies blockade the voltage-gated calcium channels at peripheral cholinergic nerve terminals. LEMS may occur with small-cell lung cancer (or other malignancies) or as a primary autoimmune disease. Brief voluntary exercise or repetitive muscle contraction produces a transient improvement in strength, and this anomalous result of formal strength testing can cause misdiagnosis of functional weakness. The distribution of the weakness involves the proximal limb muscles and axial muscles. Ptosis and occasional facial weakness occurs in this syndrome, but the severe disturbance of extraocular movements and bulbar musculature that characterizes myasthenia gravis do not. The axial weakness may cause an ataxia. In addition to weakness, patients frequently have dry mouth, abnormal pupils, impotence, and paresthesias in the thighs. The reflexes are depressed or absent. The hospital consultant may be called on when a mild case of LEMS has been exacerbated by administration of calcium channel blockers, beta blockers, quinidine, procainamide, or aminoglycoside antibiotics.

## NEUROMUSCULAR TOXINS

Consulting neurologists occasionally, though rarely, see weakness secondary to neuromuscular blockage resulting from natural or even iatrogenic intoxications.

### Botulism

Each of the distinct toxins produced by the six types of *Clostridium botulinum* blocks transmission in both nicotinic and muscarinic cholinergic nerve terminals. These heat-labile toxins usually are ingested with improperly canned foods and in severe cases can produce symptoms within a few hours. Dysfunction of the cholinergic autonomic terminals causes fixed, dilated pupils; dry mucous membranes; urinary retention; loss of peristalsis with abdominal distention; and postural hypotension. Bulbar innervated striated muscles usually develop weakness first; the patient notes diplopia, nasal voice, and difficulty chewing and swallowing. Widespread weakness followed by paralysis of respiration leads to rapid death. Treatment includes gastric lavage, which may remove unabsorbed toxin. Antitoxin is administered, and life support during the period of respiratory paralysis is crucial because full neurologic recovery can be anticipated in survivors. Importantly for correct diagnosis, mentation remains clear in botulinum poisoning (assuming that the emergency room has not paralyzed and sedated the patient before assessment!).

### Tick Paralysis

Widespread paralysis with no sensory involvement may be seen after tick infestation of the scalp. This rapid ascending paralysis is easily confused with the acute inflammatory demyelinating polyneuropathy (AIDP, also known as *Guillain-Barré syndrome* [GBS]) because both produce a distal to proximal pattern of paralysis with hypoflexia or areflexia and ataxia. A careful search of the hair, including taking apart cornrows and braids will reveal the gravid *Dermacentor andersoni*. Removal of the tick results in rapid and complete neurologic recovery. Tick infestation is an example of the kind of case in which careful history taking and a directed, meticulous physical examination can be curative. Two patients who were misdiagnosed as having GBS had the problem-causing ticks discovered by electroencephalogram technicians who were placing their electrodes.

## Prolonged Neuromuscular Blockade in Hospitalized Patients

As if the natural world is not dangerous enough, the pharmacologic poisons used within the medical system cause abundant cases of prolonged neuromuscular blockage in our hospitals. This flaccid quadriplegic syndrome has been reported in patients treated with vecuronium bromide and other neuromuscular blocking agents. These agents are widely used in medical intensive care settings with the intention of improving the efficacy of artificial ventilation during a respiratory failure. Patients given these agents cannot be weaned from the respirator, have tetraplegia, normal or reduced reflexes, no sensory loss, and normal CPK levels; but usually have abnormal renal or hepatic function with elevated active plasma metabolite of vecuronium (3-desacetyl vecuronium).

Failure to wean in the intensive care setting may also be a result of muscle disease. Acute necrotizing myopathy with tetraplegia, reduced or absent reflexes, and markedly elevated CPK levels are associated with high-dose steroids casually combined with neuromuscular blockade. Another myopathy without markedly elevated CPK levels associated with high-dose steroid therapy is marked by disappearance of myosin.

When multisystem organ failure (including encephalopathy) occurs in the intensive care unit, tetraplegia may also result from critical-illness neuropathy. Sensory abnormalities and decreased reflexes may be present, and the CPKs are normal. The help of the electrophysiologist is useful in this differential diagnostic problem. Prolonged blockade syndromes respond to supportive therapy and continued absence of the neuromuscular blocking agents.

## Bilateral Weakness Associated with Neuropathy

Since poliomyelitis has become rare in the United States, the most common acute paralytic disease of young adults is now AIDP. This disorder has been associated with infectious mononucleosis, the collagen-vascular diseases, and porphyria, but in 95% of the cases, no specific associated illness is present. In most cases there is a history of a nonspecific viral illness or surgical procedure 10–14 days before onset of the polyradiculoneuropathy.

In this syndrome, a prodrome of tingling in the extremities is followed by the appearance of a symmetric paralysis and loss of deep tendon reflexes. The pattern of evolution of the paralysis is variable, but usually the weakness appears first in the distal lower extremities, then in the thighs, forearms, proximal limb girdles, and finally in the respiratory and bulbar musculature (so-called ascending paralysis). Alternatively, a patient may develop bilateral facial paralysis at the outset, followed by "descending" spread of paralysis. This variety of paralysis must be distinguished from botulism and myasthenia gravis. The usual onset is acute or subacute, with maximal paralysis developing within a few hours to 6 weeks. Progression may cease at any state, but about one-half of patients will develop severe weakness of the respiratory muscles. Sphincter function is spared in 90% of patients. Though rare, chronic and relapsing forms of this syndrome have been delineated.

An axonal form of the disease has been described with severe muscular atrophy, and a poorer prognosis is anticipated. This axonal type often follows infection with *Campylobacter jejuni*. Examination reveals symmetric weakness, loss of deep tendon reflexes, and normal or enhanced direct muscle excitability in paralyzed muscles. The degree of weakness between the sides of the body may be different, but the pattern of weakness is symmetric. Fasciculations are absent, and wasting occurs only in proportion to disuse, because the demyelinated but otherwise preserved axons maintain trophic influence on muscle, even though the conduction of impulses is blocked. Although early sensory symptoms are common, the sensory examination is normal or reveals only a moderate loss of vibration and position sense.

In these cases, the spinal fluid is clear, colorless, and acellular. A significant elevation of cerebrospinal fluid protein (80–250 dl) occurs within 21 days, but even when the cerebrospinal fluid protein is quite elevated, xanthochromia is nearly always absent.

The most common misdiagnosis in the hyperacute phase of AIDP is of a psychiatric problem in an apparently healthy patient with "floppy legs" or bizarre gait. Intravenous immunoglobulin, plasmapheresis, and meticulous supportive care are the mainstays of treatment.

## Diphtheritic Neuropathy

Diphtheria toxin may cause paralysis of individual or multiple specific peripheral nerves or nerve roots but infrequently causes an acute or subacute largely demyelinating polyradiculoneuropathy with widespread proximal and distal weakness. More intense sensory loss to all modalities is present than is usually seen in AIDP. Early paralysis of the palate and ocular accommodation are highly characteristic of diphtheria. If the patient survives the bout of diphtheria, the prognosis for nerve recovery within several months is excellent.

## Paralytic Shellfish Poisoning (Red Tide)

Marine protozoans of the genus *Gonyaulax* proliferate massively when certain temperature, salinity, and nutrient conditions occur in the sea and cause a reddish luminescent discoloration on the surface of the water. These organisms produce a poison known as *saxitoxin*, which is ingested by clams, oysters, snails, cockles, and starfish. Lobsters and finned fish do not retain the poison. The shellfish themselves are not harmed, but birds and mammals feeding on the contaminated shellfish suffer an acute and potentially fatal illness. The lethal dose of saxitoxin in humans has been estimated to be 1–2 mg. The toxin prevents propagation of nerve impulses by interfering with neuronal membrane permeability to sodium ions. Within 30 minutes to 4 hours after

ingestion of saxitoxin, the patient experiences a prodrome of intense paresthesias in the distal extremities that rapidly spread proximally, along with vertigo and numbness of the scalp and mouth. Examination at this stage shows
severe sensory loss (especially in relation to position and vibration sense),
dysarthria, dysphagia, and intention tremor. In severe cases, the sensory symptoms are soon followed by flaccid quadriplegia and respiratory paralysis. The
spinal fluid is normal. Treatment is supportive; most patients surviving the
first 24 hours of the illness will improve.

## PORPHYRIA

Widespread polyneuropathies usually have a distal to proximal pattern. These
neuropathies are usually symmetric and slowly progress more proximally at
such a rate that office consultation is the more common venue for diagnosis of
these diseases. Occasionally, hospital consultation is requested in the case of
the unusual polyneuropathy pattern associated with porphyria. Porphyria has
six known varieties of hereditary disease, three of which have neurologic features: variegate porphyria, acute intermittent porphyria, and hereditary copro-
porphyria. In general, the porphyric neuropathies are dominated by sensory
and autonomic dysfunction as well as occasional and early intense proximal
paralysis accompanied by a proximal bathing trunk pattern of sensory loss.
Porphyric neuropathy with this proximal predilection pattern of deficits also
features abolition of upper extremity and patellar reflexes with intact Achilles
reflexes. In general, evidence shows that the short motor and sensory nerves
are first affected, followed by longer nerves. A curious additional paralysis
noted in porphyria is the use-related paralysis, in which selective weakness is
found in muscles that are used excessively during the prodrome to an acute
attack. A specific case has been reported in a woman who was redecorating a
room during the prodrome and developed severe paralysis in the right serratus,
anterior triceps, and the finger-thumb extensors that had been used vigorously
during redecorating. The features of neuropathic, proximal to distal grading of
motor, reflex, and sensory deficits along with a history of ingestion of a drug
that induces porphyria attack must be considered when consulted to evaluate
an atypical weakness pattern.

## UNILATERAL WEAKNESS ASSOCIATED WITH
## INVOLVEMENT OF THE NERVES AND ROOTS

The motor nerve roots emerge from the ventrolateral sulcus of the spinal cord
and extend through the subarachnoid space into the root sleeves of the
meninges. The most common problem affecting nerve roots is impingement on
the individual nerve roots by ruptured intervertebral lumbar or cervical disks.
The so-called acute disk syndrome involves a herniation of a disk, usually lumbar, with generally unilateral weakness, sensory changes, and reflex decrease.

*Table 3.3*  Differences in diagnosis of brachial plexus lesion

| Neoplastic infiltration | Radiation plexopathy |
| --- | --- |
| Severe pain | May or may not be accompanied by pain |
| Horner's syndrome | — |
| Lower plexus (C8, T1) | Upper plexus |
| Seen on magnetic resonance imaging | Not seen on magnetic resonance imaging |
| — | Myokymic discharges on electromyelogram |
| Rapid progression | Onset usually at least 12 months after radiation therapy |

If the spinal cord is not affected, these radiculopathies fall into unilateral specific patterns of weakness.

## ASYMMETRIC NEUROPATHIES

In hospital settings, invasive procedures and general medical illness of patients can lead to monoparesis. The brachial plexus is frequently damaged after intravascular line placement, and localization for the hospital consultant in a brachial plexopathy is often necessary on clinical grounds because of the difficulties in demonstrating electrophysiologic abnormalities in the acute setting.

In addition to damage to the brachial plexus from local infection, infiltration, and thrombosis secondary to intravascular line placement, important differences exist between a radiation effect versus a neoplastic infiltration of the brachial plexus. Both pathogenetic mechanisms are often seen in acute care wards, especially oncology services. The differences are listed in Table 3.3.

Differentiating among pattern-specific neuropathies, which can be separated into radiculopathies and specific mononeuropathies, is crucial. To correctly diagnose the problem, the examiner must understand and demonstrate the differential innervation of muscles (Table 3.4), which can be done easily at the bedside.

Lower motor neuron weakness is characterized by flaccid weakness, decreased reflexes, atrophy, and fasciculations. The following are the most dependable muscle groups to examine for these diagnostic patterns of weakness:

- C2, C3, C4: weakness in neck movement, shoulder shrugging
- C5–6: weakness in retraction (rhomboid), abduction (deltoid), and extension rotation of shoulder (infraspinatus), and flexion and supination (biceps, brachioradialis) of forearm
- C7: weakness in the extension of forearm (triceps) and extensors of wrist and fingers depressed triceps jerk
- C8-Tl: weakness in long flexors of fingers and intrinsics of hand (abduction of fingers, opposition of thumb)
- Torso: difficult to find motor levels from only one or two affected segments

*Table 3.4*   Bedside hints for differentiating weakness in root versus nerve patterns

C7 and *radial nerve* are similar, but the root lesion can also weaken the brachioradialis muscle, whose action can best be demonstrated when the patient attempts to flex the forearm while it is held midway between pronation and supination.

C8-T1 weakness of hand intrinsics will include opposition and palmar abduction of the thumb, but only the thumb adductor will be weakened by an *ulnar* nerve lesion.

L4 weakness may include internal rotation of the thigh (gluteus medius and minimus), hip abduction (gluteus medius and minimus plus tensor fascia latus), and foot inversion, whereas *femoral nerve* weakness is limited to leg extension. Associated hip-flexion and adduction weakness localizes the lesion in the plexus and roots proximal to the formation of the femoral nerve.

L5 weakness includes the action of the gluteal muscles and the extensor hallucis longus, along with the other foot and toe dorsiflexors, but *peroneal* nerve weakness is limited to the ankle and toe extensors and evertors of the foot, while *posterior* tibial nerve lesions may cause weakness detectable in the foot invertors.

- T10: Beevor's sign occurs when patient performs a sit-up and umbilicus is pulled upward because musculature below T10 is weak
- Ll: depressed cremasteric reflex (elevation of testicle with scratch of inner thigh)
- L2: weakness in hip flexion, thigh adduction
- L3: weakness in thigh adduction and knee extension
- L4: weakness in knee extension, ankle dorsiflexion, depressed knee jerk
- L5: weakness in extension of great toe, foot eversion, knee flexion, thigh extension
- Sl: similar to L5, but now weakness in plantar flexion of foot predominates; depressed ankle jerk
- S2: weakness limited to foot intrinsic muscles; cupping and fanning of toes weak
- Below S2: no weakness in lower extremities; but there is impaired vesicle, anal, and sexual function—anal scratch and bulbocavernosus reflexes depressed

## BILATERAL WEAKNESS WITH NERVE ROOT DISORDERS

AIDP is among the most commonly encountered polyradiculopathies of this type. Cases of diffuse polyradiculopathy secondary to lymphomatous and carcinomatous meningitis are increasingly common, as well as cytomegalovirus polyradiculopathy in the human immunodeficiency virus-infected patient. These patients are often in significant pain, with a diffuse areflexic weakness pattern and random sparing of certain root distributions.

Midline protrusion of a lumbar disk that impinges on the cauda equina may also cause bilateral radiculopathies. The patient experiences low back pain and radicular radiation of pain into the perineal region, as well as acute paralysis of bladder and rectal sphincters. Examination reveals a patulous anal sphincter, loss of the anal scratch and bulbocavernosus reflexes, and a sensory loss in the "saddle" region. The prognosis for recovery from this syndrome is strongly dependent on how rapidly surgical decompression of the roots can be accomplished.

## BILATERAL WEAKNESS ASSOCIATED WITH PYRAMIDAL TRACT DISEASE

Damage to the pyramidal system results in the characteristic weakness, spasticity, hyperreflexia, and Babinski's response of the upper motor neuron lesion. When pyramidal tract damage is partial, only certain movements may become weak; others may remain normal. This predilection pattern produces most marked weakness in the extensors and abductors of the upper extremity and the flexors (including dorsiflexion of the foot) and abductors of the lower extremity. For this reason, the common practice of screening for weakness by testing the hand grips should be abandoned. Initially, acute extensive damage to the pyramidal system presents with a flaccid, areflexic paralysis. The resemblance to a lower motor neuron type of weakness is not confusing when the patient is hemiplegic, but when weakness develops bilaterally with acute spinal cord damage, an incorrect diagnosis may easily be made.

## PARAPARESIS AND QUADRIPARESIS

Bilateral limb weakness resulting from pyramidal-system damage may result from bilateral lesions in the cerebral hemispheres or brain stem, but when neurologic function rostral to the medulla is normal, spinal cord disease is most likely. Bilateral paralysis is the most common feature of spinal cord disease With compressive lesions at the spinomedullary junction, the unusual pattern of bilateral upper motor neuron deficits in the upper extremities with sparing of the lower extremities may be encountered. However, spinal cord disease may present without weakness; weakness may be unilateral (as in Brown-Séquard syndrome) or predominantly of the lower motor neuron type, as in poliomyelitis or some types of motor neuron disease. Early spinal cord compression may present with a nondescript ataxia and bladder dysfunction. When strength is normal, sensory, pain, or autonomic dysfunction alone may direct attention to spinal cord disease.

## SPINAL CORD COMPRESSION

Spinal cord compression is a true emergency, and the consultant may need to make this diagnosis at the initial phone contact. The duration of the patient's history depends on the underlying disease process. If an inflammatory or neoplastic lesion involves the vertebrae, local pain at the level of the lesion may be prominent. This pain may worsen at night and change with posture. When nerve roots are also compressed, radicular pain may occur. This pain may be an important clue to the level of a compressive lesion. Radicular pain radiates out into the region of sensory distribution ordinarily supplied by that root and is often exacerbated by coughing, sneezing, or the Valsalva maneuver. Compression of the cord itself causes difficulty in urination and defecation and sensory-motor signs that begin in the distal lower extremities and progress up to the level of the lesion as the spinal cord is further compromised. For obscure reasons, some patients with rapidly evolving quadriparesis show a relative indifference to this calamity, and the misdiagnosis of hysteria is not uncommon.

The neurologic examination seeks to determine the longitudinal and transverse extent of cord dysfunction. Signs related to the dorsal columns (ipsilateral position and vibratory loss), lateral spinothalamic tracts (contralateral pin and temperature loss), and corticospinal (ipsilateral weakness) tend to begin in the distal lower extremities and ascend toward the level of the lesion. The upper level of these tract signs may therefore be significantly below the actual level of a compressive lesion. However, segmental signs, such as an absent deep tendon reflex, focal atrophy, and fasciculations or radicular sensory loss, accurately determine the true level of a compressive lesion. General medical examination may uncover signs of lung, breast, prostatic, or other neoplastic disease that may have metastasized to the epidural space. A healing furuncle may indicate the presence of an epidural abscess. Emergency imaging of the spinal cord and surrounding tissues must be performed in the patient with progressing spinal cord signs consistent with cord compression. Magnetic resonance imaging usually reliably demonstrates whether the mass is extradural (disk, spondylosis, abscess, metastasis, lymphoma), extramedullary, intradural (meningioma, neurofibroma), or intramedullary (glioma, ependymoma, syrinx).

Decompression of the cord is nearly always accomplished by immediate neurosurgical intervention. With certain cancers, however, in which the longitudinal extent of disease and associated destruction of vertebrae make surgery technically inadvisable, emergency radiation or chemotherapy may be tried. Steroids are used to reduce edema of the cord and tumor during initial radiotherapy.

## NONCOMPRESSIVE ACUTE SPINAL CORD SYNDROMES

Compressive myelopathy does not encompass all the urgent or treatable disorders of the spinal cord. The subacute combined systems disease of vitamin $B_{12}$ deficiency should be regarded as an emergency. Patients with this disorder complain of intense tingling paresthesias in the hands and show loss of position and vibration sense, with pyramidal weakness in the lower extremities. The knee and ankle jerks are lost, but Babinski's response is present. A serum vitamin $B_{12}$ level should be drawn, and the patient should be given parenteral vitamin $B_{12}$ immediately. A Schilling test also serves both to treat and to diagnose the disorder. Acute postinfectious or postimmunization transverse myelitis should be treated with steroids. Meningovascular syphilis, Lyme disease, and schistosomiasis are additional causes of treatable acute myelopathy.

## LOCALIZATION OF WEAKNESS ON ONE SIDE OF THE BODY

Hemiplegia can effectively be parsed into weakness as well as alterations in tone and clumsiness out of proportion to weakness. Other signs beyond the motor examination alone are often essential to localize the lesion, but a few helpful diagnostic principles, based on the nature of the weakness alone, do exist. First, a predilection pattern of weakness may be present, which is practically very useful, even though it may be an artifact of the way the physical examination is conducted. Weakness in the extensors and abductors of the upper extremity and the flexors and abductors of the lower extremity is easiest to find with upper motor neuron lesions. When pure motor hemiplegia occurs acutely, the most likely diagnosis is a lacunar infarction affecting the internal capsule. When a monoplegia is present, the places of greatest separation of representation of the limbs and the motor pathways are the most likely sites of lesions. The separation is largest in the motor cortex, and there is some separation in the internal capsule. The head and the face are represented at the knee of the internal capsule, and the leg is represented at the posterior end of the posterior limb of the internal capsule. A fairly wide separation once again occurs in the pons, and the face is spared because of the more posterior course of the corticobulbar fibers at this level. The corticospinal fibers are also dispersed among the nuclei pontis and corticopontine fibers, and thus a monoplegia is possible with lesions in the basis pontis.

The cortical border zone is ordinarily 1.5 gyri from the midline, which means the maximum weakness tends to be in the shoulder or the hip. Paralysis in the leg alone very likely indicates an anterior cerebral artery infarct has injured the motor cortex on the medial wall of the hemisphere. One of the subtlest signs of upper-extremity weakness is a tendency for the outstretched weak arm to drift slightly down and show minimal pronation. The obtunded patient with an underlying hemiparesis often shows outward rotation of the affected lower limb and foot, similar in appearance to a hip fracture. Unilateral hemiparesis is otherwise sorted out by examining associated deficits that pinpoint the lesion in the neuraxis.

In the acute care setting, the neurologist who is able to take an intelligent history and perform a focused, hypothesis-driven physical examination can, along with a carefully chosen laboratory test, provide an accurate confirmation of the diagnosis and provide proper counsel toward therapeutic intervention.

## SUGGESTED READING

Ackerman MJ, Clapham DE. Ion channels—basic science and clinical disease. N Engl J Med 1997;336: 1575–1585.

Amato AA, Grouseth GS, Jackson CE, et al. Inclusion body myositis: clinical and pathological boundaries. Ann Neurol 1996;40:581–586.

Dalakas MC. Polymyositis, dermatomyositis, and inclusion-body myositis. N Engl J Med 1991;328: 1487–1498.

Haymaker W, Woodhall B. Peripheral Nerve Injuries. Philadelphia: Saunders, 1953.

Kori SH, Foley KM, Posner JB. Brachial plexus lesions in patients with cancer: 100 cases. Neurology 1981;31:45.

Lennon VA, Kryzer TJ, Griesmann GE, et al. Calcium-channel antibodies in the Lambert-Eaton syndrome and other paraneoplastic syndromes. N Engl J Med 1995;332:1467–1474.

Sabin TD. Clinical implications of retrograde neuronal suicide transport. Neurologist 1996; 2:176–184.

Sandrock AW Jr (discussant). Case records of the Massachusetts General Hospital: case #11. N Engl J Med 1997;336:1079–1088.

Stewart JD. Focal Peripheral Neuropathies. New York: Raven, 1993.

Thomas CE, Mayer SA, Gungor BS, et al. Myasthenic crises: clinical features, mortality, complications, and risk factors for prolonged intubation. Neurology 1997;48:1253–1260.

Yuk N, Takahashi M, Tagawa Y, et al. Association of *Campylobacter jejuni* serotype with antiganglioside antibody in Guillain-Barré syndrome and Fisher's syndrome. Ann Neurol 1997;42:28–33.

# 4
# Behavioral Disturbances

Jonathan H. Pincus

All behavioral disorders arise in the brain, and it is only a convention that some affected patients are referred to neurologists and some to psychiatrists. Nonetheless, identifying medical illnesses requiring neurologic referral, many of which can be life threatening, is of great practical importance. Thus, disturbances in the behavior of inpatients usually raise two relatively simple questions: (1) Is the problem one for which a neurologist or a psychiatrist should be called? (2) If the problem is neurologic, is it the result of a diffuse encephalopathy or of a focal lesion? In general, the following two major principles can help physicians avoid misdiagnoses. First, most behavioral deviations can be caused by neurologic disease. Second, psychiatric referrals are inappropriate if they are purely based on the referring physician's inability to imagine a neurologic disease that could be responsible for the clinical picture. If the behavior is atypical of neurologic disease, it is not necessarily of psychiatric origin. In fact, the converse is true: If the clinical picture is not typical of psychiatric disease, it is likely to be neurologic.

A physician trying to determine whether a neurologic or psychiatric consult is necessary should consider several factors, including the actual behavioral symptomatology and its history, the rapidity of the onset of the symptoms, the family history of similar disorders, the neurologic examination, the results of tests, and the response of the patient to treatment. These factors are discussed *ad seriatim*.

## BEHAVIORAL SYMPTOMS

Behavioral symptoms are often alarming, mysterious, and bizarre. They may be so dramatic that medical physicians in charge panic when confronted with them and desperately seek a psychiatric referral without careful consideration. Yet, some of the most dramatic behavioral symptoms are completely nonspecific and are seen in many neurologic as well as many psychiatric disorders. In a general hospital, alarming behavioral symptoms are much more commonly properly referred to neurologists than to psychiatrists. Curiously, delusions (including paranoid delusions), agitation, inappropriate affect, violent behavior, excitement, withdrawal, and catatonia do not necessarily signify psychiatric disorders. All are symptoms that may often be encountered in neurologic illnesses, and therefore in themselves do not necessarily indicate the existence of disease(s) of the brain that fall within the province of psychiatrists.

Acute confusional states and agitated delirium are usually the result of metabolic encephalopathy. Drug intoxication, organ failure, and electrolyte imbalance are common causes of confusion and delirium in a general hospital. Complete blood count, toxicology screen, blood urea nitrogen, creatinine, electrolytes, sugar, blood gases, and liver function tests are usually appropriate to rule out these causes. Epilepsy, either complex partial status epilepticus or postictal encephalopathy, can mimic metabolic encephalopathy, as can acute subarachnoid pathologies such as hemorrhage and meningitis. Electroencephalogram, computed tomography, and lumbar puncture can confirm these diagnoses.

Focal disease of the brain rarely causes acute confusional states or agitated delirium, but infarction in the distribution of the right- or left-middle cerebral arteries can produce either or both. Often, the only clinical clue to a right parietal infarct is the patient's inattention to the left visual field. This can be difficult to demonstrate in a confused patient. Aphasia is the hallmark of left-hemisphere disease. Computed tomography or magnetic resonance imaging can help diagnosis but may not become abnormal for 24–72 hours after the onset of symptoms.

Imagine a paranoid individual in the emergency room, agitated, speaking, but only intermittently understandably. The patient's paranoia, other delusions, tangentiality, and excitement are nonspecific symptoms, though they may be overwhelmingly dramatic and the cause of admission to the emergency room. Uninitiated physicians prematurely make the diagnosis of schizophrenia on encountering these symptoms. Indeed, paranoia and tangentiality can be seen in schizophrenia but are completely nonspecific and may also be encountered in other psychiatric illnesses such as manic states, depression, and certain personality disorders. They may also be encountered in any neurologic disorder that causes an organic brain syndrome, including encephalitis, brain tumors, epilepsy, stroke, hydrocephalus, and hypothyroidism.

Catatonia is another dramatic behavioral symptom, but it is much less commonly encountered than paranoia or agitation. It consists of catalepsy, waxy flexibility, negativism, mutism, muscular rigidity, and bizarre mannerisms. This behavioral syndrome generally is considered to represent a psychiatric condition only, especially schizophrenia. Many physicians, in my experience, are unable to provide a differential diagnostic list for this symptom. While it may be encountered in schizophrenics, most catatonics in psychiatric hospitals have affective illness and a family history of affective illness. When seen in schizophrenics, it is always associated with other pre-existent classic features of schizophrenia. Catatonia may be encountered in dissociative states.

The development of catatonia in a patient who has received neuroleptics should raise the possibility of the potentially fatal neuroleptic malignant syndrome (NMS). Serum creatine kinase levels are usually very high in NMS. Catatonia has also been encountered in virtually every condition that can induce an organic brain syndrome (Gelenberg, 1976). For example, the author has encountered catatonia in hydrocephalus, in frontal infarctions after aneurysm surgery, in encephalitis, and in postanoxic encephalopathy. In each instance, the referring doctor had first called a psychiatrist in the mistaken belief that the patient had suddenly become schizophrenic.

A relevant factor to the determination of whether a neurologist or psychiatrist should be called is the type of hallucinations that the patient is having. Auditory hallucinations suggest schizophrenia or alcoholic hallucinosis. Tactile and visual hallucinations are encountered in drug intoxications and in sedative withdrawal states. Visual hallucinations may have many other causes that are almost always neurologic, including degenerative illnesses involving the parietal region such as Alzheimer's disease and vascular disease of the upper basilar artery (peduncular hallucinosis). Visual field cuts can be complicated by visual hallucinations within the defective field. Temporal lobe lesions can cause palinopsia and metamorphopsia. Any illness that significantly decreases vision including intraocular conditions, retinal disorders, or optic neuropathy can give rise to "release" visual hallucinations. Olfactory and gustatory hallucinations are nearly always the result of temporal lobe lesions and, according to pre–computed tomography era neurologic folklore, suggest the presence of a temporal lobe tumor when encountered in epileptics.

Much has been written about the frontal lobe and its functions that is not repeated here, except that disorders of the frontal lobe can give rise to tremendous abnormalities of judgment and, consequently, of behavior. Such abnormalities may occur in the absence of disorientation, dyscalculia, or dysmnesia, which are correctly considered the hallmarks of an organic brain syndrome.

Frontal lesions may produce less imagination, less desire for human association and sexual activity, along with the passive acceptance of circumstances and a lack of aspiration. When mild, such symptoms can mimic depression, and indeed, patients with slight brain damage often are depressed; the depression may be a reaction to or part of a neurologic deficit. When the frontal damage is severe, inability to express needs may even extend to such basics as food, shelter, and warmth.

Frontally damaged individuals have a decreased ability to anticipate either dangerous or propitious circumstances, plan, arrange, invent, postpone, modulate, or discriminate in achieving goals. Business failure, irritability, and unwise sexual liaisons may occur in the course of advancing disease and may cause great distress to the patient's family, especially when the patient seems normal in other ways.

Deficits in socially appropriate reactions of defense under stress and the capacity to recover promptly from the effects of stress can lead to the catastrophic reaction described by Goldstein (1948) in World War I veterans who had brain damage. When confronted, for example, with an arithmetic problem that they once could have solved easily, patients became "dazed, agitated, anxious, started to fumble; a moment before amiable, they became sullen, evasive, and exhibited temper." Often the best level of performance such a patient can achieve is not achieved during a catastrophic reaction.

The onset of symptoms is a very important factor in determining the cause of aberrant behavior. Contrary to popular understanding, the existence of stress and precipitating psychological elements are irrelevant to the determination of whether a neurologist or a psychiatrist is needed. Difficult life circumstances are very common and can coincidentally precede any illness, neurologic or otherwise. Unmarried people may have problems seeking a spouse. Married people frequently have marital difficulties. Married people without children may wish to have them. Couples with children have problems with their children. Jobs may change, responsibilities increase, and incomes drop; parents may become ill, and life and limb may be threatened. Once the diagnosis of psychiatric illness has been established, these factors may be important in psychotherapy, but their presence or absence is irrelevant when determining whether an illness is psychiatric or neurologic in origin.

Highly relevant to determining whether a neurologist or psychiatrist is required are abrupt changes in the patient's personality, mood, and ability to function at work and at home. Rapid incapacitation in less than 6 months, in the presence of a good premorbid social history, points to neurologic illness. Affective disorder is the only psychiatric condition that can appear de novo in a background relatively clear of behavioral abnormalities, though even affective disorder usually is manifest before age 30. Because a patient has a psychiatric history does not mean that he or she cannot become seriously ill, and the development of a behavioral decline should be assessed to rule out a neurologic origin.

The onset of symptoms of behavioral disturbance and psychosis after drug use, whether prescribed or not, is highly relevant in the assessment of etiology. The examiner should assume a relation exists between drug use and behavioral aberration if the drug was started shortly before the behavioral change. Virtually every drug that affects the central nervous system—the brain, the mind—has caused, in some case or another, a puzzling and abrupt change in behavior. It is important to know which drugs are within the purview of a toxicology screen and which are not.

Depression (unipolar or bipolar), suicide, schizophrenia, cyclothymia, hypomania, and obsessive-compulsive disorder are usually the result of genetically based conditions, and a positive family history can be most helpful in establishing a presumptive diagnosis. A family history of drug abuse, especially alcoholism, generally supports the diagnosis of bipolar disorder or unipolar depression.

Although the patient's history and symptomatology are important in providing clues to differentiate neurologic and psychiatric disease, they are almost always insufficient alone, because both neurologic and psychiatric conditions arise from the same organ, the brain. Neurologic disease is likely to be the cause of behavioral disturbances if the latter are associated with specific physical signs of cortical dysfunction.

The presence of seizures, myoclonus, asterixis, tremor, paresis, inattention to one half of the body or visual field, and Babinski's sign alone or in combination are overwhelmingly strong indicators of the neurologic origin of behavioral symptoms. Yet, even such signs are frequently insufficiently weighted by internists, family physicians, and emergency physicians in the face of florid psychosis.

The formal mental status examination is extremely helpful in the identification of neurologic disorders. In the examination, a patient's disorientation to time or place, loss of memory, inability to calculate, and aphasia all indicate a neurologic origin of symptoms. Disorientation to person always indicates a psychiatric illness.

Although the formal mental status examination (i.e., Mini-Mental Status Examination) is a useful screening tool, most of the functions assayed in this test are posterior brain functions. Very roughly, disorientation to time and place, dyscalculia, and difficulty reading are ascribed to the parietal lobes. Loss of memory is generally a medial temporal or diencephalic dysfunction. Aphasia usually arises from a lesion in the posterior dominant temporal lobe. Although this is a gross oversimplification of the correlation of structure and function, it is also true that the Mini-Mental Status Examination does a rather inadequate job of assessing dysfunction in the frontal lobes, which, after all, account for almost 40% of the total cortical mass.

How does a clinician assess the frontal lobes? The patient's behavior is first assessed. An inappropriate tendency toward jocularity (i.e., *Witzelsucht*) as well as inappropriate ill humor may exhibit themselves in a patient with damaged frontal lobes. Emotional incontinence with easy, sometimes rapidly alternating, crying or laughing or both, may occur. A dulling of subjective emotionality, with poor self-control, an inability to understand the consequences of actions, and an inability to orient actions to the social and ethical standards of the community may be present. When frontal lesions are extensive, dulling may give way to torpor and apathy and sometimes to a state of akinetic mutism close to catatonia. The patient may be able to move and to speak but prefers not to move, even in reaction to a painful stimulus, instead lying still, speechless, and open-eyed. Occasionally, the patient speaks or moves, giving the naive observer the false impression of a voluntary or psychogenic disorder. Even though the patient looks awake and is awake and is therefore not in coma, the patient has little more cognitive function than a comatose patient. When the withdrawal is severe, this state is called *coma vigil*.

Unfortunately, the most important function of the frontal lobes, judgment, is difficult to test in a standardized manner. Consequently, neurologists must rely on a series of reflexes and responses that, when present, reflect cortical or subcortical dysfunction primarily in the frontal lobes. An isolated frontal sign can be seen in 5% or so of normal adults under 70 years of age. After 70, the prevalence of frontal signs rises, but three or more signs virtually always reflect abnormality of the nervous system and, therefore, a panel of such tests should be routinely performed.

Frontal signs include snout, suck, and grasp reflexes, paratonia, jerky eye movements in visual pursuit, oculomotor impersistence, abnormal word fluency, and an abnormal response to the test assessing reciprocal coordination of the movements of the hands (a simultaneous change of position, a clenched fist with outstretched hand). Other signs include abnormal nucho-cephalic reflex, persistent glabellar blink, limited upward and downward conjugate gaze, and limb placement. The presence of three or more of these signs correctly predicted abnormal cortical function on neuropsychological tests in 64% of those who were mildly impaired, in 96% of moderately impaired subjects, and in 100% of markedly impaired subjects (Jenkyn et al., 1977, 1985).

## Psychological Tests

IQ tests, personality inventories, and even neuropsychological testing, including the Halstead-Reitan battery, de-emphasize frontal functions and concentrate on posterior brain functions. Like the neurologic examination, psychological tests do not directly assess the deficit of judgment that results from frontal dysfunction. Tests that reflect frontal function but do not measure judgment are used, but are almost routinely omitted from formal psychological assessments and, by an odd convention, psychologists often report only their own interpretation of the results rather than the results themselves. Frontal tests must specifically be requested when frontal lobe dysfunction is suspected. The most sensitive frontal tests include the Wisconsin Card Sorting Test, the Trail Making Test Parts A and B, and the Category Test.

## Laboratory Tests

In the differentiation of neurologic and psychiatric disease, a most helpful test is the electroencephalogram, which points to neurologic disorders when the results are abnormal. In addition, appropriate blood studies and imaging tests of the brain should be considered. If the imaging tests are normal, a lumbar puncture may be indicated, certainly if the patient is febrile or if inflammation or neoplastic involvement of the meninges is a real possibility.

Sometimes a therapeutic trial can provide diagnostic information. In general, the psychiatric disorders that give rise to psychosis are effectively managed with dopamine-receptor blockers. Responses to therapy can be seen within hours. Depression can be effectively managed with antidepressants. Tricyclic antidepressants and selective serotonin reuptake inhibitors require about 3 weeks for their effect to become manifest. The response of depression to amphetamines is more rapid and can be helpful diagnostically. Mania responds to valproic acid within 2–3 days; lithium is also effective but takes longer. The results of therapy of psychiatric disorders are usually quite obvious within just a few days. Patients who have been treated for a psychiatric disorder and have failed to respond should be suspected of having a neurologic problem.

In the dementia (or pseudodementia) of depression, signs of cognitive dysfunction may appear abruptly and advance rapidly, and within a few days or at most a few weeks, the patient's mental disability is obvious and severe. Usually there will be a history of attacks of depression, mania, or both and a family history of the same. Usually, patients with the pseudodementia of depression will be over 60 years old at the onset of this syndrome, and depression with vegetative features is marked. The dementia, such as it is, improves as the depression lifts.

A few caveats are appropriate: virtually all the drugs used to treat serious psychiatric disturbances can produce subtle abnormalities in the neurologic examination. The dopamine-receptor blockers all can produce a full Parkinson's syndrome and, even in the absence of obvious Parkinson's signs, can produce grasp, suck, and snout reflexes, paratonia, difficulty with smooth ocular pursuit, and hyperreflexia. Unfortunately, such signs persist for weeks after the medication has been withdrawn. Using frontal signs to distinguish neurologic and psychiatric disease is, therefore, not possible in patients who have been treated with neuroleptic medications. Tricyclic antidepressants can produce atropinism with dilated pupils, hyperreflexia, rapid pulse, dry mouth, constipation, urinary retention, and psychosis. Lithium in toxic doses can produce a very dramatic organic brain syndrome that is sometimes expressed through drug-induced hypothyroidism and may be accompanied by tremor, myoclonic jerks, and asterixis.

## PSYCHOPHYSIOLOGIC RESPONSES

Hyperventilation syndrome, headache, hysteria, and hypochondriasis may seem quite disparate, but often coexist. They are often encountered in depression and in patients with neurologic disease.

### Hyperventilation Syndrome

Of all psychological reactions, probably the most commonly seen by neurologists is hyperventilation syndrome. Because its manifestations in different body systems can mimic other conditions, this syndrome is frequently unrecognized, and patients are often shunted from doctor to doctor undergoing numerous unnecessary and upsetting diagnostic tests. Often the result of anxiety, hyperventilation produces changes in body functions that themselves become the focus of anxiety. Fear and confusion are compounded when a doctor tells the patient that the symptoms are factitious or "all in your nerves." The patient knows the symptoms are not imagined and supposes he or she has a life-threatening illness. The symptoms of the hyperventilation syndrome include faintness, visual disturbances, inability to concentrate, nausea, vertiginous instability, headache, fullness in the head, chest, and epigastrium, breathlessness, palpitations, hot flushing, cold sweating, paresthesias, and occasionally vomiting. This panoply of symptoms results from physiologic alterations caused simply by overbreathing.

I performed a study of the hyperventilation syndrome in neurologic practice and showed that hyperventilation syndrome was seen mainly in young women 15 to 30 years old, 77% of whom had a history of other psychophysiologic reactions, hypochondriasis, or conversion reactions. The prevalence of these associated conditions was three times higher than in controls. The study group's chief complaints were often multiple, involving at least two organ systems in one-third of the patients.

Hyperventilation is a common, almost universal, human response to anxiety, because it is part of the autonomic response to threatening situations. In patients predisposed to seek medical attention, it becomes a symptom. Three-fourths of the hyperventilation syndrome patients have a history of conversion reaction, hypochondriasis, or psychosomatic illnesses, and young women seem to be particularly susceptible, whereas preadolescents and patients at retirement age are less so.

A minority of patients with the syndrome had organic medical diseases as well, including regional ileitis, arthritis, adrenal insufficiency, carpal tunnel syndrome, orthostatic hypotension, and endometriosis. The majority of patients with coexistent medical illnesses were over 30 years old. For this reason, it is prudent, especially in patients over 30, to consider the possibility of associated medical illnesses even in the presence of hyperventilation syndrome.

### Headache

Determining the cause of headache is one of the most critical diagnoses a physician has to make. Headache can be a symptom of anxiety or depression, or it can be the first symptom of a brain tumor. Three historical criteria are helpful in distinguishing a dangerous headache from a benign one.

If the headache is the *worst* headache ever experienced by the patient, if it is a *new* headache, or if it is associated with *neurologic signs*, the physician must assume that the situation might be acute or life-threatening, and a full investigation should be promptly initiated. A computed tomography scan should be the first test. If it is normal, a lumbar puncture should follow. When tests are performed in this order, the diagnoses of subarachnoid hemorrhage, meningitis, encephalitis, or brain tumor will not often be overlooked. For teaching purposes, we advise medical students to fully investigate any headache that is "the worst, the first, or cursed (by neurologic abnormalities)." Conversely, any headache that has been present for more than a year, almost irrespective of its character, is rarely caused by a serious or progressive disorder. New headaches in older people demand, in addition, examination of sedimentation rate and consideration of temporal arteritis. A new headache around the eye may indicate glaucoma.

## Hysteria

Hysteria is a much-abused word. It can be used to refer to a personality type, to a psychosomatic reaction (i.e., conversion reaction) or, in a pejorative way, to a generalized disorganized response to stress.

The hysterical personality has been described as vain, egocentric, labile, excitable, dramatic, attention-seeking, overly conscious of sex, provocative but frigid, dependent, and demanding. Although this label can be applied to both men and women, it is most often attached to women.

The hysterical personality type is encountered only in a minority of patients manifesting hysterical (conversion) symptoms. Conversion symptoms are probably more prevalent among people with hysterical personalities than in the general population, but the association is by no means obligatory.

Conversion reactions involve loss or impairment of such normal neurologic functions as seeing, moving, feeling, swallowing, and so on, that does not result from physiologic abnormalities. The differentiation of conversion symptoms from neurologic disease is a frequent problem in neurologic, medical, and psychiatric practice.

Perley and Guze (1962) proposed an elaborate and restrictive system for diagnosing hysteria (Briquet's syndrome). They assigned the diagnosis if patients had (1) a dramatic or complicated medical history before age 35, (2) a minimum of 15 symptoms (out of 45) distributed in at least nine of 10 categories defined by the authors, and (3) no medical diagnosis that adequately explained their symptoms. For 6–8 years, Perley and Guze studied a group of 39 patients in whom these criteria were met. Of these patients, 90% did not develop any other illness that might have explained their symptoms. The patients' tendency to develop further psychosomatic complaints continued over the years. Thus, the criteria established by Perley and Guze for diagnosing hysteria were fully validated. This study called attention to the importance of a thoroughly detailed history in establishing a correct diagnosis for patients suspected of hysterical conversion reaction.

On examining the criteria used by Perley and Guze, however, one finds that hyperventilation syndrome could cause 18 of the symptoms distributed in seven of their 10 categories. With the addition of only a few other complaints, the hyperventilation syndrome, which is a psychophysiologic reaction, could thus satisfy their strict criteria for hysteria. One-third of my patients with hyperventilation syndrome had seen gastroenterologists and cardiologists for their related symptoms and had excessive bodily concerns manifested by frequent visits to physicians for minor problems and menstrual and sexual difficulties (i.e., they had histories resembling those of hysterical patients).

Some physicians believe that hysteria, as defined by the Perley and Guze criteria, can be differentiated from "isolated" conversion symptoms. In my experience, conversion symptoms rarely occur in isolation. When doctors label unexplained findings "conversion reaction" in patients lacking a history of hypochondriasis, psychophysiologic reactions (chief among which is hyperventilation syndrome), and other conversion reactions, their diagnoses are almost invariably wrong. I have found that two criteria are extremely important in making a positive diagnosis of conversion reaction. Unless both are present, the diagnosis should be held in doubt. These criteria are that (1) no medical diagnosis explains the patient's symptoms, and (2) a past history exists (even in children) of psychosomatic illness (conversion reaction, hypochondriasis, or psychophysiologic reaction).

Roy (1979) reported that 14 of 22 patients with hysterical seizures had on one or more occasions attempted suicide, and that 19 of 22 were clinically depressed at the time of their presentation. This finding suggests that depression may often occur in patients who manifest conversion symptoms. There is a high prevalence of the experience of physical and sexual abuse in childhood in patients with nonepileptic (pseudo)seizures (Alper 1993).

The two classic hallmarks of hysteria, la belle indifférence and secondary gain, have been, in my experience, more often misleading than helpful in establishing the diagnosis. Apparent indifference is often a sign of stoicism, and stoic hospitalized patients are more often seriously ill than hysterical. Indifference to illness is also a common sign of brain damage. This indifference is the basis of the "therapeutic" effect of frontal lobotomy. Many patients with progressive brain disease are mercifully indifferent to their desperate condition. Conversely, hysterical individuals may be excited and anxious when they develop conversion symptoms. A minority do manifest la belle indifférence

*Secondary gain* refers to a reward for the patient resulting from a conversion reaction and is often difficult to identify. Sometimes it is no more than staying in the hospital and avoiding contact with the family; sometimes it is a more subtle or even a fantasized gain. On the other hand, patients injured in automobile or industrial accidents often have lawsuits or compensation claims pending that are justified but that could be mistaken as secondary gain by their physicians. There are no established criteria to distinguish a legitimate from a secondary gain. After the diagnosis is established, secondary gain may be quite clear, but as a diagnostic aid, it is almost useless.

It has been my experience that most medical doctors consider a patient hysterical either when the physician cannot imagine an organic lesion that could explain the symptoms or when a patient with a well-known history of psychosomatic illnesses is being examined. Because the physician's diagnostic acumen is naturally a function of previous experience and knowledge, misdiagnoses can occur. No one can know everything, and peculiar facets of difficult cases of organic disease that even the most experienced clinician has not encountered before are hard to recognize.

Certain organic neurologic diseases seem predisposed to producing conversion in patients. Patients whose judgment is impaired by mental retardation, intoxication or other encephalopathies, encephalitis, brain tumor, or multiple sclerosis may exaggerate or even fabricate symptoms and signs. This behavior may draw attention away from the real disease, sometimes with tragic results.

Considering some of the conversion symptoms that mimic neurologic conditions may be worthwhile. In doing so, I wish to demonstrate that symptoms that cannot be easily ascribed to an organic lesion constitute an inadequate basis for the diagnosis of hysteria. The diagnosis requires such symptoms in addition to a past history of psychosomatic illnesses. *Both are necessary: Neither is sufficient alone.*

## Globus Hystericus

Inability to swallow or feeling a lump in the throat is typical of globus hystericus. When direct examination of the nasal and oral pharynx and barium swallow studies yield normal results, most lesions that could cause similar symptoms can be ruled out. On the other hand, both myasthenia gravis and polymyositis may begin with intermittent weakness of the swallowing mechanism. At the time of examination, the patient may be able to swallow normally and appear to be well even if one of these conditions is present. Similarly, pseudobulbar palsy, which interferes with swallowing, may wax and wane in severity. When unassociated with other signs of neurologic disease, such symptoms may be mistaken for hysteria.

## Hemisensory Loss

Hysterical hemisensory loss usually involves half of the entire body from head to feet and from the extremities to the midline. A pinprick felt normally on one side of the linea alba will not be felt on the other side. Sensory splitting at the exact midline and a shift of perception toward the side of normal sensation are considered by many to be hard-and-fast signs of hysteria: organic hemisensory deficits typically appear 1 or 2 cm toward the anesthetic side of the midline. This overlap is because segmental sensory nerve fibers extend 1 or 2 cm across the midline. Some believe that the diagnosis of hysteria can be confirmed by testing vibratory sensation on the skull. A tuning fork placed on the skull or the sternum to one side of midline should be felt by neurologic patients no matter which side the hemisensory loss is on because the oscillations of the tuning fork are transmitted throughout the entire bone. A patient who claims not to feel vibrations may be considered hysterical.

Unfortunately, sensory signs of hysteria are rather unreliable because some patients with neurologic diseases report what they think their examiner wishes them to report, for instance claiming that a change in sensation occurs at the midline when in fact this may not be so. In addition, a minority of patients could possibly have a physiologically variant pattern of sensory function in which the anesthesia caused by a brain lesion does, in fact, change at the midline or to the "wrong" side of the midline. Patients who report absent vibratory sensation on the anesthesia side of their skull or sternum may in fact feel the vibrations less on that side, but report to the examiner that they feel nothing to be "consistent."

Whatever the reason, it is an empirical fact that patients with undeniably organic lesions, such as strokes, tumors, demyelinating disease, have reported sensory changes with characteristics considered to be typical of hysteria. Conversely, the sensory examination is inherently unreliable. A patient's complaint of feeling "pins and needles" and burning pain is almost as reliable as an indicator of real sensory pathology as a Babinski's sign is an indicator of motor pathology. It is rare in medicine for symptoms to be more reliable indicators than signs, though sensory symptoms can be more reliable than sensory signs. Patients with tingling and burning usually have lesions even if the sensory examination is normal.

## Hysterical Hemiplegia

Hysterical hemiplegia may be diagnosed in the following way: Placing his or her hands underneath the patient's paralyzed heel while the patient is supine, the examiner asks the patient to raise the other, normal leg. The examiner can thereby determine whether or not the patient is actually able to move the paralyzed leg, because the normal response while raising one leg is to push down with the other. If the patient pushes down with the "paralyzed" leg, the factitious nature of the paralysis should be clear. By reversing the process and asking the patient to raise the paralyzed leg, the examiner can determine whether the patient is actually trying to lift it. If the patient does not push down with the good leg, the examiner can conclude that the patient is not trying to raise the paralyzed leg. This test is only useful in cases of complete hemiplegia, however, and does not help distinguish hysterical hemiparesis (which is more common than hysterical hemiplegia) from true hemiparesis. The presence of unilateral changes in deep tendon reflexes, spasticity, and Babinski's sign provides objective evidence indicating neurologic disease. The absence of these alterations, however, cannot conclusively establish the diagnosis of hysteria.

## Paralysis of the Extraocular Muscles

Paralysis of the extraocular muscles (i.e., those of the face and the tongue) does not occur in conversion syndromes. Paresis of the cervical muscles, with the patient showing difficulty elevating the head from a pillow or drooping of the head onto the chest, is extremely rare. Paralysis of the trunk muscles is also rare. Thus, hysterical paralysis or paresis usually involves one or more of the extremities. Weakness of the leg is more frequently encountered than weakness of the arm.

For ambulatory patients, the manner in which they move, dress, undress, and mount the examining table should be noted, because hysterical paralysis mainly consists of paralysis of movements as opposed to paralysis of individual muscles. For example, the hysteric may complain that all movements at one joint are affected, but during the examination the physician should note the distribution of the paralysis as well as the muscles affected and determine if the patient can still unknowingly use the affected muscles to perform movements that entail their use. Hysterical weakness involves simultaneous and equal contraction of agonistic and antagonistic muscles.

## Hysterical Hemiparesis

Hysterical hemiparesis is characteristically associated with "give-way" weakness (i.e., discontinuous resistance during direct muscle testing). Give-way weakness is absolutely diagnostic of factitious weakness, but occasionally a patient will exaggerate mild real weakness in order to convince the examiner that weakness is in fact present. In such cases, the patient may feel that the examiner is going to miss the diagnosis and so tries to "help out." Reflex abnormalities, when present, can rule out hysteria, but the absence of such abnormalities alone does not establish the diagnosis of hysteria.

## Hysterical Gait

Astasia-abasia, or hysterical gait, can sometimes be extremely difficult to differentiate from movement disorders. Physicians routinely place emphasis on the following indications that a disordered gait is hysterical: The patient walks well when unaware that he is being observed, never falls, and does not injure himself. The hysterical gait is usually recognized by its bizarre character and its dissimilarity from any gait disorder produced by organic disease. In hysterical hemiplegia, the affected leg is dragged along the ground and not circumducted as in organic hemiplegia. When severe, astasia-abasia will be manifested by the patient's attempting to fall as opposed to the organic patient who tries hard to avoid falling. Some patients who walk with great difficulty, clinging to walls and furniture and to the examiners, manifest normal power and coordination while lying in bed, an inconsistency that suggests hysteria.

Because almost all movement disorders are worsened by anxiety, it is not wise to accept without reservations reports by nurses and other staff to the effect that the patient is able to walk nearly normally when unaware of being observed. A patient who is made nervous by an examiner or a large group of physicians on rounds is likely to show worsening of his movement disorder. Patients with hysterical gait problems sometimes do, in fact, fall and may accidentally hurt themselves. A history of falls with occasional scrapes and bruises, therefore, does not necessarily rule out hysteria.

Inconsistency of gait disturbance is common in gait apraxia caused by frontal or diffuse cerebral disease. Peculiarities of affect in patients showing such inconsistency and an absence of the Babinski sign may lead to an incorrect diagnosis of hysteria. Formal mental status evaluation and search for frontal signs in patients are helpful in identifying gait apraxia.

Most movement disorders are organic, and as few as 1% are hysterical. Tics, chorea, myoclonus, and tremors all disappear in sleep, improve as emotional tension is relieved, and worsen with stress. Most are not associated with reflex changes, magnetic resonance imaging abnormalities, or electrical abnormalities.

Amytal infusion and hypnosis are relatively safe and fairly objective tests for organic movement disorders. Amytal is infused intravenously at a rate of 100 mg in 30 seconds until nystagmus develops. This usually requires 250–500 mg. As soon as nystagmus develops, the infusion is stopped and the patient is asked to perform the motor task previously found difficult. If a substantial improvement in gait occurs, the diagnosis of hysteria is supported. If the gait deteriorates, the diagnosis of organicity is supported. This test is often extremely helpful but it can be misinterpreted. When anxiety is responsible for marked worsening of an organic movement disorder, Amytal or hypnosis might occasionally improve the gait by relieving anxiety. When neither deterioration nor improvement is clear cut, no inference about etiology of the gait disturbance can be made.

It is probably fair to say that hysterical dystonia and chorea virtually never occur. Certain inconsistencies can be misleading, and some "inconsistencies" are virtually diagnostic. For example, in torticollis the examiner may not be able to straighten the patient's head even by exerting maximal effort, and yet the patient can often straighten the head considerably by merely touching the forehead with an index finger on the side toward which the head is tilted. This apparent examination inconsistency is unexplained but is characteristic of organic dystonia.

## Hysterical Rigidity

Hysterical rigidity increases in proportion to the effort made by the examiner to move the rigid extremity. This feature, which is also present in the frontal lobe disorders that lead to *gegenhalten* or paratonia, is a semivoluntary resistance the patient increasingly offers to the passive movement of the limbs. When the examiner attempts to extend the patient's elbow, for example, the patient resists, and the resistance increases as the elbow is extended further. Forced grasping may be seen in response to tactile stimulation of the patient's palm by the examiner's fingers. When the examiner attempts to extend the patient's fingers while disengaging his or her own from the patient's grip, counterpull may be encountered in frontal lobe disorders.

## Visual Hysterical Symptoms

Visual hysterical symptoms include monocular diplopia, triplopia, tunnel vision, and blindness. Although monocular diplopia is in most cases caused by hysteria, it can be caused by ocular pathologies such as dislocated lenses, cataracts, and parietal lobe lesions. Triplopia, theoretically a physiologic impossibility, was reported by a patient under my care who was recovering from well-documented disseminated leukoencephalitis.

The basis for a test for hysterical etiology in tunnel vision is the fact that the normal visual fields expand in a cone of vision as the distance from the target to the patient is increased. If the patient's field deficit is the same at 2 m as it is at 1 m, the inconsistency suggests hysteria.

Patients who are blind as a result of neurologic disease usually have no pupillary response to light. In disease of the parietal or occipital lobes, however, cortical blindness may be present and pupillary reflexes remain normal. If a patient with blindness and normal pupillary responses is presented with a slowly rotating, vertically striped drum and develops involuntary tracking movements (optokinetic nystagmus), the blindness can be considered factitious.

Two useful tests exist for detecting unilateral hysterical blindness. The patient is asked to read a line of alternating black and red letters while a red glass is held over the "good" eye. In hysterical blindness, the patient is able to see the red letters with the "bad" eye and reads all the letters in the line. Also, a distorting prism can be placed over the "good" eye, and the patient still is able to perform tasks requiring intact vision. Convergence spasms and blepharospasm (the result of spasm of the orbicularis oculi) can be manifestations of hysterical disturbances of ocular movements. Defects in the lateral and vertical planes of gaze caused by hysteria may induce a kind of coarse nystagmus. Blepharospasm can also be a sign of Meigs' syndrome, however, which is an organic involuntary-movement disorder.


Hysterical Deafness

Hysterical deafness can easily be demonstrated by awakening the patient from sleep with sound. A hysterical reduction of hearing (as opposed to deafness) is difficult to distinguish from organic disease of the ears. Variability of responses to audiological tests can reflect an organic brain syndrome as well as hysteria. Brain stem auditory evoked responses can provide objective evidence of neurologic dysfunction.

Dissociative states may partially mimic epilepsy and can be mistaken for it. True frontal seizures produce such bizarre behaviors and pseudoseizures can be so convincing that I no longer have any confidence in my clinical ability to distinguish real seizures from pseudoseizures. The electroencephalogram performed during the episode and elevated serum prolactin levels estimated immediately after the episode that fall an hour later both can provide objective evidence of real seizures.

Patients with psychogenic amnesia or dissociative states rather than neurologic conditions can be identified by the following characteristics. In hysterical states, patients are able to carry out complex functions during the time of amnesia. Memory loss and shift of identity to another person or personality are usually sudden and often associated with severe headache. Patients' behavior is fairly well integrated (e.g., they usually have enough money to get where they are going and take time to eat and drink). Loss of memory usually affects a specific section of life or ability (e.g., patient exhibits inability to recognize certain relatives). The transition to a normal state is abrupt. There is no history or physical evidence of neurologic disease. Even if all the characteristics of amnesia indicate hysteria, unless the patient's past history indicates a psychosomatic tendency, the diagnosis should be held in doubt.

Transient global amnesia, a condition that can be mistakenly considered hysterical, is marked by periods of confusion and disorientation to time and place that usually last a few hours. Patients have no recollection of events and describe themselves as feeling strange during the episodes of amnesia. Although patients do not lose their identity, they are unable to retain new information during these episodes. In contrast to hysterical amnesia and fugue state, which usually affect individuals in their third or fourth decade, transient global amnesia affects the middle-aged or elderly who have a history of hypertension or atherosclerosis.


Hysterical Pain

Complaints of pain are rarely hysterical. Patients with hysterical pain syndromes complain of severe pain, but exhibit none of the physical reactions associated with pain having organic origin and thus present an appearance that belies their allegations of intense pain. Some of the most common syndromes ascribed to hysteria are headaches, low back pain, abdominal pain, and atypical facial pain.

Many physicians regard low back pain as a common hysterical syndrome and are likely to consider that diagnosis if there is no muscle spasm, if the neurologic examination is normal, and if the magnetic resonance imaging is unremarkable. Complete investigation might also include pelvic and rectal examination, and prostate-specific antigen and alkaline phosphatase determinations. Most low back pain is of muscular or tendinous origin and can be relieved (not cured) by physical means (e.g., support, heat, exercises) and analgesics. Worsening of pain does not mean worsening of the condition. Most patients do not understand this and may fear paralysis. Reassured that they are not worsening, even if the pain exacerbates, they are better able to endure it.

Four diagnostic myths have been perpetuated about pain: (1) *Continuing pain in patients who have undergone multiple surgical procedures for pain without improvement indicates that the pain is either psychogenic or an undesirable side effect of surgery.* Often, the pain is musculoskeletal and has not been correctly diagnosed or treated. (2) *A high intake of analgesics, or patient requests for analgesics more often than every 4 hours, indicate that the patient's problem is not pain but addiction.* In fact, some analgesics such as meperidine (Demerol) have a shorter duration of action than 4 hours. This drug, the most widely used narcotic analgesic in the United States and prescribed by 60% of physicians for acute painful conditions and by 22% for chronic conditions associated with pain, induced excitatory effects ranging from mild nervousness to seizures in 47 of 67 cancer patients receiving the drug acutely (Kaido et al., 1983). Mood changes such as apprehension, sadness, and restlessness occurred in some patients who were repeatedly given meperidine. These side effects correlated with the buildup of the metabolite normeperidine. Therefore, chronic pain patients being treated with increasing doses of meperidine and manifesting nervousness, depression, and tolerance may not be addicted but rather may be suffering from normeperidine toxicity. (3) *A lawsuit combined with an undiagnosable pain problem is a sure sign of psychogenic origin. If the lawsuit is settled, the pain will disappear.* The data supporting this common assumption are lacking. Lawsuits are often justified and patients who settle them do not necessarily improve. (4) *Negative findings on repeated tests and bizarre complaints with no physical finding indicate pain is psychogenic.* Some of the most bizarre head pains we have seen were easily diagnosed as temporomandibular joint syndromes, though repeated computed tomography scans, electroencephalograms, and standard neurologic examinations revealed no abnormalities in these cases. Few physicians routinely palpate the head and face in headache patients, which is essential for the diagnosis of temporomandibular joint syndrome. Pain syndromes in other parts of the body may also be diagnosed when the correct test is done.

What I have tried to demonstrate with these examples is that the diagnosis of hysteria can be made in error, even when the conversion symptoms are classic. It is exceedingly rare for conversion reaction to be the first manifestation of a psychosomatic tendency. Conversion reactions are nearly always preceded, even in children, by other psychosomatic symptoms, many of which have not resulted in a visit to the physician. Symptoms including stomachaches and headaches, frequent school absences, sleep disturbances, and school phobia precede conversion hysteria by many months or years in childhood. Unless a patient has a history of previous psychosomatic disorders, a diagnosis of conversion reaction should remain open to question. In addition, because psychosomatic illness is so common, particularly in young women, its presence should not blind the physician to the possibility of organic disease.

Behavior is a major output of the brain. Every thought, feeling, memory, and mood is as much the result of brain activity as movement, sensation, and speech. The best diagnostic approach to behavioral changes is to disregard the possibility that nonneurologic illnesses are present and concentrate on organic neurologic hypotheses to explain the abnormal behavior. Though a correct psychiatric diagnosis does actually identify a disease of the brain, as neurologists we must recognize that our degree of competence is likely to be inversely proportional to the number of times we make psychiatric diagnoses. Unrecognized neurologic problems are more likely to be fatal than psychiatric problems, and it is therefore safer to err on the side of a neurologic diagnosis.

## SUGGESTED READING

Alper K, et al. Nonepileptic seizures and childhood physical and sexual abuse. Neurology 1993;43:1950.

Gelenberg AJ. The Catatonia Syndrome. Lancet 1976;1:1339.

Goldstein K. After-Effects of Brain Injuries in War: Their Evaluation and Treatment. New York: Grune & Stratton, 1948.

Jenkyn LR, Reeves AG, Warren T, et al. Neurologic sign in senescence. Arch Neurol 1985;42:1154.

Jenkyn LR, Walsh DB, Culver CM, Reeves A. Clinical signs in diffuse cerebral dysfunction. J Neurol Neurosurg Psychiatry 1977;40:956.

Kaiko RF, Foley KM, Grabinski PY, et al. Central nervous system excitatory effects of meperidine in cancer patients. Ann Neurol 1983;13:180.

Perley MJ, Guze SB. Hysteria: the stability and usefulness of clinical criteria. A quantitative study based on a follow-up of six to eight years in 39 patients. N Engl J Med 1962;266:421.

Pincus JH. Hyperventilation syndrome. Br J Hosp Med 1978;19:310.

Roy A. Hysterical seizures. Arch Neurol 1979;36:447.

# 5
# Seizures

Edward B. Bromfield

Hospital consultations for seizures fall into three broad categories: (1) new-onset seizures in systemically or neurologically ill patients, (2) transient events in admitted patients that could represent seizures and that are as yet undiagnosed, and (3) management of established epilepsy in patients being treated for other medical and surgical problems.

A seizure is the clinical manifestation of an intense, uncontrollable, paroxysmal discharge of a population of abnormally hyperactive cortical neurons. Given sufficient physiologic stress, anyone can have a seizure, and indeed the lifetime prevalence of one or more seizures is approximately 9%. About one-third of this group are young children with benign febrile convulsions; another one-third are people with a tendency toward recurrent, unprovoked seizures (i.e., epilepsy). The remaining one-third, who have one or more seizures resulting from an acute systemic or neurologic insult (i.e., acute symptomatic seizures), prompt the largest number of seizure-related neurologic consultations. In this context, the role of the consulting neurologist is to (1) verify that a seizure has occurred, (2) identify the inciting cause(s), and (3) provide guidance regarding treatment.

An acute symptomatic seizure may be caused by any condition that directly or indirectly promotes abnormal neuronal excitation or interferes with normal neuronal inhibition. A study of the Mayo Clinic database by Annegers et al. yielded a 3.6% calculated lifetime risk of such a seizure. As with epilepsy, a high incidence of acute symptomatic seizures was present in the first year of life, with a gradual decline and leveling off during young adulthood, followed by an increase with advancing age, particularly in males. Although the etiologies varied with age, overall the most common causes were trauma and stroke, followed by (in order) drug withdrawal, central nervous system infection, drug intoxication, metabolic perturbation, central nervous system tumor, and hypoxia-ischemia. These causes are reasonably reflective of the conditions present in general hospital patients for whom a neurologic consultation is requested because of seizures. In the intensive care unit, drug-related and other metabolic causes are most common.

Table 5.1 is a more detailed list of the systemic and neurologic perturbations that clinically are associated with increased seizure risk. Some are fully reversible

*Table 5.1*   Conditions associated with acute symptomatic seizures

I. Systemic
   A. Drug related (see Table 5-2)
      1. Intoxication, especially stimulants
      2. Withdrawal, especially sedatives
   B. General
      1. Fever (not a sole cause in adults)
      2. Electrolyte imbalance
         a. Decreased $Na^+$, $Ca^{++}$, $Mg^{++}$
         b. Increased $Na^+$
      3. Glucose disturbance
         a. Hypoglycemia
         b. Hyperglycemia/hyperosmolar state
   C. Cardiovascular
      1. Global ischemia
      2. Embolic disease
      3. Acute hypertension
   D. Renal
      1. Uremia
      2. Dialysis dysequilibrium/dementia
      3. Electrolyte imbalance (see I.B. General)
      4. Coagulopathy
   E. Gastrointestinal/hepatic
      1. Diarrhea/vomiting (electrolyte imbalance)
      2. Hepatic failure/coagulopathy
   F. Hematologic
      1. Coagulopathy
      2. Hypercoagulable state
   G. Oncologic
      1. Metastatic disease
      2. Treatment related
      3. Paraneoplastic
   H. Endocrine/metabolic
      1. Glucose disturbance
      2. Thyrotoxicosis/myxedema
      3. Adrenal disease (electrolyte disturbance)
      4. Pheochromocytoma
      5. Parathyroid disturbance (decreased $Ca^{++}$)
      6. Porphyria
   I. Pulmonary
      1. Hypoxemia
      2. Syndrome of inappropriate antidiuretic hormone (decreased $Na^+$)
      3. Treatment related
   J. Rheumatologic
      1. Collagen-vascular diseases, e.g., systemic lupus erythematosus
      2. Vasculitis, e.g., polyarteritis nodosa
   K. Obstetric
      1. Toxemia
      2. Embolic disease
      3. Coagulopathy
      4. Hypercoagulable state

II. Neurologic
- A. Vascular
  1. Hemorrhagic
  2. Ischemic
  3. Hypertensive
- B. Inflammatory/infectious
  1. Parenchymal
  2. Meningeal
  3. Parameningeal
- C. Traumatic
  1. Hematoma
  2. Contusion
- D. Neoplastic
  1. Primary
  2. Metastatic
  3. Treatment related
- E. Congenital
  1. Diffuse
  2. Localized

---

conditions, though others can produce permanent changes in neuronal excitability, leading to the tendency toward recurrent unprovoked seizures that constitutes epilepsy.

As alluded to earlier, drugs, both prescribed and illicit, are an important cause of acute symptomatic seizures. The list of drugs linked at least anecdotally with a lowered seizure threshold is long (many are listed in Table 5.2). Important considerations in determining whether it is likely a given drug has caused a seizure include serum levels (affected by both drug dose and patient metabolism) and associated systemic and neurologic conditions.

## APPROACH TO THE HOSPITALIZED PATIENT WITH A POSSIBLE FIRST SEIZURE

### Classification

The neurologic consultant must first determine whether a seizure has occurred. If one has occurred, he or she must then attempt to classify it (Table 5.3). Partial seizures (including secondarily generalized seizures) are the most common type. Drug intoxication or withdrawal, or metabolic perturbations, typically cause primarily generalized tonic-clonic seizures or, less commonly, myoclonic seizures. Other generalized seizure types usually do not occur de novo except in pediatric patients, in whom an acute illness may allow a latent seizure tendency to be expressed.

The consultant first must determine whether the event in question was a seizure, as opposed to another type of transient episode, and then whether an underlying neurologic illness predisposing the patient to seizures is present. In the case of a

*Table 5.2*   Drugs that may lower the seizure threshold

Antiasthmatics: theophylline (usually but not always with levels above therapeutic range)
Antibiotics
    Isoniazid (especially without vitamin $B_6$ supplements)
    Lindane
    Metronidazole
    Penicillin (especially with breakdown of blood-brain barrier, renal failure)
    Acyclovir
    Quinolones
Antidepressants
    Tricyclics (rarely a clinical problem)
    Serotonin-specific reuptake inhibitors (rarely a clinical problem)
    Bupropion
Hormones
    Insulin (if hypoglycemia produced)
    Prednisone (with hypocalcemia)
    Estrogen (especially when unopposed by progesterone)
Immunosuppressants
    Cyclosporine A
    Tacrolimus
Anesthetics
    Lidocaine (especially at high levels)
    Enflurane
    Ketamine
Narcotics
    Meperidine
    Pentazocine
Stimulants
    Amphetamines
    Cocaine
    Methylphenidate (rarely a clinical problem)
    Phenylpropanolamine (rarely a clinical problem)
    Phencyclidine
Neuroleptics
    Clozapine
    Phenothiazines
    Butyrophenones
Other
    Anticholinergics
    Anticholinesterases
    Antihistamines
    Baclofen
    Lithium
    Oral hypoglycemics
    Heavy metals
    Mexiletine

*Table 5.3*   Classification of epileptic seizures

---

  I. Partial (beginning focally)
    A. Simple partial (consciousness not impaired)
      1. Motor
      2. Somatosensory or special sensory
      3. Autonomic
      4. Psychic-cognitive
    B. Complex partial (consciousness impaired)
    C. Partial secondarily generalized
  II. Generalized (bilaterally symmetric and without local onset)
    A. Absence
    B. Myoclonic
    C. Clonic
    D. Tonic
    E. Tonic-clonic
    F. Atonic
 III. Unclassified epileptic seizures

---

witnessed convulsive event, diagnosis may be straightforward, although convulsive syncope (see the next section) can be difficult to differentiate. Nonconvulsive seizures are more problematic and more likely to be missed by the referring clinician, who may describe confusion or memory loss rather than seizures.

## Syncope

Differentiating syncope from seizure is a particularly common clinical problem. Possible pathophysiologies and predisposing factors for syncope include hypovolemia (from blood loss, diuretics), decreased arterial or venous tone (from vasodilators, autonomic dysfunction), limited cardiac output (from aortic stenosis, arrhythmias), and inappropriate baroreceptor reflexes (from emotional situations, Valsalva maneuver). Upright posture at onset and typical warning symptoms of lightheadedness, nausea, warmth, and fading vision and hearing are common but not universal. Cardiac arrhythmias, in particular, may occur in any position and without warning; palpitations may or may not be noted. With syncope, a few myoclonic jerks are commonly seen, and more complex movements as well as tonic stiffening can also occur. Convulsive manifestations are more likely if the head is kept upright. Postictal confusion should be absent or very brief, not more than a few seconds, unless head trauma or more prolonged ischemia occurs. Typical convulsive syncope represents a brain stem release phenomenon rather than the electrocortical hypersynchrony of an acute symptomatic seizure; cortical seizures caused by cerebral hypoperfusion can occur but are extremely rare.

## Migraines

Migraines are distinguished from seizures by their more gradual warnings and longer duration of neurologic symptoms. Warnings usually last more than 5 minutes and are primarily visual but may be somatosensory (e.g., tingling) or motor; an olfactory component, in particular hypersensitivity, is not rare, and olfactory precipitants have been noted. Headache usually, but not always, follows. A personal or family history of more typical bilateral or unilateral periorbital, throbbing headaches, with photophobia and abdominal symptoms, may be present before the index event, which typically includes altered mental status or sensorimotor symptoms. Loss of consciousness is rare but may occur with so-called basilar migraine. Individuals with migraine may also have a more general predisposition toward syncope. That migraine and epilepsy can coexist, that migraines can on occasion trigger seizures in susceptible individuals (particularly children with "benign occipital epilepsy"), and that migrainous headaches may follow epileptic seizures must be recognized.

## Transient Ischemic Attacks

Transient ischemic attacks (TIAs) have characteristic symptoms and (if prolonged enough to persist to the time of evaluation) signs consistent with known vascular territories. They typically evolve over minutes and last for minutes to hours. Unlike seizures, which generally manifest positive symptoms, such as stiffening or shaking in the motor system or hallucinations in the special sensory systems, ischemic symptoms are usually negative (e.g., hemiparesis, sensory loss). Exceptions include a tingling sensation as part of a TIA and limb-shaking TIAs, which are rare manifestations of severe carotid stenosis distinguishable from motor seizures mainly by (1) their consistently postural character, usually occurring promptly on standing, and (2) their involvement of exclusively the arm and leg, sparing facial muscles and cognition. On the other hand, rare seizure types, such as ictal amaurosis (total or hemianopic, not monocular) or aphasic status epilepticus (SE), require an electroencephalogram (EEG) to be distinguished from TIAs. Vascular risk factors are common in elderly patients presenting with new-onset seizures as well as with TIAs, and so are of limited help in differential diagnosis. Strokes and seizures may occur contemporaneously, as 4–14% of strokes are followed within 1–2 weeks by seizures, and rarely, even a TIA without infarction can precipitate a seizure.

## Movement Disorders

Movement disorders can usually be readily distinguished from seizures; they are typically long lasting, associated with preserved consciousness, and bilateral. The main exceptions are paroxysmal kinesogenic dyskinesias, seen mainly in children; precipitation by movement distinguishes these from most seizures. Interestingly, they usually respond to antiepileptic drugs. Difficulties may arise in patients with depressed mental status from other causes, such as toxic or metabolic encephalopathies, which may at times produce such movement disorders as extrapyramidal reactions to neuroleptics. Multifocal myoclonus in uremia and other encephalopathies presents a special challenge. Although the multifocality is not typical of seizures, and the movements are not time-locked to epileptiform discharges on the EEG, such discharges are often present and imply cortical irritability. In addition, clear-cut seizures may occur in the same patients as the condition evolves. This condition, therefore, though it may be considered a movement disorder, likely overlaps with seizures pathophysiologically. Asterixis often occurs in patients with depressed mental status resulting from hepatic or other encephalopathies, but can usually be distinguished from seizures by its positional nature, even when unilateral. Such negative motor rhythmic activity is extremely rare but can occur in epilepsy. When distinguishing between seizures and movement disorders, it is important to keep in mind the possibility that antiepileptic drugs, especially at toxic levels, can produce involuntary movements, such as dystonia with phenytoin or tremor with valproate.

## Sleep Disorders

Sleep disorders may cause brief "microsleeps" or more prolonged sleep attacks. These can be a result of any cause of hypersomnolence, most commonly disrupted sleep from obstructive sleep apnea. Although microsleeps may occur without warning, distinct sleep attacks are usually preceded by a subjective feeling of sleepiness; eyes are usually closed, and the patient may be awakened with stimulation. Periodic limb-movement disorder of sleep is also common, often associated with restless legs syndrome, and may be responsible for nonrestorative sleep and daytime hypersomnolence. Of note is that many hospitalized patients are hypersomnolent because of poor nocturnal sleep as well as sedative medications. Narcolepsy is a more dramatic but much less common cause of hypersomnolence. Associated symptoms of hypnagogic/hypnopompic hallucinations, sleep paralysis, and especially cataplexy are usually present. Onset is rare after early adulthood.

Parasomnias can be difficult to distinguish from nocturnal seizures. The classic parasomnias of slow-wave sleep, sleepwalking and night terrors, are conditions of childhood, though the former may rarely persist into adulthood. Patients may wander, perform complex behaviors, and then return to sleep, with no recollection in the morning. In adults, such complex nocturnal behavior can represent a dissociative, psychogenic event, but postictal wandering may also occur after a nocturnal complex partial seizure; this usually shows a progressive return to normal awareness, with memory and complexity of behavior at a given moment corresponding to the degree to which postictal confusion has resolved. Rapid eye movement (REM) behavior disorder, a recognized parasomnia of REM sleep, by contrast, typically begins late in life and may be associated with extrapyramidal syndromes such as Parkinson's disease. In this disorder, partial arousals from REM sleep occur, but without the usual muscle atonia of REM, resulting in "acting out" of dreams, often in a violent manner that may reflect defensive behavior prompted by a frightening dream. The timing of the spells in the later sleep cycles, when REM periods are longer, can be a useful clue in distinguishing this from other parasomnias, which often occur in earlier cycles when there is more slow-wave sleep. Polysomnography with a full set of EEG electrodes may be necessary to distinguish parasomnias from nocturnal partial seizures.

Toxic-Metabolic Disturbances

Altered behavior resulting from toxic-metabolic disturbances usually lasts much longer than changes resulting from seizures. The possibility of certain causes of encephalopathy (such as hyper- or hypoglycemia, hyponatremia, hypocalcemia, hypomagnesemia; see Table 5.1) precipitating seizures can, however, confuse the picture. The EEG, though typically showing diffuse slowing, can at times show multifocal sharp waves or the triphasic wave pattern, which can be difficult to distinguish from the generalized sharp-slow complexes of nonconvulsive generalized SE (see the section on Other Types of Status Epilepticus). Benzodiazepine infusion, which would be expected to worsen or have no effect on encephalopathies, can be diagnostic of SE if both the patient and the EEG improve. Myoclonus, discussed above, may be associated with encephalopathies and with epileptiform activity on the EEG.

Psychogenic Nonepileptic Seizures

Distinguishing psychogenic nonepileptic seizures (NES) (i.e., pseudoseizures) from epileptic seizures is the purpose of specialized epilepsy-monitoring units; the lone neurologic consultant, however, is often asked to make this distinction in patients ill with other medical and surgical conditions, as well as in those hospitalized for psychiatric disorders. In general, compared with epileptic seizures, psychogenic NES display less stereotypy, longer duration, a greater waxing and waning nature, and a less physiologic-anatomic progression of manifestations. Eyes are more likely to be closed during unresponsiveness. Precipitation by environmental factors is more likely and resulting injuries less likely in NES, although there are many exceptions. Unlike epileptic seizures, NES do not arise from sleep, although they may arise from "pseudosleep," a distinction that may be difficult to make without prolonged EEG monitoring. If the patient cannot be moved to a monitoring unit and no portable video EEG unit is available, a standard paper or digital EEG machine can be left at the bedside for nurses or other personnel to turn on during a spell. Even though the physician does not observe the EEG at the onset of the event, the presence of a reactive alpha rhythm during apparent unresponsiveness or the absence of postictal slowing after an apparent convulsion provides strong evidence against an epileptic etiology.

It should be mentioned that psychogenic NES in most cases represent dissociative states or other manifestations of a conversion disorder and are not under the patient's conscious control. The availability of compassionate psychiatric intervention in this setting is critical, and other personnel involved in the patient's care should be educated about the involuntary nature of the episodes, unless there is positive evidence of malingering.

**Evaluation**

With these differential points in mind, the examiner should evaluate the hospitalized patient with a possible first seizure by taking a history, performing an examination, and ordering a laboratory evaluation.

## History

A subjective warning, if present, may be critical in establishing the partial onset of a seizure and in providing a clue as to its anatomic origin. Although the specific phenomenology of the warning can vary enormously from patient to patient, and encompasses virtually every aspect of subjective experience, each patient's aura is usually quite consistent and in many cases has occurred many times as an isolated simple partial seizure before a complex partial or secondarily generalized event occurs. Duration is also important to note, as auras rarely last longer than a minute or two, usually 15–30 seconds. After awareness is lost or impaired, as with a complex partial or secondarily generalized seizure, witness accounts are necessary for understanding abnormal motor activity or other behaviors. A reliable description of the duration and evolution of the event can be extremely useful, as can an assessment of postictal confusion, somnolence, or focal features. A history of a previous neurologic insult that may predispose the patient to seizures can be suggestive but is not diagnostic. Additional risk factors such as a history of febrile seizures or a family history of epilepsy are less important in the hospitalized patient than in the ambulatory patient, because the former often has acute medical or neurologic predisposing factors. Probably the most important historical item is the list of current and recent medications (see Table 5.2), with an emphasis on stimulant intoxication or sedative withdrawal.

## Examination

The general examination usually reflects the underlying medical conditions associated with hospitalization. Occasionally, new signs such as meningismus or previously undocumented focal findings may suggest an undiagnosed neurologic condition as the cause of the seizure. The most important aspect of the neurologic examination is the level of consciousness and mentation. Somnolence or confusion may be transient, particularly if the patient is seen relatively soon after the seizure, or may be more persistent. If it persists for more than an hour, impairment is likely to be attributable to the underlying systemic or neurologic condition responsible for the seizure. It is imperative, however, to rule out continuing seizures, that is, SE, as the cause of a persistently depressed mental status. Convulsive SE, though usually clinically obvious, can be subtle in a deeply comatose person after prolonged seizures, and nonconvulsive SE is virtually always clinically subtle, requiring EEG for diagnosis. As several series suggest, nonconvulsive SE (see the section on Other Types of Status Epilepticus) is probably significantly underdiagnosed in ill patients. Transient focal signs may represent a Todd's or postictal paralysis, which is often reliable in lateralizing (less often in localizing) the site of seizure onset.

## Laboratory Evaluation

Serum chemistries, particularly sodium, calcium, magnesium, glucose, and renal indices, should be measured. Levels of potentially offending drugs (see Table 5.2), such as theophylline or the normeperidine metabolite of meperidine, can sometimes be obtained rapidly enough to be useful. Blood and urine toxic screens are helpful in assessing the possibility of illicit drug use. Neuroimaging is indicated in any ill patient with a first seizure, particularly if there are focal features. A computed tomographic (CT) scan can be performed if the examiner suspects an acute stroke, especially one accompanied with hemorrhaging, or if gross mass effect must be quickly ruled out prior to lumbar puncture when meningoencephalitis is suspected. If no metabolic cause of the seizure can be established or focal features are present, magnetic resonance imaging (MRI) should be performed. If the patient's condition does not suggest an acute hemorrhage or need for emergency lumbar puncture, MRI can be performed instead of CT scan. EEG should generally be obtained as early as possible, although arguably can be deferred if an unequivocal metabolic cause for the seizure can be determined, no focality is present, and rapid, complete recovery occurs. If the patient has not returned to baseline when evaluated, or is under neuromuscular blockade, the EEG is essential to rule out ongoing seizure activity of SE. The EEG can also confirm suspicion of a toxic-metabolic disturbance or of a focal neurologic abnormality. Rarely, a specific diagnosis, such as herpes simplex encephalitis, may be suggested by the EEG. If it is not certain whether a seizure has occurred, the presence of interictal epileptiform discharges may aid in diagnosis; the likelihood of obtaining such information is highest within 1–2 days of the seizure. Occasionally, long-term video-EEG monitoring may be necessary to determine whether repeated events are epileptic.

## Treatment

Although effective treatment of seizures often depends on reversal of the underlying cause, which may be beyond the scope of the consultation, in most cases the use of antiepileptic drugs must be considered. The urgency and aggressiveness of treatment are often determined by the perceived risk of morbidity and mortality posed by further seizures. No consensus yet exists on whether a single unprovoked seizure should be treated with antiepileptic drugs; data suggest, however, that the 2-year recurrence risk of another seizure is 25–50%, and can be cut in half with appropriate treatment. Long-term treatment is likely to be less strongly indicated in the hospitalized patient because the seizure often has a treatable or preventable cause; short-term treatment, however, is generally instituted unless the cause is unequivocally known and rapidly reversible. Furthermore, the risk of injury from a second seizure is often higher in hospitalized patients. For example, increased cerebral blood flow as a result of a seizure can cause a further increase in intracranial pressure in a patient with a mass lesion, and a convulsion may constitute a dangerous cardiovascular stress in a cardiac patient.

Phenytoin

The choice of an appropriate antiepileptic drug depends on potential routes of administration, interactions with other medications, and specific medical conditions such as renal or hepatic impairment. Because of its relative lack of sedation and ease of loading by a parenteral route, the mainstay of acute seizure treatment remains phenytoin, although it is not clearly efficacious in all circumstances, for example, in hypoglycemia or alcohol withdrawal. The availability of fosphenytoin provides more flexibility, mainly by allowing intramuscular administration in those without adequate intravenous access. Although it can also be given more quickly intravenously than phenytoin (and more safely in those perceived to be at risk of extravasation), adequate brain phenytoin levels may not be achieved more quickly than with phenytoin administered at the fastest recommended rate because of the time taken to dephosphorylate the molecule. Fosphenytoin is dosed in *phenytoin equivalents*, rather than in actual quantities of fosphenytoin itself. In nonemergent settings, phenytoin may be loaded orally, but in the inpatient setting, some or all of the loading dose is usually given parenterally.

Several important pharmacokinetic factors should be kept in mind when dosing phenytoin. One is the volume of distribution, which is 0.8 liters/kg in adults; when recommending an intravenous loading dose, the consultant should determine the desired phenytoin level, subtract that from the current level (0 if the patient is just starting on the drug), and multiply the result by 0.8 times the patient's weight (kg). For example, to obtain a level of 15 mg/liter in a patient weighing 80 kg, one must give $15 \times 0.8 \times 80 = 960$ mg. The loading dose is independent of metabolic factors; these affect the amount and frequency of maintenance doses. On the other hand, systemic factors affecting the free to total ratio (typically 1 to 10), such as hypoalbuminemia, affect the target level and therefore size of the loading dose. For convulsive SE, an initial loading dose of 18–20 mg/kg (not the familiar "gram of phenytoin" for most adults) should be given at the maximal rate of 50 mg per minute of phenytoin or 150 mg per minute of fosphenytoin (in phenytoin equivalents). Because of the possibility of decreases in pulse rate and blood pressure, cardiovascular monitoring is mandatory, sometimes necessitating slowing the rate of infusion, administration of fluids, or, less commonly, pressors. Because of the slow absorption of 100-mg or 30-mg extended-release capsules of phenytoin, oral loading is affected by metabolism, so that the dose to obtain a given peak level must be higher than for intravenous loading, approximately 1 mg/kg for each desired 1-mg/liter rise in level. Peak oral level is reached more quickly if the 50-mg chewable tablet is used. Of note is that the mg content of phenytoin is also higher in this preparation, which contains the acid form rather than the sodium salt; the difference is 8%, meaning that five and a half rather than six of the 50-mg tablets is the equivalent of three of the 100-mg capsules. The 125 mg/5 ml suspension also contains the acid form. Although this may be convenient to use in patients receiving tube feedings, the bottle must be vigorously shaken to avoid phenytoin precipitating in the bottom of the bottle, yielding doses that are either lower (if from the full bottle) or higher (if from the bottom of the bottle) than intended.

Important interactions with other drugs follow from two characteristics of phenytoin. First, as noted, it is highly protein bound, causing mutual displacement from binding sites when given with several other drugs, most notably aspirin. Increase in the free level results initially in increased brain levels and therefore increases in both the therapeutic and central nervous system–toxic effects. The increased free level, however, also results in faster metabolism. Therefore, within a period of days there is a new steady state characterized by lower total levels but a return to approximately the baseline free level, as a result of the higher free fraction. The toxicity resulting from such interactions is usually transient and can be clarified by measuring the free and total levels. Second, phenytoin is, like carbamazepine and phenobarbital, a potent

*Table 5.4*    Substrates for the P-450 mixed function oxidase system (levels lowered by the addition of an inducing drug such as phenytoin, carbamazepine, or phenobarbital)

---

Steroid hormones
Acetaminophen
Carbamazepine
Cyclosporine A
Digoxin
Doxycycline
Folic acid
Lamotrigine
Meperidine (increase in normeperidine)
Neuroleptics
Theophylline
Tricyclic antidepressants
Valproate
Vitamin D (25- and 1,25-hydroxycalciferol)
Warfarin

---

inducer of the P-450 mixed-function oxidase system of hepatic enzymes, which is responsible for the metabolism of many important drugs (Table 5.4). When phenytoin is added to these drugs, their doses typically must be increased if the therapeutic effect is to remain constant; careful monitoring of levels and therapeutic effects is necessary (e.g., prothrombin time if the patient is on warfarin). This interaction may take days to weeks to develop fully.

The situation most commonly necessitating phenytoin discontinuation is development of a rash, which occurs in 5–10% of patients; less common idiosyncratic reactions such as fever, lymphadenopathy, and hepatic dysfunction may also occur. Although rash may resolve even without discontinuation, most clinicians elect not to continue treatment, particularly in ill, hospitalized patients. In the latter situation, the presence of many other drugs, particularly antibiotics, that can also cause rash further complicates this decision. No evidence exists that sudden discontinuation of phenytoin causes withdrawal seizures per se, but if it is needed for seizure control, prudence dictates coverage with adequate doses of an alternative antiepileptic drug when phenytoin is withdrawn. The two most commonly used alternatives, phenobarbital and carbamazepine, may cause allergic cross-reactivity with phenytoin as often as 20% of the time. If the reaction is not severe, however, this risk may be acceptable.

## Phenobarbital

Phenobarbital offers the advantage of parenteral (i.e., intravenous or intramuscular) administration. As with phenytoin, loading doses may be given but they increase the likelihood and severity of sedation, depending on dose, rate, and route. Many laboratories consider the therapeutic range to be 15–40 mg/liter, although levels greater than 10 mg/liter or even 5 mg/liter may be enough to control seizures in some individuals. The target level depends on the perceived risk of adverse effects, principally sedation, versus the risks of another seizure and of suffering a significant injury from it. Because the volume of distribution in adults is approximately 0.5 liters/kg, a loading dose of 2 mg/kg is needed to raise the level by 1 mg/liter. In SE, 10–20 mg/kg or more can be given at up to 100 mg per minute, but again, cardiovascular depression is a significant risk, especially in the elderly. Respiratory suppression in this setting is virtually universal, particularly if benzodiazepines have been given first. At more modest doses, sedation is the most common adverse effect, although patients with neurologic impairments can sometimes have paradoxical agitation, probably resulting from disinhibition of behavioral control.

Discontinuation of phenobarbital, at least in patients on chronic treatment, has been linked to withdrawal seizures, with partial seizures increasing in frequency as the level falls between 15 and 20 mg/liter, and tonic-clonic seizures between 5 and 10 mg/liter. Like phenytoin and carbamazepine, phenobarbital is a potent inducer of the hepatic P-450 enzyme system and increases metabolism of many important drugs (see Table 5.4).

## Carbamazepine

Because of the lack of availability of a parenteral form and the difficulty of oral loading, carbamazepine, though considered along with phenytoin to be the first-choice drug for chronic treatment of partial or secondarily generalized seizures, has a smaller role to play in hospitalized patients. Loading doses, or even an average maintenance dose such as 800 mg per day in an adult, are poorly tolerated when therapy is initiated, leading to dizziness, diplopia, and malaise. On the other hand, because of slow metabolism before autoinduction of appropriate hepatic enzymes, which takes 2–6 weeks, loading doses may not be needed; typically, a well-tolerated starting dose of 100 mg bid may produce levels in at least the low end of the therapeutic range of 4–12 µg/liter, and provide some protection against seizure recurrence. Important considerations in the ill, elderly patient, in addition to drug interactions such as those described for phenytoin and phenobarbital, are the possibilities of bradyarrhythmias resulting from slowed conduction at the atrioventricular node and of hyponatremia resulting from renal insensitivity to antidiuretic hormone. These effects are more likely to occur at high carbamazepine levels.

## Valproate

Valproate or its dimeric form, divalproex, is less commonly used in the treatment of new seizures in hospitalized patients, but it offers a useful alternative to the above drugs. It has a broad spectrum, effective against not just the partial and secondarily generalized seizures most common in hospitalized patients but also absence and myoclonic seizures. Because of its short half-life (12–16 hours without concomitant administration of P-450 inducing drugs, 5–10 hours with such drugs), a steady state is reached rapidly at maintenance doses of 15–30 mg/kg; higher loading doses may also be used, although they may cause gastrointestinal upset. A liquid form is available, and the development and approval of an intravenous form further broadens potential loading options (although this has not yet been adequately studied in the treatment of SE). It should be recognized that the enteric-coated, divalproex preparation, though less likely than valproic acid or sodium valproate to produce gastrointestinal upset, has a delayed absorption resulting in peak levels 4–6 hours after administration; therefore the standard tablet or liquid preparation is preferable if a faster therapeutic effect is desired.

One advantage of valproate is its lack of cross-reactivity with phenytoin, phenobarbital, and carbamazepine; rashes and other overt allergic reactions are uncommon. Although idiosyncratic hepatic dysfunction and pancreatitis are the most severe adverse reactions, these are extremely rare after infancy in the absence of pre-existing organ dysfunction. A potentially more important risk in the hospitalized patient, particularly the neurosurgical patient, is the possibility of thrombocytopenia or thrombocytopathy. Although in part idiosyncratic, this reaction is more common at high doses and levels. Bleeding time is usually but not always abnormal in patients at risk, and aspirin can potentiate this effect. Aspirin also potentiates the therapeutic effects of valproate by displacing it from binding sites, thereby elevating free levels; as with phenytoin, the total level may be unchanged or even decline slightly because of increased free drug as a substrate for metabolism.

## Other Drugs

Among the new antiepileptic drugs that have become available in the United States, gabapentin is the one most likely to be of value to the consultant. Although it has not been approved as monotherapy and there is no evidence that it is any more effective, or even as effective, as the drugs previously described when used alone, it has the advantages of being well tolerated at rapid titration rates, of bypassing hepatic metabolism, and of not interacting pharmacokinetically with other drugs. The lack of hepatic metabolism may make it the drug of choice in such rare conditions as the porphyrias, although clinical data are sparse. There is no parenteral form, but the capsules or their contents may be administered through feeding tubes. Its spectrum of action, encompassing partial seizures with and without secondary generalization, is appropriate for most hospitalized patients with new-onset seizures. Patients with refractory epilepsy and no renal impairment usually have a dose-related improvement in seizure control between 900 and 1,800 mg per day; higher doses of up to 3,600 mg per day or more have led to improved control in some patients. For the hospitalized patient with a first seizure, initiation at 300 mg tid is reasonable; if tolerated and necessary, the dose can be increased over 1–3 days to 600 mg tid. In patients with impaired renal function, these doses may be scaled back in proportion to creatinine clearance. Side effects are usually transient and mild, and include fatigue, dizziness, and sedation; hypotension or thrombocytopenia may occur rarely.

Because of the slow titration necessary when introducing lamotrigine, topiramate, or tiagabine, these new drugs presently have little place in the initial treatment of seizures in hospitalized patients. Felbamate may be titrated more rapidly but is rarely used outside the context of longstanding, refractory epilepsy because of the associated risks of aplastic anemia and hepatic failure.

Benzodiazepines have a limited but important role in the treatment of seizures in hospitalized patients. Parenteral administration allows onset of activity within minutes, which is useful especially in the treatment of SE. However, duration of action is short, particularly for diazepam, which is redistributed out of the brain into other fatty tissues within 15–20 minutes; the parent compound, however, or its long-acting metabolite, nordiazepam, may still produce sedation for hours or even days if a high dose is given or metabolism slowed. Lorazepam, by contrast, remains active for 4–12 hours. Clonazepam has an even longer half-life but is not usually used parenterally in the United States. Midazolam has the shortest half-life of the benzodiazepines, 1–6 hours, which is useful for minimizing prolonged sedation, but mandates frequent boluses or continuous drip if prolonged effect is needed, as in SE.

## DIAGNOSIS AND TREATMENT OF STATUS EPILEPTICUS IN THE HOSPITALIZED PATIENT

SE may be colloquially defined as seizures that do not stop; formally, the accepted criterion has become at least 30 minutes of either continuous seizures or intermittent seizures without recovery between them. In the case of generalized convulsive SE (GCSE), recovery implies return to consciousness. Furthermore, studies demonstrating that isolated primarily or secondarily generalized tonic-clonic seizures rarely last longer than 2 minutes have led many clinicians to initiate treatment for GCSE after a much shorter period of 5–10 minutes.

Although any type of seizure may evolve into SE, the types of greatest importance for the consultant, either because of need for aggressive treatment, difficulty in diagnosis, or both, include GCSE (including secondarily generalized), myoclonic SE, generalized nonconvulsive SE, complex partial SE, epilepsia partialis continua, and aphasic SE.

Recognition of the importance of treating GCSE dates back largely to a series of classic studies performed in the 1970s by Meldrum and colleagues, who found that sustained generalized convulsions in baboons produced a variety of systemic and neuropathologic changes, and that the latter could be modified but not eliminated by treating the former. These findings have subsequently been extended to other species and experimental models. Because a predictable change in systemic and neurologic function seems to take place within 30–60 minutes of onset of GCSE, these changes are generally divided into early (within less than 30–60 minutes of onset) and late categories. Early changes include severe lactic acidosis, arterial hypertension, and increased cerebral venous pressure. Hyperglycemia occurs after a lag of 15 minutes or more, but later may evolve to hypoglycemia, often accompanied by hyperthermia and hypotension. Cerebral blood flow is elevated, especially early.

Pathologically, neuronal loss is noted in the small pyramidal neurons of neocortical layers 3, 5, and 6 throughout the cortex, the pyramidal neurons of CA 1 and 3 (often asymmetrically) and end folium of the hippocampus, and the anterior and dorsomedial thalamus. Without neuromuscular paralysis and mechanical ventilation, the cerebellum and amygdala also suffer neuronal loss. On a cellular level, neuropathologic changes resemble those of ischemia, but are not explained by global or regional changes in cerebral blood flow. Possible explanations include "ischemia of excess demand," or a more direct effect of excitotoxins such as glutamate, probably mediated through $Ca^{++}$ influx. In human neuropathologic studies, contributing systemic insults include cardiac arrhythmias, aspiration pneumonia, neurogenic pulmonary edema, and rhabdomyolysis with hyperkalemia and renal failure.

## Clinical Features and Diagnosis

Individual generalized tonic-clonic (GTC) seizures are more variable than commonly believed. The tonic or, less often, clonic phase may be fragmentary, and both phases may be asymmetric. Variability is increased when the seizures are secondarily generalized (as is usually the case in hospitalized patients); use of antiepileptic drugs may also modify the clinical appearance of GTC seizures. Most important is the observation that motor activity can become markedly attenuated in the context of prolonged SE. For diagnostic and therapeutic purposes, any seizure involving loss of consciousness and some bilateral rhythmic motor activity may be regarded as a GTC seizure if it does not fit into another well-defined category.

Furthermore, an observer who witnesses a single GTC seizure cannot know whether it is an isolated event or part of SE; this is true even in the hospital unless the patient is under nearly continuous observation in an intensive care unit. One should try to estimate as closely as possible the time of onset of unconsciousness and generalized motor activity, at least documenting the last time the patient was seen before seizure onset. If another GTC seizure is observed before the patient regains consciousness, or if the patient cannot be aroused to at least partial responsiveness within several minutes of evaluation, SE should be suspected and treatment begun. As noted above, it is rare for a single GTC seizure in an adult to last longer than 2 minutes, so that even a single seizure exceeding this duration should raise the suspicion of incipient SE.

Other relevant features of the examination include focal signs either during or after an observed seizure. Especially in the setting of new focal findings, neuroimaging is indicated, but not before SE has been adequately treated. An EEG can be helpful, particularly when the convulsive activity is subtle, but treatment should not be delayed to obtain this study unless the diagnosis is in doubt. (Among the most important alternative diagnoses is psychogenic nonepileptic status; stability of vital signs and respiratory status including arterial blood gases may allow delaying treatment until after EEG verification if the suspicion of nonepileptic status is high.)

Important causes of SE in patients without previous epilepsy parallel that of first seizure, and include withdrawal of alcohol or other sedatives, drug toxicity, trauma, stroke, central nervous system infection, and neoplasm. In patients with a focal brain lesion or with known partial epilepsy, a frontal focus appears most likely to be associated with SE. In children, febrile seizures may present with SE; these patients may be at relatively high risk for the later development of epilepsy.

Older studies estimate mortality from SE at 32–50%. This has declined in more recent series to 3–35%, with death usually attributable to the underlying disease rather than to uncontrolled seizures themselves. Children consistently have lower mortality than adults. With respect to etiology, the best prognosis is associated with antiepileptic drug or alcohol withdrawal and the worst with anoxia. Duration of SE beyond 1–4 hours has also been clearly linked to higher mortality, even in a multivariate analysis controlling for age, etiology, and other variables (DeLorenzo, 1992). Neurologic morbidity is more difficult to quantify, but most clinical studies have associated significant deficits up to and including the persistent vegetative state with prolonged SE; again, however, the underlying illness often contributes significantly to the negative outcome.

**Treatment of Generalized Tonic-Clonic Status Epilepticus**

Because of the risk of significant morbidity and mortality with prolonged SE, a pre-established time-based treatment plan is recommended. Several appropriate protocols have been published, including a consensus document (Working Group, 1993), on which the following is based:

- 0–10 minutes: Assess and support cardiorespiratory function (ABCs: airway, breathing, circulation). Give nasal oxygen and insert airway if necessary. Obtain history (especially duration of seizure, prior seizures, drugs used, etc.) and perform physical and neurologic examination. Insert intravenous tube (with normal saline) and draw blood for antiepileptic blood levels, toxic screen, complete blood cell count, glucose, electrolytes including calcium and magnesium, and hepatic and renal function tests. Give B vitamins and 50 ml of 50% glucose intravenously. Call for EEG monitoring but do not delay treatment.
- 11–30 minutes: Begin phenytoin infusion at 50 mg per minute (or fosphenytoin at 150 mg phenytoin equivalents per minute) to 18–20 mg/kg. In patients known or suspected to be on antiepileptic drugs, do not wait for levels before beginning infusion. Monitor electrocardiogram and blood pressure. Simultaneously, give lorazepam at 1–2 mg per minute up to 0.1 mg/kg through a separate intravenous tube, or diazepam at 2–4 mg per minute up to 20 mg. (Be prepared to assist ventilation immediately when pushing benzodiazepines.) Treat fever with antipyretics and cooling.
- 31–60 minutes: If seizures persist, give additional 5–10 mg/kg phenytoin or fosphenytoin. If SE continues, give phenobarbital at 50–100 mg per minute to a maximum of 20–25 mg/kg. If phenobarbital does not terminate SE, intubate patient and proceed to the next step on the list.
- >60 minutes: Barbiturate anesthesia with pentobarbital, 5- to 15-mg/kg load given at 25 mg per minute, until burst-suppression appears or epileptiform activity is clearly suppressed. Maintain 0.5–5.0 mg/kg per hour drip for at least several hours before tapering to look for seizure recurrence. If seizures recur, give a bolus sufficient to produce burst-suppression (50-mg increments) and increase drip by 0.5–1.0 mg/kg per hour. (An alternative for management of barbiturates is to use pentobarbital directly after phenytoin, skipping phenobarbital, or conversely using repeated phenobarbital boluses of 5–10 mg/kg at 20-minute intervals rather than pentobarbital. Benzodiazepine infusions may also be used, as outlined later.)

Maintain high therapeutic levels of either phenytoin (18–30 mg/liter) or phenobarbital (25–40 mg/liter) or both during pentobarbital or benzodiazepine infusion to protect against recurrent seizures during taper.

Hypotension during infusion of any of the above drugs should be treated by slowing or stopping the infusion and giving fluids and pressors (e.g., dopamine) as needed.

Administration of sodium bicarbonate may be necessary to prevent circulatory collapse from severe acidosis, but overcorrection should be avoided because alkalosis renders neurons hyperexcitable and mild acidosis may be protective.

If phenytoin is contraindicated because of cardiac status or allergy, alternatives include phenobarbital (although there is some risk of allergic cross-reactivity, as previously mentioned) or lorazepam, which remains effective for several hours and can be used as a maintenance drug in the short term. As noted earlier, diazepam is rapidly redistributed from the central nervous system and cannot be used without another longer-acting drug.

Paraldehyde is still sometimes used before institution of barbiturate coma. The parenteral solution is not now available in the United States, but this drug may be given rectally as 0.10- to 0.50-ml/kg boluses of a 4% solution diluted 2 to 1 in mineral oil or normal saline. Onset of action is approximately 20 minutes, and duration is 6 hours. Because it is eliminated by the lungs, paraldehyde may be valuable in renal or hepatic failure.

A possible alternative to barbiturate anesthesia is benzodiazepine infusion. Lorazepam and diazepam infusions have not been widely studied, but midazolam appears promising. Midazolam may be started immediately after failure of lorazepam or diazepam bolus and high-dose phenytoin infusion, or after failure of phenobarbital. It is given as a loading dose of 0.15–0.20 mg/kg followed by infusion of 0.05–0.30 mg/kg per hour. The EEG should be monitored and infusion stopped at least temporarily after 12 hours to check for seizure recurrence. Both hypotension and respiratory depression seem to be less problematic than with alternative regimens for refractory status.

Thiopental has also been suggested as an alternative to pentobarbital, but may have more cardiovascular side effects and less predictable pharmacokinetics. Use of inhalation anesthetics (e.g., halothane, isoflurane) instead of or after failure of barbiturate coma is controversial, but is an alternative if anesthesiology assistance is available. Propofol is a promising intravenous anesthetic that has also been used.

## Other Types of Status Epilepticus

Myoclonic SE is another form of convulsive SE which may occur in several different settings. First, repeated myoclonic jerks with preserved or clouded consciousness may occur in patients, usually in children or adolescents, with idiopathic or symptomatic generalized epilepsy. This form of SE is relatively rare and usually responds to benzodiazepines and valproate. A more common and problematic form of myoclonic SE occurs in comatose patients and consists of repeated and often massive myoclonic jerks. EEG shows diffuse periodic or semiperiodic discharges, usually on an attenuated background approaching burst-suppression. This is usually associated with severe metabolic insults, particularly global hypoxia-ischemia, but may occur in the setting of hepatic or renal failure or other disorders such as spongiform encephalopathies or neurolipidoses. The myoclonus may be stimulus sensitive or spontaneous. The utility of treatment has been questioned, especially in the setting of anoxic coma; clinical and EEG characteristics are often resistant to all treatment, and the outcome is almost uniformly poor.

In generalized nonconvulsive SE, also termed *absence SE* or *spike-wave stupor*, there is nearly continuously diminished responsiveness with bilaterally synchronous spike-wave discharges on the EEG. Although the sensorium is clouded, the degree of impairment may be quite subtle. In children, absence SE may occur in either symptomatic or (less commonly) idiopathic generalized epilepsy. It may also present as an acute confusional state in adults, often without apparent cause, but diffuse insults such as metrizamide myelography, electroconvulsive therapy, or benzodiazepine withdrawal may be associated. In some circumstances, the EEG findings may be difficult to distinguish from triphasic waves, and the distinction between this form of SE and a metabolic encephalopathy, particularly in those with identifiable metabolic impairments, may be problematic. Benzodiazepine infusion, such as a 1- to 2-mg injection of lorazepam, may be diagnostic if both the patient and the EEG improve.

Especially in adults, symmetry and rhythmicity on the EEG are variable, and the distinction from complex partial SE cannot always be made. An attempt to make this distinction is important because the latter presents a higher risk of neurologic complications and therefore demands more aggressive treatment. Absence SE is usually terminated readily by intravenous benzodiazepines, with maintenance therapy provided by either valproate or ethosuximide or both. Characteristically, response to treatment is rapid, with minimal postictal confusion. In cases difficult to distinguish from complex partial SE, including most adults, phenytoin or carbamazepine may be used.

Complex partial SE is an important syndrome, more common than suggested by the older literature, and likely underdiagnosed, especially in medical and neurosurgical intensive care units. At highest risk are those with a pre-existing history of partial epilepsy, but it may be the initial presentation of epilepsy or of an acute neurologic insult. Clinically, there is prolonged clouding of consciousness, usually with cycling over minutes corresponding to ictal and postictal phases of discrete complex partial seizures. Duration may be hours to days or longer. The epileptogenic region is usually frontal or temporal, but may be occipital or parietal. The EEG shows rhythmic activity beginning focally, followed by variable but usually bilateral spread and then by postictal slowing.

Because of reports of prolonged memory disorders and other sequelae after complex partial SE, and animal studies demonstrating hippocampal neuronal loss after partial seizures, many authorities recommend aggressive treatment. Intravenous benzodiazepines, phenytoin, and  phenobarbital may be given as recommended for GCSE, though sedative medications are usually not pushed fast and far enough to require assisted ventilation. An aggressive approach is reasonable in cases characterized by more severe alteration in consciousness before treatment and in those with a pattern of increasing frequency or severity of seizures despite initial treatment.

Simple partial SE with motor manifestations may occur either with or without a jacksonian march, reflects the cortical motor homunculus in distribution, and generally is associated with structural lesions in the central region. Eventually, semirhythmic myoclonus may develop between discrete seizures; this is called *epilepsia partialis continua*. Simple partial somatomotor SE may be very difficult to treat. Benzodiazepines are sometimes effective, and one of the first-line antiepileptic drugs should be given to prevent generalization. Treatment of the underlying lesion, often neurosurgically, may be required to alleviate this condition.

Other forms of simple partial SE present primarily a diagnostic dilemma and are revealed by EEG when no other explanation is available for aphasia or for affective or sensory disturbances. The clinical and EEG findings may be either intermittent or variably continuous, depending on duration and degree of postictal impairment after each discrete seizure. Oculoclonic and adversive status are more closely related to somatomotor SE, but involve either parieto-occipital or frontal regions important to eye movement rather than rolandic areas. If consciousness is not preserved with these movements, subtle GTC-SE, which would require much more vigorous treatment, should be suspected and treated, with EEG guidance provided as early as possible.

## SEIZURES OCCURRING IN SPECIAL SETTINGS

### Cardiac

Seizures in patients with cardiac disease are presumed to result from cerebrovascular lesions until proven otherwise. These are usually ischemic in origin, although patients treated with anticoagulants or thrombolytic agents are at risk for hemorrhage. The causative lesions usually involve cortex, often in the periolandic region, and seizures often have contralateral motor manifestations, although secondary generalization is common. Partial or secondarily generalized SE may occur rarely and should be treated as in other settings, although hypotension may be more problematic in this group. Overall, seizures occur within the first 2 weeks of ischemic insult in 4–14% of patients, and later seizures, usually indicative of chronic epilepsy, in 3–10% of patients (including perhaps one-third of those with early seizures). Risk of seizures and epilepsy in hemorrhagic stroke depends largely on size and cortical involvement and may affect 20% or more of those with large cortical lesions. The presence of epileptiform activity on the EEG, particularly periodic lateralized epileptiform discharges, may indicate a higher risk of seizures.

Cardiac medicines, particularly antiarrhythmics at high doses and levels, can precipitate seizures. These include lidocaine, mexiletine, and tocainide. Much less commonly, high doses of beta blockers, digoxin, and disopyramide may cause seizures.

Cardiac patients who have experienced global hypoxia-ischemia present a special problem, because the contribution to coma of epileptic activity, as manifested in subtle or massive clinical myoclonus and rhythmic or periodic discharges on the EEG, is difficult to evaluate. Phenytoin treatment is often given, although it is rarely effective in this setting even at high doses and levels. More aggressive treatment with sedating agents such as barbiturates can complicate assessment because of superimposed central nervous system depression, although it can be justified for a period of days, especially if the underlying insult is not believed to be sufficient to produce the observed level of coma. Benzodiazepines can treat myoclonus symptomatically, although an effect on prognosis has not been demonstrated.

Hypertensive encephalopathy, and the related condition of toxemia of pregnancy, is often associated with seizures. Simple partial seizures consisting of unformed or formed visual hallucinations or distortions may reflect the predilection of these conditions for the occipital lobes, although secondarily generalized seizures are probably more common. Control of blood pressure is critical to treatment, but phenytoin and other antiepileptic drugs are also of value, particularly in preventing secondary generalization.

### Obstetric

Some studies have suggested that parenteral magnesium is superior to phenytoin for the treatment and prevention of eclamptic seizures, perhaps through a direct effect on blood pressure or other vascular pathophysiology. Magnesium can also have anticonvulsant and antiexcitotoxic effects; its ability to cross the blood-brain barrier, minimal under normal circumstances, may be increased in this pathologic condition. The combination of magnesium and phenytoin has not been systematically studied but may be superior to either used alone.

In the obstetric patient with a first seizure apart from toxemia, the consultant's first responsibility is to determine the cause. The long list of medical conditions and drugs that could be responsible (see Tables 5.1 and 5.2) should be considered. Also, women with a genetic predisposition toward seizures could be "unmasked" by the sleep deprivation and nutritional and other stresses related to pregnancy. The history at times reveals an undiagnosed pre-existing condition, such as juvenile myoclonic epilepsy, in a woman who has dismissed years of morning myoclonus as "shakiness" or "nerves." An EEG is a simple and noninvasive means of evaluating the possibility of underlying idiopathic epilepsy and of obtaining information about focal cortical dysfunction. If the latter is suggested by seizure history, neurologic examination, or EEG, then neuroimaging is mandatory, because such lesions as brain tumors or arteriovenous malformations can influence the course of obstetric management. Such lesions should be ruled out, even if the examination and EEG are negative, in essentially all cases of first seizure without a definite, nonstructural cause. Although treatment of a first convulsive seizure in general remains controversial, as outlined, the risks to the fetus posed by convulsions usually prompt antiepileptic drug treatment in the pregnant woman. Although all antiepileptic drugs are known or presumed to be teratogenic, the issue of major malformations is moot beyond the late first trimester, by which time major organ formation is complete. Because minor anomalies and perhaps even minor effects on intellectual development may still occur, however, it is important to discuss risks and benefits with the patient and obstetrician. Adequate intake of folic acid and other nutrients must be assured. Seizures during the early postpartum period may be a result of eclampsia, or less common conditions such as amniotic fluid embolus or cerebral venous thrombosis. Again, treatment is directed toward the underlying condition, with antiepileptic drugs used at least until the condition resolves. More prolonged treatment is indicated if another seizure occurs after that time. If not, the EEG may be used as a surrogate indicator of risk, although its utility in this and similar situations has not been established.

## Surgical

Depending on the nature of surgery, postoperative patients may be at increased risk of seizures, especially those undergoing neurosurgical or cardiac procedures. Brain tumors and other structural lesions present with seizures approximately one-third of the time; low-grade gliomas or other slow-growing tumors, when located supratentorially, especially near the rolandic fissure, are most likely to present in this way. Nearly two-thirds of patients with brain tumors eventually have seizures, which may be simple or complex partial, or secondarily generalized with or without obvious focal onset. Metastatic tumors are often located at the junction of gray and white matter, and therefore commonly cause seizures. Hemorrhagic tumors, as are common in melanoma, are especially epileptogenic. The postoperative period carries a high risk of seizures, perhaps because of anesthesia withdrawal and often low levels of antiepileptic drugs, even when the patient was treated with them preoperatively or intraoperatively. The metabolism of phenytoin, in particular, is accelerated after surgery, and parenteral or oral boluses are routinely required to maintain adequate levels. Carbamazepine metabolism may actually slow postoperatively, but this is often counterbalanced early by poor oral intake or absorption of the medicine. Clinical toxicity rarely results when the level increases on postoperative day 2 or 3, perhaps because of lower levels of the unmeasured epoxide metabolite. In patients who cannot take or absorb oral medications, or who cannot tolerate parenteral phenytoin or phenobarbital, lorazepam offers a short-term alternative. Of note is that the 5–10% risk of rash with phenytoin may be doubled in patients undergoing radiotherapy for brain tumors, perhaps because of depletion of suppressor T cells or steroid withdrawal.

Seizures occur within 2 weeks of carotid endarterectomy in approximately 1% of patients. In many cases, this is part of the *hyperperfusion syndrome*, when systemic hypertension coexists with impaired cerebral autoregulation in the operated vascular bed; headaches are usually also present, and localized cerebral edema and sometimes hemorrhage are observed on neuroimaging studies. Blood pressure control and short-term use of antiepileptic drugs are the mainstays of treating this lateralized analogue of hypertensive encephalopathy. In the other main cause of postendarterectomy seizures, intraoperative embolic stroke, a higher likelihood of later development of epilepsy and concomitant need for long-term antiepileptic drug therapy exist.

Cardiac surgery also poses risks of embolic stroke as well as global hypoxia-ischemia. Seizures in these settings should be treated as in medical causes of these conditions. Cardiac and other transplant surgeries raise the additional possibility of seizures caused by immunosuppressant, neurotoxic drugs such as cyclosporine and FK-506, perhaps through a mechanism analogous to hypertensive encephalopathy. More chronically, such patients are also at risk of seizures resulting from bacterial (*Listeria*) or fungal opportunistic infections, viral meningoencephalitis, or brain abscess.

## Acquired Immunodeficiency Syndrome

Patients with the acquired immunodeficiency syndrome (AIDS) are also subject to these and other infectious processes. Depending on degree and location of cortical involvement, seizures may be the presenting feature or a later complication of toxoplasmosis, central nervous system lymphoma, or, to a lesser degree, progressive multifocal leukoencephalopathy. Some patients with AIDS-dementia complex develop seizures without apparent superimposed focal lesions, and SE may even be seen in this setting. Prescribed and illicit drugs (see Table 5.2) may also contribute to seizures, as can metabolic abnormalities such as uremia or hypoglycemia, the latter being a known complication of pentamidine given for *Pneumocystis* pneumonia. Reports of rare seizures with antiretroviral drugs such as zidovudine, foscarnet, or ganciclovir are difficult to evaluate given the other seizure risk factors present in this population.

## Oncologic

Patients with cancer other than primary and metastatic brain tumors may also experience seizures. Chemotherapeutic and other drugs should be assessed, particularly if other signs of central nervous system toxicity are present. Chlorambucil, busulfan, and possibly cisplatin have been associated with seizures. Carcinomatous meningitis may occur without parenchymal brain lesions and be difficult to diagnose. Seizures are uncommon manifestations of paraneoplastic syndromes, except for limbic encephalitis often associated with small-cell lung cancer and anti-Hu antibodies.

## Metabolic

Of patients with chronic metabolic disease, those with uremia are at greatest risk of seizures. These can include partial and primarily or secondarily generalized seizures, or myoclonic seizures as well as nonepileptic myoclonus. The frequency of electrolyte imbalance sufficient to cause seizures has declined with improvement in dialysis techniques. Abnormalities of magnesium, sodium, or calcium still occur, however, as do central nervous system lesions related to coagulopathy or immunosuppression. In patients requiring chronic or acute treatment with antiepileptic drugs, renal failure and dialysis pose several unique problems. First, with regard to phenytoin, the free fraction is often significantly higher than the normal value of 10%. This results not just from low albumin levels, but also from "idiopathic osmoles" displacing phenytoin from the albumin-binding sites that are present. Therefore, target levels (except in GCSE) should be lower than the usual 10–20 mg/dl, and loading and maintenance doses should reflect the lower levels. On the other hand, the higher free fraction means that, in the absence of coexisting hepatic impairment, the metabolic rate of phenytoin is actually accelerated, and tid or more frequent administration may be necessary. With phenobarbital, protein binding is of minor importance; the main problem is drug removal with dialysis. Levels obtained before and after dialysis can help the clinician estimate the amount of phenobarbital to administer after each treatment.

Seizures are much less common in the setting of hepatic disease, but may result from acute metabolic abnormalities such as hypoglycemia or coagulopathies leading to intracranial hemorrhage. With low albumin levels, the free fraction of strongly protein-bound drugs such as phenytoin may be elevated as in renal failure. In the absence of end-stage liver disease, metabolism of many drugs is slowed less than might be expected, and doses may not require significant reduction. The risk of administering drugs that can possibly (though rarely) cause idiosyncratic liver failure, such as valproate and, to a lesser extent, phenytoin or carbamazepine, has not been established, but valproate is usually avoided in this setting. Phenobarbital is considered to be safer, but data are limited. As mentioned earlier, gabapentin may present a useful alternative, especially in patients without coexisting renal impairment.

Among other metabolic impairments, hyponatremia is probably the most important. Seizures are not well documented until levels fall below 125 mEq/dl unless seizure threshold is already low for other reasons. Antiepileptic drug treatment is generally not indicated as long as the underlying abnormality can be corrected; too-rapid correction, however, should be avoided because of the risk of central pontine myelinolysis, and lorazepam or a more standard antiepileptic drug may be used for a few days. Some combination of low magnesium, calcium, and phosphate may coexist and lead to seizures in a variety of gastrointestinal and other medical illnesses; treatment again depends on correcting the electrolyte imbalance as well as the underlying condition.

Hypoglycemia, usually drug induced (rarely from hepatic disease or insulinoma), commonly causes generalized convulsions, usually preceded by a hyperautonomic prodrome of anxiety, tremor, sweating, and perhaps depressed consciousness. Nonketotic hyperglycemia frequently involves and may present with seizures. These are often focal, even in the absence of definable structural lesions, and epilepsia partialis continua may result. Hydration is the cornerstone of treatment; phenytoin may even worsen the situation by interfering with insulin secretion, and thus phenobarbital, carbamazepine, and valproate are alternatives. Diabetic ketoacidosis much less rarely involves seizures, perhaps because of the protective effects of acidosis or of ketone bodies themselves (as suggested by the term *ketogenic diet*, which may be effective in treating selected cases of refractory epilepsy). Thyroid disease, especially myxedema coma (now rare) can also result in seizures, the treatment of which depends on treating the underlying condition.

## Rheumatologic

Collagen vascular diseases, such as systemic lupus erythematosus, and less often, rheumatoid arthritis or Sjögren's syndrome, may cause seizures. These usually occur in the setting of systemic, especially renal, exacerbations, as well as other neurologic insults. Microvascular infarcts may be present and difficult to document, but larger ischemic or hemorrhagic strokes as well as central nervous system infections should be ruled out. Treatment with immunosuppressants as well as standard antiepileptic drugs is usually indicated; even drugs that can rarely cause a lupus-like syndrome, such as phenytoin and carbamazepine, may generally be used safely. Similar approaches apply to the systemic vasculitides, such as polyarteritis nodosa, Wegener's granulomatosis, and Churg-Strauss syndrome.

## Psychiatric

Consultations for seizures in a psychiatric unit present unique challenges. First, this population is at higher risk for nonepileptic seizures, and diagnosis may at times require specialized monitoring. This possibility should be considered before initiating treatment for apparent seizures. Second, treatment of psychiatric illness may require the use of drugs known to lower the seizure threshold. Clozapine is probably the most important of these; seizures may occur early at low doses or later at high doses. Focal and generalized epileptiform activity can be seen on the EEG. Data on its newer analogue, olanzapine, are thus far limited. Lower but still elevated risks have been reported for neuroleptics (lowest for molindone) and antidepressants (highest for bupropion). For patients with seizures requiring use of these drugs, treatment with a standard antiepileptic drug (perhaps one with psychotropic effects such as valproate, carbamazepine, or perhaps one of the newer agents) is indicated. Prophylactic use of antiepileptic drugs is generally not indicated, although patients on high doses with epileptiform activity on EEG may be exceptions.

Electroconvulsive therapy (ECT) produces its effect by means of an electrographic seizure; nevertheless, spontaneous seizures after ECT are rare. Prolonged confusion after ECT, however, should prompt an EEG, because nonconvulsive SE has rarely been reported in this setting.

## Toxic

Drug-induced seizures (see Table 5.2) have been mentioned in many of the above situations. Both prescribed and illicit stimulants, such as theophylline, phenylpropanolamine, cocaine, and phencyclidine, are important causes of partial and generalized seizures and, sometimes, SE in selected individuals. Isoniazid is a nonstimulant with similar effects, perhaps because of antagonism of vitamin $B_6$, necessary for gamma-aminobutyric acid (GABA) synthesis; vitamin $B_6$ can prevent or treat seizures in this setting, although usually antiepileptic drugs such as phenytoin (whose metabolism is slowed by isoniazid) are also required. Except for insulin, the other such drugs lack a specific antidote and usually require administration of standard antiepileptic drugs. Physostigmine may reverse many central nervous system effects of tricyclic antidepressants and other anticholinergic drugs, but potential cardiovascular toxicity as well as the possibility of producing seizures generally contraindicate this therapy. Methods to promote elimination of the offending agent are important and may include alkalinization for tricyclics, acidification for phencyclidine, or dialysis for theophylline.

Withdrawal of sedative medications is another important cause of acute symptomatic seizures. Many of these, including alcohol, barbiturates, and benzodiazepines, work via the GABA system, and administration of benzodiazepines, which are then gradually reduced in a controlled manner, is the usual treatment. Seizures may be preventable if benzodiazepines are given during the early withdrawal phase of insomnia, tremor, anxiety, anorexia, and tachycardia. The effectiveness of other drugs such as phenytoin is questionable in these settings, although it should be used if SE develops. For alcohol withdrawal seizures, usually developing within 6–48 hours of the last drink, provision of thiamine, glucose, magnesium, and fluids is important. Particularly if the seizures are focal, it is also important to consider the possibility of an underlying infectious, traumatic, or other condition requiring specific treatment. Finally, the benzodiazepine antagonist flumazenil can precipitate seizures in patients on chronic benzodiazepine therapy.

## NEUROLOGIC CONSULTATION FOR THE HOSPITALIZED PATIENT WITH EPILEPSY

Patients with epilepsy develop most medical and surgical conditions at the same frequency as others of similar age and background. One goal of the consultant is to ensure that no increase in frequency or severity of seizures occurs during hospitalization. Clarifying the patient's seizure type(s) and frequency, and if possible, the underlying epilepsy syndrome is crucial. The possibility

*Table 5.5*   Medications that lower levels of valproate and possibly lamotrigine, phenytoin, and carbamazepine (via enzyme induction or interference with absorption)

Antacids (stagger doses by 1–2 hrs)
Carbamazepine
Phenobarbital
Phenytoin
Rifampin
Sucralfate
Theophylline

of performing or repeating such studies as EEG or MRI should be considered, although it is rarely necessary. Occasionally, the consultant may question the diagnosis of epilepsy; therapeutic changes are usually not indicated, but referral to a specialized epilepsy center after discharge may be suggested. A similar approach may be appropriate for a patient with intractable epilepsy who could benefit from experimental drug or surgical treatment. More commonly, the consultant's role is to assist the primary physician in maintaining adequate drug treatment in the setting of changes in absorption, metabolism, or comedication.

For patients who cannot adequately take their usual medications orally, parenteral administration is possible with phenytoin, phenobarbital, and now valproate; equivalent doses may be used, although the schedule may need to be changed (in the absence of a slow-release phenytoin preparation, e.g., once-daily administration is no longer appropriate). Phenobarbital or lorazepam may also be substituted for other barbiturates or benzodiazepines. Lorazepam offers an attractive short-term alternative in many situations. Because the anticonvulsant effect lasts for hours, single 1-mg doses (either intravenous or sublingual) can be substituted on a twice-daily or three-times-daily basis for 1–2 days until oral intake is re-established. If oral intake will be inadequate longer than that, substitution of one of the parenterally administered drugs is probably indicated. Alternatively, a commercially prepared diazepam gel formulation is now available. It is marketed as treatment for acute repetitive seizures and offers a compromise between the fast onset and short duration of intravenous diazepam and the slow onset and intermediate duration of oral administration. Another alternative is a carbamazepine suppository specially prepared by a pharmacist.

Effects of comedications on antiepileptic drugs usually result from interactions with protein-binding sites or with hepatic metabolic enzyme systems, as described. Introduction of a new nonantiepileptic drug into a patient's treatment should prompt changes in dose as indicated by expected interactions (Tables 5.5 and 5.6) or changes in levels; the consultant should not wait for an increase in seizure frequency or severity, or for clinical toxicity, to occur.

Consultative care of the pregnant patient with epilepsy is generally provided in the outpatient setting. Seizure exacerbations in the puerperium are handled as in the postoperative patient, by use of intravenous formulations of established antiepileptic drugs, intravenous or sublingual lorazepam, or rectal diazepam. Although levels of most antiepileptic drugs fall after delivery and boluses may be required, the consultant should recognize that the metabolic changes that usu-

*Table 5.6*   Medications that increase levels of carbamazepine, phenobarbital, phenytoin, and lamotrigine (via enzyme inhibition)

Chloramphenicol
Cimetidine (more than other $H_2$ blockers)
Diltiazem
Erythromycin (especially carbamazepine)
Fluoxetine
Isoniazid
Metronidazole
Propoxyphene
Valproate
Verapamil
Warfarin (variable)

ally dictate increased doses during pregnancy reverse in days to weeks. Postpartum doses must be adjusted accordingly, with frequent measurement of levels (perhaps weekly for 2 weeks and then every 2 weeks for 2 months).

## SUGGESTED READING

Annegers JF, Hauser WA, Lee SR, Rocca HA. Incidence of acute symptomatic seizures in Rochester, Minnesota, 1935–1984. Epilepsia 1995;36:327–333.

Boggs JB. Seizures in medically complex patients. Epilepsia 1996;38(suppl 4):S55–S59.

Bromfield EB. Epilepsy and the Elderly. In D Schomer, S Schachter (eds), The Comprehensive Evaluation and Treatment of Epilepsy. New York: Academic Press, 1997;233–254.

DeLorenzo RJ, Towne AR, Pellock JM, Ko D. Status epilepticus in children, adults, and the elderly. Epilepsia 1992;33(suppl 4):S15–S25.

Fountain NB, Lothman EW. Pathophysiology of status epilepticus. J Clin Neurophysiol 1995;12:326–342.

Garcia PA, Alldredge BK. Drug-induced seizures. Neurol Clin 1994;12:85–99.

Lowenstein DH, Alldredge BK. Status epilepticus. N Engl J Med 1998;338:970–976.

Messing RO, Simon RP. Seizures as a manifestation of systemic disease. Neurol Clin 1986;4:563–584.

Wen PY. Clinical Presentation and Diagnosis of Brain Tumors. In MA Samuels, S Feske (eds), Office Practice of Neurology. New York: Churchill Livingstone, 1996;813–817.

Working Group on Status Epilepticus. Treatment of convulsive status epilepticus. JAMA 1993;270:854–859.

# II
# SPECIAL ISSUES

# 6
# Drugs and Toxins
## John C.M. Brust

Neurologic symptoms and signs are associated with the use of recreationally abused drugs; prescription and over-the-counter pharmaceuticals; household, industrial, and agricultural products; and animal and plant toxins. A neurologist asked to assess a patient with neurologic symptoms or signs may or may not be aware of the toxic origin of the findings. If the responsible agent is known, the principal task is to anticipate the course of illness and manage it accordingly, keeping in mind the possibility of additional toxins or confounding illnesses (including, in the case of drug dependence, simultaneous intoxication with one agent and withdrawal from another). If the responsible agent is unknown or if neurotoxicity has not been considered, a thorough history and examination are often more revealing than random toxicologic screening.

## DRUG DEPENDENCE

### Types of Drugs: Intoxication and Withdrawal

Table 6.1 lists the major categories of substance abuse encountered in industrialized countries. Global communication and travel ensure that this list will expand to include exotic new drugs. For example, khat, a shrub containing an amphetamine-like psychostimulant that is widely used recreationally in eastern Africa and Arabia, has begun to appear in Europe and the United States.

Recreationally abused agents differ widely in their ability to produce psychic dependence (i.e., addiction), their intended effects, and their syndromes of overdose and withdrawal. Opioid agonist overdose (most often from parenteral heroin; Table 6.2) produces the triad of coma, respiratory depression, and miosis, and treatment includes an opioid antagonist such as naloxone or nalmefene plus ventilatory support. Opioid agonist withdrawal produces intense craving and a flu-like syndrome, which does not (at least in adults) include seizures or delir-

*Table 6.1*    Major categories of substance abuse

Opioids
Psychostimulants
Sedatives/hypnotics
Marijuana
Hallucinogens
Inhalants
Phencyclidine
Anticholinergics
Ethanol
Tobacco

*Table 6.2*    Major opioids

Agonist
    Powdered opium
    Tincture of opium
    Camphorated tincture of opium (paregoric)
    Morphine
    Heroin
    Methadone
    Fentanyl
    Hydromorphone
    Oxymorphone
    Codeine
    Oxycodone
    Meperidine
    Levorphanol
    Propoxyphene
Antagonist
    Naloxone
    Nalmefene
    Naltrexone
Mixed agonist-antagonist or partial agonist
    Pentazocine
    Butorphanol
    Nalbuphine
    Buprenorphine

ium and is easily treated with a substitute agonist such as methadone. (An exception is neonatal opioid withdrawal, which if untreated carries a high mortality.)

As with ethanol, sedative/hypnotic drugs (Table 6.3) produce coma and respiratory depression, and treatment depends on sustained respiratory support. Benzodiazepines are much less likely than barbiturates or other sedatives to produce respiratory depression, and whereas no specific antidote exists for barbitu-

*Table 6.3*    Major sedatives/hypnotics

Barbiturates
    Amobarbital
    Butalbital
    Pentobarbital
    Phenobarbital
    Secobarbital
Benzodiazepines
    Alprazolam
    Chlordiazepoxide
    Diazepam
    Lorazepam
    Oxazepam
    Flurazepam
    Triazolam
Nonbarbituates/nonbenzodiazepines
    Chloral hydrate
    Ethchlorvynol
    Glutethimide
    Meprobamate
    Methaqualone
    Methyprylon
    Paraldehyde

*Table 6.4*    Major psychostimulants

Dextroamphetamine
Methamphetamine
Methylphenidate
Phenmetrazine
Diethylpropion
Fenfluramine
Phenylpropanolamine
Ephedrine
Pseudoephedrine
Cocaine

rate or other sedative poisoning, the benzodiazepine antagonist flumazenil reverses symptoms of benzodiazepine overdose. (The short biological action of flumazenil, however, makes it more useful for diagnosis than for treatment.) Withdrawal from barbiturates and other sedatives can cause hallucinations, seizures, and life-threatening delirium tremens.

Psychostimulant overdose (Table 6.4)—usually associated with parenteral use or smoking of methamphetamine (popularly known as *ice*) or alkaloidal cocaine (known as *crack*)—causes varying combinations of headache, chest pain, para-

*Table 6.5*   Major categories and examples of hallucinogenic drugs

Ergot-derived: D-lysergic acid diethylamide (LSD)
Indolalkylamines: psilocin, psilocybin (from mushrooms)
Phenylalkylamines: mescaline (from peyote cactus), methylenedioxyamphetamine,
  methylenedioxymethamphetamine ("ecstasy")

*Table 6.6*   Household products subject to inhalant abuse

Aerosols (refrigerants, frying pan cleaners, hair sprays, shampoos, deodorants, antiseptics)
Dry-cleaning fluids, spot removers
Furniture polish
Glues, cements, rubber patching
Lighter fluid
Fire extinguishing agents
Bottled fuel gas
Typewriter correction fluid
Marker pens
Paints, enamels, lacquers, paint and lacquer thinners
Petroleum
Anesthetics, whipped cream canisters (nitrous oxide)
Room deodorizers (amyl, butyl, and isobutyl nitrite)

noia, excitement, psychosis, delirium, hallucinations, dyskinesias, seizures, severe hyperthermia, hypertensive crisis, cardiac arrhythmia, myoglobinuria, metabolic acidosis, coma, and death. Treatment includes sedatives, oxygen, bicarbonate, cooling, antihypertensives, anticonvulsants, and cardiorespiratory monitoring. Withdrawal from psychostimulants produces fatigue, depression, and craving but few measurable signs.

High doses of marijuana cause hallucinations and excitement or panic, but fatal overdose has not been documented and treatment is seldom necessary. Withdrawal from marijuana produces nervousness, headache, and craving, but objective signs are not evident.

High doses of hallucinogenic agents (Table 6.5) can produce paranoia or panic as well as tremor, tachycardia, hypertension, and fever, and death may result from accidents or suicide. Withdrawal symptoms do not occur. The phenylalkylamine drugs methylenedioxyamphetamine and methylenedioxymethamphetamine have amphetamine-like as well as D-lysergic acid diethylamide (LSD)-like properties.

Recreationally inhaled household products contain a variety of compounds, including halogenated hydrocarbons, toluene, n-hexane, naphthanes, butane, nitrites, and nitrous oxide (Table 6.6). They can produce death as a result of suffocation, aspiration of vomitus, accidents, or cardiac arrhythmia, but the ethanol-like intoxication produced is usually short-lived and does not require acute treatment. Withdrawal signs are not observed, but psychic dependence is common.

Phencyclidine (known as *angel dust* or *PCP*) overdose produces the full clinical spectrum of schizophrenia, including hallucinatory paranoid psychosis and catatonia; there are also abnormal movements, myoclonus, seizures, myoglobinuria, stupor, and cardiorespiratory collapse. Treatment includes forced diuresis, cardiorespiratory monitoring, and, as needed, antihypertensives, anticonvulsants, sedatives, or neuroleptics. Abstinence produces craving, but there is little evidence of physical dependence.

Anticholinergic poisoning, usually encountered in children and adolescents who recreationally ingest the jimson weed *Datura stramonium*, causes hallucinations, seizures, delirium, or coma with decreased sweating, fever, tachycardia, large unreactive pupils, and urinary retention. Treatment includes physostigmine, cooling, and cardiorespiratory monitoring. Withdrawal symptoms are unusual but include tremor and craving.

## Medical and Neurologic Complications

Trauma

Intoxication with any of the described agents can cause trauma involving the central or peripheral nervous system, and the simultaneous presence of drug overdose and traumatic injury complicates diagnosis and management. Ethanol or drug intoxication should be considered in the case of anyone involved in motor vehicle accidents (whether driver or pedestrian), assault or attempted homicide (whether assailant or victim), and suicide. Sedatives should be especially suspected in the case of elderly patients with falls or fractures. Violence associated with illicit drugs is much more often related to the socioeconomics of their illegality than to their psychopharmacologic effects, but paranoia induced by agents such as cocaine and phencyclidine can make users a danger to others, and inhalant and hallucinogen users may commit self-mutilation and suicide.

Infection

Alcoholics and drug abusers are often immunosuppressed, even in the absence of human immunodeficiency virus (HIV) exposure, and parenteral drug abusers are at particular risk for an array of infections involving the nervous system (Table 6.7). Acute meningitis is sometimes overlooked in delirious or stuporous patients whose symptoms are attributed to intoxication or withdrawal.

Nonhomosexual drug abusers comprise about 25% of acquired immunodeficiency syndrome (AIDS) cases reported to the U.S. Centers for Disease Control and Prevention, and an additional 7% are homosexual or bisexual drug users. The majority of female patients with AIDS in the United States either are drug abusers or have contracted the infection through sexual contact with a drug abuser. Even in the absence of parenteral drug use, female crack-cocaine smokers are at risk for HIV infection as a result of sexual promiscuity and coexisting sexually transmitted diseases. In New York City, roughly two-thirds of subjects receiving methadone maintenance therapy are HIV-seropositive. Drug abusers are subject

*Table 6.7*   Infectious complications of parenteral drug abuse

Hepatitis
Skin abscesses, cellulitis, pyomyositis, fasciitis
Pneumonia, sepsis, meningitis
Infected venous pseudoaneurysm
Endophthalmitis, chorioretinitis, episcleritis
Pyogenic arthritis, osteomyelitis (especially vertebral)
Endocarditis, brain abscess, mycotic aneurysm
Malaria
Tetanus
Botulism
Human immunodeficiency virus and acquired immunodeficiency syndrome
Human T cell lymphotropic virus type 1 myelitis

to the same spectrum of AIDS-related illnesses that afflict other risk groups, especially syphilis and tuberculosis, the latter frequently involving drug-resistant strains. Drug abuse should be suspected in any AIDS patient, and HIV infection should be suspected in any drug abuser.

In addition to various HIV-related myelopathic syndromes, parenteral drug abusers may develop spastic paraparesis secondary to infection with human T cell lymphotropic virus type 1 (HTLV-1).

## Seizures

As with alcoholics, seizures in drug abusers require investigation for acute or remote head injury, central nervous system infection, and stroke. In both epileptics and nonepileptics, illicit drugs cause seizures either as a feature of intoxication or during withdrawal.

Opioid agonists lower seizure threshold, but seizures as a feature of heroin overdose are unusual and require a search for alternative causes. Seizures and myoclonus are more readily produced by meperidine, propoxyphene, and fentanyl, and they are commonly encountered in parenteral abusers of pentazocine combined with the antihistamine tripelennamine (known as *T's and blues*). As noted, seizures are not a feature of opioid withdrawal except possibly in newborns.

Amphetamine-like psychostimulants produce seizures usually in association with other signs of overdose, and in such a setting they carry a poor prognosis. By contrast, perhaps related to its local anesthetic properties, cocaine is more likely to precipitate seizures in the absence of other symptoms. Status epilepticus as a feature of cocaine intoxication can be very difficult to control. The threat of seizures is well recognized in users of the over-the-counter diet preparation and decongestant phenylpropanolamine.

Seizures occur during withdrawal from large doses of barbiturates or benzodiazepines. As with ethanol, symptoms can progress to delirium tremens.

Seizures may complicate acute intoxication with glutethimide, perhaps related to its anticholinergic properties.

Marijuana has reportedly either precipitated seizures or improved seizure control in epileptics. Seizures in marijuana users require a full diagnostic workup. Although phencyclidine is a glutamate-receptor blocker, myoclonus and seizures are features of severe overdose. Seizures sometimes occur during intoxication from hallucinogens, inhalants, or anticholinergics.

## Stroke

Current epidemiologic evidence suggests that moderate doses of ethanol are protective against ischemic stroke but that heavy doses confer risk. For hemorrhagic stroke, any dose lowers the threshold. Similar epidemiologic evidence points to tobacco as a risk factor for both occlusive and hemorrhagic stroke. By contrast, the association of stroke with illicit drugs is largely anecdotal. Most convincingly causal is cocaine, especially crack. Of the more than 200 reported cases of stroke, about half were occlusive and half hemorrhagic, and of those patients with hemorrhagic stroke who received cerebral angiography, about half demonstrated intracranial saccular aneurysms or vascular malformations. A thorough diagnostic workup, including consideration of cerebral angiography, is therefore warranted in any cocaine user with a stroke.

Parenteral drug abusers develop strokes secondary to bacterial or fungal endocarditis, and whether occlusive or hemorrhagic, their occurrence mandates a search for septic (i.e., mycotic) cerebral aneurysms. Strokes in parenteral drug abusers are also attributed to injection of foreign material and to cerebral vasculitis. LSD, an ergot, may cause hemorrhagic stroke in association with severe delayed hypertension.

## Altered Mentation

As with ethanol, the practitioner must always consider the possible coexistence of a life-threatening condition such as head injury, meningitis, or metabolic derangement in a patient with altered mentation in association with intoxication or withdrawal from illicit drugs.

Whether recreational drugs directly produce long-term adverse effects on cognition is (as with ethanol) controversial. Claims for such effects include depression or intellectual loss in psychostimulant users, so-called antimotivational behavior in heavy marijuana users, social deterioration in barbiturate addicts, and persistent schizophrenia-like symptoms in phencyclidine users. Confounders include lack of psychometric testing before drug use and the frequent coexistence of alcoholism, polysubstance abuse, or other drug-related illness. Sniffers of toluene (present in glues, cements, paints, lacquers, and paint and lacquer thinners) do develop dementia and cerebral white matter changes, and gasoline sniffers develop lead encephalopathy. Chronic use of opioids, benzodiazepines, hallucinogens, or anticholinergics has not been associated with long-term cognitive or behavioral change. A substance abuser with unexplained neurobehavioral symptoms merits a comprehensive workup.

*Table 6.8*    Miscellaneous neurologic complications and the illicit drugs that cause them

Peripheral neuropathy: heroin, n-hexane (glue), nitrous oxide
Myopathy/rhabdomyolysis: heroin, cocaine, amphetamine, phencyclidine, toluene, gasoline
Myelopathy: heroin, nitrous oxide
Parkinsonism: methylphenyltetrahydropyridine, a by-product in the synthesis of a heroin
    substitute
Blindness: quinine (in heroin mixtures)
Dyskinesias, including dystonia and exacerbation of Tourette's syndrome: cocaine, other
    psychostimulants
Cerebellar ataxia: toluene (paint, lacquer, paint and lacquer thinners)
Impotence, sterility, menstrual irregularity: marijuana

## Fetal Effects

In contrast to ethanol and tobacco, each of which convincingly causes fetal damage, the effect of in utero exposure to illicit drugs on neurodevelopment is uncertain. Confounders include poor prenatal care, ethanol or tobacco use, and inadequate parenting. Considerable media attention has focused on a supposed epidemic of cognitively impaired so-called cocaine babies. Prospective studies suggest that such fears, though not groundless, are exaggerated.

As noted above, neonatal withdrawal from heroin or methadone can be life threatening, and such newborns are often small for gestational age and subject to respiratory distress and sudden infant death. Cognitive impairment later in life has been reported. Other investigators maintain that such abnormalities tend to be outgrown.

## Miscellaneous Effects

Table 6.8 lists a number of neurologic conditions associated with one or more illicit drugs. For detailed information on the neurologic complications of illicit drugs, see Brust, 1993.

## PRESCRIPTION AND OVER-THE-COUNTER PHARMACEUTICALS

Neurologists are often asked to assess patients whose symptoms are secondary to drugs they have been prescribed or have purchased over the counter. Such patients may be unable to provide an adequate history, or they may deliberately withhold crucial information; it may not have occurred to either the patient or the physician that the symptoms are in fact drug related. A neurologic consultation must always consider that the symptoms in question might signify neurotoxicity. A careful drug history is an appropriate starting point.

Because it is the symptoms and signs rather than the drug or drugs per se that the consultant is usually asked to assess, Tables 6.9–6.22 categorize by symptom rather than by drug. Assigning the cause of neurologic symptoms to particular

*Table 6.9*   Drugs associated with cognitive impairment, abnormal behavior, or hallucinations

Acyclovir
Adrenocorticosteroids, adrenocorticotropic
  hormone
Aldesleukin
Allopurinol
Alpha-adrenergic agonists
Alpha-adrenergic blockers
Aluminum-containing antacids
Amantadine
Amiloride
Aminocaproic acid
Amiodarone
Amphetamine-like psychostimulants
Amphotericin B
Androgens
Anesthetics: local amide type
Angiotensin-converting enzyme inhibitors
Antimuscarinic anticholinergics
Aprotinin
L-Asparaginase
Baclofen
Barbiturates
Benzodiazepines
Benzonatate
Benzquinamide
Beta-adrenergic blockers
Bismuth subsalicylate
Bromocriptine
Bumetanide
Bupropion
Buspirone
Butyrophenones
Caffeine
Calcium channel blockers
Calcium preparations
Carbamazepine
Carbonic anhydrase inhibitors
Carisoprodol
Carmustine
Chloral hydrate
Chlorambucil
Chloramphenicol
Chlormezanone
Chloroquine
Chlorprothixene
Clofibrate
Clozapine
Cocaine
Colchicine
Cyclobenzaprine
Cyclosporine
Cytarabine
Dantrolene
Dapsone

Diclofenac
Digitalis
Diphenidol
Disopyramide
Disulfiram
Doxazosin
Domperidone
Dronabinol
Ergotamine
Etodolac
Ethacrynic acid
Ethambutol
Ethchlorvynol
Ethosuximide
Felbamate
Fenoprofen
Flavoxate
Flecainide
Fluconazole
Flucytosine
Fludarabine
Flumazenil
Fluoride
5-Fluorouracil
Flurbiprofen
Furosemide
Gabapentin
Ganciclovir
Gemfibrozil
Glutethimide
Gold salts
Gonderelin
Granisetron
Griseofulvin
Guanabenz
Guanadrel
Guanethidine
Guanfacine
Histamine $H_1$-receptor antagonists
Histamine $H_2$-receptor antagonists
Histrelin
3-Hydroxy-3-methylglutaryl coenzyme A-
  reductase inhibitors
Hydralazine
Hydroxychloroquine
Hydroxyurea
Ibuprofen
Idarubicin
Ifosfamide
Indomethacin
Insulin
Interferon alfa-2a, alfa-2b
Interferon beta-1b
Iron preparations

*Table 6.9*   (continued)

| | |
|---|---|
| Itraconazole | Pentostatin |
| Ketoconazole | Pentoxifylline |
| Ketoprofen | Phenacemide |
| Ketorolac | Phenothiazines |
| Lamotrigine | Phensuximide |
| Lansoprazole | Phenylbutazone |
| Levamisole | Phenytoin |
| Levodopa, levodopa/carbidopa | Phosphate salts |
| Lidocaine | Piroxicam |
| Lithium | Prazosin |
| Lomustine | Primaquine |
| Macrolide antibiotics | Procaine amide |
| Mechlorethamine | Procarbazine |
| Meclofenamate | Propafenone |
| Mefloquine | Propofol |
| Melarsoprol | Quinacrine |
| Meprobamate | Quinidine |
| Mesalamine | Quinine |
| Methotrexate | Quinolone antibiotics |
| Methsuximide | Reserpine |
| Methyldopa | Rimantadine |
| Methysergide | Salicylates |
| Metoclopramide | Saquinavir |
| Metronidazole | Selegiline |
| Metyrosine | Serotonin uptake inhibitors |
| Mexiletine | Spironolactone |
| Miconazole | Sulfonamides |
| Mitotane | Sulfonylurea hypoglycemics |
| Monoamine oxidase inhibitors | Sulindac |
| Moricizine | Sumatriptan |
| Muromonab-CD3 | Tacrine |
| Nabilone | Tacrolimus |
| Nabumetone | Terazosin |
| Nafarelin | Theobromine |
| Naproxen | Theophylline |
| Nicotine | Thiabendazole |
| Nifurtimox | Thiazide diuretics |
| Nitrofurantoin | Thiothixene |
| Nitroprusside | Tocainide |
| Olsalazine | Tolmetin |
| Omeprazole | Tranexamic acid |
| Opioid agonists and mixed agonist/ antagonists | Trazodone |
| | Triamterene |
| Orphenadrine | Tricyclic and tetracyclic antidepressants |
| Oxamniquine | Trimethadione |
| Oxaprozin | Trimethobenzamide |
| Oxybutinin | Valproate |
| Paraldehyde | Vasopressin |
| Paramethadione | Vigabatrin |
| Pegaspargase | Vinca alkaloids |
| Penicillamine | Vitamin D preparations |
| Penicillins | Zidovudine |
| Pentamidine | Zolpidem |

*Table 6.10*   Drugs associated with myoclonus or seizures

| | |
|---|---|
| Acyclovir | Dopamine |
| Adrenocortical steroids, adrenocorticotropic hormone | Ergotamine |
| | Erythropoietin |
| Albendazole | Estrogens |
| Aldesleukin | Ethacrynic acid |
| Alpha-adrenergic agonists | Ethionamide |
| Altretamine | Ethosuximide |
| Amantadine | Etodolac |
| Aminocaproic acid | Etomidate |
| Aminoglycoside antibiotics | Etretinate |
| Amphetamine-like psychostimulants | Felbamate |
| Amphotericin B | Fenoprofen |
| Anesthetics: local amide type | Flecainide |
| Angiotensin converting enzyme inhibitors | Floxuridine |
| Antimuscarinic anticholinergics | Fluconazole |
| Aprotinin | Flumazenil |
| Baclofen | Fluoride |
| Barbiturates | Foscarnet |
| Bumetanide | Furosemide |
| Benzodiazepines | Glutethimide |
| Beta-adrenergic blockers | Gold salts |
| Bethanechol | Gonadorelin |
| Bismuth subsalicylate | Granisetron |
| Bromocriptine | Guanadrel |
| Bupropion | Guanethidine |
| Buspirone | Histamine $H_1$-receptor antagonists |
| Busulfan | Histrelin |
| Butyrophenones | Hydroxychloroquine |
| Caffeine | Hydroxyurea |
| Calcitonin | Ibuprofen |
| Carbamazepine | Idarubicin |
| Carbonic anhydrase inhibitors | Ifosfamide |
| Carboprost | Indomethacin |
| Carmustine | Insulin |
| Cephalosporins | Interferon alfa-2a, alfa-2b, alfa-n3 |
| Chlorambucil | Iron preparations |
| Chloroquine | Isoniazid |
| Chlorprothixene | Isotretinoin |
| Clozapine | Itraconazole |
| Cocaine | Ketoconazole |
| Cyclobenzaprine | Ketoprofen |
| Cycloserine | Ketoralac |
| Cyclosporine | Levodopa, levodopa/carbidopa |
| Cytarabine | Lidocaine |
| Danazol | Lindane |
| Dantrolene | Lithium |
| Dextromethorphan | Meclofenamate |
| Diclofenac | Mechlorethamine |
| Digitalis | Mefenamic acid |
| Dinoprostone | Mefloquine |
| Dobutamine | Melarsoprol |
| Domperidone | Methocarbamol |

*Table 6.10*   (continued)

| | |
|---|---|
| Methsuximide | Praziquantel |
| Methotrexate | Procarbazine |
| Methysergide | Propafenone |
| Metoclopramide | Propofol |
| Metronidazole | Pyrimethamine |
| Mexiletine | Quinacrine |
| Miconazole | Reserpine |
| Mitoxantrone | Rimantadine |
| Moricizine | Salicylates |
| Muromonab-CD3 | Saquinavir |
| Nafarelin | Selegiline (deprenyl) |
| Naproxen | Serotonin uptake inhibitors |
| Nicotine | Sulfinpyrazone |
| Nifurtimox | Sulfonamides |
| Ondansetron | Sulfonate |
| Opioid agonists and mixed agonist- | Sulfonylurea hypoglycemics |
|   antagonists | Sulindac |
| Orphenadrine | Sumatriptan |
| Osmotic diuretics | Theobromine |
| Oxamniquine | Theophylline |
| Oxytocin | Thiabendazole |
| Paclitaxel (Taxol) | Thiazide diuretics |
| Papaverine | Thiothixene |
| Penicillamine | Tocainide |
| Penicillins | Tolmetin |
| Pentoxifylline | Tranexamic acid |
| Phenothiazines | Tricyclic and tetracyclic antidepressants |
| Phensuximide | Trimethobenzamide |
| Phenytoin | Vasopressin |
| Phosphate salts | Vinca alkaloids |
| Physostigmine | Vitamin A |
| Piperazine | Zidovudine |

*Table 6.11*   Drugs associated with peripheral neuropathy

| | |
|---|---|
| Allopurinol | Ifosfamide |
| Altretamine | Indomethacin |
| Amiodarone | Isoniazid |
| Amphotericin B | Levodopa, levodopa/carbidopa |
| Angiotensin-converting enzyme inhibitors | Lithium |
| Aminoglycoside antibiotics | Melarsoprol |
| Carboplatin | Mesalamine |
| Chlorambucil | Metronidazole |
| Chloramphenicol | Mitotane |
| Chloroquine | Monoamine oxidase inhibitors |
| Cisplatin | Nifurtimox |
| Clofibrate | Nitrofurantoin |
| Colchicine | Olsalazine |
| Cytarabine | Paclitaxel (Taxol) |
| Danazol | Penicillamine |
| Dapsone | Phenytoin |
| Didanosine | Polymyxins |
| Dideoxycytidine | Probucol |
| Dimercaprol | Procarbazine |
| Disulfiram | Pyridoxine |
| Ethambutol | Quinolone antibiotics |
| Ethchlorvynol | Stavudine |
| Ethionamide | Succimer |
| Flucytosine | Sulfasalazine |
| Foscarnet | Sulfonamides |
| Glutethimide | Suramin |
| Gold salts | Tacrine |
| Griseofulvin | Fibrinolysin (Thrombolysin) |
| Hydralazine | Ticlopidine |
| 3-Hydroxy-3-methylglutaryl coenzyme A- | Vinca alkaloids |
|    reductase inhibitors | Zolpidem |

*Table 6.12*   Drugs associated with myopathy

| | |
|---|---|
| Abciximab | Dantrolene |
| Acetaminophen | 3-Hydroxy-3-methylglutaryl coenzyme A- |
| Adrenocortical steroids, adrenocorticotropic |    reductase inhibitors |
|    hormone | Magnesium-containing antacids |
| Allopurinol | Nicotinic acid |
| Aminocaproic acid | Nifurtimox |
| Amiodarone | Penicillamine |
| Amphetamine-like psychostimulants | Procaine amide |
| Amrinone | Spironolactone |
| Aprotinin | Succinylcholine |
| Carbenoxolone | Thiazide diuretics |
| Carbonic anhydrase inhibitors | Ticlopidine |
| Carboplatin | Tranexamic acid |
| Cisplatin | Triamterene |
| Clofibrate | Tricyclic and tetracyclic antidepressants |
| Cocaine | Trientine |
| Colchicine | Zidovudine |
| Cytarabine | |

*Table 6.13*   Drugs associated with myasthenia or neuromuscular blockade

| | |
|---|---|
| Aminoglycoside antibiotics | Metrifonate |
| Anticholinesterase agents | Nondepolarizing neuromuscular |
| Bacitracin | blocking agents |
| Beta-adrenergic blockers | Paramethadione |
| Botulinum-A toxin | Penicillamine |
| Busulfan | Penicillins |
| Butyrophenones | Phenothiazines |
| Cephalosporins | Polymixin antibiotics |
| Clindamycin | Quinidine |
| Chloroquine | Quinolone antibiotics |
| Chlorprothixene | Serotonin uptake inhibitors |
| Clozapine | Succinylcholine |
| Lincomycin | Tetracyclines |
| Lithium | Thiothixene |
| Macrolide antibiotics | Trimethadione |
| Magnesium sulfate | |

*Table 6.14*   Drugs associated with impaired vision, optic neuropathy, or retinopathy

| | |
|---|---|
| Adrenocortical steroids, adrenocorticotropic hormone | Fluorouracil |
| Allopurinol | Griseofulvin |
| Aminocaproic acid | Ibuprofen |
| Amiodarone | Indomethacin |
| Aprotinin | Interferon alfa-2a, alfa-2b |
| Butyrophenones | Iodoquinol |
| Carboplatin | Isotretinoin |
| Carmustine | Ketoprofen |
| Chloramphenicol | Ketorolac |
| Chloroquine | Meclofenamate |
| Chlorprothixene | Mefenamic acid |
| Cisplatin | Mitotane |
| Clofazimine | Muromonab-CD3 |
| Clofibrate | Nabumetone |
| Clozapine | Naproxen |
| Cyclosporine | Nicotinic acid |
| Cytarabine | Nitrofurantoin |
| Deferoxamine | Paramethadione |
| Diclofenac | Penicillamine |
| Didanosine | Phenothiazines |
| Diethylcarbamazine | Piroxicam |
| Digitalis | Procarbazine |
| Ethambutol | Propofol |
| Etodolac | Quinacrine |
| Etoposide | Quinidine |
| Etretinate | Quinine |
| Fenoprofen | Quinolone antibiotics |
| | Succimer |

Sulfonamides
Sulindac
Suramin
Tamoxifen
Thiabendazole
Thiazide diuretics
Thiothixene

Tolmetin
Tranexamic acid
Trimethadione
Vinca alkaloids
Vitamin A
Vitamin D preparations
Zidovudine

*Table 6.15* Drugs associated with tinnitus or hearing loss

Allopurinol
Aminocaproic acid
Aminoglycoside antibiotics
Amphotericin B
Angiotensin-converting enzyme inhibitors
Aprotinin
Bumetanide
Beta-adrenergic blockers
Bromocriptine
Buspirone
Caffeine
Capreomycin
Carbonic anhydrase inhibitors
Carboplatin
Chloramphenicol
Chloroquine
Cholestyramine
Cisplatin
Clindamycin
Cyclobenzaprine
Cyclosporine
Dapsone
Deferoxamine
Diazoxide
Diclofenac
Ethacrynic acid
Etodolac
Fenoprofen
Flucytosine
Furosemide
Gonadorelin
Histamine $H_2$-receptor antagonists
Histrelin
Hydroxychloroquine
Ibuprofen
Indomethacin
Ketoprofen
Ketorolac
Lamotrigine
Lansoprazole

Lidocaine
Lincomycin
Macrolide antibiotics
Mechlorethamine
Meclofenamate
Mefenamic acid
Mefloquine
Mexiletine
Misoprostol
Mitotane
Monoamine oxidase inhibitors
Moricizine
Muromonab-CD3
Nafarelin
Naproxen
Omeprazole
Penicillamine
Piroxicam
Probucol
Propofol
Quinidine
Quinine
Quinolone antibiotics
Rimantadine
Salicylates
Saquinavir
Serotonin uptake inhibitors
Succimer
Sulfonamides
Sulindac
Thiabendazole
Ticlopidine
Tocainide
Tolmetin
Tricyclic and tetracyclic antidepressants
Vancomycin
Vitamin D preparations
Zidovudine
Zolpidem

*Table 6.16*    Drugs associated with dizziness or vertigo

| | |
|---|---|
| Angiotensin-converting enzyme inhibitors | Mechlorethamine |
| Altretamine | Mefenamic acid |
| Amphotericin B | Mefloquine |
| Bromocriptine | Methocarbamol |
| Capreomycin | Methysergide |
| Carbonic anhydrase inhibitors | Metronidazole |
| Carisoprodol | Mitotane |
| Cholestyramine | Muromonab-CD3 |
| Clindamycin | Nabumetone |
| Cyclobenzamine | Naproxen |
| Cycloserine | Nitrofurantoin |
| Dapsone | Omeprazole |
| Diclofenac | Paramethadione |
| Ergotamine | Phenylbutazone |
| Etodolac | Piroxicam |
| Fenoprofen | Polymixin antibiotics |
| Finasteride | Quinidine |
| Flucytosine | Quinine |
| Gabapentin | Quinolone antibiotics |
| Histamine $H_2$-receptor antagonists | Salicylates |
| 3-Hydroxy-3-methylglutaryl coenzyme A-reductase inhibitors | Serotonin uptake inhibitors |
| | Sulfonamides |
| Ibuprofen | Sulindac |
| Indomethacin | Tacrine |
| Ketoprofen | Tetracyclines |
| Ketorolac | Thiazide diuretics |
| Lansoprazole | Trimethadione |
| Lincomycin | Vancomycin |
| Macrolide antibiotics | Vitamin D preparations |
| Meclofenamate | Zidovudine |

*Table 6.17*    Drugs associated with ataxia and nystagmus

| | |
|---|---|
| Baclofen | Methysergide |
| Barbiturates and other sedatives/hypnotics | Metronidazole |
| Benzodiazepines | Mitotane |
| Carbamazepine | Nabilone |
| Carbonic anhydrase inhibitors | Nitrofurantoin |
| Cyclobenzaprine | Paclitaxel (Taxol) |
| Cytarabine | Paramethadione |
| Dronabinol | Phenacemide |
| Ergotamine | Phensuximide |
| Ethosuximide | Phenytoin |
| Felbamate | Procarbazine |
| Floxuridine | Pyrimethamine |
| Fluorouracil | Quinolone antibiotics |
| Foscarnet | Selegiline (deprenyl) |
| Gabapentin | Tacrine |
| Idarubicin | Trimethadione |
| Lamotrigine | Valproate |
| Lithium | Zolpidem |
| Methsuximide | |

*Table 6.18*　Drugs associated with tremor parkinsonism or abnormal movements

| | |
|---|---|
| Amiodarone | Ketorolac |
| Amphetamine-like psychostimulants | Lamotrigine |
| Angiotensin-converting enzyme inhibitors | Levodopa, levodopa/carbidopa |
| L-Asparaginase | Lithium |
| Baclofen | Meclofenamate |
| Beta-adrenergic blockers | Mefenamic acid |
| Bromocriptine | Methsuximide |
| Bupropion | Methyldopa |
| Buspirone | Metoclopramide |
| Butyrophenones | Mexiletine |
| Caffeine | Metyrosine |
| Calcium channel blockers | Milrinone |
| Carbamazepine | Mitotane |
| Chloroquine | Monoamine oxidase inhibitors |
| Chlorprothixene | Moricizine |
| Chlorzoxazone | Nabumetone |
| Cisapride | Naproxen |
| Clonidine | Nicotine |
| Clozapine | Ondansetron |
| Cocaine | Pegaspargase |
| Diclofenac | Phenothiazines |
| Digitalis | Phensuximide |
| Domperidone | Phenytoin |
| Estrogens | Piperazine |
| Ethosuximide | Piroxicam |
| Etodolac | Procaine amide |
| Etomidate | Reserpine |
| Felbamate | Ritodrine |
| Fenoprofen | Selegiline (deprenyl) |
| Flecainide | Serotonin uptake inhibitors |
| Flucytosine | Sulindac |
| Gabapentin | Sumatriptan |
| Granisetron | Tacrine |
| Guanabenz | Tamoxifen |
| Guanadrel | Thiothixene |
| Guanethidine | Tocainide |
| Guanfacine | Tolmetin |
| Histamine $H_2$-receptor antagonists | Trazodone |
| Hydralazine | Tricyclic and tetracyclic antidepressants |
| Hydroxychloroquine | Trimethobenzamide |
| Ibuprofen | Valproate |
| Indomethacin | Vigabatrin |
| Ketoprofen | |

*Table 6.19*   Drugs associated with increased intracranial pressure

| | |
|---|---|
| Adrenocortical steroids | Osmotic diuretics |
| Aminoglycoside antibiotics | Penicillins |
| Amiodarone | Quinolone antibiotics |
| Danazol | Somatotropin, somatrem |
| Etretinate | Sulfonamides |
| Isotretinoin | Tetracycline |
| Lithium | Thyroid |
| Nitrofurantoin | Vitamin A |
| Nitroprusside | |
| Opioid agonists and mixed agonist-<br>antagonists | |

*Table 6.20*   Drugs associated with aseptic meningitis

| | |
|---|---|
| Adrenocortical steroids, adrenocorticotropic<br>hormone | Methotrexate |
| Albendazole | Naproxen |
| Amphotericin B | Polymixin antibiotics |
| Carbamazepine | Praziquantel |
| Cytarabine | Sulindac |
| Fenoprofen | Sulfonamides |
| Ibuprofen | Trimethoprim |

*Table 6.21*   Drugs associated with myelopathy

| | |
|---|---|
| Anesthetics: local amide type | Iodoquinol |
| Cyclosporine | Leuprolide |
| Cytarabine | Mesalamine |
| Fluorouracil | Mitoxantrone |
| Gold salts | Olsalazine |
| Goserelin | Sulfasalazine |

*Table 6.22*   Drugs associated with disulfiram-ethanol–like reaction

| | |
|---|---|
| Cephalosporins | Itraconazole |
| Chloramphenicol | Ketoconazole |
| Disulfiram | Metronidazole |
| Fluconazole | Miconazole |
| Furazolidone | Procarbazine |
| Griseofulvin | Quinacrine |
| Isoniazid | Sulfonylurea hypoglycemics |

agents is often problematic, especially when based on a small number of anecdotal reports, and some associations are a good deal more convincing than others. For example, seizures are very likely a true side effect of beta-lactam
antibiotics and isoniazid; the cause of seizures associated with other antimicrobials is less certain, and in some instances—for example, acyclovir, zidovudine,
and praziquantel—seizures probably are related more to the condition being
treated than to the drug itself. Drugs precipitate seizures through a variety of indirect mechanisms, for example thiazide diuretics do so by causing hyponatremia
and L-asparaginase by causing stroke.

The tables do not include vague or nonspecific symptoms such as fatigue,
headache, nonvertiginous dizziness, so-called paresthesias, altered taste, decreased
libido, myalgia, blurred vision, irritability, insomnia, diplopia, or photophobia.
Such symptoms may signify true neurotoxicity (e.g., headache with indomethacin),
but in most instances, descriptions are too limited to tell.

As noted, drug complications are sometimes secondary to cerebrovascular effects and also vary in mechanism (e.g., procaine amide and lupus anticoagulant, warfarin and bleeding, estrogen/progestin and coagulopathy,
monoamine oxidase inhibitors and hypertensive crisis, ergot alkaloids and
vasoconstriction).

For detailed information on the neurotoxic side effects of prescription drugs,
see Brust, 1996.

## HOUSEHOLD AND OCCUPATIONAL TOXINS

Environmental toxins include metals, organic solvents, gasoline, gases, and
organophosphates. Except when exposure is obvious, environmental poisoning
does not usually head the list of diagnostic possibilities in patients with such
nonspecific symptoms and signs as altered mental status, seizures, ataxia, optic
neuropathy, or peripheral neuropathy. When the diagnosis is uncertain, however,
unsuspected poisoning (including suicide or homicide) must be considered.

Table 6.23 lists those metals most often associated with neurologic symptoms.
Sources of exposure and clinical features are incompletely listed, and special
diagnostic and treatment options are not included. For particulars, see Goetz and
Cohen, 1989, and Goldfrank et al., 1990.

Methyl alcohol (widely used in manufacturing), ethylene glycol (used as an
antifreeze), and isopropyl alcohol (available as rubbing alcohol) are occasionally
ingested as ethanol substitutes. Methyl alcohol, through its toxic metabolite
formaldehyde, causes metabolic acidosis, delirium, seizures, coma, and cranial
neuropathies. Retinal toxicity can result in permanent blindness, and some survivors are left with dementia and extrapyramidal signs. Treatment includes alkalinization, ethanol, and in severe cases, dialysis.

Ethylene glycol causes metabolic acidosis, ataxia, cranial neuropathies,
myoclonus, seizures, stupor, and coma; the metabolite ethylene oxylate chelates
calcium, producing tetany. Treatment also includes alkalinization and ethanol, as
well as forced diuresis and possibly dialysis.

*Table 6.23*    Metal poisoning

| Agent | Source | Systemic symptoms and signs | Neurologic symptoms and signs |
|---|---|---|---|
| Lead | Atmospheric pollution, especially gasoline additives<br>Paints, dyes<br>Pottery, glass<br>Bullets<br>Storage batteries<br>Welding<br>Industrial and agriculture exposure | Nausea, vomiting, constipation, abdominal pain, colic<br>Fever<br>Slow irregular pulse, hypertension | Tremor of face, tongue, and limbs<br>Irritability, memory impairment, drowsiness, delirium, coma<br>Seizures<br>Ptosis, strabismus<br>Hemianopia, blindness, papilledema<br>Myelopathy<br>Sensorimotor polyneuropathy, especially wristdrop |
| Mercury | Antiseptics<br>Fossil-fuel burning<br>Seafood<br>Antifungal products<br>Thermometers, dentistry<br>Dyes, paints<br>Industrial and agricultural exposure | Inflammation of buccal mucosa, salivation<br>Diarrhea, colic, metallic breath | Irritability, behavioral change, neurasthenia, lethargy, hallucinations, coma<br>Tremor, dyskinesias, parkinsonism<br>Vertigo, nystagmus, ataxia<br>Optic neuropathy, blindness<br>Seizures<br>Sensorimotor polyneuropathy<br>Deafness |
| Arsenic | Insecticides<br>Disinfectants<br>Paints, enamels<br>Pharmaceuticals<br>Industrial and agricultural exposure | Inflammation of buccal mucosa<br>Abdominal pain, nausea, vomiting<br>Fever<br>Labored breathing<br>Skin rash, Mees' lines in nails<br>Hepatic, renal, and hematopoietic involvement | Headache, nervousness, excitement, lethargy, coma<br>Seizures<br>Vertigo, nystagmus<br>Myelopathy<br>Optic neuropathy<br>Sensorimotor polyneuropathy |
| Thallium | Depilatories<br>Rodenticide, insecticide | Alopecia<br>Hepatic and renal toxicity | Limb pain, sensorimotor polyneuropathy<br>Irritability, depression, lethargy, coma<br>Chorea, myoclonus, seizures<br>Optic neuropathy, blindness<br>Ptosis, strabismus, facial or vocal cord palsy |

| | Sources | | |
|---|---|---|---|
| Manganese | Mining<br>Fungicide<br>Gasoline additive<br>Paints, dyes<br>Industrial and agricultural exposure | Sialorrhea, sweating | Weakness, fatigue, lethargy<br>Personality change, emotional lability<br>Tremor, retropulsive gait, masked facies |
| Iron | Pharmaceuticals | Bloody vomiting and diarrhea | Coma<br>Seizures |
| Phosphorus | Matchheads<br>Fireworks<br>Insecticides<br>Industrial exposure | Nausea, vomiting, diarrhea, abdominal pain, thirst<br>Bleeding<br>Hepatic and renal toxicity | Delirium, coma<br>Seizures |
| Antimony | Pharmaceuticals | Vomiting, diarrhea, abdominal pain | Weakness, lethargy, coma<br>Seizures |
| Zinc | Sheet metal manufacture<br>Storage batteries<br>Paints<br>Emetics, astringents<br>Industrial exposure | Nausea, vomiting, bloody diarrhea<br>Chills, fever | Headache<br>Muscle cramps<br>Apathy, mutism, irritability, coma<br>Tremor, ataxia |
| Gold | Pharmaceuticals | Skin rash<br>Fever<br>Nausea, vomiting, diarrhea<br>Bone marrow depression<br>Renal toxicity | Sensorimotor polyneuropathy<br>Brachial plexopathy<br>Depression, psychosis, delirium<br>Ptosis, anisocoria, unreactive pupils<br>Ataxia<br>Aphasia<br>Aseptic meningitis |
| Aluminum | Household utensils<br>Deodorants<br>Paints<br>Explosives<br>Pharmaceuticals<br>Industrial exposure | "Bauxite lung" | Dialysis encephalopathy: speech apraxia/dysarthria myoclonus, seizures, gait ataxia, progressive dementia, coma |

*Table 6.23*  (continued)

| Agent | Source | Systemic symptoms and signs | Neurologic symptoms and signs |
|---|---|---|---|
| Barium | Ceramics, glass<br>Automobile parts<br>Paints<br>Food contamination<br>Industrial exposure | Nausea, vomiting, diarrhea, abdominal pain | Myopathy, flaccid paralysis<br>Seizures |
| Bismuth | Pharmaceuticals<br>Industrial exposure | Stomatitis<br>Renal toxicity<br>Obstructive jaundice | Headache, asthenia<br>Dementia, delirium, hallucinations, coma<br>Myoclonus, seizures<br>Tremor, ataxia |

*Table 6.24*  Miscellaneous industrial and agricultural toxins

| | |
|---|---|
| Acetone | Organophosphates |
| Benzene | Triorthocresyl phosphate |
| Toluene | Organochloride insecticides |
| Methyl-*N*-butyl ketone | Methyl bromide |
| n-Hexane | Acrylamide |
| Gasoline, naphtha | Hydrazine |
| Pinenes, turpenes | Cyanide |
| Trichloroethane | Camphor |
| Trichloroethylene | Dioxin |
| Carbon tetrachloride | Polychlorinated biphenyls |
| Methyl chloride | Phenol |
| Carbon disulfide | Styrene |
| Ethylene oxide | |

Isopropyl alcohol usually causes ketosis without lactic acidosis. Symptoms (ataxia or coma) are treated supportively; dialysis is used in severe cases. Because isopropyl alcohol is itself the neurotoxin, ethanol is not given.

Table 6.24 lists a number of other compounds used in industry or agriculture and capable of damaging the peripheral or central nervous systems. As noted, some of these agents are also used as recreational inhalants.

## ANIMAL AND PLANT TOXINS

Weakness progressing to respiratory paralysis is the major neurologic symptom in most snakebite victims; coagulopathy can result in intracranial hemorrhage. The fish toxin ciguatera (produced by an ingested dinoflagellate) also affects the neuromuscular junction, causing weakness and respiratory compromise; visual symptoms include transient blindness. Tick paralysis usually begins a few days after a tick becomes attached and then progresses over days, eventually affecting cranial muscles and respiration. Death can result, but if the tick is removed in time, improvement begins within hours.

In contrast to these animal toxins, which affect mainly the peripheral nervous system, mushroom poisoning directly or indirectly affects the central nervous system. Mushrooms that cause hallucinations are ingested recreationally; overdose causes delirium and coma. Most mushroom poisoning is caused by *Amanita* species, which produce neurologic symptoms (and death) indirectly through liver damage.

## SUGGESTED READING

Bost RO. 3,4-Methylenedioxymethamphetamine (MDMA) and other amphetamine derivatives. J Forensic Sci 1988;33:576.

Brust JCM. Neurological Aspects of Substance Abuse. Boston: Butterworth–Heinemann, 1993.

Brust JCM. Neurotoxic Side-Effects of Prescription Drugs. Boston: Butterworth–Heinemann, 1996.

Brust JCM. Seizures Secondary to Substance Abuse. In H Luders (ed), The Epilepsies: Etiology and Prevention. In press.

Brust JCM, Richter RW. Quinine amblyopia related to heroin addiction. Ann Intern Med 1971;74:84.

Caplan LR, Thomas C, Banks G. Central nervous system complications of addiction to "T's and blues." Neurology 1982;32:623.

Chiriboga CA. Fetal effects. Neurol Clin 1993;11:707.

Chiriboga CA, Bateman DA, Brust JCM, Hauser WA. Neurological outcome of neonates exposed in utero to cocaine. Pediatr Neurol 1993;9:115.

Des Jarlais DC, Friedman SR, Novick DM, et al. HIV-1 infection among intravenous drug users in Manhattan, New York City, from 1977 through 1987. JAMA 1989;261:1008.

Earnest MP. Seizures. Neurol Clin 1993;11:563.

Goetz CG, Cohen MM. Neurotoxic Agents. In R Joynt (ed), Clinical Neurology, vol 2. Philadelphia: Lippincott, 1989;1–101.

Goldfrank LR, Flomenbaum NE, Levin NA, et al. (eds). Toxicologic Emergencies (4th ed). Norwalk, CT: Appleton & Lange, 1990.

Goldfrank LR, Hoffman RS. The cardiovascular effects of cocaine. Ann Emerg Med 1991;20:165.

Holman BL, Carvalho PA, Mendelson J, et al. Brain perfusion is abnormal in cocaine-dependent polydrug users: a study using technetium Tc 99m, HMPAO, and ASPECT. J Nucl Med 1991;32:1206.

Hormes JT, Filley CM, Rosenberg NL. Neurologic sequelae of chronic vapor abuse. Neurology 1986;36:698.

Howrie DL, Wolfson JM. Phenylpropanolamine-induced seizure. Pediatrics 1983;102:143.

Kelly T. Prolonged cerebellar dysfunction associated with paint sniffing. Pediatrics 1975;56:605.

Levine SR, Brust JCM, Futrell N, et al. Cerebrovascular complications of the "crack" form of alkaloidal cocaine. N Engl J Med 1990;323:699.

Lolin Y. Chronic neurological toxicity associated with exposure to volatile substances. Hum Toxicol 1989;8:293.

McCarron MM, Schultz BW, Thompson GA, et al. Acute phencyclidine intoxication: incidence of clinical findings in 1000 cases. Ann Emerg Med 1981;10:237.

Mikolich JR, Paulson GW, Cross CJ. Acute anticholinergic syndrome due to jimson seed ingestion. Ann Intern Med 1975;83:321.

Pascual-Leone A, Anderson DC. Cerebral atrophy in habitual cocaine abusers: a planimetric CT study. Neurology 1991;41:34.

Pascual-Leone A, Dhuna A, Altafallah I, Anderson DC. Cocaine-induced seizures. Neurology 1990;40:404.

Weinreib RM, O'Brien CP. Persistent cognitive deficits attributed to substance abuse. Neurol Clin 1993;11:663.

# 7
# Stroke

Albert Pall Sigurdsson and Edward Feldmann

Stroke is an *acute* neurologic disorder produced by ischemia (80%) or hemorrhage (20%). Each year approximately 500,000 Americans suffer new or recurrent stroke and nearly one-fourth of those die. Among stroke survivors, 10% return to normal, 48% are hemiparetic, and 22% are unable to walk. One-fourth to one-half are dependent and one-third are clinically depressed. Diagnosis of stroke is aggressively pursued to determine stroke mechanism, as it affects options and prognosis.

## EMERGENCY DEPARTMENT EVALUATION

Patients in the emergency room with suspected ischemic stroke may be candidates for tissue plasminogen activator (t-PA). Criteria for the use of t-PA are listed in Table 7.1. Patients with more severe deficits (those with a National Institutes of Heath Stroke Scale [NIHSS] score greater than 22) are at a higher risk of intracerebral hemorrhage (ICH) when given t-PA. For NIHSS scoring see Table 7.2. Hypodensity and edema in more than one-third of the middle cerebral artery (MCA) distribution is also associated with higher rate of ICH when t-PA is administered. These patients still benefit, however, when treated with t-PA.

Eligible patients should receive 0.90 mg/kg (90-mg maximal dose) of t-PA; 10% should be given as a bolus over 1 minute, followed by continuous infusion over 60 minutes. During the infusion and for the first 24 hours after the infusion, no heparin, warfarin, or antiplatelet drugs should be given. Computed tomographic (CT) scan of the brain should be repeated in 24 hours. If no sign of ICH is present on the CT scan at that time, one may consider using heparin without bolus or aspirin as indicated.

*Table 7.1*    Tissue plasminogen activator (t-PA) inclusion and exclusion criteria

Inclusion criteria
    1.  Time of acute ischemic stroke symptoms ≤3 hrs
    2.  Baseline computed tomographic (CT) scan does not show intracranial hemorrhage
       (ICH) or tumor
Exclusion criteria
    1.  Patient has only:
      a. minor stroke symptoms, or
      b. rapidly improving neurologic deficits
    2.  Clinical presentation suggestive of subarachnoid hemorrhage, even if the initial CT
       scan is normal
    3.  History of ICH, arteriovenous malformation, aneurysm, or cerebral neoplasm
    4.  Prior stroke or serious head injury within the past 3 mos
    5.  Active internal bleeding (in the previous 3 wks)
    6.  Known bleeding diathesis including but not limited to:
      a. Current use of oral anticoagulants with prothrombin time >15
      b. Administration of heparin within 48 hrs preceding the onset of stroke and an ele-
         vated partial thromboplastin time at presentation
      c. Platelet count <100,000
    7.  Systolic blood pressure >185 mm Hg or diastolic blood pressure >110 mm Hg on
       repeated measurement, despite acute treatment
    8.  Major surgery in the previous 2 wks
    9.  Seizure at symptom onset
   10. Pregnancy, lactation, or parturition within 30 days
   11. Major surgery in the previous 2 wks
   12. Arterial puncture at a noncompressible site or a lumbar puncture in the previous 7 days
   13. Blood glucose <40 or >400 mg/dl

## INTRAVENOUS HEPARIN

The risks and benefits of acute anticoagulation with heparin in patients with ischemic stroke are still being weighed. Clinical trials of acute heparin therapy for stroke have been small or uncontrolled and have generated conflicting results. The largest modern study of intravenous heparin for stroke enrolled only 212 patients. Neither stroke progression nor neurologic improvement was significantly influenced by heparin in that trial. This result was confirmed in the International Stroke Trial, where aspirin but not heparin, given early after stroke onset (less than 48 hours) reduced the risk of subsequent strokes. The Trial of ORG 10172 in Acute Stroke Treatment, which used low-molecular-weight heparin within 24 hours after stroke onset, also failed to show a benefit. Despite the lack of data supporting its effectiveness, heparin continues to be used in selected stroke patients.

Hemorrhagic transformation associated with heparin use appears to be most common in patients with large infarcts and uncontrolled hypertension. Excessive prolongation of the partial thromboplastin time and heparin boluses have also been associated with an increased risk of brain hemorrhage.

At present no definite recommendation regarding the use of heparin in acute stroke can be made; rather, it is used at the discretion of the physician. Heparin should be

*Table 7.2*  National Institutes of Health Stroke Scale

1a. Level of consciousness (LOC)
    0 = Alert; keenly responsive
    1 = Not alert, but arousable by minor stimulation to obey, answer, or respond
    2 = Not alert, requires repeated stimulation to attend, or is obtunded and requires strong or painful stimulation to make movements (not stereotyped)
    3 = Responds only with reflex motor or automatic effects or totally unresponsive, flaccid, areflexic
1b. LOC questions (What month is it? Patient's age?)
    0 = Answers both questions correctly
    1 = Answers one question correctly
    2 = Answers neither question correctly
    (Intubated, severe dysarthria or language barriers—score 1)
1c. LOC commands (Open and close eyes and grip and release with nonparetic hand—only first attempt is scored)
    0 = Performs both tasks correctly
    1 = Performs one task correctly
    2 = Performs neither task correctly
2. Best gaze
    0 = Normal
    1 = Partial gaze palsy
    2 = Forced deviation, or total gaze paresis not overcome by the oculocephalic maneuver
3. Visual fields
    0 = Normal
    1 = Partial hemianopia
    2 = Complete hemianopia
    3 = Bilateral hemianopia (blind including cortical blindness)
4. Facial palsy
    0 = Normal symmetric movement
    1 = Minor paralysis (flattened nasolabial fold, asymmetry on smiling)
    3 = Complete paralysis of one or both sides (absence of facial movement in the upper and lower face)
5. Motor in arms (5a. Left arm. 5b. Right arm—score for both)
    0 = No drift, limb holds 90 degrees (if sitting) or 45 degrees (if supine) for full 10 secs
    1 = Drift, limb holds 90 degrees or 45 degrees, but drifts down before full 10 secs; does not hit bed or other support
    2 = Some effort against gravity, limb cannot get to or maintain (if cued) 90 degrees or 45 degrees
    3 = No effort against gravity, limb falls
    4 = No movement
    9 = Amputation, joint effusion (not included in the scoring )
6. Motor in leg (6a. Left leg. 6b. Right leg—score for both)
    0 = No drift, leg holds 30-degree position for full 5 secs
    1 = Drift, leg falls by the end of the 5-sec period but does not hit bed
    2 = Some effort against gravity; leg falls to bed by 5 secs, but has some effort against gravity
    3 = No effort against gravity; leg falls to bed immediately
    4 = No movement
    9 = Amputation, joint fusion (not included in the scoring)
7. Limb ataxia (finger-nose-finger and heel-knee-shin tests)
    0 = Absent
    1 = Present in one limb

*Table 7.2* (continued)

---

    2 = Present in two limbs
    Only scored if the ataxia is out of proportion to the weakness
    Not scored if patient cannot understand or is hemiplegic
  8. Sensory
    0 = Normal; no sensory loss
    1 = Mild to moderate sensory loss; patient feels pinprick is less sharp or is dull on the affected side; or there is a loss of superficial pain with pinprick but patient is aware he or she is being touched
    2 = Severe to total sensory loss; patient is not aware of being touched in the face, arm, and leg
  9. Best language
    0 = No aphasia, normal
    1 = Mild to moderate aphasia
    2 = Severe aphasia
    3 = Mute, global aphasia
10. Dysarthria (patient is asked to read or repeat words)
    0 = Normal
    1 = Mild to moderate; patient slurs at least some words and, at worst, can be understood with some difficulty
    2 = Severe; patient's speech is so slurred as to be unintelligible, or patient is mute or anarthric
    9 = Intubated or other physical barriers (not included in the scoring)
11. Extinction and inattention
    0 = No abnormality
    1 = Visual, tactile, auditory, spatial, or personal inattention or extinction to bilateral simultaneous stimulation in one of the sensory modalities
    2 = Profound hemi-inattention or hemi-inattention to more than one modality; does not recognize own hand or orients to only one side of space

---

considered for acute cardioembolic stroke patients who are at high risk of early recurrent embolization (e.g., patients with mechanical heart valves, established intracardiac thrombi, or atrial fibrillation with concomitant valvular disease or significant congestive heart failure), especially if the patient has no significant risk factors for brain hemorrhage. In addition, short-term heparin is a reasonable choice for patients with progressing ischemic stroke, particularly in the vertebrobasilar circulation.

## HEMORRHAGIC STROKES

### Subarachnoid Hemorrhage

Pathophysiology

In 85% of cases, subarachnoid hemorrhage (SAH) results from bleeding from a saccular aneurysm located at the bifurcation of the large arteries at the base of the brain. Although autopsy studies estimate that 5% of the population harbors an aneurysm, the incidence of rupture is only 4–10 per 100,000 each year. The greatest incidence is in the fifth, sixth, and seventh decade. Women are affected more than men. Aneurysms usually bleed into the subarachnoid space or less commonly into the brain or ventricular system or both, resulting in ICH, intraventricular hemorrhage, or acute hydrocephalus.

Approximately 85% of ruptured saccular aneurysms occur in the anterior circulation (30% at the junction of the internal carotid artery [ICA] and posterior communicating artery, 30% in the anterior communication artery, and 25% in the proximal MCA), and 15% in the posterior circulation; 12–31% of patients have multiple aneurysms. Approximately 10–15% of patients with saccular aneurysms have a family history of SAH or intracranial aneurysm.

Cigarette smoking, use of oral contraceptives, acute hypertension, use of stimulating drugs, physical stress, and alcohol consumption may increase the risk of aneurysmal SAH. Medical conditions associated with formation of intracranial aneurysm include autosomal dominant polycystic kidney disease, intracranial arteriovenous malformation (AVM), coarctation of the aorta, Marfan syndrome, Ehlers-Danlos syndrome, fibromuscular dysplasia, pseudoxanthoma elasticum, moyamoya disease, neurofibromatosis, and pituitary tumors.

## Clinical Presentation

Aneurysms are usually asymptomatic until they rupture. Rarely, patients suffer short-lived "sentinel" or warning headaches. Rupture occurs while the patient is active and produces sudden, severe headaches with or without loss of consciousness. The cardinal symptom is headache that varies from the classic severe, striking, generalized headache with meningismus to a much milder headache resolving within 24–48 hours. Focal signs such as hemiparesis are unusual. Many patients have impaired consciousness, nuchal rigidity, subhyaloid or preretinal hemorrhages, and fever during the first week.

Complications are common and serious. Rebleeding is unpredictable, but often occurs between days 2 and 19 after the initial rupture. Nearly 40% of patients rebleed, approximately 50% of whom die. If the aneurysm is not clipped and the patient survives, the long-term rebleeding rate is 3% per year.

Vasospasm occurs in approximately 30% of patients and is defined angiographically as severe narrowing of intracranial arteries. Symptoms of vasospasm include headache, ischemia, and raised intracranial pressure. However, not all patients with angiographically proven vasospasm have symptoms. Vasospasm frequently occurs between days 4 and 14 and is associated with the presence of a thick clot in the subarachnoid space.

Hydrocephalus occurs after the formation of blood breakdown products, which block the drainage of cerebrospinal fluid (CSF), in the subarachnoid space. It may occur any time after the bleeding and produces progressive ventriculomegaly and impairment of gait and consciousness.

## Diagnosis

The diagnosis of SAH requires a high degree of suspicion on the part of the examining medical personnel. Although abrupt onset of headache is a common presentation, less-severe headaches with or without an associated brief loss of consciousness, nausea, or vomiting may also be seen. In any patient with new onset of an unusually severe or atypical headache, particularly if associated with a brief loss of consciousness, nausea, vomiting, stiff neck, or any focal neurologic finding, the diagnosis of SAH should be suspected. CT scan obtained within 24 hours reveals blood in the subarachnoid space in about 90% of patients with SAH. Magnetic resonance imaging (MRI) is much less sensitive early in the progression of the condition.

If CT shows no blood, and clinical suspicion for SAH is high, a lumbar puncture should be performed. Typically, the tap reveals grossly bloody CSF if SAH is present. The diagnosis of traumatic lumbar puncture must be excluded, however. If successive tubes of CSF show progressively fewer red blood cells, a traumatic puncture should be suspected. Clotting of the specimen virtually never occurs with true SAH. Xanthochromia occurs within hours of SAH and remains in the spinal fluid for an average of 2 weeks. Erythrocytes often disappear within several days after SAH. The CSF may not show xanthochromia if small amounts of erythrocytes are present from SAH (approximately less than 400/ml). On the other hand, xanthochromia has been reported in rare instances of traumatic lumbar puncture when the erythrocyte count is very high (greater than 200,000/ml). In true SAH, cerebral angiography is indicated, both for diagnosis and for surgical planning.

## Treatment

Hypertension must be acutely controlled in an effort to prevent rebleeding. Nimodipine or labetalol are commonly used. Although seizures are not common in SAH, phenytoin is used to prevent seizures that would increase blood and intracranial pressure. Administration of nimodipine is considered routine to prevent vasospastic deficits in stable patients. Transcranial Doppler (TCD) imaging should be performed routinely to assess for the development of vasospasm. As the flow velocity increases, medical treatment for spasm, including volume expansion, hemodilution and induced hypertension, may be intensified. Attention must also be given to electrolyte balance, as some patients may develop hyponatremia. If neurologic deficit attributable to vasospasm occurs despite maximal medical therapy, angioplasty or intra-arterial papaverine infusion should be considered.

Early aneurysm operation within the first 3 days after hemorrhage is indicated for patients who are alert, have little or no neurologic deficit (i.e., Hunt and Hess grade of 1, 2, or 3; the Hunt and Hess scale is given in Table 7.3), have no CT evidence of brain swelling, have an aneurysm that can be approached without excessive retraction, and are considered medically stable. Surgical options include clipping the aneurysm or wrapping it. For those that are inoperable, treatment may involve embolizing the aneurysm with metallic coils during angiography.

It is impossible to determine which aneurysms are likely to rupture, though limited data suggest that size is an important factor. Those larger than 7 mm may warrant prophylactic microsurgical obliteration.

## Prognosis

The Hunt and Hess scale grades the clinical severity of SAH. The patient's grade at the time of arrival to the hospital is the best predictor of survival. The mortal-

*Table 7.3*   Hunt and Hess scale for subarachnoid hemorrhage

| Grade | Criteria |
|---|---|
| 1 | Asymptomatic or minimal headache or stiff neck |
| 2 | Moderate to severe headache, stiff neck, no neurologic deficit other than cranial nerve palsy |
| 3 | Drowsiness, confusion or mild focal signs |
| 4 | Stupor, moderate to severe hemiparesis, possibly early decerebrate signs |
| 5 | Deep coma |

ity of SAH ranges from 5% to 95%, depending on the Hunt and Hess grading. Patients who show extensive alteration in consciousness with or without focal neurologic deficits (i.e., Hunt and Hess clinical grade 4 or 5) have an 80–90% mortality rate in the first 30 days. Alternatively, patients with little or no neurologic deficit (i.e., Hunt and Hess grade 1, 2, or 3) have a more favorable prognosis, with 10–30% mortality at 30 days. Many of the deaths in this group result from rebleeding in the first 2 weeks after initial SAH.

## Intracerebral Hemorrhage

Pathophysiology

ICH is responsible for about 10% of all strokes. Half are caused by hypertension, though its importance has declined during the last several decades. The mechanism of hypertensive hemorrhage is unclear. Hypertension is believed to chronically damage the small penetrating arteries in the brain (50–200 μm in diameter). These vessels are thought to bleed if blood pressure or blood volume rises abruptly. Pathologic support for this hypothesis lies in the detection of lipohyalinosis and microaneurysms of small penetrating arteries in the brains of patients with hypertensive ICH. The distribution of these lesions mirrors the predominant sites of ICH: putamen and internal capsule (40%), lobe (frontal, parietal, temporal, or occipital) (30%), cerebellum (15%), thalamus (10%), and pons (5%).

Nonhypertensive causes of ICH include cerebral amyloid angiopathy, which presents as lobar hemorrhage in elderly patients who do not have hypertension. Anticoagulants cause 10% of ICH. The relative risk of ICH is estimated to be nearly eightfold compared with nonanticoagulated patients. Nearly one in every 100 patients treated with anticoagulants has ICH. The risk of ICH increases when the underlying parenchyma is diseased (e.g., after acute ischemic stoke) or when the degree of systemic anticoagulation is high. Low-dose chronic anticoagulation is less risky. Patients are typically on anticoagulation for years before hemorrhages occur. Compared with ICH caused by hypertension, the duration of bleeding in anticoagulation-associated ICH may be many hours. The cellular or vascular events that lead to bleeding and the precise artery that bleeds have not been identified. ICH related to the administration of thrombolytic agents such as urokinase, streptokinase, or t-PA has been documented in nearly 1% of patients who received them for acute myocardial infarction. Hemorrhages are lobar and increase in frequency as the dose of thrombolytic agent is increased. ICH, in addition to SAH, occasionally occurs in patients with aneurysms and AVMs. Because AVMs are located within the brain parenchyma, and aneurysms lie in the subarachnoid space, ICH is more common with the bleeding of AVMs. Clues to the diagnosis of AVM-associated ICH include presentation early in life, lobar hemorrhage, a history of inherited malformation, or radiologic features suggestive of an underlying vascular lesion. Angiography usually confirms the diagnosis, but angiographically occult lesions may require MRI or surgical exploration for diagnosis. In young patients with typical clinical presentation, surgical exploration can be curative if the offending lesion is removed, thereby preventing recurrence of ICH.

## Clinical Presentation

The neurologic deficits associated with ICH are focal and rapid in onset, usually occurring when patients are active. Most patients attain their maximal deficit over a period of minutes or hours. The specific symptoms depend on the location of ICH. Bleeding closer to the midline produces brain stem compression and a more dire prognosis. If the blood extends to the cortex, an epileptogenic scar may occur. The breakdown products of blood in the spinal fluid may lead to hydrocephalus. Small ICH mimics the clinical picture of ischemic stroke.

## Diagnosis

A noncontrast CT scan is usually sufficient to diagnose all but the smallest ICH, in which case an MRI may be helpful. MRI, magnetic resonance angiography (MRA), and invasive angiography are performed when hypertension is absent or when the hemorrhage occurs in an atypical location. In young patients in whom an underlying vascular malformation is suspected, despite a negative angiogram, surgical exploration may be required.

## Therapy

The first step in the management of ICH is treatment of life-threatening raised intracranial pressure, which includes elevation of the head to 30 degrees above the horizontal, hyperventilation with maintenance of the carbon dioxide partial pressure between 25 and 30 mm Hg, avoiding hypotonic intravenous solution, and fluid restriction. Mannitol is the most commonly used osmotic agent, and should be given as a 20% solution at 1 g/kg over 15 minutes. Its effect lasts 3–4 hours, after which the brain and plasma osmolality equilibrate, requiring increasingly higher plasma osmolality for the same effect. Serum osmolality should be monitored to avoid levels above 320 mOsm/liter. Furosemide may be used in addition to mannitol, with close observation of serum and urine

*Table 7.4* Suggested algorithm for blood pressure control in tissue plasminogen activator candidates or patients with subarachnoid hemorrhage

| | |
|---|---|
| Diastolic blood pressure >140 mm Hg | Intravenous sodium nitroprusside (0.5–10.0 μg/kg/min) |
| Systolic blood pressure >230 mm Hg or diastolic blood pressure 121–140 mm Hg | Give 20 mg labetalol IV over 1–2 mins<br>(a) The dose may be repeated or doubled every 10 mins up to 150 mg or both.<br>(b) Alternatively, following the first bolus of labetalol, an IV infusion of 2–8 mg/min labetalol may be initiated and continued until the desirable blood pressure is reached.<br>(c) If satisfactory response is not obtained, use sodium nitroprusside.<br><br>Obtain blood pressure every 15 mins<br>Observe for hypotension |
| Systolic blood pressure is 180–230 mm Hg or diastolic blood pressure is 105–120 mm Hg on two readings 5–10 mins apart | Give 10 mg labetalol IV over 1–2 mins<br>(a) The dose may be repeated or doubled every 10–20 mins up to 150 mg.<br>(b) Alternatively, following the first bolus of labetalol, an IV infusion of 2–8 mg/min labetalol may be initiated and continued until desired blood pressure is reached.<br><br>Obtain blood pressure every 15 mins<br>Observe for hypotension |

electrolytes and for signs of dehydration and prerenal oliguria. No established role exists for the immediate use of corticosteroids, barbiturates, or intracranial pressure monitoring, and corticosteroids are potentially harmful in this setting.

The next step involves reducing significantly elevated blood pressure. Blood pressure that enters the range encountered in malignant hypertension (i.e., 200/120 mm Hg) is likely to exacerbate bleeding, but less severe hypertension is not treated. For treatment suggestions, see Table 7.4.

Patients must have any coagulopathy reversed as soon as possible. Fresh frozen plasma and vitamin K are used in patients on warfarin; protamine is administered to patients on heparin. Patients with platelet disorders and elevated bleeding time receive platelet transfusion. Hemophiliacs must receive their deficient coagulation factor. Treatment of ICH after thrombolysis is discussed above.

There are few guidelines for the use of antiepileptic drugs in patients with ICH. These agents are often unnecessary in patients with deep hemorrhage who have not had seizures. Many patients with superficial hemorrhage are treated before a convulsion, although this approach is of unproven benefit.

Prognosis

The size of the hemorrhage predicts survival and functional recovery. An estimation of hematoma volume can be obtained by measuring the greatest diameter ($A$), the perpendicular diameter ($B$) of the hematoma, and the thickness ($C$), by adding the number of 10-mm CT slices visualizing the hematoma. These values are multiplied, and the product ($A \times B \times C$) is divided by 2 to yield the approximate volume (in ml) of the hematoma. Overall mortality is approximately 40%. This figure increases to nearly 90% if the hematoma is larger than 60 ml in volume. Alternatively, survival with good recovery can be expected with hematomas less than 20 ml in volume. Survival at 30 days exceeds 90% if the hemorrhage is less than half a lobe in size, the patient's Glasgow Coma Score was more than 9 at admission, and pulse pressure is less than 40 mm Hg. In contrast, the probability for 30-day survival with coma, a hemorrhage larger than a lobe, and pulse pressure greater than 65 mm Hg is less than 10%.

ICH rarely recurs if hypertension is treated. The long-term functional outlook for medically treated patients is good. In most studies only about one in five patients is left with permanent severe neurologic deficit. The remainder make a good recovery and are able to resume independent lives with a mild neurologic deficit.


## ISCHEMIC STROKES

### Cardioembolic Stroke

Pathophysiology

Brain embolism may have various origins. Brain embolism caused by thrombus or microthrombus from a diseased artery may be distinguished from cardioembolic stroke because of differences in diagnostic tests and different preventive measures taken. Cardioembolic stroke accounts for about 20% of strokes in older patients, but a larger percentage in younger patients.

Factors that predispose to intracardiac thrombus formation include intracardiac blood stasis (atrial fibrillation, acute myocardial infarction, ventricular aneurysm, and cardiomyopathy); endocardial disruption (acute myocardial infarction or a prosthetic cardiac valve); systematic coagulopathy, and valvular vegetations associated with infective endocarditis. Intracardiac tumors such as atrial myxoma may also cause emboli. Paradoxical embolism, which is an arterial embolism of venous origin that traverses an intracardiac shunt, occurs more frequently than previously believed and appears to be particularly important in younger patients.

A series of brain infarcts involving the cortex or cerebellum in several vascular territories is highly suggestive of cardioembolic stroke. Cardioembolism may also involve the origins of the perforating arteries, resulting in subcortical infarcts.

Petechial hemorrhage may occur after cardioembolic infarction, and is termed *hemorrhagic infarction* or *hemorrhagic transformation*. Its frequency after cardioembolic stroke has been reported as 51–78% in autopsy studies and 2–50% on CT studies. Most are not symptomatic. In thrombotic stroke the frequency is

2–21% in autopsy series. Distal migration of embolic fragments with reperfusion of infarcted tissue is the presumed mechanism. Larger areas of infarction and older age appear to be associated with higher incidence of hemorrhagic transformation. Massive hemorrhagic transformation causing a symptomatic globular parenchymal hemorrhage resembling primary ICH is observed in approximately 10% of hemorrhagic transformation and is more likely to occur in patients treated with anticoagulants.

Nonvalvular atrial fibrillation (NVAF) is the most common cardiac disorder responsible for cardioembolic stroke. NVAF affects 3% of the population over 65 years of age. Patients with NVAF have a fivefold increased risk of stroke or an annual stroke incidence of 5%. If untreated, approximately one-third will experience a stroke. Subgroups with increased risk of stroke are older patients, those with congestive heart failure, coronary heart disease, a history of prior stroke or silent stroke on CT scan, and those with intracardiac thrombus. In contrast, atrial fibrillation (AF) in men under age 60 at the time of diagnosis without clinical, electrocardiographic, or chest x-ray evidence of other heart disease is associated with a very low risk of stroke, about 0.5% per year.

Acute myocardial infarction causes approximately 15% of all cardioembolic strokes. Patients with acute myocardial infarction experience evidence of systemic embolism 1–6% of the time, more often after anterior wall infarction. Mural thrombus usually develops within 7 days after an acute myocardial infarction. Embolic stroke is most likely to occur within the initial 4 weeks. Although chronic myocardial infarction is less likely to cause embolization, patients with ventricular aneurysm have a long-term potential for embolic stroke of approximately 13%. Pedunculated, mobile, or heterogenous thrombi are more apt to embolize than flat homogenous thrombi and may warrant anticoagulation.

Embolism has been reported in patients with dilated cardiomyopathy who do not receive anticoagulants, up to 12% per year. Brain embolism may be the presenting feature of cardiomyopathy.

Rheumatic heart disease, particularly mitral valve disease with AF, was the most important cause of cardioembolic stroke several decades ago. About 20% of unanticoagulated patients with mitral stenosis experience embolism over their lifetimes, with 60–75% having a brain embolism. Mechanical valves, especially in the mitral position, have a higher risk of embolization. Bioprosthetic valves also have the propensity to form emboli, but usually only in the first few months after surgery.

Investigations have demonstrated several possible cardiac sources of emboli that were not previously recognized, including mitral annulus calcification, calcific aortic stenosis, atrial septal aneurysm, and idiopathic hypertrophic subaortic stenosis. Their contribution to the overall incidence of cardioembolic stroke is very low.

For mitral valve prolapse, paradoxical embolism, infective endocarditis, and nonbacterial thrombotic endocarditis, see Stroke in Young Patients

Clinical Presentation

Patients with cardioembolic stroke typically have a history of coronary artery disease, AF, rheumatic heart disease, prosthetic valves, recent myocardial infarction, or cancer. Warning transient ischemic attacks (TIAs) are unusual. The only clinical features of stroke correlating with the presence of a cardiac source of emboli are diminished level of consciousness at stroke onset and a history of systemic embolism. Approximately 5–20% of patients develop symptoms gradually or intermittently at onset, which is probably attributable to repeated embolization at short intervals or to changes in the cerebral circulatory status following distal migration of emboli.

More than 70% of cardioembolic stroke occurs in the MCA territory. The posterior branch of the MCA is more frequently involved than the anterior branch, producing receptive aphasia and visual field deficit. Other syndromes often seen with cardioembolism include global aphasia without hemiparesis, rapid recovery from major hemispheric stroke symptoms (spectacular shrinking deficit), and "top of the basilar" syndrome. Isolated (posterior cerebral artery) PCA syndromes are also most often cardioembolic.

Diagnosis

An algorithm for approaching the diagnosis of all types of ischemic strokes is illustrated in Figure 7.1. Individual neurologic features of the stroke do not usually identify the stroke mechanism. CT and MRI studies of the brain may provide suggestive evidence for a cardioembolic stroke, such as infarction in other vascular territories, visualization of embolic material in the brain vessels (known as *dense MCA sign* on CT scan), and hemorrhagic infarction.

Physicians must be careful about the interpretation of ultrasound and angiography examinations in ischemic stroke patients. These patients have prominent vascular risk factors and may harbor concomitant but unrelated atherosclerotic vascular lesions. Before ordering tests, it is extremely important to decide if the findings would alter the clinical diagnosis.

Prolonged electrocardiogram (Holter) monitoring, up to 48 hours, may detect paroxysmal AF and the sick sinus syndrome in selected patients, especially those under the age of 50. Transthoracic echocardiography (TTE) is relatively insensitive for detecting small intraventricular thrombi and evaluating the atrium. Transesophageal echocardiography (TEE) and ultrafast CT scans have been reported to be more sensitive. TEE detects cardiac sources of embolism such as patent foramen ovale with right to left shunt, segmental hypokinesis/akinesis, an enlarged left atrium or left atrial thrombus, intracardiac mass (apical thrombus or tumor), valvular disease such as mitral valve prolapse, and stenotic or regurgitating lesions of mitral and aortic valves. Other findings that may be associated with stroke are spontaneous echocardiographic contrast, aortic arch debris, and valvular strands. In 6–25% of cases, patients with suspected cardioembolic stroke have no obvious cardiac source despite an extensive search.

TTE is performed on older patients with known cardiac disease in an attempt to find potential sources of emboli. In young stroke patients or in those with ischemic events of unknown or uncertain cause in whom the detection of a cardiac source would lead to a change in therapy, TEE is indicated. TEE is more sensitive and better defines the cardiac chambers and valves, improving detection of potential paradoxical embolism. Holter monitoring is performed in patients with

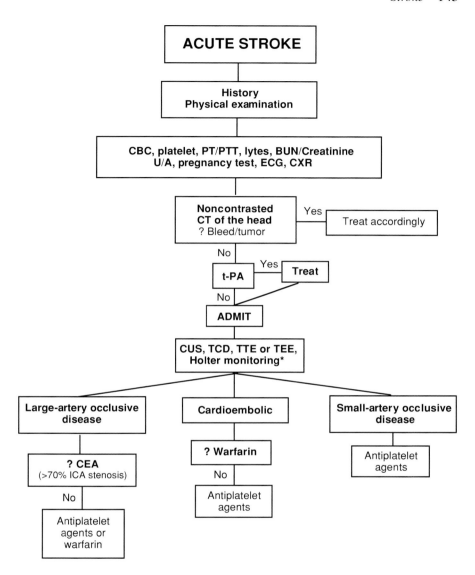

*Figure 7.1* A suggested algorithm for management of acute stroke. *All tests are not performed on all patients. (CBC = complete blood cell count; PT/PTT = prothrombin time/partial thromboplastin time; BUN = blood urea nitrogen; U/A = urinanalysis; ECG = electrocardiography; CXR = chest x-ray; CT = computed tomography; t-PA = tissue plasminogen; CUS = carotid ultrasound; TCD = transcranial Doppler; TTE = transthoracic echocardiography; TEE = transesophageal echocardiography; CEA = carotid endarterectomy; ICA = internal carotid artery.)

suspected cardiac dysrhythmia or in those who have otherwise had a normal cardiac evaluation but in whom the suspicion of cardiac embolism remains.

## Therapy

If the patient presents within 3 hours of stroke onset with no contraindication, t-PA should be considered. Intravenous hydration and immediate anticoagulation with heparin is often performed to prevent embolism within 2 weeks after stroke onset. Anticoagulation is held for the first 24 hours in patients who receive t-PA. Chronic anticoagulation is recommended for patients with cardioembolic stroke caused by rheumatic heart disease, NVAF, and other cardiac disease if there are no contraindications for anticoagulation and patients can be monitored carefully. In patients with anterior myocardial infarction, recurrent embolism is rare after several months. Long-term anticoagulation should be maintained only in those with ventricular wall motion abnormalities. Long-term anticoagulation is generally indicated, even if left ventricular thrombi are not demonstrated, in patients with non-ischemic cardiomyopathy, especially if AF is present. Patients with a mechanical valve in the mitral position have the greatest risk of emboli and need long-term anticoagulation. Anticoagulation is recommended for the first few months for patients with bioprosthetic valves, especially if they have concomitant AF.

## Prognosis

Embolism from a cardiac source often causes severe neurologic deficits or death. The stroke is often larger in size than infarction associated with other causes.

The risk of recurrence of cardioembolic stroke varies with the time after stroke onset, associated cardiac disease, as well as hematologic and hemodynamic conditions. Approximately 10% of patients with cardioembolic stroke experience a second embolic stroke within 2 weeks. Little difference in early recurrence rate is found between NVAF and other cardiac sources.

## Large-Artery Occlusive Disease

### Pathophysiology

Large-artery occlusive disease (LAOD) is primarily due to atherosclerosis. Patients often have associated coronary artery or peripheral vascular disease. Atherosclerosis located at the proximal portion of the (ICA) and the vertebral artery (VA) causes most neurologic symptoms. Atherosclerosis has a predilection for forming in the common carotid bifurcation and the first 2 cm of the ICA origin, sparing the remainder of the cervical ICA. Atherosclerosis may also affect the siphon region and the origin of the anterior cerebral artery (ACA) and MCA stem but to a lesser extent than the extracranial ICA. Atherosclerosis also affects the posterior circulation arteries. With increased use of TEE, atherosclerosis in the aortic arch has become recognized as another potential source of cerebral embolization and ischemia, although its clinical significance is still under study.

Atherosclerosis at the ICA origin is the principal underlying condition that leads to retinal and cerebral ischemia in patients with large artery occlusive disease. Two postulated mechanisms are vessel-to-vessel embolism or a low-perfusion state. These mechanisms may operate individually or concomitantly, and their impact varies based on the availability of effective collateral circulation. Plaque within the parent arteries may block or extend into a penetrator arterial branch or form microatheroma at the orifices of such a branch vessel, occluding the penetrating arteries.

Blood flow across the stenotic artery becomes impaired once more than 75% of its lumen has been lost. This narrowing may occur gradually, over years or decades, allowing for collateral blood flow to develop, thus avoiding stroke. Therefore, it is not uncommon to see asymptomatic patients with a total occlusion of one or more major cranial cervical arteries.

Coagulation disorders may lead to in situ thrombus formation in any artery, even without underlying arterial disease. This has been demonstrated in the extracranial ICA circulation. Cardiac emboli that are too large to pass the common carotid bifurcation may also block the ICA. For arterial dissection, fibromuscular dysplasia, and migraine, see Stroke in Young Patients.

## Clinical Presentation

Patients with LAOD typically have coronary heart disease, hypertension, myocardial infarction, diabetes, hyperlipidemia, or peripheral vascular disease. Men are more often affected than women. A carotid bruit is a relatively poor predictor of ICA stenosis in an asymptomatic patient and is noted in about 40% of patients with greater than 50% ICA diameter stenosis. TIAs in the territory of the diseased artery may have occurred over a period of days, weeks, or months preceding the stroke, although some strokes occur without TIAs. The stroke is maximal at onset or may be stepwise and stuttering. Headache is not uncommon, and nausea and vomiting occur, especially if the stroke is in the posterior circulation.

The location of the lesion is usually cortical and deep, suggesting a lesion larger than that produced by small-artery occlusive disease (SAOD), though individual neurologic features do not usually identify the stroke mechanism. Stroke from large artery occlusive disease varies in severity based on the size and location of the infarct.

## Diagnosis

CT scanning is often normal on the day of presentation, but reliably reveals a low-density lesion after 24 hours. The stroke is usually in the territory of one artery and is larger than a lacune. Carotid ultrasound (CUS), TCD, MRA, and invasive catheter angiography reveal the location and degree of the atherosclerosis. Compared with angiography, CUS has about 90% sensitivity for the identification of extracranial ICA disease. MRA has similar sensitivity but tends to overestimate the degree of stenosis. TCD is nearly 90% sensitive for distal ICA, siphon and proximal MCA/ACA stenosis. MRA may also be used for this purpose. Angiography confirms the presence of disease and allows precise measurements of the stenosis, as well as demonstrating carotid ulceration. Present angiographic techniques involve a 1–3% risk of stroke or death.

Every patient with a stroke should have CUS to determine whether carotid artery disease is present. TCD is helpful for evaluating the posterior circulation, as well as giving information about disease in the anterior intracranial circulation. MRA is also helpful in such patients and may be performed instead of ultrasound or to confirm ultrasound findings. Cerebral angiography is reserved for patients for whom findings on CUS, TCD, and MRA are conflicting or in preparation for surgery after ultrasound or MRA identify a surgical candidate.

## Therapy

Like patients with cardioembolic stroke, patients with LAOD should be considered for t-PA. General therapy includes keeping the patient's head level and avoiding major iatrogenic changes in blood pressure, blood volume, or cardiac output.

Randomized trials have demonstrated that carotid endarterectomy is superior to medical therapy alone for patients with greater than 70% symptomatic ICA stenosis on carotid angiography. Patients with stenosis less than 35% are, in most instances, inappropriate surgical candidates. Those with 35–70% stenosis are still under trial. Patients with no surgical lesion or who are not surgical candidates are usually treated with long-term antiplatelet agents (i.e., aspirin, ticlopidine, or clopidogrel). Warfarin may be used for patients with severe ICA disease who are unable to undergo surgery and for patients with severe intracranial stenosis.

The risk of nonfatal stroke is decreased by 23% in patients who are treated with aspirin. The appropriate dose, however, is controversial, varying from a low dose of 80 mg to a high dose of 1,300 mg per day. Most physicians prescribe 325 mg per day. Ticlopidine may be more effective than aspirin in decreasing the total number of nonfatal strokes during the first 12 months. The benefit at 2 years is minimal, however. Ticlopidine should be considered for aspirin-intolerant patients and those who have had recurrent spells during aspirin therapy, but do not have a disorder that may be more appropriately treated with warfarin. Clopidogrel has been shown to be as safe and probably slightly more effective than aspirin and clearly is safer than ticlopidine.

## Prognosis

Patients with LAOD have on average an annual risk for recurrent stroke of 5–10%, which is substantially lower than their cardiac morbidity and mortality.

## Small-Artery Occlusive Disease

### Pathophysiology

Another subgroup of ischemic stroke is caused by SAOD, accounting for approximately 15% of ischemic stroke. Almost all strokes due to SAOD occur in the territory of small penetrating arteries, the lenticulostriate, thalamoperforants, the paramedian branches of the basilar, and branches of the anterior choroidal artery.

Vessels involved by SAOD are less than 200 μm in diameter, rise directly from much larger arteries, and are unbranched end-arteries. The size of these penetrators varies. The resulting infarct is termed a *lacune*, or small fluid-filled cavity, and ranges from 0.2 to 15.0 μl in volume. Occlusion at the origin of a penetrator may yield a swath of infarction greater than 15 μl (called a *superlacune*).

Four major vascular processes are associated with lacunes: lipohyalinosis, atherosclerosis (microatheroma), presumed microembolism, and atherosclerotic plaque in the wall of the parent artery (mural plaque) that blocks the orifice of the penetrator artery. Lipohyalinosis affects small penetrating arteries, resulting in smaller lacunes, most of which are asymptomatic. This pathologic change occurs in the setting of chronic hypertension. In microatheroma, a miniature focus of atherosclerotic plaque forms in the penetrator vessel in patients with advanced hypertension. In microembolism, the vessel has a normal intrinsic pathology, but the lumen is occluded by embolus. Mural plaques may affect a penetrator at its origin, particularly in the basilar territory.

Chronic hypertension has a close relationship to in situ small-vessel diseases and is an important risk factor for lacunar stroke. A cerebral autosomal dominant arteriopathy with subcortical infarcts and leukoencephalopathy has been described. It is linked to chromosome 19q12 and is associated with recurrent stroke-like episodes, subcortical dementia, migraine-like headaches and depression. Patients with this condition do not have hypertension. Autopsy reveals nonamyloid and nonatherosclerotic angiopathy of small cerebral and leptomeningeal arteries with concentric deposition of a basophilic granulomatous material replacing smooth muscle cells of the media.

## Clinical Presentation

The essential clinical features of strokes resulting from SAOD can be attributed to their small size and unique locations. Four clinical subtypes have been described according to the associated neurologic symptoms (Table 7.5). Lacunar stroke results in restricted symptoms and a less severe outcome.

A relatively slow or stuttering mode of onset is observed in many lacunar stroke cases. As many as 30% develop over a period of up to 36 hours. The initial deficit intensifies or occasionally spreads into limbs not affected initially. A sudden onset occurs, however, in 40% of cases. TIAs are observed in 30% of patients with lacunar stroke. As compared with TIA associated with LAOD, lacunar TIAs are more likely to recur over days, rather than weeks or months.

Dementia, pseudobulbar palsy, and bilateral motor deficit caused by multiple bilateral lacunar lesions involving the basal ganglia, subcortex, and brain stem, with or without associated stroke symptoms, may occur.

## Diagnosis

The clinical diagnosis of lacunar stroke is made by the signs and symptoms that occur. Brain imaging studies may demonstrate a deep infarct in a penetrator ter-

*Table 7.5*    Classic lacunar syndrome

| Syndrome | Manifestation | Lesion sites |
|---|---|---|
| Pure motor hemiparesis | Hemiparesis in face, arm, leg | Corona radiata<br>Posterior limb of internal capsule (IC)<br>Basis pontis<br>Medullary pyramid |
| Pure sensory stroke | Hemisensory deficit | Thalamus (ventroposterior nucleus) |
| Ataxia hemiparesis | Hemiparesis + ipsilateral ataxia | Posterior limb of the IC<br>Corona radiata<br>Basis pontis |
| Dysarthria–clumsy-hand syndrome | Severe dysarthria and dysphagia + slight weakness and clumsiness of the hand | Dorsal-pontine<br>IC<br>Corona radiata |

ritory, smaller than 15 mm in diameter. Compared with CT scan, MRI is much more sensitive in detecting lacunar stroke. Brain stem lacunes can only be reliably seen with MRI, which may, however, fail to show the small infarct of pure sensory or pure motor stroke in the lowermost pons or smaller lacunes in the range of 3–4 mm. On the other hand, MRI is often sensitive enough to display asymptomatic lacunes. Therefore, a small lesion demonstrated on MRI does not always indicate a stroke.

When patients present with a lacunar syndrome, the danger exists of interpreting it as resulting from an SAOD process when in fact it is the early phase of a major carotid or basilar artery stroke. Deep brain infarcts caused by major arterial occlusive diseases should be routinely excluded, because the prognosis and therapeutic measures are different from those of SAOD. Thus, all patients are subject to CUS, TCD, or MRA evaluation. When cardioembolism or large-artery atherosclerosis is associated with a small deep infarct, the term lacune should be avoided.

## Therapy

Patients with SAOD that present within 3 hours of onset of stroke symptoms and have no contraindication should be considered for t-PA. Controlling chronic hypertension is the primary prevention of lacunar stroke. Aspirin and other antiplatelet agents also reduce the risk of recurrent stroke. Acute elevations in blood pressure are not treated, as discussed earlier.

Patients should be given appropriate hydration during the first days to avoid orthostatic hypotension and dehydration. Anticoagulant therapy is not recommended because it may cause brain hemorrhage through the arterial wall affected by lipohyalinosis. Patients with small strokes downstream from severe carotid disease or in association with atrial fibrillation are typically assumed to have suffered stroke as a result of those conditions and receive therapy directed at those disorders.

Prognosis

Patients with lacunar stroke show improvement in a large percentage of cases within days or months. The improvement in motor deficit is more rapid than in other artery occlusive diseases. In one study, 63% had no or minor residua, 26% had moderate residua, and 11% experienced severe hemiparesis. Most patients with lacunar stroke are alive 5 years after stroke onset. The recurrence rate of lacunar strokes is reported to be about 8% per year.

The following sections discuss several stroke-related syndromes, including TIA, asymptomatic carotid artery stenosis, stroke in the young, and stroke of unknown cause.

## Transient Ischemic Attacks

TIAs are abrupt, rapidly fading neurologic deficits of vascular origin. These are defined as lasting less than 24 hours, though duration is usually only 5–10 minutes. Transient monocular blindness may last as little as 10 seconds. CT scan may show small infarction in as many as 50% of TIA patients, though MRI is more sensitive in detecting these infarcts. Only 40% of thrombotic strokes are preceded by a TIA.

The two most usual causes of transient ischemia are cerebral emboli from a plaque in the extracranial cerebral arterial tree and cardiac sources of embolism. Less commonly, in the setting of a cerebral artery stenosis, a transient drop in blood pressure with associated cerebral hypoperfusion causes transient, focal neurologic symptoms.

Clinical Presentation

The symptom complex of TIAs is broad and depends on whether the episode takes place in the carotid or vertebrobasilar territories. The symptoms are identical to those of cerebral infarcts.

Diagnosis

Diagnosing TIA may be difficult as there is no satisfactory laboratory test to prove or disprove its occurrence. Conditions that mimic TIA should be excluded. TIAs do not produce unconsciousness or seizure and are almost never the cause of acute confusional states or vertigo alone. A common misdiagnosis is postictal monoparesis (Todd's paralysis), especially when the focal seizure is the result of a previous stroke. A less common alternative diagnosis is hypoglycemia following an insulin reaction in diabetics. Rarely, occult brain tumors produce transient neurologic symptoms that are indistinguishable from a TIA.

Noncontrasted CT scan of the head is obtained to rule out hemorrhage and non-hemorrhagic mass lesions. Small infarcts may produce transient symptoms and signs, though larger lesions that displace brain (e.g., subdural hematoma or brain tumors) may produce transient symptoms.

Evaluation is orderly and identical to that for LAOD, SAOD, or cardioembolism.

## Treatment

Treatment guidelines are identical to those described for LAOD, SAOD, or cardioembolism, depending on the abnormalities found by diagnostic tests. Patients with recurrent TIAs are often admitted briefly for antiplatelet therapy and further evaluation. Patients suspected of having a cardiac source of emboli are often anticoagulated with heparin while further evaluation is performed. If a cardiac source of emboli is found, they are switched to warfarin or otherwise placed on antiplatelet agents.

## Prognosis

About 33% of patients with TIAs have a stroke within 5 years; 20% occur in the first month and 50% within the first year.

## ASYMPTOMATIC CAROTID ARTERY STENOSIS

Patients who have not had ischemic symptoms may be found to have asymptomatic carotid disease when ultrasound is performed on the carotid arteries. In the Asymptomatic Carotid Artery Stenosis trial, carotid endarterectomy was performed with less than 3% perioperative morbidity and mortality. Patients with carotid artery stenosis greater than or equal to 60% had a 5-year risk for ipsilateral stroke or death of 5.1% in the surgical arm of the trial and 11% in the medical arm. Although the difference is statistically significant, the difference is not profound. Patients with good life expectancy should be fully informed of the risks and benefits and the surgical complication rate when offered carotid endarterectomy for asymptomatic ICA stenosis.

## STROKE IN YOUNG PATIENTS

Stroke in the young usually refers to stroke in patients under 45 years of age. The reported stroke incidence in young patients is much lower than that for older adults and accounts for 4–10% of all strokes. For adults 18–44 years old, however, cerebrovascular disease is twice as prevalent as multiple sclerosis.

The diagnosis and management of stroke needs to be tailored to the individual patient. Specific diagnosis for such patients is extremely important. Young patients who survive the initial injury may live for many years, and therefore the risk of recurrent stroke should be accurately defined. Because patients may be of reproductive age, genetic counseling is appropriate for inherited disorders responsible for stroke. Given the large number of possible tests and the associated risks and expense, a systematic approach is often useful. Valuable clues may be present in the history and examination (Table 7.6).

In patients over 60, 80% of strokes are ischemic, but in younger patients only 50% are ischemic. The lack of a satisfactory classification for ischemic

*Table 7.6*   Clinical clues to less common causes of stroke

| History/physical symptoms | Suspected condition | Evaluation |
|---|---|---|
| Fever | Endocarditis, meningitis | Blood cultures, cerebrospinal fluid examination, echocardiography |
| Recent neck injury or Horner's syndrome contralateral to motor or sensory deficits | Carotid dissection | Neck magnetic resonance imaging (MRI)/magnetic resonance angiography (MRA), angiography |
| History of sudden severe headache | Vasospasm after subarachnoid hemorrhage | Cerebral angiography |
| Thrombocytopenia, azotemia, purpura | Thrombotic thrombocytopenia purpura | Blood smear, conjunctival biopsy |
| Cancer | Marantic endocarditis | Echocardiography, D-dimer immunoassay |
| Evidence of systemic emboli | Cardioaortic source | Transesophageal echocardiography (TEE) |
| Sickle cell anemia | Large vessel stenosis | Carotid ultrasound, transcranial Doppler, MRA, cerebral angiography |
| Recent angiography | Cholesterol embolism | Skin and retinal examination, renal biopsy |
| Drug abuse | Endocarditis, amphetamine- and cocaine-related stroke | Toxicology screen, echocardiography, cerebral angiography |
| Chest or back pain | Aortic dissection | Chest x-ray, chest computed tomography scan, MRI |
| Recent ophthalmic zoster | Granulomatous angiitis | Cerebral angiography, meningeal biopsy |
| Livido reticularis, history of recurrent spontaneous abortion | Antiphospholipid antibody syndrome | Anticardiolipin antibody, lupus anticoagulant screening |
| Postpartum | Venous sinus thrombosis | Magnetic resonance venography, cerebral angiography |
| Deep vein thrombosis or pulmonary embolus | Paradoxical embolus | TEE |

stroke is even more of a problem for younger stroke patients than for older ones. Ischemic causes of stroke in young patients are hematologic (8%), cardiac (20%), vasculopathies (10%), dissection (15%), atherosclerosis (15%), other (12%), and undetermined (20%). ICH accounts for a large percentage of strokes in young patients.

The prognosis for recovery and the rate of recurrent stroke or death are better in younger patients. The mortality for younger stroke patients is about 5% and the overall incidence of recurrence is less than 1% per year. In most series, more than 75% of patients show significant improvement or return to normal. The more favorable outcome may be the result of higher frequency of migraine, trauma, and nonatheromatous etiologies in younger stroke patients. The prognosis and the need for secondary prevention varies widely with the stroke etiology. Therefore, a thorough evaluation for the underlying etiology is essential.

Table 7.7 provides a listing of stroke causes in young patients.

## INFARCTS OF UNKNOWN CAUSE

Patients with infarction of unknown cause present with symptoms attributable to either LAOD or cardioembolic stroke. CT scanning reveals a stroke larger than a lacune. They have normal angiography, ultrasound, Holter monitoring, and echocardiography. Normal angiography essentially rules out intrinsic atherosclerosis as the cause of the stroke. Cardioembolic stroke may be suspected, but the source of embolization cannot be detected. Treatment is based on a presumptive guess of the patient's stroke mechanism. One approach is to anticoagulate with warfarin for a short time, perhaps 3 months. The patient is then reevaluated for a source of embolus. If a source is detected, specific therapy is undertaken. Alternatively, these patients may be treated with antiplatelet agents. Some physicians may elect to evaluate the patient for unusual causes of stroke, as illustrated in Table 7.7.

## GENERAL CARE OF THE STROKE PATIENT

Medical complications of stroke are common and serious. Concomitant myocardial infarction occurs in 10% of all stroke patients. Deep venous thrombosis (DVT) and consequent pulmonary embolism are common. Measures to prevent it should be implemented soon after admission and continued until the patient is no longer at high risk. Risk factors for DVT include immobility, advanced age, congestive heart failure, lower-extremity trauma, major surgery, obesity, history of DVT, and cancer. Treatment choices include intermittent pneumatic compression stockings or low-dose unfractionated heparin (5,000 units twice a day subcutaneously) and low-molecular-weight heparin (enoxaparin, 30 mg twice a day subcutaneously).

Urinary sepsis and incontinence are common in stroke patients. Catheterization should be performed to avoid skin breakdown and keep the bladder decompressed in cases of retention. Intermittent straight catheterization is preferable to continuous catheterization. Large, unilateral hemisphere lesions may lead to urinary retention or hyperactive bladder. In those patients, postvoid residual volume should be measured by catheterization. If the volume is elevated, intermittent straight catheterization may be required. If patients remain incontinent and postvoid residuals are low, then a diaper or pharmacologic blockade of the paralyzed bladder may be needed. Urinary tract infection must be ruled out in all patients with bladder dysfunction.

Aspiration pneumonia is another frequent complication of stroke. Avoid oral feeding of patients with acute brain stem stroke, especially those with impaired gag reflexes. Patients with significant impairment of consciousness should not be fed orally. A nasogastric tube or intravenous fluid may be used acutely. If swal-

*Table 7.7* Causes of stroke in young patients

| | |
|---|---|
| **Vasculopathies** | |
| Atherosclerosis | Genetic traits associated with premature atherosclerosis, risk factors such as hypertension, diabetes, a history of smoking or lipid abnormalities. |
| Arterial dissection | Spontaneous or related to minor trauma such as vomiting, sneezing, coughing, neck movements, or other routine activities. |
| Venous occlusive disease | Associated with hypercoagulability due to pregnancy, cancer, infection, dehydration, or other hematological disorders; magnetic resonance venography is the diagnostic test of choice. |
| Fibromuscular dysplasia | Relationship to clinical symptoms controversial; angiographic patterns vary, but the "string of beads" configuration predominates, a reflection of localized, concentric, narrowing from media involvement. |
| Moyamoya | Occlusion of one or both internal carotid arteries (ICAs) (later involving proximal intracranial vessel) leads to the formation of the collateral network at the base of the brain. Symptoms vary from asymptomatic, headaches, stroke to severe mental retardation. |
| **Cardiac causes** | |
| Paradoxical embolus | Patent foramen ovale, atrial septal defect, ostium secundum, and pulmonary arteriovenous malformaion can cause stroke by bypassing the pulmonary capillary bed; anticoagulation if there is evidence for peripheral venous thrombosis; closure of the pulmonary or cardiac conduit should be considered. |
| Mitral valve prolapse | Estimated stroke risk is <0.01% per year. |
| Myxomas | Cause stroke by embolization—most often tumor fragment; surgical treatment is usually curative. |
| Nonbacterial (marantic) thrombotic endocarditis | Suspected when ischemic stroke occurs in patient with malignancy or a chronic wasting illness. |
| **Hematologic causes** | |
| Sickle cell anemia | Transfusion therapy is used both to treat acute stroke and for secondary prevention; transcranial Doppler is used for screening, as transfusion therapy lowers the risk of stroke in patients with middle cerebral artery and ICA velocities >200 cm/sec. |
| Platelet disorders | Both primary and secondary platelet abnormalities contribute to stroke in young patients due to microvascular thrombosis. |
| Activated protein C resistance | Carries sevenfold increased risk of developing deep venous thrombosis and is currently being studied as a cause for stroke; DNA analysis from a blood sample is required for diagnosis. |
| Protein C and protein S deficiency | Most deficiencies are acquired; associated with malignancies, liver disease, hemodialysis, antiphospholipid antibodies, postoperative states, disseminated intravascular coagulation, some antibiotics, and warfarin. |
| Antithrombin III | Most cases are acquired, associated with severe hepatic and renal disease and oral contraceptives. |
| Paroxysmal nocturnal hemoglobinopathy | Disorder of younger adults that may result in venous thrombosis in the brain and liver; arterial occlusion has been postulated, but is rare. |
| Polycythemias | Ischemic stroke parallels the hematocrit and occurs in 10–20% of patients; in secondary polycythemias the risk of stroke is lower. |

*Table 7.7*   (continued)

| Rheumatologic and autoimmune causes | |
|---|---|
| Antiphospholipid antibody syndrome | Check for anticardiolipin antibody and lupus anticoagulant. |
| Systemic lupus erythematosus | An association with antiphospholipid antibody as well as vascular and valvular lesions has implicated systemic lupus erythematosus as a cause of stroke. |
| Vasculitis | Many types associated with strokes; categorized as follows: (1) inflammatory (Takayasu's disease, allergic [Churg-Strauss] and granulomatous angitis), (2) vasculitis associated with infection (syphilis, mucormycosis, herpes zoster, tuberculosis, malaria, acquired immunodeficiency syndrome, and neuroborreliosis), (3) drugs (amphetamines, cocaine, and pseudoephinephrine), or (4) associated with systemic disease (systemic lupus erythematosus, Wegener's granulomatosis, rheumatoid arteritis, Sjögren's syndrome, scleroderma, acute rheumatic fever, sarcoidosis, Earl's disease, and inflammatory bowel disease); most of those diseases are associated with systemic manifestations. Another, but uncommon, form of vasculitis is isolated (granulomatous) angiitis of the central nervous system, which often occurs in younger patients; meningeal biopsy is often needed for definite diagnosis. |
| Infectious causes | |
| Endocarditis | Risk factors for infectious endocarditis are congenital or acquired heart disease, prosthetic valves, IV drug use, hemodialysis, and immunosuppression; serial blood clutters are essential for diagnosis and treatment; echocardiography can identify vegetations as small as 2 mm and thus establish the diagnosis. |
| Human immunodeficiency virus | Most common pathologic finding is multifocal microvascular disease, associated with thickening of the intraparenchymal arterioles; a nonbacterial thrombotic or an inflammatory vasculopathy is also seen secondary to cryptococcal or tuberculosis meningitis, lymphoma, or herpes zoster. |
| Hormone | |
| Birth control pills | Implicated as a cause of ischemic stroke, and possibly subarachnoid hemorrhage (SAH); risk is higher in those who also smoke or have migraine |
| Pregnancy, peripartum and postpartum period | Associated with increased incidence of stroke possibly as a result of vascular hypoplasia, hypercoagulable state, anemia, sepsis, and dehydration. Cardiomyopathy, amniotic fluid, or air may cause embolization. Arterial dissection can occur during delivery. Eclampsia and hypertension may cause superior sagittal sinus thrombosis, intracranial hemorrhage (ICH), and SAH. |
| Migraine | Most neurologists restrict the diagnosis to those with a history of classic migraine with aura; some additionally require that the deficit be similar to the migraine aura. Diagnosis should only be made after a full evaluation for other etiologies. |
| Drugs and alcohol | |
| Drugs | ICH is associated with sympathomimetics (amphetamine and phencyclidine); cocaine and crack cocaine can cause both types of strokes. Prescription drugs like phenylpropanolamine |

| | |
|---|---|
| | (Dexatrim), pentazocine lactate (Talwin-pyribenzamine), and methylphenidate (Ritalin) are associated with ICH. In most patients, hemorrhage occurs soon after the drug is ingested, regardless of whether they are habitual or first-time users. |
| Alcohol | Alcohol can lead to ischemic stroke through the induction of cardiac dysrhythmias, cardiac wall motion abnormalities, hypertension, enhanced platelet aggregation, activation of coagulation factors, vasospasm, and altered cerebral blood metabolism. Chronic abuse of alcohol can also lead to ICH, probably through its effects on the coagulation and platelets and by acutely elevating the blood pressure. |
| Miscellaneous | |
| Homocysteine | Patients heterozygous for the enzyme deficiency (as many as 1 in 70 of the population) and those with the acquired form have an increased risk of stroke; modest elevation of homocysteine levels may occur in up to 25% of young stroke patients. The heterozygous state is diagnosed by measuring homocysteine levels after methionine loading. Homocystinuria and elevated levels of homocysteine often respond to dietary manipulation and treatment with folic acid or vitamin $B_6$. |
| Mitochondrial myopathy, encephalopathy, lactic acidosis, and stroke-like episode (MELAS) | Presents in childhood; patients typically have short stature, seizures, hemiparesis, or cortical blindness. Ragged red fibers (typical for mitochondrial myopathies) are seen on muscle biopsy. Ischemic stroke has been associated with this syndrome; however, many of the "stroke-like episodes" in MELAS syndrome do not correspond to a single vascular territory. |

lowing is impaired, a rigorous evaluation by an occupational therapist or a speech therapist should be obtained.

Bed sores may be avoided by frequent position changes and the use of "egg crate" mattresses. Shoulder dislocation must be suspected if patients have severe arm weakness. The patient may complain of pain in the affected shoulder. The prudent use of physical therapy begun soon after stroke can prevent contracture. Depression should be aggressively diagnosed and treated because it can make rehabilitation difficult.

## STROKE UNITS

Trends reflect the growing interest in wards dedicated to stroke care, staffed by physicians, nurses, and therapists experienced with this disorder and following a meticulous, organized care plan. Patients treated in stroke units have better outcome compared with those treated in general medical wards, reflected in greater and more rapid functional recovery, shorter hospitalization, fewer nursing home placements, fewer medical complications, and lower mortality. Benefits may be attributed to a standardized approach, intensified observation, earlier physical and occupational therapy, and more aggressive mobilization.

## REHABILITATION

Stroke rehabilitation is the primary therapeutic intervention after the initial hospital phase. It is costly, accounting for nearly one-third of the cost of stroke treatment. Stroke rehabilitation is complex, as it coordinates medical, neurologic, physiologic, social, vocational, and physical measures for training and retraining the patient to the highest possible level of functional ability by an interdisciplinary team of physicians and nurses as well as physical, occupational, and speech therapists, recreational therapists, dietitians, psychologists, social workers, administrators, case managers, and pastoral-care providers. Rehabilitation addresses all facets of a patient's life affected by stroke. Stroke rehabilitation is effective, with an effect comparable to acute interventions such as t-PA.

Stroke rehabilitation is based on four principles: prevention of secondary complications, treatment to reduce neurologic impairment, compensation and adaptation to reduce disability, and maintaining function over the long term. Rehabilitation seeks to improve the functional independence and quality of life for the stroke patient. The domain of rehabilitation extends beyond the traditional medical mode, and is centered on the patient, his or her disabilities, and the handicap that ensues from these disabilities. This focus extends from weeks to years after the initial event.

## SUGGESTED READING

Barnett HJM, et al. Stroke: Pathophysiology, Diagnosis and Management (2nd ed). New York: Churchill Livingstone, 1992.
Fisher M. Clinical Atlas of Cerebrovascular Disorders. St. Louis: Mosby–Year Book, 1993.
Weksler BB. Hematologic disorders and ischemic stroke. Curr Opin Neurol 1995;8:38–44.
Wiebers DO, Feigin VL, Brown RD Jr. Cerebrovascular Disease in Clinical Practice. Boston: Little, Brown, 1996.

# 8
# Electrolyte Disorders

Robert Laureno

Electrolyte disorders may be manifested by neurologic problems ranging from coma to muscle cramps. On this spectrum are headache, depression, weakness, tetany, and seizures. For these and many other symptoms, the neurologist should consider electrolyte disorders in the differential diagnosis. Appropriate correction of electrolyte disorders can relieve neurologic symptoms and save lives. Correction of these disorders can be dangerous, however; rapid normalization can cause severe neurologic disease in some situations. This chapter discusses the major neurologic features and issues for each electrolyte disorder.

## HYPONATREMIA

Neurologists typically encounter hyponatremia in inpatients when they are consulted for drowsiness, obtundation, stupor, coma, delirium, confusion, or convulsions. As documented in experimental hyponatremia in normal volunteers, the chief complaint also may be cramps, weakness, decreased taste sensation, fatigue, dullness, headache, tremor, or dizziness. Nausea and vomiting may also occur. These manifestations can occur in isolation or in combination.

Hyponatremia may accentuate underlying neurologic problems. It can lower seizure threshold in an epileptic; it can worsen edema around a brain tumor and thereby cause or accentuate focal signs such as hemiparesis; and it can elicit transient hemiparesis related to a previously asymptomatic cerebral infarct. Occasionally hyponatremia can cause reversible hemiparesis in the absence of an identifiable underlying lesion.

Duration and rapidity of onset of hyponatremia are important determinants of the clinical manifestations. More than one-third of Daggett's patients with serum sodium below 120 mEq/liter were without neurologic symptoms, perhaps because the hyponatremia evolved slowly. These data imply that a relatively mild complaint of malaise, cramps, headache, or vomiting occasionally has as its basis severe hyponatremia (Na <110 mEq/liter). On the other hand, status epilepticus can be caused by a sudden drop of serum Na to 125 mEq/liter.

Brain swelling has been described in autopsied animals and humans who have died from hyponatremia. Rarely, reversible cerebral edema resulting from acute water intoxication has been demonstrated by cranial computed tomographic (CT) scans. Fatal hyponatremic cerebral edema would occur more often, were it not for the brain's compensatory mechanism.

Adaptation begins within hours of the onset of severe hyponatremia. Initially a loss of brain electrolytes occurs, primarily potassium. The resultant decrease in intracellular osmolality prevents the brain from swelling as much as it would have and is thereby protective. In addition to the electrolyte response, loss of organic osmolytes from brain cells provides protection from brain swelling by further decreasing intracellular osmolality. Loss of amino acids such as taurine, sugar alcohols such as myoinositol, and other molecules contribute. When severe hyponatremia is prolonged for 2 weeks, the brain water content returns to control levels. In other words, complete brain adaptation to chronic hypo-osmolality eventually occurs.

When compensatory mechanisms are inadequate to cope with acute water intoxication, ominous symptoms such as bizarre, agitated behavior, coma, or status epilepticus may be followed by death. On the other hand, even extreme hyponatremia, when less symptomatic, does not carry the same degree of risk. In Sterns' (1987) prospective study of 62 consecutive patients with severe hyponatremia (Na ≤110 mEq/liter), the mortality rate was only 8%. Most of the deaths were attributable to the underlying disease rather than the hyponatremia itself. In an experimental animal cohort, little morbidity results from a slow drop in mean serum Na concentration to 111.6 mEq/liter, even when severe hyponatremia is sustained for 2–5 weeks.

The poor prognosis attributed to hyponatremia in some other reports may relate to the treatment as much as the hyponatremia itself. Many reports of morbidity and mortality concern patients treated with 3% sodium chloride (NaCl) to raise the serum Na level above 130 mEq/liter. Detailed autopsy information is seldom included in such articles. Often, the patients have awakened from coma with correction of hyponatremia and then, within days, have relapsed into coma. This biphasic course is typical of myelinolysis, a disease caused by rapid correction of hyponatremia.

## Myelinolysis after Correction of Hyponatremia

Rapid correction of hyponatremia can result in neurologic worsening resulting from myelinolysis in the center of the pons and in symmetric extrapontine regions. The characteristic clinical manifestations are tetraplegia and pseudobulbar palsy. Early in the illness the neurologist may be consulted for mutism, behavioral change, or confusion.

Myelinolysis is the term selected by Adams et al. (1959) to distinguish the unique histologic features of this disorder from other demyelinative diseases. Loss of myelin and oligodendroglial cells, relative sparing of neurons and axons, and lack of inflammation are the essential microscopic features. Macrophages swollen with myelin debris permeate the lesion in recent or old lesions. In older lesions, fibrillary gliosis may develop. In the center of a lesion, axons and neurons may be severely affected.

In humans, the classic myelinolytic lesion is at the center of the basis pontis. From the symmetry and stereotyped location of this lesion, Adams et al. deduced that some metabolic cause for this disease existed. Only later reports showed the association of extrapontine lesions, which are present in about 10% of autopsied cases reported. Typically, extrapontine lesions occur symmetrically in the thalamocapsular regions and more or less symmetrically in subcortical patches. Symmetric neostriatal, mesencephalic, lateral geniculate, and cerebellar lesions may occur. Usually, extrapontine lesions accompany a sizable central pontine lesion. Cases exist, however, in which major extrapontine lesions occur with modest pontine involvement.

Typically there is a biphasic neurologic course in which there is improvement from the encephalopathy of hyponatremia, after which there is neurologic worsening resulting from myelinolysis. This new neurologic syndrome usually occurs about the third day after correction when speech difficulty and generalized weakness emerge. Over days, pseudobulbar palsy and tetraplegia develop. Many variations are seen on this standard profile of the illness. In some patients there is no perceived improvement in the hyponatremic encephalopathy before the manifestations of myelinolysis appear; in other words the two encephalopathic conditions merge. Sometimes the onset may be delayed as long as a week or more after correction. Occasionally there is transient mild neurologic worsening after correction of hyponatremia. This passing encephalopathy may have no anatomic correlate or may leave minimal lesions. Certainly it is not rare for central pontine myelinolysis to be found at autopsy when the medical record shows no evidence of a related neurologic event. These are so-called asymptomatic lesions.

Classic central pontine myelinolysis (CPM) can cause tetraplegia and pseudobulbar palsy. In extreme cases, the locked-in syndrome may occur. The tetraplegia may be flaccid or spastic. Tendon reflex hyperactivity and Babinski's signs are typically present. Rarely, the paresis is asymmetric enough to be described as hemiparesis. At times, the arms are affected more than the legs because the lesion is in the midline of the pons, where the corticospinal fibers for the arms are more medial than those for the legs. The pseudobulbar features include dysarthria, dysphagia, emotional lability, and facial paresis; dysarthria and muteness are common features. When the pontine lesion extends from the rostral basis pontis to the caudal pons, unilateral or bilateral sixth-nerve palsy may occur. With tegmental involvement, internuclear ophthalmoplegia, Horner's syndrome, and other neuroophthalmic features may occur. When the pontine lesion extends into the tegmentum, damage to the reticular activating system may result in coma.

Clinicopathologic correlation is less simple when extrapontine lesions are also present. Subcortical, thalamocapsular, and neostriatal lesions all may be factors contributing to coma. Extrapontine lesions may also cause emotional disorders and cognitive problems. The thalamocapsular lesions can contribute as much to paralysis as the pontine lesion. Subcortical lesions may result in seizures. Neostriatal lesions cause movement disorders, and cerebellar lesions can cause tremor. Lateral geniculate lesions have been reported to cause homonymous "hourglass" visual field defects.

Recovery from myelinolysis is variable. No evidence exists for benefit from treatment with steroid medication given after myelinolysis is clinically manifest. Patients may remain comatose and tetraplegic until death. On the other hand, locked-in patients may improve dramatically. Some patients regain satisfactory use of the limbs but continue to have severe speech problems. Any feature that appears in the initial days or weeks may be persistent. Sometimes gradual improvement of tetraparesis allows the appearance of dystonic or ataxic features not previously evident.

Central pontine and extrapontine myelinolysis may appear on CT brain scans as radiolucent lesions. On magnetic resonance imaging (MRI), the lesions may show increased signal intensity on the T2-weighted images and decreased signal intensity on the T1-weighted images. Lesion size on imaging does not always correlate with the severity of neurologic signs. Relatively asymptomatic patients may have sizable lesions on imaging. On the other hand, a tetraplegic patient with myelinolysis may have no abnormality on repeated CT scans. MRI scans are clearly more sensitive than CT scans. Early in the disease, however, MRI as well as CT scanning often fail to detect lesions that repeat scans show 1–2 weeks later. CT and MRI images of myelinolytic lesions often improve on sequential studies over the first year.

Other diagnostic tests are much less specific. Cerebrospinal fluid (CSF) protein may be normal or elevated. The CSF cell count is usually normal. Myelin basic protein has been found to be elevated in a few patients. The electroencephalogram (EEG) typically shows diffuse slowing which may last for weeks, months, or even years depending on the severity and location of lesions. In other cases the EEG may show paroxysmal features, burst suppression, low voltage, or focal slowing. Brain stem auditory evoked potentials may indicate a pontine lesion before imaging studies disclose abnormality. Typically, prolongation of the wave I–V interpeak latency or I–III latency are described. Similar to the EEG abnormalities, these findings may improve over time, sometimes when there is no improvement in imaging or neurologic state.

How rapid correction of hyponatremia causes myelinolysis is unknown. Rapid correction of sustained severe hyponatremia causes brain dehydration. The concentrations of brain K and nonelectrolyte solutes (organic osmolytes) decline in the process of adaptation to hyponatremia and cannot return quickly to normal levels. Thus, during rapid correction of hyponatremia, the brain cells are hypotonic to the normalizing extracellular fluid, which by osmosis draws water from the brain. Nevertheless, it is unclear how brain dehydration or related chemical changes of rapid correction results in damage to specific brain regions such as the center of the basis pontis.

## Treatment of Hyponatremia

Moderating the rate of correction of hyponatremia lessens the incidence of myelinolysis. On the other hand, acute water intoxication can itself cause death; thus the physician must weigh the risks of hyponatremia against the risks of too-rapid correction. If the patient is not convulsing, conservative measures such as water restriction and discontinuation of diuretics or other drugs allow the serum Na to rise slowly. Saline administration may be considered if the patient is convulsing or highly agitated. If hypertonic saline is prescribed, it should be given in 100-ml bottles to avoid any possibility of accidental infusion of a large volume. Caution is also necessary when a large amount of isotonic saline is given, as this method may also result in myelinolysis. Saline treatment should be reassessed as soon as the convulsions are terminated and the patient is stable. Whenever possible, serum Na should be elevated less than 10 mEq/liter over any 24-hour period.

When prescribing saline, the physician must remember that a saline dose will not necessarily raise the serum Na to the target. Administering an amount of 3% saline calculated to increase serum Na to a target level is a reliable method only in the statistical sense; the mean postcorrection level will approximate the target. There is marked individual variation in response to therapy, however. The unpredictability of the individual's response necessitates frequent monitoring of serum Na during the correction. When the Na rises to an unexpectedly high level, relowering of the Na has been shown to be beneficial in experimental animals and should be considered in humans. Deamino-8-D-arginine vasopressin (DDAVP), hypotonic fluid administration, or both may be administered with careful monitoring of serum Na.

## HYPERNATREMIA

Symptoms of hypernatremic encephalopathy may range from mild confusion to stupor and coma. When serum Na exceeds 160 mEq/liter, only 11% of hypernatremic patients are fully alert. Agitation is an occasional feature of this condition, and seizures or even status epilepticus may occur. Occasionally tremor, chorea, or myoclonic jerks are seen. The CSF protein is often elevated; the EEG can be surprisingly normal. The neurologic manifestations are more severe when hypernatremia is extreme or when it develops acutely. In chronic hypernatremia, symptoms may be absent even at a level of 175 mEq/liter.

In acute hypernatremia, brain shrinkage and a variety of cerebrovascular pathologies may occur. Subdural hemorrhage, subarachnoid hemorrhage, cerebral hemorrhages, and petechiae are typical; cerebral vein or sinus thrombosis with cerebral infarction may occur. Much of the cerebral bleeding has been attributed to a sudden drop in intracranial pressure with acute hypernatremia. Those patients, who die in hypernatremia but have no hemorrhage at autopsy, usually have developed hypernatremia less rapidly. A few case reports suggest that hypernatremia may cause symmetric myelinolytic lesions, but this has yet to be experimentally confirmed.

The neurologic manifestations of hypernatremia are minimized by osmoprotective mechanisms. Because NaCl is primarily an extracellular salt, hypernatremia results in osmotic movement of intracellular water to the extracellular compartment. The brain, however, in acute hypernatremia does not lose as much water as expected. Even during the first hours of acute hypernatremia, uptake of plasma K by brain cells increases intracellular osmolality, thereby lessening brain cell shrinkage. In addition to K, a variety of organic osmolytes accumulate intracellularly to provide osmotic protection. These include glutamine, taurine, myoinositol, trimethylamines, and betaine.

Unfortunately the increased intracellular amines and polyols, which have accumulated for osmoprotection, do not diminish quickly. As extracellular osmolality rapidly declines during therapy for the hypernatremia, the brain's elevated organic osmolytes draw water intracellularly, and the brain swells. This brain edema correlates with neurologic deterioration during rehydration. Focal and generalized seizures occur with rehydration but can be avoided if the decline in serum Na is less than 0.5 mEq/liter per hour.

Some texts suggest normalizing hypernatremia over 48 hours. This method is satisfactory for moderate to severe hypernatremia. For extreme hypernatremia, however, the guideline of 12 mEq/liter every 24 hours is safer.

## HYPOKALEMIA

Generalized weakness is the primary neurologic manifestation of hypokalemia. Weakness may be episodic but typically is subacute or chronic. Occasionally, the weakness is acute, evolving over hours.

When K is greater than 2.5 mEq/liter, prominent weakness is rare. Some patients, however, with minimal depression of serum K (3.0–3.5 mEq/liter) have malaise, muscle weakness, fatigue, or restless legs. The author has seen mildly hypokalemic patients with muscle cramps or myalgia that respond to K supplementation. When the K is less than 2.0 mEq/liter, weakness to some degree is usually present. In a series of six patients with K depletion myopathy (Comi et al., 1985), the K ranged from 1.1 to 2.3 mEq/liter. The weakness affects the limbs more proximally than distally. When weakness is severe, toe and finger wiggling may be the only retained extremity movements. Muscles of respiration and neck flexor muscles may be involved. Rarely are facial muscles affected; extraocular muscles are spared. Although quadriparesis may occur in patients with a K level of 2.0 mEq/liter or less, other patients are able to walk despite K at that level. There is a case on record with serum K as low as 1.4 mEq/liter with leg pain as the only major complaint. Another documented patient had remarkable sparing of arm strength with K of 0.8. There is no simple correlation between severity of weakness and severity of hypokalemia. Deep tendon reflexes are often retained, but areflexia may accompany severe weakness. In the latter case the neurologist in the emergency room may suspect Guillain-Barré syndrome. There is no sensory involvement in hypokalemic weakness, however.

Sometimes the serum creatine phosphokinase is elevated when the K level falls below 3.0 mEq/liter. As a rule, however, muscle enzyme elevation does not occur until the serum K falls below 2.5 mEq/liter. When rhabdomyolysis occurs, light microscopy shows focal fiber necrosis with phagocytosis and fiber regeneration. Vacuoles are occasionally seen.

Electromyographic findings in hypokalemic weakness include abundant brief, small, polyphasic motor unit potentials. Moderate numbers of fibrillations are commonly seen and pseudomyotonic discharges occur. Electrical inexcitability of muscle is present.

The mechanism of hypokalemic weakness is unknown. Acute weakness is believed to relate to alterations in muscle membrane polarization. Once rhabdomyolysis has occurred, the weakness is in part the result of muscle necrosis. Rhabdomyolysis in K deficiency may be precipitated by muscular exertion, convulsions, fasting, or fever.

In the presence of alkalosis, hypokalemia can cause tetany. In one case, hypokalemia was reported to cause tetany in the absence of alkalosis. Paradoxically, hypokalemia protects against tetany in the presence of hypocalcemia. Thus, when hypocalcemia is undiagnosed, the correction of coexistent hypokalemia can precipitate hypocalcemic tetany.

## HYPERKALEMIA

Although weakness almost always occurs when the serum K exceeds 9 mEq/liter, exceptions to this rule may exist. Usually no weakness is present unless the serum K exceeds 7 mEq/liter, but rarely weakness does occur with K less than 6 mEq/liter. Weakness may be gradually progressive or may occur in intermittent episodes. Such episodes typically last for hours, but they may be less than an hour or more than a day in duration. Flaccid tetraplegia can occur, and weakness of this severity also may be episodic. Proximal muscles may be disproportionately affected. Typically, cranial nerves are spared; however, facial weakness, dysarthria, and dysphagia may occur. Respiration may be so affected as to require mechanical ventilation; death from respiratory arrest has been reported. Deep tendon reflexes are usually depressed or absent. The patient often complains of numbness or burning paresthesias, but position and vibratory sense loss in the lower extremities are only inconsistently reported.

Not surprisingly, this constellation of symptoms and signs sometimes results in an incorrect diagnosis of Guillain-Barré syndrome; the paresthesias and the areflexia do suggest peripheral nerve involvement. Consistent is the retained mechanical irritability of muscle (contraction in response to percussion), suggesting that muscle is not inexcitable. This combined evidence points to the peripheral nerve as the primary site of physiologic dysfunction.

Severe symptomatic hyperkalemia may be treated immediately by infusing calcium to antagonize the membrane effects and thereby prevent arrhythmia. Additional treatments are intended to increase the transfer of extracellular K from the body (e.g., cation exchange resin, dialysis, or diuretic) or to reverse the specific cause of the hyperkalemia.

## HYPOCALCEMIA

The neurologic manifestations of hypocalcemia include tetany, obtundation, confusion, seizures, increased intracranial pressure, and other features. These phenomena may occur separately or in various combinations in the same patient.

Tetany is a syndrome of sensory symptoms and painful muscle contractions that occur and abate in a characteristic sequence. When tetany is mild, only the earlier stages of the sequence may be manifest. The earliest symptoms are a generalized ill feeling with paresthesias of the hands, feet, and perioral region. The initial involuntary muscle contractions occur in the distal muscles. As a rule, upper extremities are affected first. The stronger muscles predominate and thereby determine the postures assumed. Initially, adduction of the thumbs occurs; followed by flexion at the metacarpophalangeal joints and extension of the fingers. Eventually sequential flexion of the wrists, bending of the elbows, adduction of the arms, and supination of the forearms occur. The contorted hands are brought in front of the chest.

All regions of the body may be affected. Tetanic extension of the legs and plantar flexion of the toes can be very painful. In more severe cases opisthotonos may result.

Tetanic contractions may be very brief. Untreated patients may have intermittent brief episodes of stridor or carpopedal spasm for many years. On the other hand, tetanic contractions can persist for days at a time. As tetanic cramps clear, the muscles relax in reverse order of the sequence of contraction. Consciousness and clarity of thought are unaffected with uncomplicated tetanic episodes.

Tests are available to demonstrate latent tetany. Chvostek's sign is present when contraction of the facial muscles follows percussion of the ipsilateral facial nerve anterior to the external auditory meatus. In severe cases, the entire side of the face may contract. Unless the periocular muscles contract, the test should be considered negative. Approximately 8% of normal individuals have Chvostek's sign. Trousseau's sign is much more specific for latent tetany, occurring in only 1% of normal individuals. Trousseau reported paresthesias and muscle contractions typical of tetany in an arm to which he had applied a tourniquet. Today, to duplicate this phenomenon, a pneumatic cuff is inflated on the upper arm to a level about 20 mm Hg above systolic pressure. When the sign is positive, the hand develops characteristic paresthesias and muscle contractions within 3 minutes.

The phenomena of latent and overt tetany result from hyperirritability of the peripheral nerves. Erb first deduced this localization when he demonstrated a decreased threshold of peripheral nerves to galvanic stimulation in tetany. Subsequent electrophysiologic study of Chvostek's sign and Trousseau's phenomenon have confirmed a peripheral nerve origin for tetany. Kugelberg elicited Trousseau's phenomenon below a peripheral nerve block indicating that only the peripheral nerve distal to the cuff need be intact for Trousseau's phenomenon to be manifest. The electromyographic manifestation of this peripheral nerve irritability is repetitive discharge of a single motor unit potential. As a tetanic spasm develops, the individual motor unit potentials often appear as doublets or multiple action potentials. These multiplets are triggered by short bursts of action potentials in fast-conducting, thickly myelinated nerve fibers. The paresthesias of tetany also originate in the peripheral nerves.

Seizures are as common as tetany in idiopathic hypoparathyroidism or pseudo-hypoparathyroidism. There is a wide range of hypocalcemic seizures, focal and generalized, convulsive and nonconvulsive. In addition, patients with underlying epilepsy are more vulnerable to seizures when they are hypocalcemic. EEG abnormalities include paroxysmal slowing, slowing of background rhythms, and focal or generalized epileptiform discharges.

Altered mental status in the form of depression, confusion, dementia, or personality change can occur in hypocalcemia. Even coma may result.

With coma, there may be papilledema, which is a result of increased intracranial pressure. Aside from the raised pressure, the CSF shows no consistent abnormality. In some patients, the increase in intracranial pressure may be manifest by headache and papilledema without altered mentation. In the author's experience, headache may be present in the absence of papilledema.

# HYPERCALCEMIA

Hypercalcemia can cause a wide range of mental disorders. Confusion and drowsiness are typical manifestations. Obtundation may progress to the point of coma. Delirium may occur. Depression, a mixed picture of depression and anxiety, paranoid illness, and manic states have been reported. Such cases can be mistaken for primary psychiatric problems. Reversible myoclonus or rigidity may be features. In the author's experience, hypercalcemia may greatly and reversibly accentuate asterixis and confusion in renal failure patients. The CSF protein may be increased in hypercalcemia; levels as high as 175 mg/dl have been reported. The usual EEG correlate of these mental aberrations is slowing of background rhythms. The EEG may show focal or generalized epileptiform features, and occasionally convulsions may occur. These seizures may be generalized or focal and are resolved by normalization of the serum calcium.

Other focal signs, such as transient hemiparesis, have been reported in association with hypercalcemia. One reported patient had reversible hemiparesis with hypercalcemia. During the acute phase, cerebral arterial spasm was documented by angiography. After treatment of hypercalcemia, a repeat angiogram showed resolution of the spasm. Another reported case showed basilar artery spasm in a hypercalcemic patient who presented with a brain stem stroke. After treatment of hypercalcemia, a repeat angiogram showed resolution of the arterial spasm. Nevertheless, this patient was left with mild residual symptoms of the brain stem infarct. These cases suggest that hypercalcemic vasospasm can cause brain ischemia.

Generalized weakness, maximal in the proximal muscles, is a common but not universal feature of severe hypercalcemia. This weakness may be acute, but it is typically chronic and gradual in onset. The weakness may be so severe as to result in tetraparesis. Tendon reflexes are characteristically brisk. Muscle pains and cramps may be associated. With the exaggerated tendon reflexes, Babinski's signs and clonus may be present. Muscle atrophy may occur. This clinical syndrome can suggest the diagnosis of amyotrophic lateral sclerosis, but all neuromuscular features are reversible with correction of hypercalcemia. Short-duration polyphasic potentials have been observed on electromyography in such cases. Serum creatine phosphokinase and other muscle enzymes are normal. No consistent pattern of muscle pathology has been reported.

# HYPOMAGNESEMIA

Hypomagnesemia can cause tetany identical to that seen with hypocalcemia. In fact, hypomagnesemia may induce tetany by causing a decrease in ionized calcium levels. Whatever the mechanism, the tetany is successfully treated with magnesium. Chvostek's sign and Trousseau's phenomenon may be present.

Central nervous system effects of hypomagnesemia exist as well. Generalized convulsive seizures may occur. Focal seizures and multifocal seizures are typical, however; they may be complex partial or convulsive. In such cases the EEG shows focal epileptiform discharges. The seizures can be intractable until magnesium is administered. Mental aberrations caused by hypomagnesemia include confusion, delirium, stupor, and coma. Tremor, chorea, hyperreflexia, athetosis, myoclonus, and cramps may occur.

The common occurrence of hypomagnesemia in alcoholic patients led to the hypothesis that magnesium depletion was a major factor in the causation of delirium tremens. Delirium tremens may develop despite magnesium repletion, however. In other words, hypomagnesemia is an epiphenomenon to alcohol-withdrawal states. Nevertheless, it is important to provide magnesium to patients in alcohol withdrawal. Normalizing magnesium may elevate the seizure threshold in these patients.

## HYPERMAGNESEMIA

Although individuals vary somewhat in sensitivity to magnesium, particular signs typically appear at certain magnesium levels. Weakness and hyporeflexia emerge at levels of 7–9 mEq/liter, and areflexia is present at levels of 9–10 mEq/liter. Cardiac arrest is not unusual when the serum magnesium level reaches 15 mEq/liter. Two scientists have induced tetraplegia by intravenously infusing magnesium sulfate into each other (Somjen et al., 1966). In each subject the jaw, tongue, mouth, and pharynx muscles were paralyzed, rendering speech and swallowing impossible. Each retained phonation throughout the experiments. In one person, there was partial ptosis and some weakness of extraocular muscles. Although respiration was not affected in this study, respiratory failure may occur and artificial ventilation may be necessary. In severe cases, pupils may be fixed by autonomic involvement. Weakness resolves with normalization of serum magnesium. Edrophonium chloride (Tensilon), neostigmine bromide (Prostigmin), and physostigmine improve weakness. Mentation is unaffected unless there is severe hypotension. Paralyzing doses of magnesium sulfate have no effect on the EEG of experimental animals.

It had long been known that magnesium causes neuromuscular block when Del Castillo and Engbalk clarified the phenomenon using a frog sciatic nerve and sartorius muscle preparation. They found that a dose of magnesium that blocks neuromuscular transmission does not prevent nerve conduction or the response of muscle to direct stimulation. This neuromuscular block was largely a result of decreased acetylcholine release (i.e., a presynaptic effect).

In human paralysis, electrodiagnostic studies reveal low-amplitude compound muscle action potentials, a progressive decline in amplitude at 2-per-second repetitive nerve stimulation, an increase in compound muscle action potential after isometric exercise, and an increase in amplitude with 50-per-second nerve stimulation. These electrical abnormalities and the weakness resolve with normalization of serum magnesium. The electrical findings have been compared to those of the Lambert-Eaton syndrome.

Hypermagnesemia may accentuate pre-existing Lambert-Eaton syndrome or myasthenia gravis. Most interesting is a documented patient in whom magnesium therapy for eclampsia transiently unmasked previously asymptomatic myasthenia gravis. The patient developed severe weakness when the magnesium level was only 3.0 mEq/liter. Her tendon reflexes were brisk, a finding characteristic of myasthenia but not of hypermagnesemia. After normalization of serum magnesium, there was persistently increased jitter on single-fiber electromyographic study. This finding and the marked elevation of the acetylcholine-receptor antibody titer suggested underlying myasthenia gravis.

# HYPOPHOSPHATEMIA

Hypophosphatemia can cause obtundation or seizures in the setting of hyperalimentation. When the encephalopathy is less severe, manifestations are irritability, confusion, or dysarthria.

Neuromuscular manifestations are more common than central nervous system disorders in hypophosphatemia. Although encephalopathy and neuromuscular disorder may occur in the same patient, neuromuscular conditions usually occur without encephalopathy. The two categories of neuromuscular disorder are acute areflexic paralysis and rhabdomyolysis.

Acute areflexic paralysis was described in two patients with hypophosphatemia following hyperalimentation. Profound areflexic weakness is the core syndrome. The illness may progress rapidly, involving within days facial, extraocular, pharyngeal, and other muscles innervated by cranial nerves. The most severe cases result in ventilatory failure and may require mechanical ventilation. Patients with respiratory failure typically have levels of 0.5 mg/dl. Although respiratory failure typically occurs at such low levels, weakness can emerge when the level falls below 2 mg/dl. Edrophonium testing is negative. Sensory features are a prominent aspect of the illness. Paresthesias are an early symptom in the circumoral area and in the extremities. Recovery may be delayed for days or weeks after normalization of the phosphate level.

The most thorough electrodiagnostic report on these patients showed severely reduced motor amplitudes, mildly reduced sensory amplitudes, and normal distal conduction latencies and conduction velocities. F-wave latencies were normal in the arm and mildly prolonged or absent in the leg. There were no decremental or incremental responses to repetitive stimulation. On needle examination, motor unit potentials were reduced in number with an excess of small, polyphasic potentials. There were diffuse fibrillation potentials. The normal serum creatine phosphokinase, areflexia, sensory abnormalities, and the electrodiagnostic findings suggest that acute hypophosphatemic weakness is a result of polyneuropathy.

Knochel has suggested that hypophosphatemic weakness can also be caused by muscle injury (rhabdomyolysis), the second major neuromuscular disorder of hypophosphatemia. The usual setting is chronic alcoholism. Typically, the alcoholic patient's serum phosphorous reaches a nadir between 2 and 4 days following hospitalization. When severe and sustained for a day or two, this hypophosphatemia is followed by a sharp rise in serum creatine phosphokinase. Myalgia and weakness ensue. Knochel et al. suggest that this sequence underlies some of the acute "alcoholic" myopathies.

# CONSULTATIONS

## Medical Service

Although the entire range of electrolyte disorders are manifest on the medical wards of a general hospital, it is helpful for the neurologist to be alert to the possibility of certain electrolyte disorders in particular situations. In renal failure, hypophosphatemia can result from the use of enteric phosphate binders, and hyponatremia can result from dietary indiscretion. Dialysis patients are prone to develop hyperkalemia when there is dietary indiscretion. Treatment with vitamin D and calcium for metabolic bone disease can occasionally cause hypercalcemia. Superimposed on modest azotemia, the hypercalcemia can cause reversible obtundation and asterixis. Improper preparation of the dialysis bath can cause hypernatremia and other electrolyte disorders. In the oncology ward, encephalopathy is frequently the result of hypercalcemia in multiple myeloma, lymphoma, epidermoid esophageal cancer, epidermoid lung cancer, or other malignancies. Medication may precipitate neurologic problems. For example, cisplatin can cause hyponatremia, hypocalcemia, or hypomagnesemia, which may result in seizures and other manifestations of encephalopathy. Vincristine or cyclophosphamide (Cytoxan) can cause hyponatremia via the syndrome of inappropriate antidiuretic hormone (SIADH), as can small-cell cancer of the lung. Aggressive treatment of lymphoma can cause tumor lysis with hyperphosphatemia, hypocalcemia, and hyperkalemia. In the cardiology service, hyponatremia and hypokalemia frequently result from administration of diuretics. Uncommonly syncope can be the chief complaint when hypokalemic or hyperkalemic arrhythmia is present. In the endocrinology division, patients may develop neurologic difficulty when they cease to comply with therapy or when for some reason medication requirements increase. For example, a patient with Addison's disease may present with hyperkalemic weakness when he or she stops taking prescribed medication. A patient with hypoparathyroidism, whose capacity to absorb calcium and or vitamin D has for some reason decreased, may present with tetany. On the other hand, excessive endocrine therapy is sometimes the cause for neurologic consultation, as in the case of a patient who consumes too much calcium, vitamin D, or both, and thereby develops hypercalcemia. In the gastroenterology division one may encounter hypocalcemia or hypomagnesemia resulting from malabsorption. Naturally, diarrhea or vomiting can cause hypokalemia. The use of vasopressin to treat variceal hemorrhage or gastrointestinal bleeding can cause hyponatremia. Hepatic encephalopathy may be worsened when aggressive diuretic therapy for ascites results in depleted intravascular volume and hypokalemia. Cirrhotic patients often develop hyponatremia. Pulmonary lesions often cause hyponatremia (SIADH). In the rheumatology service, nonsteroidal anti-inflammatory drugs may cause hyperkalemia, especially when mild renal failure occurs. In the medical intensive care unit, improper formulation of hyperalimentation can cause hypophosphatemia. In the infectious disease unit, the neurologic consultant should remember that the combination of meningitis and hyponatremia suggests tuberculosis. Amphotericin B can cause hypomagnesemia and hypokalemia. Trimethoprim-sulfamethoxazole can cause hyperkalemia, especially when underlying renal dysfunction is present. In the geriatrics department, even modest hyponatremia can cause profound neurologic effects like ataxia, confusion, or obtundation.

## Surgery Service

Both renal and hepatic transplantation are followed by important metabolic changes. The hyponatremia commonly present in chronic liver disease often improves briskly with liver transplantation, and this sequence is thought to be responsible for the exceedingly high incidence of CPM during the early postoperative days and weeks. After kidney transplantation, renal tubular dysfunction can cause hyperphosphaturia. If in this setting the surgeons inadvertently continue the preoperatively prescribed enteric phosphate binders, subacute hypophosphatemia may develop. In the surgical recovery room, encephalopathy can result from postoperative hyponatremia. This condition may be more problematic in young women. Encountering such patients provides the neurologist an opportunity to educate the surgeons about the dangers of hypotonic fluid use during the preoperative and intraoperative period. On the surgical intensive care ward, it is common to encounter trauma patients whose injuries occurred as a result of neurologic impairment, one cause of which is electrolyte disorders. For example, a patient may be so confused by severe hyponatremia that he or she incurs severe burns. The routine treatment of serious burns requires a volume of intravenous fluid so large that even normal saline or lactated Ringer's solution can cause a large increment in serum Na over a 24-hour period. If consulted for the hyponatremic encephalopathy on admission, the neurologist should warn the surgeons that the risk of CPM is high and that the use of some 5% dextrose in half normal saline should be considered to minimize the rise of the serum Na. If consulted for tetraparesis days after admission, the neurologist should suspect CPM. In the urology service, hyponatremic convulsions may occur after dilute fluids have been used to irrigate the prostate during surgery. As a rule, the sodium returns to normal spontaneously without residual neurologic effect. Ureterosigmoidostomy can cause hypokalemia. In the neurosurgical service, postoperative hypernatremia resulting from diabetes insipidus is not unusual. Subarachnoid hemorrhage often causes hyponatremia, in some cases by SIADH (euvolemia or increased intravascular volume) and in other cases by cerebral salt wasting (decreased intravascular volume).

## Other Hospital Departments

In the obstetric ward, neurologic consultation is sometimes requested for generalized weakness resulting from hypermagnesemia, which can occur when magnesium is being infused for eclampsia or preterm labor. When the weakness is excessive compared with that expected at a given magnesium blood level, an underlying neurologic condition should be suspected. Hyperemesis gravidarum can result in hypokalemia or hypophosphatemia.

In the psychiatry wards, hyponatremia may result from SIADH resulting from the use of neuroleptic or antidepressant medications. Eating disorders may cause electrolyte problems; examples are hypophosphatemia in anorexia nervosa and hypokalemia in bulimia.

## GENERAL CONCEPTS

The major clinical presentations of electrolyte disorders are generalized weakness, tetany, and encephalopathy. Generalized weakness occurs in hypokalemia, hyperkalemia, hypercalcemia, hypermagnesemia, hypophosphatemia, and myelinolysis. Occasionally, generalized weakness is the main complaint in hyponatremia or hypernatremia. Tetany occurs in hypocalcemia, hypomagnesemia, and hypokalemia. Encephalopathy including seizures occurs in hyponatremia, hypernatremia, hypocalcemia, hypercalcemia, hypomagnesemia, hypophosphatemia, and after excessively rapid correction of hyponatremia or hypernatremia. Movement disorders occur in hypernatremia, hypocalcemia, hypercalcemia, hypomagnesemia, and myelinolysis.

Although most patients with metabolic encephalopathy have relatively symmetric neurologic manifestations, focal neurologic features are possible in any of these conditions. Particular electrolyte disorders have a special tendency to cause focal signs. Hypomagnesemia is especially prone to cause focal and multifocal seizures. Hypercalcemia may cause vasospasm of cerebral blood vessels and thereby result in transient brain ischemia or cerebral infarction.

Severe neurologic signs can emerge when an electrolyte disorder accentuates a mild underlying neurologic disease. Modest hypermagnesemia may greatly accentuate pre-existing Eaton-Lambert syndrome or myasthenia gravis. Hyponatremia or hypocalcemia may lower the seizure threshold in an epileptic patient. Hypokalemia or hyperkalemia may accentuate the weakness of a patient with muscular dystrophy.

For several reasons, no simple correlation exists between the severity of an electrolyte derangement and the severity of the neurologic manifestation. First, some individuals are more sensitive than others to a given metabolic insult. Second, the electrolyte level measured is sometimes not the critical physiologic parameter. Whereas ionized calcium is the stronger correlate of neurologic dysfunction, total serum calcium is often routinely measured. Third, the duration and rapidity of onset of an electrolyte derangement are major factors determining the severity of symptoms. A serum Na of 120 mEq/liter may be manifest by convulsions, when hyponatremia is acute. A serum Na of 110 mEq/liter, however, may cause no symptoms when hyponatremia has developed gradually over weeks or months. Rarely, a patient may slowly develop a serum calcium as high as 19 mg/dl without apparent symptoms. Finally, other variables may be interacting with the electrolyte in question. For example, when hypocalcemia and hypokalemia coexist, the latter disorder prevents the former from causing tetany.

Correction of electrolyte derangements can cause or precipitate neurologic disorders. Correction of hypokalemia may unmask tetany in a hypocalcemic individual. Rapid correction of hypernatremia can cause potentially lethal brain swelling with obtundation and seizures. Rapid correction of hyponatremia can cause tetraplegia as a result of central pontine myelinolysis. The incidence of these complications can be minimized by caution in therapy.

## SUGGESTED READING

Adams RD, Victor M, Mancall EL. Central pontine myelinolysis. A hitherto undescribed disease occurring in alcoholic and malnourished patients. Arch Neurol 1959;81:154.

Comi G, Testa D, Cornelio F, et al. Potassium depletion myopathy: a cranial and morphological study of six cases. Muscle Nerve 1985;8:17.

Daggett P, Deanfield J, Moss F. Neurological aspects of hyponatraemia. Postgrad Med J 1982;58(686): 737–740.

Del Castillo J, Engbaek L. The nature of the neuromuscular block produced by magnesium. J Physiol 1954;124:370–384.

Fishman RA. Neurological aspects of magnesium metabolism. Arch Neurol 1965;12:562.

Henson RA. The neurological aspects of hypercalcaemia: with special reference to primary hyperparathyroidism. J R Coll Physicians Lond 1966;1:41.

Karp BI, Laureno R. Pontine and extrapontine myelinolysis: a neurologic disorder following rapid correction of hyponatremia. Medicine 1993;72:359.

Knochel JP. The pathophysiology and clinical characteristics of severe hypophosphatemia. Arch Intern Med 1977;137:203–220.

Krendel DA. Hypermagnesemia and neuromuscular transmission. Semin Neurol 1990;10:42.

Laureno R. Neurologic Syndromes Accompanying Electrolyte Disorders. In CG Goetz, CM Tanner, MJ Aminoff (eds), Handbook of Clinical Neurology (vol. 63): Systemic Diseases, Part I. Amsterdam: Elsevier, 1993;545.

Layzer RB. Neuromuscular Manifestations of Systemic Disease. Philadelphia: FA Davis, 1985.

Lutrell CN, Finberg CN, Drawdy LP. Hemorrhagic encephalopathy induced by hypernatremia. II. Experimental observations on hyperosmolarity in cats. Arch Neurol 1959;1:153.

Macaulay D, Watson M. Hypernatremia in infants as a cause of brain damage. Arch Dis Child 1967;42:485.

Macefield G, Burke D. Paresthesiae and tetany induced by voluntary hyperventilation. Brain 1991;114:527.

Silvis SE, DiBartolomeo AG, Aaker HM. Hypophosphatemia and neurological changes secondary to oral caloric intake. Am J Gastroenterol 1980;73:215.

Somjen G, Hilmy M, Stephen CR. Failure to anesthetize human subjects by intravenous administration of magnesium sulfate. J Pharmacol Exp Ther 1966;154:652–659.

Sterns RH. Severe symptomatic hyponatremia: treatment and outcome—a study of 64 cases. Ann Intern Med 1987;107:656.

Weintraub MI. Hypophosphatemia mimicking acute Guillain-Barré-Strohl syndrome. JAMA 1976;235:1040.

Young RSK, Truax BT. Hypernatremic hemorrhagic encephalopathy. Ann Neurol 1979;5:588.

# 9
# Human Immunodeficiency Virus–Positive Patients

Igor J. Koralnik

An estimated 30 million adults and approximately 2 million children worldwide are infected with the human immunodeficiency virus type 1 (HIV-1). Since the beginning of the epidemic, more than 13 million people have developed acquired immunodeficiency syndrome (AIDS). In the United States, 1 million people are HIV-1–positive, 580,000 have been diagnosed with AIDS, and 315,000 of them have died. The prevalence of HIV-1 infection in people between 15 and 49 years old is 1 in 250. It is now the leading cause of death in men 25–44 years of age.

Neurologic manifestations are frequent in HIV-1 infection. They constitute the initial presentation in 10% of patients, and 30–50% develop neurologic complications during the course of the disease [1,2]. Autopsy shows involvement of the nervous system in more than 90% of cases.

The neurologic consultation for patients with HIV infection represents a particular challenge for the neurologist. HIV-infected individuals admitted to the hospital are often severely debilitated and present with multiple constitutional symptoms related to systemic infections or tumors, which can overshadow or mimic a primary neurologic condition.

In addition, patients with AIDS are usually treated with a combination of prophylactic drugs and a rapidly growing number of antiretroviral medications that are not familiar to the neurologist. Drug interactions and neurologic side effects of these medications are common, adding another level of complexity for the consultant neurologist. The following rules can be applied, however, to facilitate the understanding of these difficult cases:

1.  The spectrum of neurologic manifestations in HIV-1–infected individuals depends on the degree of immunosuppression. The current classification is based on the CD4$^+$ lymphocyte count, which when normal is greater than 800/μl. When minimal immunosuppression is present, and most patients are asymptomatic, the CD4$^+$ count is 500–800/μl. With marked immunosuppression, generalized lymphadenopathy, and constitutional symptoms, the CD4$^+$ count is 200–500/μl.

175

Severe immunosuppression with opportunistic infections is revealed when a $CD4^+$ count less than 200/µl is present.

The measure of the viral load is another surrogate marker of HIV disease progression with which the consultant neurologist should become familiar. It is a quantification of the number of HIV RNA genomes present in the serum or plasma using the polymerase chain reaction (PCR) or the branched-DNA signal amplification assay [3,4]. High levels, such as 100,000 copies/ml, correlate with $CD4^+$ cell count decline and clinical progression, whereas low levels characterized by less than 10,000 copies/ml are associated with long-term survival.

Thus, if the $CD4^+$ cell count represents the degree of immunosuppression of a patient, the viral load is a good estimate of the speed of HIV disease progression.

2.  Multiple pathologies can coexist in an immunosuppressed individual. A positive culture or a finding on brain imaging does not ensure that the single diagnosis has been found. The peripheral nervous system and central nervous system (CNS) are frequently affected concomitantly in HIV infection. Opportunistic infections of the CNS are usually superimposed on primary HIV-associated neurologic disorders.

3.  Potential side effects of antiretroviral medications and prophylactic drug regimens on the nervous system must always be included in the differential diagnosis.

This chapter surveys the most frequent neurologic manifestations of HIV-1 infection that are the source of consultation to the neurology service.

## PRINCIPAL NEUROLOGIC PRESENTATIONS IN HUMAN IMMUNODEFICIENCY VIRUS TYPE 1 INFECTION

### Meningismus with Normal Neurologic Examination

Patient Otherwise Asymptomatic, $CD4^+$ Cell Count Greater Than 200/µl

*Aseptic Meningitis*

Headache, stiff neck, and fever associated with nausea and vomiting can be the first presentation of HIV-1 infection. The cerebrospinal fluid (CSF) analysis shows a moderate lymphocytic pleocytosis (i.e., 10–100 cells/µl). It is a self-limited illness that subsides spontaneously after several weeks. In atypical cases, transient cranial neuropathies may develop, affecting mostly the fifth, seventh, and eighth cranial nerves. This aseptic meningitis usually occurs soon after the primary infection, when HIV-1 conventional serology is still negative. HIV-1 PCR, if available, is positive, and the HIV-1 p24 antigen might be detected in the blood. A repeat serology testing after 6 weeks will usually help clarify this situation.

Early onset of aseptic meningitis has not been associated with late neurologic manifestations in HIV-1 infection. This condition might recur at any time throughout the course of the disease, however. CSF pleocytosis becomes less common with advanced immunosuppression. Treatment is symptomatic.

## Patient with History of Other Opportunistic Infections, CD4+ Cell Count Less Than 200/µl

### *Cryptococcal Meningitis*

**Presentation.** Cryptococcal meningitis is the most common opportunistic meningitis in AIDS, affecting 10% of patients [5]. The presentation differs from aseptic meningitis in that meningismus is present in less than 40% of patients. Confusion or altered state of consciousness occurs in severe cases. Focal neurologic findings or seizures may indicate the development of a cryptococcoma or associated venous sinus thrombosis.

**Laboratory Investigations.** The detection of *Cryptococcus neoformans* antigen titers of more than 1 to 8 in the CSF provides a rapid diagnosis, which is confirmed subsequently by CSF culture. Other CSF findings include elevated opening pressure, mononuclear pleocytosis, elevated protein and decreased glucose concentration in 50% of the cases, and direct detection of the organism by India ink staining in 70% of the cases.

CSF and serum cryptococcal antigen are almost always detected in cryptococcal meningitis, and blood and urine cultures may also be positive. Brain imaging is usually negative unless an associated abscess or hydrocephalus is present. Poor prognosis factors include altered mental status, CSF opening pressure greater than 200 mm of water, absence of CSF pleocytosis, CSF antigen titer greater than 1 to 1,024, a positive blood culture, and hyponatremia.

**Treatment.** Treatment consists of amphotericin B (Fungizone), 0.5–0.7 mg/kg per day intravenously, for a minimum of 2 weeks, followed by fluconazole (Diflucan), 400 mg per os (PO) qd, for 8–10 weeks or until sterilization of the CSF [6]. Mild cases can be treated with fluconazole, 800 mg PO loading dose, then 400 mg PO qd. The outcome is generally favorable within 2 weeks, but early mortality can reach 10%. Complications such as hydrocephalus and elevated intracranial pressure should be recognized and treated aggressively with mechanical drainage, including repeated lumbar punctures, intraventricular shunt, and optic nerve sheath fenestration in cases of vision impairment [7]. To avoid 50–60% of relapses within 6 months, fluconazole, 200 mg PO qd, should be continued for life.

### *Neurosyphilis*

**Presentation.** Many HIV-infected individuals have a history of syphilis. *Treponema pallidum* infection can also occur at any time during HIV-1 infection and may mimic neurologic complications of AIDS. Both may produce acute or chronic meningitis, myelopathy, cranial or peripheral neuropathies, cerebrovascular disease, and dementia.

**Laboratory Investigations.** A persistent mononuclear pleocytosis and elevated protein concentration can be found in the CSF [8], as well as elevated immunoglobulin G (IgG) synthesis rate and oligoclonal bands. This is of no help in establishing the diagnosis of neurosyphilis, because these findings occur in 40–60% of asymptomatic HIV-1 seropositive patients.

In addition, positive results from a VDRL test of the CSF, which establishes the diagnosis of neurosyphilis, has a sensitivity of only 30–70% in HIV infection [9,10]. A reactive CSF fluorescent treponemal antibody absorption (FTA-ABS) test increases the likelihood of *Treponema pallidum* infection, but is less specific because it can result from treated neurosyphilis or from contamination of the CSF with small amounts of blood containing antibody at the time of the lumbar puncture. Moreover, neurosyphilis might be more aggressive and progress more rapidly in HIV-infected individuals than in the immunocompetent population and may not respond adequately to conventional treatment [8].

In summary, HIV-infected individuals with a positive serum VDRL test, CSF pleocytosis, and elevated protein concentration as well as symptoms consistent with neurosyphilis should be treated with intravenous penicillin, even in the absence of a positive VDRL test in the CSF.

**Treatment.**   Treatment consists of aqueous penicillin, 2–4 million units intravenously q4h, for 10–14 days (12–24 million U/day) or procaine penicillin, 2.4 million U/day intramuscularly, for 14 days plus probenecid, 500 mg PO qid. A careful follow-up in these patients is needed with repeat CSF and serum VDRL tests because the rate of relapse is unknown.

### Differential Diagnosis of Meningitis

Other less common CNS infections in AIDS include tuberculosis, histoplasmosis, aspergillosis, coccidioidomycosis, amoebiasis, *Candida albicans* infection, *Trypanosoma cruzii* infection, herpes simplex and zoster infection, and *Nocardia asteroides*. Bacterial meningitis is rare in HIV-infected patients, and the treatment is the same as in immunocompetent individuals.

## Alteration of Mental Status with a "Nonfocal" Examination

Alteration of mental status is a frequent reason for neurologic consultation in patients with AIDS. It is a challenging task for the consultant neurologist because these patients are usually admitted in the setting of other systemic illnesses, and thus are by definition acutely ill, with toxic-metabolic derangements that might overshadow or mimic a primary neurologic condition. Knowledge of the patient's baseline mental function and time course of the disease presentation obtained from family and friends is often key in establishing a diagnosis.

### HIV-1–Associated Dementia Complex

HIV-1–associated dementia complex is a common complication of HIV-1 infection that occurs in 15% of patients with AIDS and can be the first manifestation of the disease in 3–10% [11]. A less severe entity named *HIV-1–associated minor cognitive/motor disorder* can be found in another 20–25%.

*Table 9.1*　Clinical triad in human immunodeficiency virus
type 1–associated dementia complex

| Cognition | Behavioral | Motor |
| --- | --- | --- |
| Forgetfulness | Apathy | Gait instability |
| Mental slowing | Social withdrawal | Poor coordination |
| Inability to concentrate | Lack of spontaneity | Leg weakness |

Numerous groups have attempted to detect early neurologic dysfunction in HIV-1 asymptomatic individuals [12]. Subtle electrophysiologic abnormalities (e.g., in electroencephalogram, evoked potentials, and nerve conduction studies) can be found in early HIV-1 infection, but do not seem to have a predictive value for the later onset of AIDS dementia, which occurs generally when the $CD4^+$ cell count is around 100/μl or less.

The clinical characteristics of this disorder can be subdivided into three main categories: cognitive, behavioral, and motor (Table 9.1).

*Presentation*

The onset of symptoms is usually subtle. Patients often complain of difficulty with memory and note a slowness of thinking. They have trouble concentrating. Complex mental activities become more time-consuming and difficult to perform. A loss of interest in social and professional activities soon follows. This apathy and social withdrawal are frequently perceived as depression by patients' friends and relatives. Motor symptoms such as reduced coordination, altered handwriting, loss of balance, and gait instability can be elicited on detailed questioning.

During the early stages of HIV-associated dementia complex, which usually occurs when the $CD4^+$ lymphocyte count is 500–200/μl, the mental status examination might only reveal minor psychomotor slowing, inattention, decreased short-term memory, and inability to perform simple calculations. The cranial nerve examination is usually normal, except ocular movements show saccadic pursuit. Other frequent findings are brisk reflexes, frontal release signs, mild postural tremor, slowing of rapid alternating movements, and gait instability when performing half-turns.

The late stages are generally concomitant with profound immunosuppression (i.e., $CD4^+$ counts <200 μl), and dementia becomes more global, profoundly impairing orientation, memory, and cognition. Confusional or psychotic episodes can occur. Seizures are rare. Despite the extent of the cerebral involvement in HIV-associated dementia, there is usually no aphasia, apraxia, or other signs of discrete cortical dysfunction, except in the terminal stages. This syndrome has thus been classified together with the group of subcortical dementias, along with the cognitive impairment found, for example, in Parkinson's or Huntington's diseases.

This is a diagnosis of exclusion in patients with advanced immunosuppression, but it frequently coexists with opportunistic infections and tumors. Neuropsychological evaluation should include tests of attention, memory, and psychomotor speed such as trail making, digit span, verbal fluency, grooved pegboard, symbol digit modalities, and Rey auditory verbal learning tests [13].

## Laboratory Investigations

CSF analysis shows mild lymphocytic pleocytosis in 25% of cases and elevated protein in 55% [14], which can also be present in nondemented patients. Elevated beta$_2$-microglobulin and neopterin levels have been reported, but their usefulness in clinical practice has not been demonstrated. Because HIV-1–associated dementia complex is a diagnosis of exclusion, bacterial, fungal and acid-fast bacteria (AFB) cultures, cryptococcal antigen, VDRL test, and CSF cytology should be negative.

## Imaging Studies

Computed tomographic (CT) scan and magnetic resonance imaging (MRI) often show subcortical and cortical atrophy, which is not proportional to the degree of dementia. The MRI can demonstrate multiple hyperintense signals in T2-weighted images, nonenhancing, and localized bilaterally in the subcortical white matter (Figure 9.1). MRI is superior for distinguishing these abnormalities from confounding illnesses such as progressive multifocal leukoencephalopathy.

## Brain Biopsy

Brain biopsy is not indicated in HIV-1–associated dementia complex unless imaging studies are atypical. Histologic examination reveals white matter pallor, multinucleated giant cells, and microglial nodules, as well as astrocytosis and perivascular mononuclear cell infiltrates. HIV-1 is probably transported across the blood-brain barrier by infected monocytes. In the brain, HIV-1 has been found in microglial nodules and multinucleated giant cells as well as in few epithelial cells. HIV-1 does not infect neurons or glial cells in adults, and only a limited expression of viral regulatory gene products has been demonstrated in glial cells from children with AIDS encephalopathy [15].

Potential pathogenetic mechanisms include (1) indirect toxicity of the viral protein gp120, which promotes calcium influx in neuronal cells in vitro; (2) production of cytokines such as tumor necrosis factor–alpha and interleukin-6 by infected microglial cells; and (3) production of toxins responsible of the activation of the $N$-methyl-D-aspartate (NMDA) receptors that mediate the excitatory transmission in the brain [16]. Nimodipine, a calcium channel blocker, and memantine, an NMDA-receptor antagonist, are currently being evaluated as adjuncts to antiretroviral therapy in the treatment of HIV-1–associated dementia.

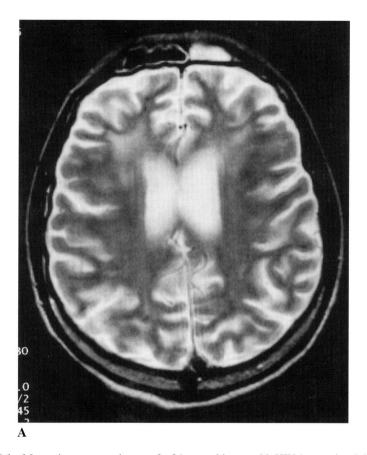

*Figure 9.1* Magnetic resonance image of a 34-year-old man with HIV-1–associated dementia complex. The T2-weighted image **(A)** shows bilateral symmetric hyperintense signal in the frontal periventricular white matter, which does not enhance with gadolinium injection on the T1-weighted image **(B)**. A marked cortical and subcortical atrophy is present.

## Treatment

Zidovudine (AZT) penetrates the CSF, but its effect in preventing HIV-1–associated dementia remains controversial [11,14,17]. The early use of this medication may allow the development of resistant isolates. The available information suggests that neuroprophylaxis should consist of at least 600 mg of zidovudine per day. Zidovudine, 600–1,000 mg per day, has been shown to produce clear improvement in at least 50% of patients with HIV-1–associated dementia after 6–8 weeks of treatment [18].

The appropriate treatment of HIV-1–associated dementia that develops while patients are already on zidovudine is unknown. Other types of nucleoside ana-

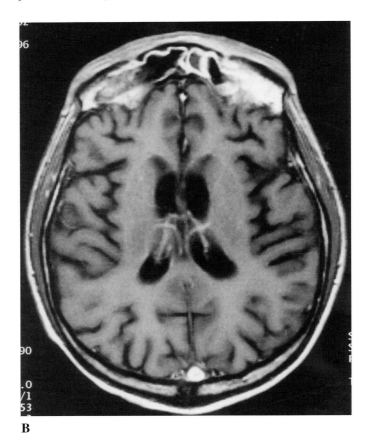

**B**

*Figure 9.1*   (continued)

logue reverse transcriptase inhibitors include didanosine (ddI), zalcitabine (ddC), and stavudine (d4T), which all cause peripheral neuropathy, as well as lamivudine (3TC) (Table 9.2). These medications have poor penetration into the CSF. Nevirapine, delavirdine, and efavirenz are non-nucleoside reverse transcriptase inhibitors. They are used in combination with other antiretroviral drugs. The protease inhibitors saquinavir, ritonavir, indinavir, and nelfinavir are the newest class of anti-HIV drugs (see Table 9.2). They have been shown to have dramatic effect in reducing the viral load in limited human studies, but penetration into the CSF has not been well demonstrated. At the present time, the efficacy of these drugs in treating dementia is unknown. There are, however, theoretical reasons to believe that reducing viral load and restoring immune function will have some beneficial effect on the nervous system. Other experimental drugs include the NMDA antagonist memantine. Antiretrovirals awaiting FDA approval include adefovir (Preveon), abacavir (Ziagen), and amprenavir.

*Table 9.2*    Antiretroviral medications

Nucleoside reverse transcriptase inhibitors
    Zidovudine (AZT, Retrovir)
    Didanosine (ddI, Videx)
    Zalcitabine (ddC, Hivid)
    Stavudine (d4T, Zerit)
    Lamivudine (3TC, Epivir)
Non-nucleoside reverse transcriptase inhibitors
    Nevirapine (Viramune)
    Delavirdine (Rescriptor)
    Efavirenz (Sustiva)
Protease inhibitors
    Saquinavir (Invirase)
    Ritonavir (Norvir)
    Indinavir (Crixivan)
    Nelfinavir (Viracept)

## Mass Lesions of the Central Nervous System

The neurologist is often asked to consult on HIV-infected patients presenting with change of mental status or an abnormal neurologic examination who have brain lesions on CT scan or MRI. These can be quite extensive and may represent life-threatening emergencies. A brain biopsy is often the only way to ascertain the diagnosis. Because of the risks inherent to this procedure in profoundly debilitated patients, or because of the localization of the lesions, this is often not an option. The radiologic appearance and the distribution of the lesions as well as the response to empiric therapy are often the only way to establish the diagnosis.

### Toxoplasmosis

Cerebral toxoplasmosis is the most common cerebral mass lesion in patients with AIDS. In the United States, where the incidence of seropositivity for *Toxoplasma gondii* is below 30% in the adult population, toxoplasmic encephalitis (TE) develops in 3–10% of patients with AIDS [19]. In Europe and Africa, where the overall seroprevalence is higher, 25–50% of patients with AIDS may develop this condition.

#### Presentation

Almost 90% of patients have CD4$^+$ cell counts of less than 200/μl, and 75% have CD4$^+$ counts less than 100/μl at the time of presentation. The most common symptoms include headache, confusion, fever, and lethargy. Up to 30% of patients develop seizures [20,21]. Seventy percent of patients have focal signs such as hemiparesis, cranial nerve palsies, ataxia, and sensory deficits on the neurologic examination. The presentation is usually subacute, ranging from a few days to 1 month.

## Laboratory Investigations

As is the case in the general population, serum antitoxoplasma IgG antibodies can be detected in patients with TE, whereas IgM antibodies are rarely found, supporting the notion that most cases represent a reactivation of latent infection. A rise in IgG titers occurs in less than half of the cases [20]. By immunofluorescence, up to 16% of patients had nondetectable antibodies at the time of presentation [21]. However, using the newer enzyme-linked immunosorbent assay, only 7% of patients known to be seropositive for *T. gondii* had lost their antibodies at the time of presentation [20]. Therefore, a negative toxoplasmic serology points to another diagnosis, whereas a positive serology is not diagnostic.

A mild elevation of CSF protein and a moderate mononucleated pleocytosis (<60 cells/µl) are common but nonspecific and may be a result of the underlying HIV infection.

A slight decrease of the CSF glucose has been reported, but is not a constant finding. In patients with a CT scan or MRI suggestive of TE but with negative serum titers, CSF serology might be negative as well and cannot be used to rule out the diagnosis. The PCR technique has been used to detect *T. gondii* DNA in the CSF, showing a sensitivity of 44–65% and a specificity of 100% [22,23]. CSF analysis is therefore more useful to exclude other infectious processes than to confirm the diagnosis of CNS toxoplasmosis.

## Imaging Studies

Head CT scan and MRI demonstrate CNS lesions in almost all cases, with the exception of the rare diffuse encephalitic form of toxoplasmosis. Lesions are multiple in two-thirds of the cases, and display ring enhancement in approximately 90%. The MRI has been shown to be more sensitive than the CT scan to detect multiple lesions. These are generally localized at the cortico-medullar junction, in the white matter, or in the basal ganglia, and are surrounded by edema, with possible mass effect on surrounding structures (Figure 9.2). Unfortunately, the neuroradiologic characteristics of TE are not pathognomonic, and may be observed in other conditions, particularly lymphoma.

## Brain Biopsy

Because of the good response to therapy, tissue diagnosis is not required for the diagnosis of CNS toxoplasmosis, and an empiric therapeutic trial is recommended when the clinical and radiological findings are consistent with this diagnosis.

The meta-analysis of 200 cases reported in nine different series in which patients underwent a brain biopsy after failure of 2 weeks of antitoxoplasma treat-

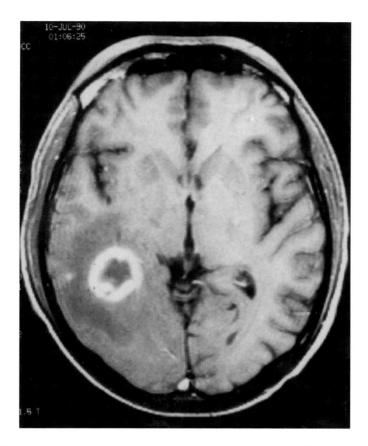

*Figure 9.2*   Magnetic resonance image of a 29-year-old man with AIDS and toxoplasmic encephalitis. The T1-weighted image with gadolinium injection shows a ring enhancing lesion in the right hemisphere, surrounded by swelling and mass effect on the surrounding structures.

ment indicates that the second most frequent diagnosis was toxoplasmosis, in 23.4% of cases [24]. Histologic examination shows mainly necrotic abscesses with blood vessel thrombosis and necrosis. The wall of the abscess is composed of a dense collection of mononuclear cells and newly formed blood vessels surrounded by reactive gliosis. Cysts containing bradyzoites, the dormant form of *T. gondii,* coexist with numerous active tachyzoites.

## Treatment

Treatment consists of a combination of pyrimethamine and sulfadiazine, which cause a synergistic and sequential block on the folic acid metabolism necessary for the development of the parasite. Standard acute therapy is 200 mg of pyrimethamine PO on the first day of treatment, followed by 50–75 mg per day PO; sulfadiazine, 4–6 g per day per PO intravenously; and folinic acid, 7.5 mg per day PO for 6 weeks.

Alternatives are pyrimethamine and folinic acid (same doses) and clindamycin, 2.4–3.6 g per day for 6 weeks, which is an adequate combination for patients allergic to sulfonamides. Side effects, which consist of cytopenia, rashes, diarrhea, and elevated liver enzymes, have been reported in 40–70% of patients receiving pyrimethamine and sulfadiazine and in 36% of those receiving pyrimethamine and clindamycin [20]. These can cause early discontinuation of therapy. Although corticosteroids are frequently prescribed to diminish cerebral edema, their use has not been shown to be either beneficial or harmful in TE [25]. Because high doses of steroids might help reduce the size of CNS lymphomas, their use should be limited only to cases of impending cerebral herniation during the initial medical treatment of presumed TE, in order not to confuse the diagnosis.

Neurologic improvement is clinically apparent in more than half the cases by day 3 of therapy [19], and in most cases by day 7. A failure to improve or a worsening of the symptoms should prompt repeat imaging studies by days 10–14 to consider the possibility of brain biopsy.

**Secondary Prophylaxis.**   *T. gondii* is only sensitive to treatment when in tachyzoite form. Because dormant cystic forms may rupture and reinitiate the infectious process at any time, maintenance therapy is thought to be necessary indefinitely to prevent a relapse, which is likely to occur after a delay of 6–8 weeks of interruption of treatment. Standard maintenance therapy consists of pyrimethamine, 50 mg per day, and either sulfadiazine, 2–3 g per day, or clindamycin, 1.2–1.8 g per day. Intermittent doses of pyrimethamine (25 mg twice a week), sulfadiazine (5 g twice a week), or clindamycin (2.4 g twice a week) are also reportedly effective [26].

Median survival after diagnosis of TE is difficult to evaluate, because most of the prospective studies were performed before the determination of adequate maintenance drug regimen and before the availability of antiretroviral medications such as protease inhibitors. In one series, median survival was 310 days, but patients who were also on zidovudine did significantly better than those who were not. If the diagnosis is made in a timely fashion and the patient does not become intolerant to the treatment, TE is an opportunistic infection with a relatively high therapeutic success rate, and death is usually caused by other complications of AIDS.

**Primary Prophylaxis.**   Prevention of exposure to *T. gondii* is an important prophylactic measure for HIV-infected individuals. HIV-infected persons should have serologic testing for *T. gondii*, to detect latent infection. The life cycle of this intracellular parasite requires an obligatory passage in the intestinal epithelium of cats. Humans and animals are infected either by ingestion of sporozoites after contact with cat feces or contaminated soil or by eating undercooked meat containing tissue cysts. All patients, but particularly those who lack IgG antibody to *T. gondii,* should be advised not to eat raw or undercooked meat and to wash their hands after contact with raw meat and after gardening or other contact with soil. Fruits and vegetables should be washed thoroughly before being eaten raw.

Patients should avoid contact with cat litter or should wash their hands thoroughly after contact.

*Toxoplasma*-seropositive patients with CD4$^+$ lymphocyte count of less than 100 µl should receive prophylactic treatment. The dosage of trimethoprim-sulfamethoxazole (TMP-SMZ), one double-strength tablet PO qd, recommended for *Pneumocystis carinii* pneumonia (PCP) prophylaxis is also effective for TE. If patients cannot tolerate TMP-SMZ, the regimen including dapsone, 100 mg per day; pyrimethamine, 50 mg per week; and leucovorin, 25 mg per week, is effective for both TE and PCP.

## Primary Central Nervous System Lymphoma

Primary CNS lymphoma affects 2% of patients with AIDS, and its radiographic appearance makes it the principal differential diagnosis of cerebral toxoplasmosis. It is a separate entity from systemic lymphoma seen in patients with AIDS, which does not metastasize to the brain.

### Presentation

The onset of symptoms is generally subacute, lasting weeks to months. Confusion, lethargy, memory loss, and headache are the most frequent symptoms. As the disease progresses, hemiparesis, aphasia, seizures, and cranial nerve palsies can occur [27]. Fever and constitutional symptoms are generally absent, unless another systemic infection develops concomitantly. At the time of diagnosis, the average CD4$^+$ cell count in one series was 40/µl (range: 6–189).

### Laboratory Investigations

A mild mononuclear pleocytosis (<30 cells/µl) and elevation of the protein concentration in the CSF is a common finding in patients with CNS lymphoma, but is nonspecific and might be a result of the underlying HIV infection. High protein levels (up to 590 mg/dl) have been reported in patients with extensive lymphomatous infiltration of both cerebral hemispheres [27]. Hypoglycorrhachia is a rare finding.

It is important to perform cytologic analysis of the CSF because the presence of atypical or malignant lymphomatous cells can establish the diagnosis. Systemic extracerebral lymphoma seen in AIDS patients can also cause lymphomatous meningitis, however, but does not generally spread to the brain itself. Similarly, primary CNS lymphoma does not metastasize systemically.

The Epstein-Barr virus (EBV) genome can be detected in tumor cells of nearly all primary CNS lymphomas, but only in some systemic lymphomas of AIDS patients, and rarely in primary brain lymphoma tissue from patients without known immunodeficiency [28]. EBV DNA has been detected by PCR in the CSF of 100% of AIDS patients with CNS lymphoma, but was undetectable in the CSF of patients with other CNS pathologies.

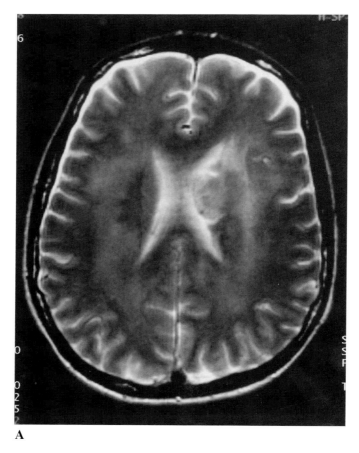

A

*Figure 9.3*   Magnetic resonance image of a 38-year-old man with primary central nervous system lymphoma. A 2-cm lesion with high T2 signal is present in the left periventricular white matter (**A**), with minimal enhancement in the T1-weighted image after administration of gadolinium (**B**).

## Imaging Studies

The head CT scan or MRI in most cases shows findings consistent with CNS tumor. Solitary mass lesions are about as frequent as multiple lesions [27]. The majority display some degree of enhancement, most commonly nodular or patchy. Ring enhancement, identical to that commonly seen in TE can occur. These correlate with central tumor necrosis. Subependymal enhancement seems more specific of CNS lymphoma. The usual periventricular location of CNS lymphoma seen in non-AIDS patients, however, does not apply, and most lesions are localized in the cortex or deep structures. Lesions can be surrounded by edema and produce variable mass effect on neighboring structures (Figure 9.3).

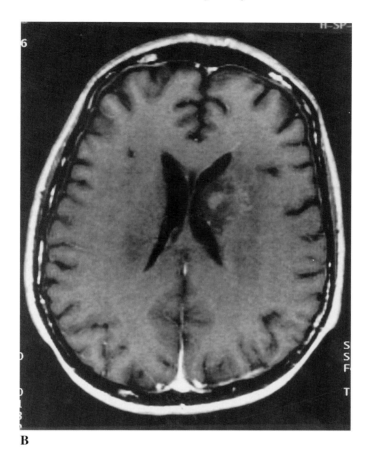

**B**

MRI is more sensitive than CT scanning in revealing multiple lesions, which can be useful if a biopsy is considered. It has been suggested that thallium-201 single photon emission computed tomography shows an accumulation of isotope in the tumor resulting from increased metabolic activity [29,30]. The usefulness of this method in differentiating CNS lymphoma from opportunistic infection remains to be demonstrated in larger series.

## Brain Biopsy

If the CSF cytology fails to reveal lymphomatous cells, an image-guided–stereotactic brain biopsy using CT scan or MRI is the only way to ascertain the diagnosis. This is not often feasible, however, because of the localization of the lesions in vital centers or because the patient is too debilitated to sustain the procedure.

The rate of success of this technique ranges from 50% to 96% [31–33]. Sometimes, two different pathologies are found to coexist within the same lesion [33].

This variability in the success rate of stereotactic biopsy can be explained in part by the surgical approach. To avoid the sampling of necrotic, nondiagnostic tissue frequently found in the center of an enhancing mass, it is crucial to target the periphery of the lesion as well. In addition, series showing the greatest rate of diagnosis were using a comprehensive protocol for histopathologic studies including specific immunochemical staining techniques and electron microscopy in addition to light microscopic evaluation. The complication rate from brain biopsy approaches 8% [32] and consists mainly of hemorrhage. These occurred within the tumor bed of 3 of 14 patients with CNS lymphoma and produced permanent deficit in one. The fragile, abnormal vascularity of these tumors may place them at greater risk of biopsy-associated hemorrhage.

The macroscopic appearance of these tumors is generally that of a multifocal, diffusely infiltrating, and expanding nonhemorrhagic mass, without well-demarcated borders, simulating the appearance of an infiltrating glioma.

Well-circumscribed, largely necrotic masses, however, can also look like abscesses [34]. Microscopic analysis reveals a variety of patterns, including large cells, large-cell immunoblasts, small noncleaved cells, or mixed [27,34]. These are generally of B cell lineage. The presence of EBV in tumor cells has been demonstrated using a variety of techniques [28,34,35], and EBV genome has been found in tumor cell as well as in the CSF of these patients, suggesting that this virus may serve as an effector in tumorigenesis, as is the case in Burkitt's lymphoma and in nasopharyngeal carcinoma.

*Treatment*

The response to steroids seen in lymphomas of non-AIDS patients is not always present [36]. In patients with altered mental status, debilitating focal symptoms, or impending herniation, dexamethasone, 10 mg intravenously or PO followed by 4 mg every 6 hours, can provide a temporary amelioration. The treatment of CNS lymphoma in AIDS consists of 4,000 cGy of whole brain irradiation over a 3-week period. Steroids are added to decrease peritumoral edema and mass effect. Twenty percent of patients progress rapidly and die before completing therapy. Those who receive irradiation have a complete remission of their tumor in 20–50% of cases and live an average of 4 months, compared with 1 month if left untreated. Survival for longer than 1 year, however, has been reported [37]. Up to two-thirds of patients treated with irradiation die of tumor progression or relapse.

A trial combining systemic and intrathecal methotrexate, thiotepa, and procarbazine before radiation therapy in 10 patients showed a global median survival of 3.5 months and median survival of 7 months in the patients who completed therapy (with a range of 2–54 months) [36]. Granulocyte colony–stimulating factor (G-CSF) should be administered to prevent leukopenia. Two of eight deaths were attributed to treatment-related infections. Other trials combining various chemotherapies and radiation therapy are being performed.

## Progressive Multifocal Leukoencephalopathy

Before the AIDS era, progressive multifocal leukoencephalopathy (PML) was a rare disease affecting mainly patients with chronic lymphocytic leukemia, non-

Hodgkin's lymphoma, or tuberculosis. Up to 4% of patients with AIDS develop this condition [38]. PML is caused by the polyomavirus JC. This double-stranded DNA virus infects 90% of the normal adult population worldwide and is not linked to any disease in the immunocompetent host. In the setting of immuno-suppression, JC virus is reactivated and replicates within the nuclei of oligoden-drocytes, causing multifocal demyelination of the CNS.

## Presentation

PML develops in the setting of profound immunosuppression, with CD4$^+$ cell counts usually below 100/μl [39]. The most common presenting symptoms are limb weakness (hemi- or monoparesis), altered mental status, gait ataxia, and visual symptoms, including hemianopsia, diplopia, and third-nerve palsy.

About 80% of patients have focal neurologic findings [38]. Because PML lesions can occur anywhere in the CNS white matter, however, particularly at the subcortical level, presentations implying cerebral cortical dysfunction such as aphasia, apraxia, memory loss, visual agnosia, or seizures do not rule out this diagnosis. One has also to bear in mind that some symptoms can be a result of HIV-associated dementia, which is often superimposed on other CNS pathologies in the end stages of AIDS.

## Laboratory Investigations

Conventional CSF analysis is either normal or shows a moderate increase of pro-tein concentration and a mild mononucleated pleocytosis (<25 cells/μl), which is nonspecific in the context of HIV infection. The detection of JC virus in the CSF by PCR has been shown to be 74–92% sensitive and 92–96% specific for the diagnosis of PML [40,41]. Although the brain biopsy remains the gold standard for diagnosis, it is not always possible to perform if lesions are localized in vital centers or the patient is too debilitated to withstand the procedure. Because it is a rapid, relatively cheap, and noninvasive test, JC virus PCR deserves a wider use than in selected research laboratories.

## Imaging Studies

The hallmark of PML is patchy or confluent areas of low attenuation on CT scans, or hyperintensity of T2-weighted images on MRI (Figure 9.4). MRI is twice as sen-sitive as CT in distinguishing multiple lesions [42]. These are generally not con-trast-enhancing and are not surrounded by edema, and hence, substantial mass effect on surrounding structures is absent. However, 8% of lesions can show faint, peripheral, and irregular enhancement. Lesions are usually bilateral, asymmetric, and localized preferentially to the periventricular areas and the subcortical white matter [42]. Involvement of the deep gray structures including basal ganglia and thalamus can nevertheless be found in up to 17% of cases. Normal CT scan or MRI does not rule out PML because microscopic lesions might be smaller than the power of resolution of these tests. One such case showed multiple, small foci of demyelination disseminated among the cortical U fibers at autopsy [43].

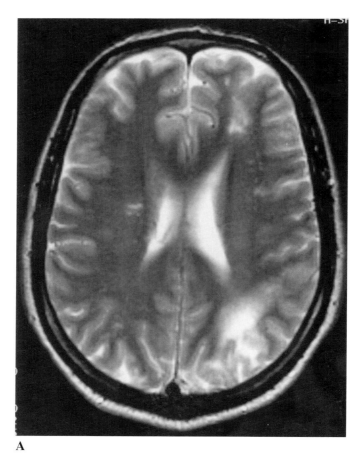

**A**

*Figure 9.4*   Magnetic resonance image of a 42-year-old man with progressive multifocal leukoencephalopathy. Patchy areas of high T2 signal can be seen in the left subcortical white matter at the level of the left parietal and frontal lobes, as well as in the right periventricular white matter (**A**). There is no enhancement in the T1-weighted image after injection of gadolinium (**B**).

## Brain Biopsy

The brain biopsy shows areas of demyelination as well as large, hyperchromatic oligodendrocytic nuclei that are positive for JC virus by immunoperoxidase and contain large amounts of virion detectable by electromicroscopy. Large, bizarre astrocytes with lobulated nuclei are also frequent and may be undergoing mitosis. Lipid-laden macrophages are scattered throughout the affected areas and are engaged in removing the affected oligodendrocytes and myelin breakdown products. Rarely, a significant perivascular lymphocytic infiltrate can be seen in cases that tend to have a more protracted course.

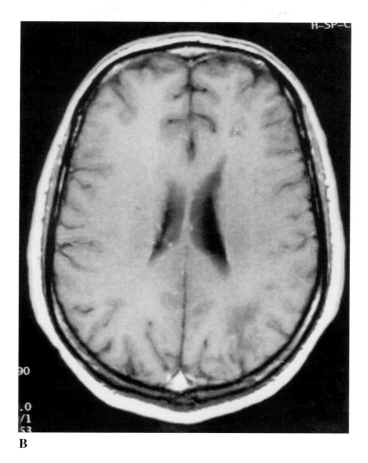

**B**

## Treatment

Multiple treatments have been tried for PML, including steroids, nucleoside analogs (cytosine arabinosine, cytosine adenosine, iododeoxyuridine), interferons, and heparin sulfate. Case reports show mixed but mostly negative results. Prolonged survival of more than 4 years, however, has been reported in some cases [44]. The first prospective controlled study comparing intrathecal or intravenous Ara-C with AZT or AZT alone in the treatment of PML was stopped after showing no difference in outcome between groups [45].

There is a large diversity in the natural evolution of PML. In non-AIDS patients with transient immunosuppression induced by chemotherapy, PML may have a prolonged course, lasting several years once immunocompetence is restored. In patients with AIDS who are profoundly immunosuppressed, the course of the disease is usually rapidly progressive, leading to death within 2–4 months from the time of symptom presentation [38]. In rare cases, PML can stabilize without specific treatment, with prolonged survival.

Caution should be used in the interpretation of case reports using a given treatment regimen. There is no proven therapy for this condition. The effects on the immune system of decreasing the HIV viral load with a combination of nucleoside analogues and protease inhibitors, however, might improve the overall outcome of this deadly disease.

## Cytomegalovirus Encephalitis

Cytomegalovirus (CMV) may cause necrotizing focal encephalitis and ventriculoencephalitis [46,47]. It occurs in patients with CD4+ counts of less than 50 cells/μl and is often concomitant with CMV infection of other organs, including retinitis, adrenalitis, and pneumonitis. Because CMV infection of the brain often coexists with HIV encephalopathy, it remains a problematic clinical diagnosis.

### Presentation

Patients with CMV encephalitis show similar features to those with HIV-1–associated dementia but tend to have a more acute onset with shorter duration of presentation and more prominent confusion and disorientation or apathy and withdrawal. Hyponatremia and cranial nerve involvement, which are usually not present in HIV-associated dementia, are also helpful for establishing the diagnosis.

### Laboratory Investigations

The conventional CSF examination is generally nonspecific, because it is either normal or shows a mild protein elevation and mononucleated pleocytosis. CMV culture often remains negative. The detection of CMV DNA by PCR in the CSF, however, seems to be both very sensitive and specific [48,49].

### Imaging Studies

MRI is much more sensitive than CT for detecting this condition. Focal necrotizing lesions are frequently associated with periventricular and meningeal enhancement or hydrocephalus [50].

### Brain Biopsy

Microglial nodule encephalitis with cytomegalovirus inclusions can be diagnosed at autopsy in 6–40% of patients with AIDS and dementia [46]. Autopsy findings of CMV infection of the brain, however, do not always correlate with the presence of clinical manifestations.

*Treatment*

The management of CMV encephalitis is difficult. In one autopsy-confirmed series, half of the patients were taking maintenance doses of ganciclovir for treatment of CMV retinitis. CMV encephalitis developed in others during first full-dose inductions with ganciclovir or foscarnet [51]. Ganciclovir penetrates the blood-brain barrier, and treatment failures might be caused by acquired viral resistance to the medication.

The treatment is similar to that for CMV retinitis, with induction of ganciclovir, 5 mg/kg per day intravenously q12h for 14–21 days, followed by maintenance 6 mg/kg intravenously qd 5 days per week indefinitely, or foscarnet induction, 60 mg/kg intravenously q8h for 14–21 days, followed by maintenance 90 mg/kg per day indefinitely. The prognosis is usually poor, with median survival not exceeding 5 weeks. Therefore, a combination therapy with ganciclovir and foscarnet at the doses mentioned above is justified.

## Miscellaneous Mass Lesions and Rationale for Brain Biopsy

A meta-analysis was performed regarding the outcome of brain biopsies in a total of 200 AIDS patients reported in nine retrospective studies of patients who underwent a brain biopsy after failing a 2-week trial of antitoxoplasmosis therapy [24]. This analysis revealed in order of frequency the following diagnoses: lymphoma (32.8%), toxoplasmosis (23.4%), PML (21.4%), nondiagnostic (10.4%), other treatable (e.g., infections, tumors) (8%), and other untreatable (e.g., HIV, encephalitis, infarction) (4%). In the above meta-analysis, the 8% of cases with treatable lesions other than lymphoma, toxoplasmosis, or PML included mycotic abscess, bacterial abscess, tuberculous, and atypical mycobacterial lesions, tumor metastasis, primary CNS glioma, and herpes or CMV encephalitis. Tertiary syphilis lesions have also been reported.

The mortality rate related to the procedure was 1.5%, and the morbidity rate was 4.2%, leaving permanent sequelae in only one case. Based on these data, a decision-analysis model indicated that the life expectancy of patients undergoing brain biopsy was 98 days, compared to 67 days for those who did not, with a net survival benefit of 31 days. The technical skills of those performing and analyzing brain biopsies in various institutions become of paramount importance. In hospitals where the likelihood of obtaining a diagnosis from brain biopsy is only 60%, the net survival advantage might be reduced to 20 days.

These numbers might seem dismal, but they do not take into account the improved quality of life of patients in whom a treatable diagnosis has been uncovered by brain biopsy. In addition, one hopes that the overall survival of patients with AIDS will improve with the antiretroviral medications available such as the protease inhibitors.

## Spinal Syndrome

Myelopathy is a frequent finding at autopsy in patients with AIDS and is probably underrecognized clinically. It can be primarily HIV-associated, or caused by other opportunistic infections or tumors.

## Vacuolar Myelopathy

Vacuolar myelopathy (VM) is present in 17–46% of patients with AIDS at autopsy [52–54]. This disorder occurs with advanced immunosuppression, and the symptoms are often overlooked or attributed to the debilitation related to intercurrent illnesses.

### Presentation

Symptoms are often overshadowed by coexisting central or peripheral nervous system impairment. Usually, patients complain of progressive, painless gait disturbance; weakness and sensory disturbances in the legs; and bowel and bladder incontinence. Neurologic signs include spastic paraparesis, hyperreflexia, extensor plantar responses, and mild sensory impairment with vibratory and position sense being disproportionately affected. There is usually no associated sensory level. Seventy percent of cases have concomitant HIV-associated dementia [53].

### Laboratory Investigations

CSF analysis is either normal or demonstrates the mild elevation of protein and lymphocytosis frequently seen in HIV infection. It is, however, a useful test to rule out other treatable infections.

### Imaging Studies

The MRI of the spinal cord is usually normal in patients with VM. This examination is, however, useful to exclude the possibility of a mass lesion, such as lymphoma or epidural abscess.

### Histologic Studies

Because an anatomic diagnosis is not possible, VM remains a clinical diagnosis of exclusion. At autopsy, discrete or coalescent vacuoles containing cellular debris or macrophages, and, rarely, axonal swellings, can be seen in the white matter of the spinal cord, involving principally the posterior columns, lateral columns, or both [53,54]. These lesions are usually symmetric and more frequent at the middle to lower thoracic levels. These vacuoles appear to be the result of focal swellings within the myelin sheath. Axonal destruction is seen only in areas of intense vacuolation. The etiology of VM is still unknown. Histologic findings are similar to those of subacute combined degeneration of the spinal cord, although serum levels of vitamin $B_{12}$ and folic acid are generally normal.

*Treatment*

There is currently no specific treatment for VM. Other toxic/metabolic or infectious causes should be ruled out. Patients should receive appropriate antiretroviral medication according to their state of immunosuppression.

## Differential Diagnosis of a Noncompressive Myelopathy

Other etiologies of noncompressive myelopathy in patients with advanced HIV infection include other viral infections such as CMV, varicella zoster, and herpes simplex virus (HSV) types 1 and 2, as well as human T cell leukemia/lymphoma virus type I (HTLV-I). HTLV-I is also transmitted sexually or through transfusion of cellular blood products and is the agent of a chronic spastic paraparesis called *HTLV-I–associated myelopathy* [55]. Syphilitic meningomyelitis and rare fungal or parasitic infections are diagnosed by appropriate serologies and cultures.

An algorithm for the clinical management of HIV-1–infected patients with central nervous system symptoms is provided in Figure 9.5.

## **Peripheral Syndrome**

Up to 50% of HIV-infected individuals are affected by peripheral neuropathy. Although some of these might result from medications, metabolic disorders, concomitant infections, or nutritional deficiencies, three major groups have been associated with HIV-1 infection.

## Inflammatory Demyelinating Polyneuropathy

Inflammatory demyelinating polyneuropathy (IDP) can occur at the time of seroconversion, but is generally diagnosed in seropositive patients who are otherwise asymptomatic and not yet profoundly immunosuppressed. Its clinical features are similar to Guillain-Barré syndrome (GBS). Sensory symptoms such as paresthesias may precede an acute, progressive weakness of distal and proximal muscles of two or more limbs, associated with areflexia. Respiratory muscles may be involved, and patients sometimes require assisted ventilation [56]. Sensory signs are usually mild, even in the setting of severe weakness. The nadir of strength is usually reached within the first 4 weeks. Patients with a more protracted course are affected by the chronic form of inflammatory demyelinating polyneuropathy (CIDP), which may be monophasic or relapsing [57].

*Laboratory Investigations*

The CSF analysis differs from HIV-seronegative patients with GBS by the presence of a mononuclear pleocytosis of 20–50 cells. The CSF protein concentra-

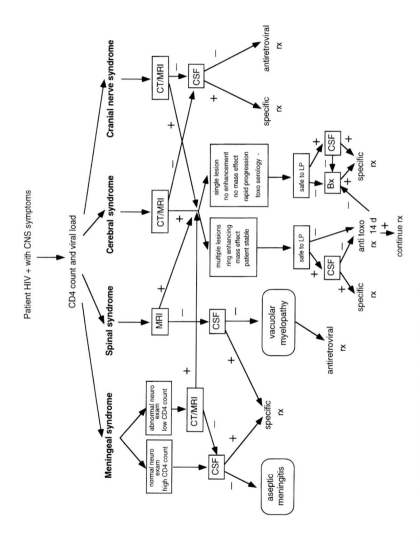

*Figure 9.5*  Management of the HIV-1-infected patient with central nervous system (CNS) symptoms. Knowledge of the CD4+ cell count provides information on the degree of immunosuppression, while measuring the viral load indicates the speed of disease progression (see text for details). (HIV = human immunodeficiency virus; CT = computed tomography; MRI = magnetic resonance imaging; CSF = cerebrospinal fluid; bx = biopsy; LP = lumbar puncture; rx = treatment.)

tion is usually elevated to levels up to 250 mg/dl [56], and a polyclonal gamma-globulinemia can be detected.

## *Electrophysiologic Studies*

Demyelination is demonstrated by reduced motor nerve conduction velocities or prolonged distal latencies and minimum F-wave latencies in two or more nerves. Conduction block is often prominent.

## *Nerve Biopsy*

Sural nerve biopsy generally demonstrates the presence of a perivascular and endoneural mononuclear cell infiltrate with macrophage-mediated segmental demyelination. In severe cases, wallerian-like degeneration of axons can be seen. Similar to GBS, the etiology of inflammatory demyelinating polyneuropathy is thought to be autoimmune. Antiperipheral nerve myelin antibodies have been found in HIV-1–positive patients with GBS, as well as increased levels of soluble CD8 and neopterin in the CSF, indicating an abnormal immune activation.

## *Treatment*

Spontaneous recovery is usually the outcome of GBS, although patients who develop this condition in the setting of HIV-1 infection tend to have a more severe course with a slower recovery. Plasmapheresis is indicated if the illness is sufficiently severe to warrant treatment. Patients with CIDP benefit from treatment with prednisone or plasmapheresis [57,58]. Prednisone should, however, be used with great caution in patients with immunosuppression. Other treatments such as intravenous Ig have also been used successfully in HIV-positive patients with IDP, sometimes in combination with plasmapheresis [59].

## Distal Symmetric Polyneuropathy

Distal symmetric polyneuropathy (DSP) is the most common cause of peripheral neuropathy in HIV-1 infection, which can be diagnosed clinically and electrophysiologically in more than one-third of patients [60] and may be detected at autopsy in most patients dying with AIDS [61]. It occurs generally in patients with advanced immunosuppression and is often associated with HIV-1–associated dementia.

## *Presentation*

DSP is characterized by symmetric paresthesia, numbness, and painful dysesthesia of the lower extremities distally. Pain, temperature, and vibration sense are usually more affected than light touch and proprioception. Hyporeflexia of the lower extremities is a common finding. Weakness is apparent only in advanced cases.

## Laboratory Investigations

CSF analysis shows only nonspecific findings with mild elevation of protein concentration and mononucleated pleocytosis, which is common in HIV infection.

## Electrophysiologic Studies

Nerve conduction studies show low-amplitude or absent sural nerve action potentials. Sensory and motor nerve conduction velocities are normal or only mildly reduced. Electromyogram (EMG) studies demonstrate acute denervation and chronic reinnervation in distal leg muscles. These findings are consistent with a distal symmetric degeneration of sensory and motor axons.

## Nerve Biopsy

Sural nerve biopsy confirms the diagnosis of axonal degeneration of myelinated and unmyelinated axons. A mild perivascular mononucleated infiltrate is present in one-third of the cases, and some demyelination can be seen.

Because this type of polyneuropathy is common in the HIV-1–seronegative population, other etiologies such as vitamin $B_{12}$ deficiency, neurotoxins, alcoholism, or diabetes mellitus should be ruled out. Direct infection of the peripheral nerve by HIV-1 has been suggested [62], but has not been confirmed by other investigators [61,63]. CMV inclusions or antigens have been identified in the peripheral nerves or dorsal root ganglia of some patients with DSP, but this virus has been mainly implicated in cases of progressive polyradiculopathy. Thus, the etiology of DSP in HIV-1 infection remains unclear. AIDS patients treated with didanosine, stavudine, and zalcitabine can present with a similar type of polyneuropathy. Other drugs frequently prescribed are listed in Table 9.3. In drug-induced DSP, clinical improvement should occur within 12 weeks of the drug withdrawal, and patients should be treated with another, nonneurotoxic, antiretroviral medication.

## Treatment

Symptomatic treatment includes tricyclic antidepressants, gabapentin, lamotrigine, carbamazepine, transcutaneous electrical nerve stimulation, or topical capsaicin.

## Mononeuritis Simplex or Multiplex

Patients with previously asymptomatic HIV-1 infection and CD4+ cell counts above 200/µl, as well as patients with AIDS and profound immunosuppression, can be affected by mononeuritis simplex or multiplex (MM).

*Table 9.3* Neurotoxic drugs used in human immunodeficiency virus infection

| Drug | Presentation |
|---|---|
| Nucleoside analogs | |
|     Zidovudine (AZT) | Myopathy |
|     Zalcitabine (ddC) | Distal sensory polyneuropathy (DSP) |
|     Didanosine (ddI) | DSP |
|     Stavudine (d4T) | DSP |
| Antiviral agents | |
|     Foscarnet | Seizures |
| Antibacterial agents | |
|     Isoniazid (INH) | DSP |
|     Dapsone | Distal sensory motor polyneuropathy (DSMP) |
|     Metronidazole* | DSP |
|     Thalidomide | DSP |
| Antineoplastic agents | |
|     Vincristine | DSMP, cranial neuropathy |
|     Cisplatin | DSP |

*High doses only.

## Presentation

Patients present with acute onset of sensory or motor deficit limited to one or more peripheral nerves. Involvement of a facial or laryngeal nerve has also been reported. The course can be self-limited in early HIV-1 infection [64], or more severe in patients with advanced disease.

## Laboratory Investigations

CSF analysis is nonspecific and shows only a mild elevation of protein concentration and a mononuclear pleocytosis.

## Electrophysiological Studies

Nerve conduction studies reveal a reduction of the amplitude of sensory nerve action potentials and compound muscle action potentials as well as a mild reduction in nerve conduction velocities in the distribution of single nerves. The EMG examination is also consistent with focal or asymmetric multifocal axonal degeneration, although considerable overlap may exist with DSP and IDP.

## Nerve Biopsy

Similar to its clinical presentation, the nerve biopsy specimens of patients with MM show a spectrum of pathologies rather than a single pattern. Axonal degeneration and perivascular inflammatory infiltrates are found in patients with early HIV-1 infection and limited clinical involvement. Patients with AIDS and CMV infection have usually mixed axonal and demyelinating lesions with inflammatory infiltrates containing also polymorphonuclear cells, as well as, sometimes, characteristic cytomegalic inclusion bodies. The most aggressive form consists of a necrotizing arteritis with necrosis of endoneural or epineural vessels and might be caused by circulating immune complexes.

*Treatment*

Mild forms of MM developing in patients who are otherwise asymptomatic might improve without specific treatment. Others might benefit from therapies such as plasmapheresis or intravenous Ig. Corticosteroids and cyclophosphamide are reserved for aggressive cases of MM with vasculitis proved by nerve biopsy. In late HIV-1 infection, especially in patients with concurrent systemic CMV infection, empiric therapy with ganciclovir for CMV should be considered.

Progressive Polyradiculopathy

Because it occurs late in the course of HIV-1 infection in patients with low CD4+ cell count and concurrent systemic illnesses, progressive polyradiculopathy is often underrecognized.

*Presentation*

Patients complain initially of lower extremities and sacral paresthesia, and sometimes, radicular pain in the cauda equina distribution. These symptoms are followed by a rapidly progressive areflexive paraparesis and ascending sensory loss, often accompanied by urinary retention. The upper extremities are relatively spared. A thoracic sensory level, if present, indicates concomitant medullary involvement, but other features indicating upper motor neuron damage such as spasticity and hyperreflexia are usually absent. A systemic infection with CMV, mainly retinitis, esophagitis, or colitis is conspicuously present in a majority of cases.

*Laboratory Analysis*

In contrast to other peripheral nervous system diseases associated with HIV-1 infection, the CSF analysis is useful in establishing the diagnosis. A marked polymorphonuclear cell pleocytosis, elevated protein concentration, and hypoglycorrhachia are the hallmark of this syndrome [65]. CSF cultures demonstrate the presence of CMV in 60% of the cases [66]. Cultures may take up to 2 weeks, and CSF samples have to be kept on ice immediately after the lumbar puncture. As is the case with CMV encephalitis, CMV DNA might be detectable in the CSF by PCR. Because of the frequent concomitant systemic infection with CMV, blood culture may also be positive for this virus. Urine culture is nonspecific, because many AIDS patients shed CMV in the urine without being acutely ill from it. Cytologic studies can reveal cytomegalic cells with intranuclear and intracytoplasmic CMV inclusions.

### Electrophysiologic Studies

The EMG examination is useful to differentiate this syndrome from acute IDP. Severe and widespread proximal axonal damage in lumbar nerve root distribution is correlated by fibrillation potentials, complex repetitive discharges, and motor unit recruitment patterns in lower extremities muscles. Motor nerve conduction velocities are minimally altered, but affected muscles will display prolonged or absent F-waves. These findings are consistent with extensive denervation of the lower extremities muscles, which is characteristic in this syndrome.

### Nerve Biopsy

Because of the radicular localization of the lesions, a nerve biopsy is not helpful for diagnosis. Autopsy studies reveal a severe inflammation associated with necrosis of the ventral and dorsal nerve roots [65–67]. Cytomegalic inclusions can be detected within the nucleus and cytoplasm of Schwann, ependymal, and endothelial cells, which are also positive for CMV by in situ hybridization studies. Similar findings have been reported in cranial nerves at the site of exit from the brain stem.

CMV infection is frequent in HIV-1–infected patients and affects multiple organs such as the lungs, intestine, adrenals, and eyes as well as the nervous system. Its actual role in causing specific disease depends, however, on its localization. There is no doubt that CMV is the agent of a retinitis, but CMV pneumonitis is mostly asymptomatic. As reviewed in the earlier section of this chapter on CMV, the presence of CMV in the brain does not necessarily correlate with clinical evidence of encephalopathy. In polyradiculopathy, however, the overwhelming viral presence associated with inflammation and necrosis of the cauda equina strongly advocates for a causal mechanism, which is further supported by a response to specific antiviral treatment.

Despite the strong association of polyradiculopathy and CMV in patients with AIDS, other possibilities include neurosyphilis and lymphomatous meningitis, which should be ruled out on the CSF analysis.

### Treatment

The treatment of CMV infection consist of intravenous ganciclovir (DHPG, Cytovene) or foscarnet (PFA, Foscavir). Ganciclovir, 5.0–7.5 mg/kg intravenously q12h, as induction therapy for a minimum of 2 weeks is followed by a lower maintenance dose of 5 mg/kg qd, while a foscarnet induction regimen of 90 mg/kg intravenously q12h for a minimum of 2 weeks is followed by 90 mg/kg qd for maintenance. The clinical response is variable, but usually is best if therapy is started within days after the onset of symptoms.

Because culture for CMV can take 2 weeks, empiric treatment can be justified, especially if the workup reveals a polymorphonuclear pleocytosis in the CSF or widespread systemic infection with this virus. The rationale is to prevent irreversible necrosis of the nerve roots. In patients who are already paraplegic several weeks after the onset of their symptoms, treatment can achieve stabilization, but no real improvement should be expected.

Treatment of CMV represents a considerable burden for patients with AIDS, because it commits them to long-term, and possibly lifelong, daily intravenous therapy, necessitating a permanent central line. Neutropenia is the most common dose-limiting toxicity of ganciclovir, and may preclude concomitant use of other myelotoxic drugs such as AZT. Concomitant treatment with G-CSF may become necessary in such a setting. Ganciclovir has also been shown to raise the plasma level of ddI, thus increasing the risk of pancreatitis. Foscarnet side effects include nephrotoxicity, electrolyte abnormalities, anemia, and central nervous system toxicity responsible for seizures. The treatment with oral ganciclovir, 1,000 mg tid, has been approved as an alternative maintenance therapy for CMV retinitis, after 2 weeks of intravenous induction as noted above. There are no data regarding oral ganciclovir therapy in patients with polyradiculopathy, but drug levels achieved by using this route of administration are unlikely to be sufficient. Finally, patients who present with progressive polyradiculopathy in the setting of specific treatment of other systemic CMV infection will continue to deteriorate. Double therapy with ganciclovir and foscarnet can be justified because viral resistance may be responsible. Cidofovir (HPMPC) is a new anti-CMV medication that has obtained FDA approval for use in CMV retinitis. There are no data at present regarding its efficacy in patients with polyradiculopathy.

An algorithm for the clinical management of HIV-1–infected patients with peripheral neuropathy is presented in Figure 9.6.

## Muscular Syndrome

Muscular disorders have been described in HIV-1–infected individuals and are sometimes the presenting symptoms but occur predominantly in late stages of the disease.

## Myopathy

### Presentation

Patients complain principally of lower extremity weakness, characterized by difficulty in rising from a chair or climbing stairs as well as fatigue. Myalgias are present in up to half the cases [68], and the neurologic examination reveals proximal symmetrical weakness, predominant at the level of the hip flexors. This syndrome has to be differentiated from HIV wasting syndrome, although some overlap can occur. It might happen simultaneously with other central or peripheral nervous system complications of HIV-1 infection.

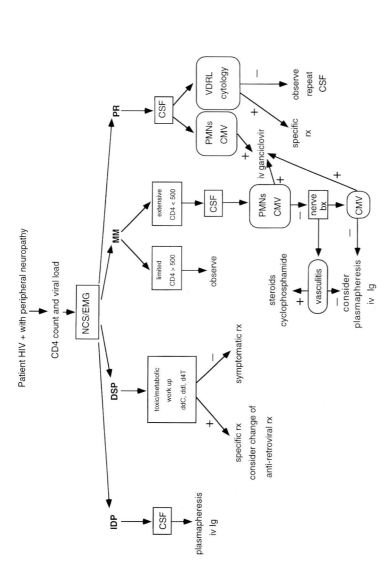

*Figure 9.6* Management of the HIV-1–infected patient with peripheral neuropathy. The nerve conduction studies and electromyographic examination (EMG) are indicated to help differentiate the pattern of peripheral nerve involvement when the clinical examination shows overlap between different entities or when patients are not able to collaborate during the examination. (HIV + = human immunodeficiency virus–positive; NCS = nerve conduction studies; IDP = inflammatory demyelinating polyneuropathy; DSP = distal sensory polyneuropathy; MM = mononeuritis multiplex; PR = polyradiculopathy; CSF = cerebrospinal fluid; PMNs = polymorphonuclear cells; CMV = cytomegalovirus; iv Ig = intravenous immunoglobulins; bx = biopsy; rx = treatment.)

206 Hospitalist Neurology

## Laboratory Investigations

A mild elevation of creatine phosphokinase (CPK) in the serum (median around 500 IU/liter) is the rule, and may be an incidental finding that orients toward a diagnosis in cases where muscle strength is still intact. The level correlates with the degree of myonecrosis seen on muscle biopsy but not necessarily with weakness.

## Electrophysiologic Studies

EMG testing reveals myopathic motor unit potentials with early recruitment and full interference patterns, predominantly in proximal muscles [69]. In half of the cases, NCS show concurrent DSP.

## Muscle Biopsy

The etiology of myopathy in AIDS is a matter of debate [70], because both HIV itself and zidovudine have been incriminated as causative factors. In patients not treated with zidovudine presenting with myopathy, the most common finding is scattered myofiber degeneration, fibrosis, necrosis, and phagocytosis of muscle fibers associated occasionally with an inflammatory infiltrate similar to the one seen in idiopathic polymyositis. The incidence of HIV-1–associated myopathy has not been determined prospectively, but retrospective studies indicate that this is rather a rare event, occurring in around 0.15% of patients. HIV-1 does not seem to infect muscle fibers, and opportunistic organisms have been detected only exceptionally.

Zidovudine therapy has been associated with the occurrence of myopathy in 17% of patients treated for periods over 270 days [71]. Biopsies reveal numerous ragged-red fibers and abnormal mitochondria [72]. Zidovudine-induced mitochondriotoxicity seems to be mediated through the inhibition of the enzyme DNA gamma-polymerase, which is responsible for the replication of mitochondrial DNA. This induces an energy shortage within the muscle, which results in overt myopathy over time.

## Treatment

As in idiopathic polymyositis, immune mechanisms have been proposed in HIV-1 myopathy, and some patients have had a favorable response with corticosteroids [67]. Because of the risks of steroid therapy in immunosuppressed individuals, however, such treatment should be reserved for patients with debilitating weakness and those without evidence of active systemic infection. Other immune-based therapies such as plasmapheresis or intravenous immunoglobulins have not been evaluated in this myopathy. In zidovudine-induced myopathy, treatment consists of zidovudine withdrawal. Objective improvement in muscle strength should occur in most patients after 8 weeks [73].

A summary of the principal neurologic complications of HIV-infection is provided in Figure 9.7.

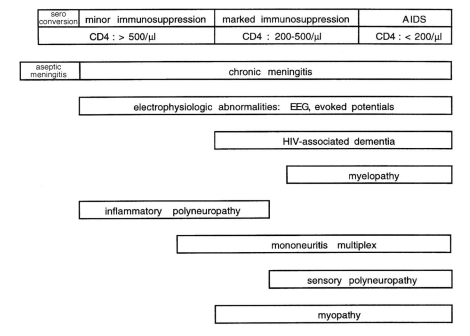

*Figure 9.7*   Occurrence of the principal neurologic complications caused by HIV-1 according to the degree of immunosuppression measured by CD4+ cell count (see text for details). (AIDS = acquired immunodeficiency syndrome; EEG = electroencephalogram; HIV = human immunodeficiency virus.)

## Acknowledgements

We are thankful to Dr. Helen Jacoby and Dr. Seward Rutkove for helpful suggestions and to Dr. Mahesh Patel for Figure 9.3.

## REFERENCES

1. Levy RM, Bredesen DE, Rosenblum ML. Neurologic manifestations of the acquired immunodeficiency syndrome (AIDS): experience at UCSF and review of the literature. J Neurosurg 1985;62: 475–495.
2. Brew BJ, Sidtis JJ, Petito CK, et al. The Neurologic Complications of AIDS and Human Immunodeficiency Virus Infection. In F Plum (ed), Advances in Contemporary Neurology, vol 29. Philadelphia: Davis, 1988;1–49.
3. O'Brien T, Blattner WA, Waters D, et al. Serum HIV-1 RNA levels and time to development of AIDS in the multicenter hemophilia cohort study. JAMA 1996;276:105–110.
4. Mellors JW, Rinaldo CR, Gupta P, et al. Prognosis of HIV-1 infection predicted by the quantity of virus in plasma. Science 1996;272:1167–1170.
5. Powderly WG. Cryptococcal meningitis and AIDS. Clin Infect Dis 1993;17:837–842.
6. Saag MS, Powderly WG, Cloud GA, et al. Comparison of amphotericin B with fluconazole in the treatment of acute AIDS-associated cryptococcal meningitis. N Engl J Med 1992;326:83–89.

7. Johnston SR, Corbett EL, Foster O, et al. Raised intracranial pressure and visual complications in AIDS patients with cryptococcal meningitis. J Infect 1992;24:185–189.
8. Johns DR, Tierney M, Felsenstein D. Alteration in the natural history of neurosyphilis by concurrent infection with the human immunodeficiency virus. N Engl J Med 1987;316:1569–1572.
9. Musher DM, Hamill RJ, Baugh RE. The effect of human immunodeficiency virus (HIV) infection on the course of syphilis and on the response to treatment. Ann Intern Med 1990:113:872–881.
10. Feraru ER, Aronow HA, Lipton RB. Neurosyphilis in AIDS patients: initial CSF VDRL may be negative. Neurology 1990;40:541–543.
11. McArthur JC, Hoover DR, Bacellar H, et al. Dementia in AIDS patients: incidence and risk factors. Multicenter AIDS cohort study. Neurology 1993;43:2245–2252.
12. Koralnik IJ, Beaumanoir A, Häusler R, et al. A controlled study of early neurologic abnormalities in men with asymptomatic human immunodeficiency virus infection. N Engl J Med 1990;323:864–870.
13. Miller EN, Selnes OA, McArthur JC, et al. Neuropsychological performance in HIV-1-infected homosexual men: the multicenter AIDS cohort study (MACS). Neurology 1990;40:197–203.
14. Portegies P, Enting RH, de Gans GJ, et al. Presentation and course of AIDS dementia complex: 10 years of follow-up in Amsterdam, The Netherlands. AIDS 1993;7:669–675.
15. Tornatore C, Chandra R, Berger JR, et al. HIV infection of subcortical astrocytes in the pediatric central nervous system. Neurology 1994;44:481–487.
16. Lipton SA, Gendelman HE. Dementia associated with the acquired immunodeficiency syndrome. N Engl J Med 1995;332:934–939.
17. Hamilton JD, Hartigan PM, Simberkoff MS, et al. A controlled trial of early versus late treatment with zidovudine in symptomatic human immunodeficiency virus infection. Results of the Veterans Affairs Cooperative Study. N Engl J Med 1992;326:437–443.
18. Sitdis FF, Gatsonis C, Price BW, et al. Zidovudine treatment of the AIDS dementia complex: results of a placebo-controlled trial. Ann Neurol 1993;33:343–349.
19. Luft BJ, Hafner R, Korzun AN, et al. Toxoplasmic encephalitis in the acquired immunodeficiency syndrome. N Engl J Med 1993;329:995–1000.
20. Renold C, Sugar A, Chave J-P, et al. Toxoplasma encephalitis in patients with the acquired immunodeficiency syndrome. Medicine 1992;71:224–239.
21. Porter SB, Sande MA. Toxoplasmosis of the central nervous system in the acquired immunodeficiency syndrome. N Engl J Med 1992;327:1643–1648.
22. Farmley SF, Goedbel FD, Remington JS. Detection of *Toxoplasma gondii* in cerebrospinal fluid from AIDS patients by polymerase chain reaction. J Clin Microbiol 1992;30:3000–3002.
23. Schoondermark-van de Ven E, Galama J, Kraaijeveld C, et al. Value of the polymerase chain reaction for the detection of *Toxoplasma gondii* in cerebrospinal fluid from patients with AIDS. Clin Infect Dis 1993;16:661–666.
24. Holloway RG, Mushlin AI. Intracranial mass lesions in acquired immunodeficiency syndrome: using decision analysis to determine the effectiveness of stereotactic brain biopsy. Neurology 1996;46:1010–1015.
25. Haverkos HW. Assessment of therapy for toxoplasma encephalitis. The TE study group. Am J Med 1987;82:907–913.
26. Pedrol E, Gonzales-Clemente JM, Gatel JM, et al. Central nervous system toxoplasmosis in AIDS patients: efficacy of an intermittent maintenance therapy. AIDS 1990;4:511–517.
27. So YT, Beckstead JH, Davis RL. Primary central nervous system lymphoma in acquired immune deficiency syndrome: a clinical and pathological study. Ann Neurol 1986;20:566–572.
28. MacMahon EM, Glass JD, Hayward SD, et al. Association of Epstein-Barr virus with primary central nervous system lymphoma in AIDS. AIDS Res Hum Retroviruses 1992;8:740–742.
29. Borggreve F, Diercks RA, Crols R, et al. Repeat thallium-201 SPECT in cerebral lymphoma. Funct Neurol 1993;8:95–101.
30. Ruiz A, Ganz WI, Donovan Post MJ, et al. Use of thallium-201 brain SPECT to differentiate cerebral lymphoma from toxoplasma encephalitis in AIDS patients. Am J Neuroradiol 1994;15:1885–1894.
31. Levy RM, Russell E, Yungbluth M, et al. The efficacy of image-guided stereotactic brain biopsy in neurologically symptomatic acquired immunodeficiency syndrome patients. Neurosurgery 1992;30:186–190.
32. Marks WJ, McArthur JC, Kumar RW. Intracranial mass lesions in AIDS: diagnosis and response to therapy. Neurology 1989;39(suppl):380.
33. Levy RM, Berger JR. Neurologic critical care in patients with human immunodeficiency virus 1 infection. Crit Care Clin 1993;9:49–72.

34. Morgello S, Petito CK, Mouradian JA. Central nervous system lymphoma in the acquired immunodeficiency syndrome. Clin Neuropathol 1990;9:205–215.
35. Rosenberg NL, Hochberg FH, Miller G, et al. Primary central nervous system lymphoma related to Epstein-Barr virus in a patient with acquired immune deficiency syndrome. Ann Neurol 1986;20:98–102.
36. Forsyth PA, Yahalom J, DeAngelis LM. Combined-modality therapy in the treatment of primary central nervous system lymphoma in AIDS. Neurology 1994;44:1473–1479.
37. Gill PS, Levine AM, Meter PR, et al. Primary central nervous system lymphoma in a homosexual man. Am J Med 1985;78:742–748.
38. Berger RJ, Kaszovitz B, Donovan Post JM, et al. Progressive multifocal leukoencephalopathy associate with human immunodeficiency virus infection. A review of the literature with a report of sixteen cases. Ann Intern Med 1987;107:78–87.
39. Fong IW, Toma E, et al. The natural history of progressive multifocal leukoencephalopathy in patients with AIDS. Clin Infect Dis 1995;20:1305–1310.
40. Fong IW, Britton CB, Luinstra KE, et al. Diagnostic value of detecting JC virus DNA in cerebrospinal fluid of patients with progressive multifocal leukoencephalopathy. J Clin Microbiol 1995;33:484–486.
41. McGuire D, Barhite S, Hollander H, et al. JC virus DNA in cerebrospinal fluid of human immunodeficiency virus-infected patients: predictive value for progressive multifocal leukoencephalopathy. Ann Neurol 1995;37:395–399.
42. Hansman Whiteman ML, Donovan Post JM, Berger JR, et al. Progressive multifocal leukoencephalopathy in 47 HIV-seropositive patients: neuroimaging with clinical and pathologic correlation. Radiology 1993;187:233–240.
43. Gray F, Geny C, Lescs MC, et al. AIDS-related progressive multifocal leukoencephalopathy confined to U fibers with subacute encephalopathy and normal CT scan findings. Arch Anat Cytol Pathol 1992;40:132–137.
44. Major EO, Amemiya K, Tornatore CS, et al. Pathogenesis and molecular biology of progressive multifocal leukoencephalopathy, the JC virus-induced demyelinating disease of the human brain. Clin Microbiol Rev 1992;5:49–73.
45. Hall CD, Dafni U, Simpson D, et al. Failure of cytarabine in progressive multifocal leukoencephalopathy associated with human immunodeficiency virus infection. N Engl J Med 1998;338:1345–1351.
46. Morgello S, Cho ES, Nielsen S, et al. Cytomegalovirus encephalitis in patients with acquired immunodeficiency syndrome: an autopsy study of 30 cases and review of the literature. Hum Pathol 1987;18:289–297.
47. Vinters HV, Kwok MK, Ho HW, et al. Cytomegalovirus in the nervous system of patients with the acquired immunodeficiency syndrome. Brain 1989;52:975–979.
48. Wolf DG, Spector SA. Diagnosis of human cytomegalovirus central nervous system disease by DNA amplification from cerebrospinal fluid. J Infect Dis 1992;166:1412–1415.
49. Cinque P, Vago L, Brytting M, et al. Cytomegalovirus infection of the central nervous system in patients with AIDS: diagnosis by DNA amplification form cerebrospinal fluid. J Infect Dis 1992;166:1408–1411.
50. Post MJ, Hensley GT, Moskowitz LB, et al. Cytomegalic inclusion virus in patients with AIDS: CT, clinical, and pathologic correlation. Am J Roentgenol 1986;146:1229–1234.
51. Holland NR, Power C, Mathews VP, et al. Cytomegalovirus encephalitis in acquired immunodeficiency syndrome (AIDS). Neurology 1994;44:507–514.
52. Henin D, Smith TW, DeGirolami U, et al. Neuropathology of the spinal cord in the acquired immunodeficiency syndrome. Hum Pathol 1992;23:1106–1114.
53. Petito CK, Navia BA, Cho ES, et al. Vacuolar myelopathy pathologically resembling subacute combined degeneration in patients with the acquired immunodeficiency syndrome. N Engl J Med 1985;312:874–879.
54. Dal Pan GJ, Glass JD, McArthur JC. Clinicopathologic correlations of HIV-1–associated vacuolar myelopathy: an autopsy-based case-control study. Neurology 1994;44:2159–2164.
55. Gessain A, Gout O. Chronic myelopathy associated with human T-lymphotropic virus type I (HTLV-I). Ann Intern Med 1992;117:933-946.
56. Cornblath DR, McArthur JC, Kennedy PGE, et al. Inflammatory demyelinating peripheral neuropathies associated with human T-cell lymphotropic virus type III infection. Ann Neurol 1987;21:32–40.
57. Miller RG, Parry GJ, Pfaeffl W, et al. The spectrum of peripheral neuropathy associated with ARC and AIDS. Muscle Nerve 1988;11:857–863.
58. Leger JM, Bouch P, Bolgert F, et al. The spectrum of polyneuropathies in patients infected with HIV. J Neurol Neurosurg Psychiatry 1989;52:1309–1374.

59. Kiprov DD, Sticker RB, Miller RG. Treatment of HIV neuropathy with plasmapheresis and intravenous gammaglobulin: an update. Int Conf AIDS 1992; abstract Pub 7281,8:95.
60. So YT, Holtzman DM, Abrams DI, et al. Peripheral neuropathy associated with acquired immunodeficiency syndrome. Arch Neurol 1988;45:945–948.
61. Griffin JW, Crawford TO, Tyor WR, et al. Predominantly sensory neuropathy in AIDS: distal axonal degeneration and unmyelinated fiber loss. Neurology 1991;41(suppl):374.
62. de la Monte S, Gabuzda DH, Ho DD, et al. Peripheral neuropathy in the acquired immunodeficiency syndrome. Ann Neurol 1988;23:485–492.
63. Mah V, Vartavarian LM, Akers MA, et al. Abnormalities of peripheral nerve in patients with human immunodeficiency virus infection. Ann Neurol 1988;24:713–717.
64. So YT, Olney RK. The natural history of mononeuropathy multiplex and simplex in patients with HIV infection. Neurology 1991;41(suppl):375.
65. Miller RG, Storey JR, Greco CM. Ganciclovir in the treatment of AIDS-related polyradiculopathy. Neurology 1990;40:569–574.
66. de Gans J, Portegies P, Tiessens G, et al. Therapy for cytomegalovirus polyradiculopathy in patients with AIDS. Treatment with ganciclovir. AIDS 1990;4:421–425.
67. Eidelberg D, Sotrel A, Vogel H, et al. Progressive polyradiculopathy in acquired immune deficiency syndrome. Neurology 1986;36:912–916.
68. Simpson DM, Tagliati M. Neuromuscular complications of HIV infection. Hosp Phys 1994;30:18–33.
69. Simpson DM, Citak KA, Godfrey MS, et al. Myopathies associated with human immunodeficiency virus and zidovudine: can their effect be distinguished? Neurology 1993;43:971–976.
70. Dalakas MC. HIV or zidovudine myopathy ? [letter] Neurology 1994;44:360–364.
71. Peters BS, Winer J, Landon DN, et al. Mitochondrial myopathy associated with chronic zidovudine therapy in AIDS. QJM 1993;86:5–15.
72. Dalakas MC, Illa I, Pezeshkpour GH, et al. Mitochondrial myopathy caused by long-term zidovudine therapy. N Engl J Med 1990;322:1098–1105.
73. Grau JM, Masanes F, Pedro E, et al. Human immunodeficiency virus type 1 infection and myopathy: clinical relevance of zidovudine therapy. Ann Neurol 1993;34:206–211.

# 10
# Ethical Questions

James L. Bernat

Neurologists frequently encounter ethical questions in the course of hospital consultations. For example, does a neurologist have an ethical duty to treat patients infected with human immunodeficiency virus (HIV) at a risk to the neurologist's own health? Can a demented patient provide valid consent for treatment? What are the limits of a neurologist's duty to maintain patient confidentiality when a third party may be harmed as a result? Should neurologists always tell patients the truth about their diagnosis and prognosis? When and how should a neurologist terminate a patient's life-sustaining therapy and institute palliative care? Is palliative care the most appropriate treatment for patients with advanced dementia? Are physician-assisted suicide and voluntary active euthanasia acceptable medical practices? How should neurologists respond to patients' requests for assistance in helping them to die? This chapter addresses these and other ethical questions arising in the course of hospital neurologic consultations. I have more thoroughly discussed the full scope of ethical issues arising in neurologic practice elsewhere [1].

## PHYSICIAN-PATIENT RELATIONSHIP

Answering ethical questions concerning neurologists' professional duties to patients first requires an understanding of the physician-patient relationship. The physician-patient relationship contains elements of both a contract and a fiduciary trust. Patients and neurologists enter an unwritten contract in which the neurologist promises to provide competent and conscientious neurologic care and to respect the dignity, privacy, confidentiality, and autonomy of the patient. The patient promises to cooperate with the mutually agreed on diagnostic and treatment plan and to tell the neurologist the truth. As a fiduciary, the neurologist promises always to place the patient's welfare above the neurologist's proprietary interests.

## Terminating the Physician-Patient Relationship

Neurologists retain the freedom to initiate or terminate the physician-patient relationship within certain bounds. Neurologists may choose whom they wish to treat, but it is unethical to refuse to treat a patient solely on the basis of a patient's gender, religion, race, nationality, or disease state, assuming the competence to treat. Once a patient has been accepted for treatment, the neurologist has an ethical obligation to maintain the relationship until one of the parties terminates it. In many cases, both parties terminate the physician-patient relationship, such as when a neurologist returns a patient's care to a primary physician. The neurologist who chooses unilaterally to terminate the relationship has a duty to assure that adequate provisions have been made for follow-up care by another physician. Neurologists who unilaterally terminate a relationship without making such provisions may be accused of abandonment [2].

## Duty to Treat

The acquired immunodeficiency syndrome (AIDS)/HIV epidemic again has raised the ancient question of the physician's duty to treat sick patients when such treatment entails personal risk to the physician. Throughout history, physicians have been exposed to personal health risks in the course of their treatment of patients. From their patients, physicians have contracted countless cases of infectious diseases such as tuberculosis, plague, hepatitis, yellow fever, and viral respiratory tract infections. Thus, the practice of medicine always has had some degree of intrinsic health risk to the practitioner that automatically was assumed by entering the profession. It would be unreasonable and foolish, however, to require physicians to assume an overwhelming personal health risk when caring for patients, although some altruistic physicians in the setting of epidemics historically have volunteered to do so.

Medicine is a learned profession and not a business or trade. The purpose of the medical profession is to provide medical care to patients, not the accumulation of wealth. The welfare of the patient remains of paramount importance. The medical profession imposes binding obligations to treat the sick that require physicians to be willing to undergo some degree of personal risk. Indeed, the implicit and explicit oaths physicians take on entering and becoming socialized into the medical profession formalize such a commitment [3].

The duty to treat AIDS and HIV patients, therefore, is clear but must be balanced against the neurologist's personal risk. The risk of a physician contracting HIV from an infected patient has been quantitated. For an internist caring for patients in a population with a 5% prevalence of HIV, there is a 0.000075 annual risk of seroconversion (i.e., about 75 cases per million), largely the result of accidental needlestick injuries. This estimated rate would be higher for a surgeon, because of greater blood and injury exposure, and higher for physicians treating patients in practices with a greater prevalence of HIV [4].

Neurologists probably have a lower rate of HIV seroconversion than internists because they perform venipuncture and arterial puncture less often and therefore are less likely to be injured by a contaminated needle. The risk of acquiring HIV by accidental needlestick injury during lumbar puncture is probably relatively small because there are fewer infectious particles present per unit of volume in cerebrospinal fluid than in blood. The risk of acquiring HIV by accidental self-puncture by electromyography needles is low because solid needles convey fewer infectious particles than hollow-bore needles. Thus, neurologists probably have an exceeding low risk of HIV seroconversion from infected patients and should not refuse to treat HIV patients based on this tiny risk.

The medical specialty societies that have studied this issue all have concurred that physicians have an ethical duty to treat HIV patients, but should act prudently to minimize their personal risk of accidental infection by observing proper universal precautions. The American Academy of Neurology, the American College of Physicians, the American Medical Association, and the Infectious Diseases Society of America all affirm the duty to treat the HIV patient and to observe universal precautions [5].

## INFORMED CONSENT

One of the defining characteristics of contemporary medical ethics is the physician's requirement to obtain a patient's informed consent before beginning a course of diagnosis or treatment. Medical ethics requires informed consent because the medical profession and society respect patients' fundamental rights of personal autonomy to decide freely what will or will not be done to their bodies. Informed consent can be abrogated only in an emergency medical situation in which a patient's consent for treatment is presumed. When the patient lacks the capacity to provide consent, physicians must obtain such consent from a proxy decision maker.

Informed consent is a process of communication between a physician and a patient during which a patient's valid approval is sought for specific types of medical care. It is not merely obtaining a patient's signature on a written consent form. Such a signature, when required, only is meant to signify that a process of communication has occurred. The signature without the preceding process of communication is insufficient for valid consent.

Contemporary medicine recognizes that consent is a process of shared decision making. Physicians and their patients both contribute unique components to the process. Physicians bring information, experience, and a learned opinion. They have a duty to educate the patient sufficiently to permit an informed treatment choice. Patients filter this information and the treatment opinion through their system of personal values and preferences. Jointly the patient and physician reach an optimum treatment choice [6].

Three elements are necessary and sufficient for informed consent to be valid: (1) the patient must be competent to provide consent, (2) the patient must be provided with information adequate to obtain consent, and (3) the physician must not coerce the patient to provide consent [7].

## Competence

In clinical ethics, the term *competence* refers to the capacity of a patient to understand and process the information provided by a physician in order to reach a health care decision. Physicians ordinarily do not use the term in its strict legal sense, in which it describes a patient's mental capacity that can be determined only by a court of law. Competence in its medical sense is a task-specific capacity. Thus, a patient may be competent to consent to treatment but not to execute a will.

Neurologists classify patients as competent, incompetent, or of unclear competence. Generally, neurologists assume patients are competent unless they have specific evidence to the contrary. Among hospitalized patients, stupor, coma, dementia, and delirium are common causes of patient incompetence. Patients with mild degrees of dementia and concomitant metabolic or toxic encephalopathies may have fluctuating states of competence. When patients lack the capacity to understand the information neurologists present to them, cannot process the information rationally, or cannot communicate a treatment decision, neurologists usually conclude that they are incompetent to provide consent. When the status of competence remains unclear after careful study, psychiatric consultation may be indicated to help further clarify the issue.

## Adequate Information

Patients need adequate information from neurologists to be able to reach a rational treatment decision. The amount and type of information simply are those that a reasonable person would require to be able to make such a decision. Reasonable people need to know (1) their treatment choices; (2) the risks and benefits of each choice, including that of no treatment; (3) the treatment course recommended by the neurologist; and (4) the reason for the neurologist's treatment recommendation [8].

Neurologists should present the first two categories of information in an unbiased manner with the neurologist taking care not to exaggerate the benefits or to minimize the risks of the favored treatment over the alternatives. Later in the discussion, the neurologist can offer his learned opinion as well as the reasons for that opinion. To the fullest extent possible during the consent process, neurologists should clearly separate facts and opinions to permit patients to disagree with treatment recommendations while agreeing about the facts.

Reasonable people want to know their range of options. The neurologist is not required to offer or discuss treatments that are of no medical benefit, however. Patients need to know the risks of treatment that are common, even if not serious, and those that are serious, even if not common. Generally, neurologists are not required to discuss risks smaller than 0.0001, such as those that are idiosyncratic, although many prudent neurologists do so when the risk is death or serious disability.

## Absence of Coercion

Neurologists should not coerce patients; their consent is valid only when it is a freely made decision. Neurologists should avoid all forms of coercion, such as threatening patients with abandonment or exaggerating the harms of not following a prescribed treatment regimen.

The framing effect can be a subtle form of coercion. Physicians know that *how* they present a topic to a patient predicts to a large extent how the patient will respond to it [9]. Some physicians wrongly frame topics in a biased way by consciously or subconsciously exaggerating the benefits and minimizing the risks of their preferred course of treatment and by using leading statements, gestures, or voice inflection in a tendentious manner. Some physicians rationalize this practice by arguing that, because the patient needs the specific treatment anyway, framing it in a biased way comforts the patient by making the best treatment choice easier to make. In fact, such manipulative behavior prevents the patient from making an informed decision. During the consent process, physicians should make a treatment recommendation. Indeed, they have the privilege to make a strong treatment recommendation if they feel it is appropriate. But by biasing the factual portion of the consent process, physicians have crossed the ethical boundary separating a strong treatment recommendation from coercion, and in so doing, they have violated one of the fundamental tenets of the doctrine of informed consent.

## CONFIDENTIALITY

Maintaining the privacy and confidentiality of patients represents an important ethical duty of neurologists. This duty encompasses the care neurologists should take in not discussing patient cases where they may be overheard and not sharing a patient's confidential medical information with anyone without the patient's consent. This duty is more complex when the written and computerized medical record must be shared with insurers and other third parties who demonstrate the "right to know." Nevertheless, strict patient confidentiality is a goal toward which neurologists and all physicians should aspire. Two ethical questions arise commonly in the course of the physician's usual attempt to protect inpatient confidentiality: (1) what are the limits of the duty to maintain confidentiality when third parties may be at risk as a result, and (2) what should physicians do about unsubstantiated "secrets" about patients told to them by relatives and friends?

### Confidentiality versus the Duty to Prevent Harm

The conflict between the duty to protect patient confidentiality and the duty to protect third parties known to be at risk of harm has arisen most recently in cases of HIV-seropositive patients whose continued unprotected sexual activity or needle-sharing drug abuse behavior is placing one or more third parties at risk of contracting HIV. If the HIV-seropositive patient refuses to notify the at-risk sexual partner or needle-sharing partner about his or her HIV status, should the physician abrogate the ordinary duty to maintain patient confidentiality and notify the health department or the third party directly without the patient's consent?

This question has become the subject of intense debate over the past decade. Most authorities have concluded that, in the case of an identifiable third party known to be at risk of harm whose risk could be lessened or prevented by disclosure, there is a strong ethical duty to notify him or her. This duty takes precedence over the usual duty to maintain patient confidentiality. First, the physician should strongly urge the HIV-seropositive patient to notify the at-risk third party directly so he or she can take appropriate safety precautions to prevent transmission. Only in the presence of a refusal to notify or inaction after agreeing to notify should the physician take specific steps without the patient's consent.

Many states have altered their HIV patient confidentiality statutes to no longer provide absolute confidentiality when a third party is in jeopardy of direct and easily preventable harm. Similarly, several medical societies, including the American Academy of Neurology, American College of Physicians, American Medical Association, and Infectious Diseases Society of America, have stated that physicians' highest ethical duty in such cases is to protect third parties known to be at risk even if that requires violating patient confidentiality [10].

### Secrets about Patients

Neurologists may sometimes be told unsolicited secrets about their patients from well-meaning or malicious friends and relatives. Such secrets may include that the patient has a covert problem with alcohol or other drug abuse, is not following prescribed medical therapy, or is engaging in various high-risk behaviors. Often the secret-teller adds a disclaimer such as "don't tell him I told you so" or the teller communicates the message anonymously by letter or telephone call. What should neurologists do with such information?

First, neurologists should encourage the secret-teller to communicate his or her concern directly to the patient and not ask the neurologist to intervene. If, as is often the case, the secret-teller is unwilling to do this, the neurologist should tell the secret-teller that physicians have an ethical obligation to share this information with patients once they have been made aware of it. Neurologists are under no obligation to withhold secret information from their patients simply because a secret-teller told them to. It may be desirable for the neurologist to communicate this information to the patient, but the neurologist should exercise judgment about whether to share the source of the information [11].

## TRUTH-TELLING

An ongoing ethical debate surrounds whether physicians always should tell patients the truth about their diagnosis and prognosis. In times past, many physicians paternalistically withheld communicating diagnostic and prognostic information from patients if they believed the information could not help and might harm the patient. These practices were most widespread in the setting of chronic, untreatable, and ultimately fatal neurologic conditions such as amyotrophic lateral sclerosis, multiple sclerosis, and Alzheimer's disease. Most Western physicians today recognize that such deception cannot be justified in the majority of circumstances, but physicians' purposely withholding information in an attempt to protect a patient remains the normal medical practice in many other cultures.

## Is Deception Justified?

Physicians who believe that it is appropriate not to communicate unfavorable diagnostic and prognostic information to patients with progressive or untreatable diseases employ a series of justifications for their practices. Their reasons include the following: (1) telling patients that they have an untreatable disease will extinguish all hope and eliminate the will to continue living; (2) patients learning bad news will develop depression that will produce great suffering; (3) it is wrong to burden patients with the knowledge that they have an untreatable disease when, in fact, no physician ever can be completely certain of medical diagnosis and prognosis; (4) many patients really do not wish to know this information and it is wrong to force it on them; and (5) many patients lack the ability to understand technical information and may not comprehend what they are being told.

The possible benefits of withholding information must be balanced against the harms that may result from doing so. One harm for patients wishing to learn their diagnosis is that they may "doctor shop" and thereby undergo painful, dangerous, expensive, wasteful, and unnecessary repeated evaluations until they finally learn their diagnosis. They may learn to mistrust all physicians once they discover that they were purposely deceived. They may develop anxiety from the fear that they have a disease that is so terrible that even their own physician cannot muster the courage to tell them what it is.

The most serious harm that befalls patients, however, is that without knowledge of their diagnosis or prognosis, they cannot plan realistically for important life events such as education, marriage, and childbearing. If patients are not told that they are dying, they may be denied the opportunity to make amends, say good-byes, resolve conflicts, and spend time with their loved ones. Despite the beneficent motives of the physician in trying to use deception to protect a patient, from a purely utilitarian perspective, more harm likely will be created than prevented. Paternalism cannot be justified in the majority of cases of deception because of this net harm and because no physician would advocate publicly for deception in all such cases. Surveys of patients with chronic illnesses such as multiple sclerosis and amyotrophic lateral sclerosis reveal that the large majority wish to be told their diagnosis and prognosis [12].

## How to Tell the Truth

Neurologists should communicate the truth to patients about their diagnosis and prognosis but should do so in a gentle, compassionate, and reassuring way. Diagnostic uncertainty can be minimized by offering to assist patients in securing a second opinion if they wish, without fear of offending the neurologist. Neurologists should make a pact with patients that they will not abandon them no matter how sick they become during course of their illness. The neurologist's continuity of care and availability for follow-up visits and telephone calls are essential features of proper chronic disease medical care [13].

One of the major roles for neurologists in the management of chronic disease is education of the patient and family. Neurologists should recommend to patients and their families one of the numerous self-help books available about their illness that can provide them additional information and coping strategies. Neurologists also can assist their patients and families to participate in community discussion groups with other patients and families with their particular disease and to receive newsletters and other information and services from the national foundations serving those with their particular disease.

Patients' hopes can be maintained by assisting them in informing themselves about and entering controlled clinical treatment trials that may be effective in ameliorating symptoms of their disease. Even if the trials do not turn out to be effective, participating in them promotes hope and provides an avenue for patients to make the ennobling gesture of helping others, an experience that often generates important personal meaning from their illness.

## TERMINATION OF LIFE-SUSTAINING TREATMENT

At some point in the treatment of the critically ill or chronically ill patient, the patient and physician both recognize that the patient is dying and that further life-sustaining treatment will act only to prolong the inevitable dying process. At this point, most patients or proxies refuse further life-sustaining treatment. In this situation, physicians should order a palliative care treatment plan to permit the patient to die of his or her underlying illness in the most comfortable manner possible.

The implementation of this decision often is stressful for neurologists and other physicians. They may resist accepting it for several reasons: (1) They may be uncertain about the patient's exact prognosis and therefore reluctant to stop life-sustaining treatment until they can be more certain; (2) they may have psychological discomfort in treating a dying patient and therefore deny that the patient is dying; (3) they may lack knowledge of how to provide palliative care; (4) they may be uncomfortable responding to patients' requests for physician-assisted suicide or voluntary active euthanasia; and (5) they may be uncertain how to plan the details of a patient's death. This section considers these and other ethical questions arising in the termination of life-sustaining treatment and management of the dying patient.

### Importance of Prognosis in Decision Making

The neurologist's shift in treatment modes from curative to palliative care first requires a clear understanding of the patient's diagnosis and prognosis. Indeed, an unambiguous statement of prognosis is a prerequisite for proper ethical decision making in critically ill patients. Although it may be appropriate medical practice to terminate life-sustaining treatment for a critically ill, dying patient, generally it is inappropriate medical practice to terminate life-sustaining therapy on a critically ill patient who has an entirely reversible underlying illness.

Many of the most vexing questions about the management of critically ill patients arise in those for whom the prognosis remains unclear or changes with time. For example, consider an elderly woman with pneumonia and respiratory failure who is admitted to an intensive care unit. On admission, there may be no reason to think that her illness is not entirely reversible. Therefore, most physicians, patients, and proxies would find an aggressive, curative approach to be the most appropriate medical care. But if subsequently she were to develop sepsis, renal failure, and disseminated intravascular coagulation, her prognosis would become much worse and her illness reversibility far less likely. At this point, a proxy decision maker appropriately may refuse further life-sustaining therapy. When her illness is viewed in retrospect, commentators may criticize the physician for being inappropriately aggressive earlier in the management of a dying patient. But as this case demonstrates, the understanding that a critically ill patient also is terminally ill often may be had more clearly in retrospect.

To help address this common problem, researchers have worked to devise and validate prognosis scales for critically ill patients. The Acute Physiology and Chronic Health Evaluation (APACHE) III scale has been tested widely and can provide instantaneous prognostic information using a set of variables measuring the functioning of multiple organ systems. APACHE III and similar scales provide a statistical estimate of survival probability at each stage of a critical illness. The Study to Understand Prognoses and Preferences for Outcomes and Risks of Treatments showed the difficulty physicians experience in incorporating this information into their practices, however [14]. For example, if a prognosis scale revealed that a patient's chances for survival in the setting of a given critical illness were 20%, should the proxy refuse further life-sustaining treatment? What treatment course should the physician recommend? Indeed, what is the precise numerical prognostic threshold for converting from curative care to palliative care?

The threshold for the ethical acceptability of terminating life-sustaining treatment and initiating only palliative care must remain a controversial issue because the threshold floats depending on a particular patient's or proxy's preferences. For example, surveys have shown that some patients refuse further life-sustaining treatment only when their chances for recovery are below 1% whereas others do so when their chances for recovery are as high as 40%. Despite the psychological difficulties involved, generally neurologists and other physicians should defer to the particular preferences of patients and their proxies regarding the delineation of such a statistical threshold.

## The Proxy Decision Maker

Patients who lack the capacity to make their own health care decisions require a proxy decision maker to act in their place. Proxies can be appointed formally or informally. Informal proxy decision making usually is performed by the next of kin or by the most interested relative or friend of the patient. If there is no disagreement among the family or between the proxy's decision and the treatment course recommended by the physician, such informal mechanisms usually are followed and work well in practice. Because the patient's family's opinion is not always unified, however, it is preferable to recommend to patients that they formally name a proxy decision maker in advance of the time that such decision making will be necessary.

Most states now have enacted formalized mechanisms for appointing a legally authorized proxy decision maker. Some states refer to the legal proxy as the *health care agent*; others as the *durable power of attorney for health care*.

When a patient legally appoints a health care agent, the agent has the same general authority to consent to or refuse treatment as does the patient. The physician must approach the health care agent for all consent questions that ordinarily would be addressed to the patient. Most states authorize health care agents to refuse life-sustaining therapy on behalf of an incompetent patient, but some states restrict that authority in those cases in which the physician recommends continued treatment [15].

## Proxy Decision-Making Standards

Proxy decision makers must reach a judgment about treatment using the proper standards of decision making. There are three general standards that should be employed. The proxy first should abide by the patient's expressed wishes if these are known. Lacking that knowledge, the proxy should use the standard of substituted judgment if possible. If this cannot be accomplished, the proxy should use the standard of best interest.

Following the patient's expressed wishes represents the highest standard of proxy decision making because it perfectly reproduces the decision that the patient would have made if the patient retained the capacity to do so. It is the most ethically powerful standard because it most highly respects the autonomy of the patient despite the patient's present incompetence.

If the patient has executed a written directive, such as a living will or terminal care document, a record of the patient's expressed wishes may be found there. Most written directives, however, are too vague and ambiguous to identify a patient's expressed wishes in any particular medical situation. If the patient earlier had held a conversation with the proxy about the specific topic in question, such a conversation would count as a less formal record of the patient's expressed wishes. Many states would not consider such informal directives to carry the same weight as written directives, however, because of the presumption that patients consider written directives more thoughtfully. Because of the complexity and variability of most medical situations, it is relatively uncommon for a proxy to know the patient's expressed wishes in any given clinical circumstance.

In the absence of knowledge of expressed wishes, the proxy should employ the standard of substituted judgment. Using this standard, the proxy employs the value system and known preferences of the patient to attempt to reproduce the decision that the patient would have made in a novel medical situation. It is important that the proxy understand that it is not *the proxy's* decision that is being requested. Indeed, a substituted judgment decision may be the opposite of that which the proxy would choose for himself or herself. Rather, the proxy is asked to make the decision the patient would have made. Such a process requires that the proxy know about and faithfully follow the values and preferences of the patient. This type of decision permits patients' autonomy to be respected despite their present incapacity.

The accuracy of substituted judgment decision making has been tested in survey studies. In one study, elderly residents of a retirement community were asked to predict the preferences of their longstanding spouses for receiving cardiopulmonary resuscitation (CPR) in the event of sudden cardiac arrest. Surprisingly, approximately one-third guessed incorrectly, mostly that their spouses would want to receive CPR when they would not. Other studies have yielded similar results [16]. These are sobering data; if long-standing spouses cannot make reliable substituted judgments, then who can? Despite the inaccuracy of substituted judgment, it probably is superior to alternative methods of decision making, such as best interests.

If proxies do not know the values and preferences of the patients they represent sufficiently to make a substituted judgment decision, they should employ a best-interest standard, which asks the proxy to consider what course of treatment he or she feels is in the best interest of the patient. This is ethically less powerful than a substituted judgment standard because the proxy is using his or her own values and preferences to reach a judgment, rather than those of the patient. Thus, the chances are less that the decision would conform to that which the patient would have made. Proxies must take special care when using this standard to balance their potentially conflicting interests against that course which is truly in the patient's best interest.

## Legal Issues

Neurologists and other physicians often wish to know the legal ramifications of their actions to terminate a patient's life-sustaining treatment. The courts have issued rulings on several relevant questions including (1) whether termination of medical treatment by a physician can be considered criminal homicide, (2) whether patients and their proxies have a legal right to terminate treatment if the patient will die as a result, and (3) whether artificial hydration and nutrition are considered medical therapies that can be refused by a patient or proxy and terminated by a physician. Elsewhere I have more thoroughly reviewed these decisions and their implications [17].

The question of criminal homicide was first considered by the *Quinlan* and *Barber* courts. Karen Ann Quinlan was a young woman in a persistent vegetative state (PVS) resulting from a presumed hypoxic-ischemic insult. Her parents requested that she be removed from the ventilator, but her physicians refused, stating that it would be unethical to do so. The homicide liability question was presumed by the court to be a factor in the physicians' reluctance to accede to the parents' wishes. The New Jersey Supreme Court ruled that if Quinlan died as the result of removal of the ventilator that she would have died of her pre-existing illness and her death would not count as criminal homicide. The same issue was litigated by the California Court of Appeals in *Barber* and the same conclusion was reached. Indeed, there has never been a case of a successful prosecution for criminal homicide of a physician discontinuing a patient's life-sustaining therapy in this circumstance.

That patients and their proxies have a legal right to refuse life-sustaining therapy even if patients will die as a result has been asserted by numerous high state courts and the U.S. Supreme Court. In the circumstance of competent patients, the amyotrophic lateral sclerosis cases of *Perlmutter*, *Farrell*, and *Requena* are illustrative. In each case, a competent dying patient refused further life-sustaining treatment and a high court ruled that they had the right to do so even if they would die as a result. The courts asserted the primacy of patients' rights of self-determination over any countervailing interests of the state to maintain their lives against their will. The

American Academy of Neurology similarly asserted the primacy of the competent, paralyzed patient to refuse life-prolonging therapy and the duty of neurologists to respect and follow the patient's treatment refusal [18].

In the circumstance of incompetent patients, a series of highly publicized decisions on patients in PVS are instructive, from *Quinlan* in the mid-1970s to *Cruzan* in 1990. In each case, the courts found that incompetent patients also enjoy the right of self-determination and that their right to refuse life-sustaining treatment may be exercised by proxy decision makers. In *Cruzan*, the U.S. Supreme Court found a constitutional basis for this right in the liberty protection provisions of the due process clause of the Fourteenth Amendment. High state courts also have examined the standards of proxy decision making and have underscored the validity of the standards of expressed wishes, substituted judgment, and best interest.

The question of whether artificial hydration and nutrition can be withheld or withdrawn was considered in several PVS cases, most notably *Cruzan*. In *Cruzan*, the Missouri Supreme Court was asked whether the parents of a young woman in a hypoxic-ischemic PVS could refuse to permit physicians to order further artificial hydration and nutrition for her. They ruled that the Missouri "clear and convincing" standard of evidence of what Nancy Cruzan wanted had not been met in this case. On appeal, the U.S. Supreme Court concurred, but also ruled that in the case of PVS, artificial hydration and nutrition should be classified as forms of medical therapy that could be withheld or withdrawn at the refusal of the proxy decision maker.

## Palliative Care

When patients or proxies refuse further life-sustaining treatment, neurologists and other physicians should order a palliative care treatment plan. Palliative care is a set of orders designed to maximize patient comfort by relieving pain and other sources of suffering and by attending compassionately to the psychological, social, and spiritual needs of the dying patient. Palliative care attempts not to cause the patient's death, but rather to permit it as painlessly as possible by attending primarily to patient comfort and by not attempting to reverse the underlying disease process. Palliative care is also known as hospice care.

The contemporary emphasis on palliative care in the United States arose from the hospice movement and from the nursing profession. Only by the 1990s had it become widely recognized as an important branch of mainstream medicine. The first comprehensive textbook of palliative medicine was not published until 1993 [19]. Palliative care can be provided in the hospital by palliative care consultation teams or hospice inpatient units, where available, if particular attending physicians are not trained sufficiently in its use. In the community, inpatient or outpatient hospices most commonly provide these services.

Physicians should write palliative care orders clearly and specifically. Physicians should not write the vague order "comfort measures only" because such an order inappropriately transfers the responsibility of deciding which therapies will and will not be given to a patient from the physician where it belongs to the nurse where it does not. Usual palliative care provisions include (1) oxygen or morphine for dyspnea; (2) atropine and suctioning to decrease secretions; (3) around-the-clock opiates for pain; (4) benzodiazepines or morphine for restlessness; (5) hygienic and comfort measures such as bathing, grooming, range of motion exercises, and attentive nursing care; (6) do-not-resuscitate orders; and (7) avoidance of hospital admissions unless they contribute directly to maintaining patient comfort.

Pain relief is an important goal of palliative care. Numerous surveys of dying cancer patients have shown that many physicians do not adequately palliate the pain of dying patients. Providing proper pain palliation requires a knowledge of opiate drug pharmacology. The right drug must be given using the right dosage via the right route at the right dosage interval. Physicians must be aware that chronic opiate use induces tolerance and that patients may require dosages that appear very large when judged by standards of patients with acute pain who have not taken opiates chronically. Fears about inducing drug addiction in dying patients are grossly exaggerated and mostly unfounded. To assist the physician in ordering a regimen of optimal pain management, the judicious use of other hospital services, including physical therapy, occupational therapy, anesthesiology, and neurosurgery should be included in a comprehensive palliative care plan [20].

Some neurologists and other physicians worry that too large a dose of morphine or other opiate may kill the patient or lead to the patient's death sooner than if the dosage were smaller. This fear contributes to physicians' undertreatment of pain in many dying patients. In fact, there are relatively few instances in which proper palliation of pain, even with seemingly large doses of intravenous morphine, has contributed to the earlier death of a patient. Even if there were such a risk, the major goal of therapy should continue to be adequate pain palliation. If, by a "double effect," the patient were to die slightly sooner than without adequate pain palliation, this small and unintended acceleration of the moment of death becomes the price physicians must pay for adequate pain control. The alternative of consigning a dying patient to an unnecessarily painful death from the fear of possibly accelerating the moment of death does not represent acceptable medical practice.

The majority of patients currently receiving palliative care in hospices and inpatient palliative care units have metastatic cancer, advanced chronic obstructive pulmonary disease, or advanced congestive heart failure. Most are admitted or cared for with the understanding that they have less than 6 months to live. Patients with Alzheimer's disease and other advanced states of dementia currently represent only a small portion of patients receiving palliative care. Palliative care is the appropriate treatment, however, for the patient with advanced dementia who no longer can eat or drink and for whom the proxy decision maker has decided should not receive artificial hydration and nutrition. The American Academy of Neurology has formally endorsed this position [21].

## PHYSICIAN-ASSISTED SUICIDE
## AND VOLUNTARY ACTIVE EUTHANASIA

Some dying patients ask their physicians to help them to die sooner by requesting physician assistance in committing suicide or by requesting the administration of a lethal injection to kill them mercifully. The topics of physician-assisted suicide (PAS) and voluntary active euthanasia (VAE) have become important ethical controversies and divisive public policy issues. Widespread public interest has placed bills for their legalization on ballots in some states. A neurologist's response to such requests requires an understanding of the definitions, morality, legality, and medical practice standards that govern these issues. I have discussed these questions in greater depth elsewhere [22].

## Definitions

PAS is defined as a physician's act, at the request of a patient, to provide the medical means for the patient's suicide, which the patient subsequently employs for a successful suicide. In PAS, the physician's act is necessary but not sufficient for the patient's death because the patient must act to commit the suicide using the medical means provided by the physician. A common example of PAS is the case of a dying patient who requests and a physician who provides a prescription for a lethal dose of barbiturate drugs for the express purpose of suicide, at the time and place of the patient's choosing, which the patient subsequently commits. In PAS, the patient's underlying illness provides the reason for the suicide, but is not a necessary physiologic factor in producing the patient's death.

VAE is defined as an act, committed by a physician at the request of a patient, to kill the patient using medical means such as a lethal injection. The patient's death usually follows immediately after the physician's act and is a direct physiologic consequence of it. In VAE, the physician's act is both necessary and sufficient for the patient's death and the patient's underlying illness provides only the setting but not the cause of death. An example of VAE is a terminally ill patient who requests a physician to kill him or her "mercifully," to which the physician complies by administering a lethal intravenous dose of rapidly acting barbiturate.

The misleading term *passive euthanasia* has been applied to the situation in which a terminally ill patient dies after refusing further life-sustaining therapy. This term should be abandoned because this situation does not represent euthanasia in any correct sense of the term. The patient validly refused life-sustaining therapy and died solely from the underlying illness. In such cases, the physician is not authorized to provide life-sustaining therapy because the patient refused to give consent for it. Referring to this situation as *passive euthanasia* unnecessarily politicizes and confuses the issue of euthanasia and should be avoided.

## Morality, Legality, and Practice Standards

The morality of PAS and VAE remains a controversial topic, with strong opinions expressed by physicians and philosophers on both sides of the debate [23,24], although there remains no serious question about the morality of withdrawing or withholding life-sustaining therapies validly refused by a patient. The legality of PAS varies among jurisdictions. It is illegal in the majority of states in the United States, but some states currently have no laws governing it. A bill specifically legalizing PAS was passed by voters in Oregon in 1994 and 1997 and remains in effect. Several other states are considering similar legislation.

By contrast, VAE remains illegal in every American jurisdiction and generally is classified as criminal homicide. Because of their usually compassionate motives, however, physicians committing VAE may not be indicted by grand juries, may be found not guilty at jury trials, or may be given light or suspended sentences even if found guilty.

Many scholars believe that, independent of the question of morality, legalizing PAS or VAE makes poor public policy because the resulting net harms that would befall society are greater than the benefits. For example, if PAS were legalized, the implicit trust that patients place in physicians could be jeopardized if physicians were known to be killers in addition to healers. Some patients might choose PAS not because they really wished to commit suicide but because they felt the duty to die and get out of the way and no longer be a burden to their loved ones. In these cases, the meaning of voluntary becomes questionable. Members of lower socioeconomic strata of our society could become selectively victimized because they may have no choice other than PAS when they are terminally ill given their often poor access to medical care. Analyses of the wide experience of legalized PAS and VAE in the Netherlands have shown that cases of *involuntary* euthanasia followed PAS and VAE legalization despite the fact that it was and remains expressly forbidden [25].

A number of medical societies including the American College of Physicians, the American Geriatric Society, the American Medical Association, and the British Medical Association have stated that PAS and VAE are not acceptable medical practices. They argue that the harms to patients and society of PAS and VAE outweigh any benefits and that the principal duty of physicians to their dying patients should be to provide them with excellent palliative care.

## Patient Refusal of Hydration and Nutrition

When a dying patient asks a physician for PAS or VAE, the request should cause the physician to reflect on the reasons the patient made such a request. The physician should explore the sources of the patient's suffering and should redouble efforts to provide excellent palliative care through all available means. If this effort does not succeed and the patient continues to express the wish to die sooner, the physician can notify the patient that, although PAS and VAE are not acceptable medical practices, there is a legally acceptable alternative. The dying patient can refuse to eat or drink and can refuse artificial hydration and nutrition.

The practice of patient refusal of hydration and nutrition (PRHN) has received more scholarly attention as an alternative to PAS and VAE because hospice physicians and nurses have reported widely that terminally ill patients who died without eating or drinking rarely suffered if given proper palliative care [26]. Indeed, the deaths, which usually take place within a week or so of the total cessation of hydration and nutrition, appear to be comfortable in approximately 90% of the cases, because of the normal involution of thirst and hunger drives that accompanies the process of dying.

PRHN is morally and legally acceptable. Patients have the right to refuse to eat or drink and to refuse parenteral hydration and nutrition without creating any changes in current law or current roles of the physician. It is unlikely that any physician would regard it as proper medical care to involuntarily admit such a dying patient and insert a feeding tube against the patient's will in an attempt to prevent his or her inevitable death.

Physicians have the duty to prevent any suffering that might accompany PRHN by the judicious ordering of a palliative care plan. Palliation in this setting should include mouth care, using methylcellulose drops and ice chips, morphine for pain and restlessness, and light sedation using benzodiazepines. As is true in any palliative care plan, the goal remains to promote patient comfort during the dying process.

## REFERENCES

1. Bernat JL. Ethical Issues in Neurology. Boston: Butterworth–Heinemann, 1994.
2. Bernat JL, Beresford HR. The American Academy of Neurology code of professional conduct. Neurology 1993;43:1257–1260.
3. Emanuel EJ. Do physicians have an obligation to treat patient with AIDS? N Engl J Med 1988;318:1686–1690.
4. Henderson DK, Fahey BJ, Willey M, et al. Risk for occupational transmission of human immunodeficiency virus type 1 (HIV-1) associated with clinical exposures: a prospective evaluation. Ann Intern Med 1990;113:740–746.
5. Bernat JL. Ethical Issues in Neurology. Boston: Butterworth–Heinemann, 1994;60 [note 7].
6. Brock DW. The ideal of shared decision making between physicians and patients. Kennedy Inst Ethics J 1991;1:28–47.
7. Culver CM, Gert B. Basic ethical concepts in neurologic practice. Semin Neurol 1984;4:1–8.
8. Gert B, Culver CM. Moral theory in neurologic practice. Semin Neurol 1984;4:9–13.
9. Tversky A, Kahneman D. The framing of decisions and the psychology of choice. Science 1981;211:453–458.
10. Bernat JL. Ethical Issues in Neurology. Boston: Butterworth–Heinemann, 1994;63 [note 36].
11. Burnham JF. Secrets about patients. N Engl J Med 1991;324:1130–1133.
12. Elian M, Dean G. To tell or not to tell the diagnosis of multiple sclerosis? Lancet 1985;291:27–28.
13. Quill TE, Townsend B. Bad news: delivery, dialogue, and dilemmas. Arch Intern Med 1991;151:463–468.
14. SUPPORT Principal Investigators. A controlled trial to improve care for seriously ill hospitalized patients: the study to understand prognoses and preferences for outcomes and risks of treatments (SUPPORT). JAMA 1995;274:1591–1598.
15. Schneiderman LJ, Arras JD. Counseling patients to counsel physicians on future care in the event of patient incompetence. Ann Intern Med 1985;102:693–698.
16. Suhl J, Simons P, Reedy T, et al. Myth of substituted judgment: surrogate decision making regarding life support is unreliable. Arch Intern Med 1994;154:90–96.
17. Bernat JL. Ethical Issues in Neurology. Boston: Butterworth–Heinemann, 1994;157–165, 215–216, 234–236.
18. American Academy of Neurology Ethics and Humanities Subcommittee. Position statement. Certain aspects of the care and management of profoundly and irreversibly paralyzed patients with retained consciousness and cognition. Neurology 1993;43:222–223.
19. Doyle D, Hanks GWC, MacDonald N (eds). Oxford Textbook of Palliative Medicine. New York: Oxford University Press, 1993.
20. American Academy of Neurology Ethics and Humanities Subcommittee. Palliative care in neurology. Neurology 1996;46:870–872.
21. American Academy of Neurology Ethics and Humanities Subcommittee. Ethical issues in the management of the demented patient. Neurology 1996;46:1180–1183.
22. Bernat JL. Ethical Issues in Neurology. Boston: Butterworth–Heinemann, 1994;313–332.
23. Pellegrino ED. Doctors must not kill. J Clin Ethics 1992;3:95–102.
24. Weir RF. The morality of physician-assisted suicide. Law Med Health Care 1992;20:116–126.
25. Hendin H, Rutenfrans C, Zylicz Z. Physician-assisted suicide and euthanasia in the Netherlands: lessons from the Dutch. JAMA 1997;277:1720–1722.
26. Bernat JL, Mogielnicki RP, Gert B. Patient refusal of hydration and nutrition: an alternative to physician-assisted suicide or voluntary active euthanasia. Arch Intern Med 1993;153:2723–2728.

# TWO

## MAJOR NEUROLOGIC CONSULTATION PROBLEMS SEEN IN VARIOUS HOSPITAL SERVICES

# I
# MEDICINE

# 11
# Nephrology
## Charles F. Bolton and G. Bryan Young

In the United States, more than 100,000 persons at any given moment are being treated for end-stage renal disease: 80% by various types of dialysis, a few by continued conservative treatment, and the rest by transplantation. Nervous system complications are common in all groups.

This chapter concentrates on the principal neurologic complications of renal failure and its treatment as they would present in neurologic consultations, usually when the consultant is near a major hemodialysis and transplant center. Comments concerning the general principles of the clinical and laboratory approach are followed by a review of the main disorders of the central and peripheral nervous systems.

## GENERAL PRINCIPLES

### Central Nervous System

Clinical Evaluation

Mental status changes are generally the earliest and most common central nervous system effects of renal failure or its treatment. The consultant should ask the patient's companion, either directly or by telephone from the hospital, about changes in behavior, speech, memory, and intellectual capabilities. The time course of such changes should be established. For example, progressive dialysis encephalopathy tends to fluctuate at first, then steadily progress, and slowly resolve with effective treatment. Stroke, transient ischemic attacks, and seizures are of sudden onset and resolve quickly. A simple mental status examination, such as the Mini-Mental State Examination (Table 11.1), serves both to document specific deficits and to quantify the dysfunction for follow-up purposes.

*Table 11.1*   Mini-Mental State Examination

| Maximum score | Test |
| --- | --- |
| | Orientation |
| 5 | What is the (year) (season) (day) (month)? |
| 5 | Where are we (state/province) (country) (city) (building) (floor)? |
| | Registration |
| 3 | Name three objects (1 sec to say each), then ask the patient to repeat all three. Give 1 point for each correct answer. Repeat until the patient learns all three. Count trials and record. |
| | Attention and concentration |
| 5 | Serial 7s (counting backwards by 7 from 100). Stop after five answers. Alternatively, spell *world* backwards. |
| | Recall |
| 3 | Ask for the three objects repeated above. Give 1 point for each correct answer. |
| | Language |
| 9 | Name a pencil and a watch (2 points). Repeat the following: "No ifs, ands, or buts" (1 point). Follow a three-stage command: "Take a paper in your right hand, fold it in half, and put it on the floor" (3 points). Read and obey: "Close your eyes" (1 point). Write (not copy) a sentence (1 point). Copy a design (1 point). |

Source: Reprinted with permission from MF Folstein, SE Folstein, PR McHugh. Mini-Mental State: a practical guide for grading the cognitive state of patients for the clinician. J Psychiatr Res 1975;12:189–198.

## Investigative Tests

Which investigative tests to have done is dependent on the history and physical examination. The indications and limitations of tests of function and structure should be clearly understood.

Electrophysiologic tests of brain function include electroencephalography (EEG) and evoked responses. EEG is useful in assessing uremic encephalopathy, the adequacy of dialysis, and seizure disorders, and in making the specific diagnosis of progressive dialysis encephalopathy. It is particularly valuable in the intensive care unit where clinical assessment is difficult and metabolic encephalopathy may be a result mainly of sepsis and slowly cleared drugs rather than renal failure. Quantitative tests, including frequency analysis and middle-latency auditory evoked responses, are useful in assessing the adequacy of dialysis.

Tests of brain structure include computed tomographic (CT) scan and magnetic resonance imaging (MRI). These can detect specific structural lesions such as subdural hematomas, abscesses, or neoplasms. Because of the presence of bony artifact in posterior fossa structures and the temporal lobes on CT scan, MRI is a more sensitive examination.

*Table 11.2*  Main disorders of the peripheral nervous system in the management of stages of uremia

| Conservative management | Dialysis | Renal transplantation |
|---|---|---|
| Developing uremic poly- neuropathy | Stabilizing uremic poly- neuropathy | Recovery from uremic poly- neuropathy |
| Diabetic mononeuropathy and polyneuropathy | Persisting diabetic neuropathy | Persisting diabetic neuropathy |
| Subacute diabetic and uremic polyneuropathy | Improvement with high- flux hemodialysis? | ? |
| Pressure palsies | Carpal tunnel syndrome and amyloidosis | — |
| Cachectic myopathy | Ischemic neuropathy and shunts or fistulas | — |
| | Primary myopathy and bone disease | |

## Peripheral Nervous System

Clinical Evaluation

Neuromuscular conditions associated with acute renal failure are uncommon and are usually confined to muscle weakness induced by disturbances of water and electrolyte metabolism. On the other hand, such conditions are common in chronic renal failure. The nature of these neuromuscular disorders varies depending on the stage of renal failure: during the conservative treatment, during hemodialysis, or following successful renal transplantation (Table 11.2). These facts should be kept in mind, because they will help focus questioning during history taking and aid in selection of the most appropriate tests on physical examination.

In taking a history, one should ask about muscle weakness or fatigue, cramps, the presence or absence of sweating in the hands and feet, disorders of bowel and bladder function, and problems in standing or walking. Impotence in the male can be clarified from the observation that it is probably psychogenic if early morning penile erections regularly occur, but it is probably organic in their absence.

The patient's own words for describing symptoms should be noted and are important diagnostically. Thus, the sensory symptoms of neuropathy are characteristically not only numbness and tingling, but a tight or bandlike feeling about the ankles, a sensation on the soles of the feet as if the patient were wearing tight socks, and, rarely, pain or burning. The restless legs syndrome, which may or may not be associated with peripheral neuropathy, is often an indescribably unpleasant sensation in the legs that is relieved only by movement of the legs.

On physical examination, one should observe the location and type of surgical scars, particularly those related to the creation of arteriovenous fistulas in the

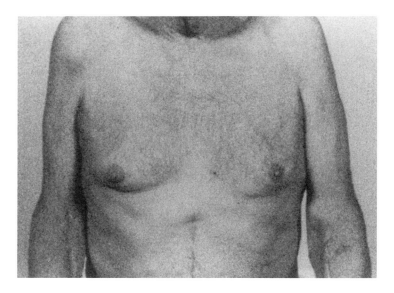

*Figure 11.1*   Severe muscle wasting in a 67-year-old man receiving maintenance hemodialysis for 7 years. It was associated with underlying pain secondary to progressive bone disease. He also had a progressive dementia, but aluminum intoxication was never proven. Although he had a mild uremic polyneuropathy, needle electromyography of shoulder girdle muscles revealed only an increased proportion of polyphasic units, consistent with a primary myopathy. (Reprinted with permission from CF Bolton, GB Young. Neurological Complications of Renal Disease. Boston: Butterworth, 1990.)

upper limbs for access during long-term hemodialysis, because they may play a role in the development of upper limb mononeuropathies. The type and severity of muscle wasting are important diagnostically. Diffuse muscle wasting may be a result of disuse, secondary either to the cachexia associated with chronic renal failure or to diffuse pain from underlying bone or joint disease. In the bone disease induced by hyperparathyroidism or the toxic effects of aluminum, muscle pain and wasting are characteristically more severe in the proximal lower limbs but occasionally involve the proximal upper limbs as well (Figure 11.1). Focal wasting may occur in the distribution of the nerves that are subject to compression or entrapment. In carpal tunnel syndrome there is wasting of the thenar eminence due to compression of the median nerve in the wrist; in compressive neuropathy of the ulnar nerve at the elbow there is wasting of the ulnar-innervated intrinsic hand muscles; in compression of the common peroneal nerve at the fibular head there is anterior compartment wasting. Fasciculations are not a major manifestation of neuromuscular disease in renal failure.

Many patients in chronic renal failure are frail, and excessive force should be avoided when testing muscle strength. The deep tendon reflexes are usually preserved in primary myopathies and defects in neuromuscular transmission, and are characteristically decreased in neuropathy. Reduced or absent ankle jerks are one of the early signs of uremic polyneuropathy. In eliciting deep tendon reflexes, it is important to use a hammer that is of sufficient length and mass to effectively move the tendon but that has a soft enough rubber not to cause undue discomfort.

In testing sensation, one should first ask the patient to outline carefully with a finger the areas of impaired sensation that he or she has experienced. This procedure is often more reliable than formal sensory testing in delineating areas of sensory loss. Sensitivity to light touch should be tested with a tissue, and sensitivity to pain should be tested with a sharp splinter from a tongue depressor. The splinter should later be disposed of, to avoid transmitting an infectious agent. Vibratory sensation is tested with a 128-Hz tuning fork. Position sense first becomes abnormal at a distal digital joint in the hands or feet and is normally sensitive enough that the patient can detect even the smallest movement. Two-point discrimination can be measured with an instrument that has two well-defined, but not excessively sharp, points. Values on the fingertips greater than 3 mm in patients of all ages, and on the feet greater than 1 cm in the young and greater than 3 cm in the elderly, should be considered abnormal. Testing of temperature sensation has little practical value in this group of patients.

In testing stance and gait, one should look for a steppage gait resulting from predominant weakness of the feet and ankles. In proprioceptive loss involving the lower limbs, the gait is ataxic, and this phenomenon will be worse with the eyes closed. Early distal weakness in the lower limbs can be identified by asking the patient to walk on either the toes or heels; proximal weakness can be detected by having the patient attempt to rise from the squatting position.

Postural hypotension caused by fluctuations in fluid volume is common in patients on long-term hemodialysis. However, postural hypotension resulting from an autonomic neuropathy is observed only rarely. One can test clinically for autonomic insufficiency by observing blood pressure and pulse in the recumbent position and then on standing. A significant postural hypotension is present if there is a drop in the systolic pressure of 30 mm Hg or more. The heart rate should normally increase by a factor of at least 1.04. Sweating can be crudely assessed by palpating the skin surfaces. Sweating in the axilla is mediated by apocrine glands, which are stimulated by circulating catecholamines and, hence, are not affected by neuropathy.

## Neurophysiologic Studies

After the history is taken and the physical examination is performed, the nature of the underlying neuromuscular disorder is often still in doubt. Here, electrophysiologic studies are of great value. They are of particular value in the intensive care unit, where critical-illness polyneuropathy—a complication of sepsis and multiple organ failure—is a common cause of difficulty in weaning the patient from the ventilator. Such studies clearly identify the presence and severity of uremic polyneuropathy and are valuable in following the course of this neuropathy during the various stages of chronic renal failure (see Table 11.2). They are also valuable in detecting the presence and severity of mononeuropathies, such as carpal tunnel syndrome, and compressive neuropathy of the ulnar nerve at the elbow and of the common peroneal nerve at the fibular head. For example, in carpal tunnel syndrome, symptoms may be strongly suggestive of the disorder but the physical examination is negative. No evidence of muscle weakness or sensory loss is found. Phalen's and Tinel's signs are unreliable. In cases of primary myopathy, if the cause is simply disuse atrophy, electrophysiologic studies will be entirely normal. Repetitive nerve stimulation studies will rule out neuromuscular transmission defects induced by antibiotic drugs.

Patients on long-term hemodialysis are understandably reluctant to undergo unnecessary painful procedures. However, standard motor and sensory nerve conduction studies cause little discomfort, particularly when performed by a sensitive and experienced electromyography technician. On the other hand, needle electromyography of muscle is clearly more uncomfortable, and thus this type of testing should be reserved for patients who have moderate or severe polyneuropathies and are likely to have evidence of denervation. Moreover, abnormal spontaneous activity, a sign of denervation, may be peculiarly absent in uremic neuropathy. (See the section Uremic Polyneuropathy for a discussion of this rather interesting aspect of uremic polyneuropathy.)

### Nerve and Muscle Biopsy

Nerve and muscle biopsy may be necessary in only a few instances, when history, physical examination, and electrophysiologic studies are still inconclusive. This circumstance is most likely to occur in cases of primary myopathies. Electrophysiologic studies may be normal when there are metabolic disturbances of muscle or equivocal in other types of primary myopathies. In patients in endstage renal failure, the usual indications for nerve biopsy are suspicion of underlying vasculitis or amyloidosis.

In most instances, if nerve biopsy is decided upon, it is best to take a longitudinal section of the entire cross section of a sural nerve. The biopsy should include adjacent muscle, subcutaneous tissue, and skin, which are particularly important when one is looking for a vasculitis. Special stains have to be performed when amyloidosis is suspected. In cases of muscle biopsy, the muscle should be chosen from a muscle that is moderately weak and one that has not been needled by a previous electromyographic examination.

These biopsies should be performed only by an experienced and skilled surgeon. The neuropathologist should also be competent and should be informed in advance about the nature of the suspected disorder, so that the tissue can be received in optimal condition and the appropriate testing and analysis can be conducted.

## PRINCIPAL DISORDERS OF THE NERVOUS SYSTEM

### Central Nervous System

#### Acute Uremic Encephalopathy

Acute renal failure (ARF) can be divided into prerenal failure (i.e., circulatory failure), postrenal failure (i.e., obstructions to outflow), and failure resulting from specific renal causes. At least 40% of ARF cases occur in an acute care medical setting. Most cases are a result of renal ischemia with either systemic hypotension or local ischemia related to aortic disease. Nephrotoxic medical materials such as aminoglycosides and radiographic contrast agents are more common causes than the organic solvents, heavy metals, and glycols of the past. Massive release of myoglobin into the circulation (as in crush injuries, ischemia to muscle, alcoholism, and malignant neuroleptic and malignant hyperthermia syndromes), massive hemolysis, and complications of pregnancy may produce acute tubular necrosis.

There are few specific features that differentiate uremic encephalopathy from other metabolic encephalopathies. However, the following combination suggests uremia, once exogenous agents have been excluded: (1) an encephalopathy with hyperventilation from a metabolic acidosis, and (2) excitability, including prominent myoclonus or seizures.

As with other metabolic encephalopathies, early changes include lethargy, irritability, problems with concentration and attention, disorientation, omissions in speech, and sleep disturbances. Patients are usually subdued, but delirium, or an agitated confusional state, may be found. There may be periods of profanity, euphoria, depression, or catatonic stupor. Coma from acute uremia is found when the patient is in extremis, or in association with complications, for example, seizures, strokes, subdural hematomas, malignant hypertension, systemic infections, intoxications, or electrolyte imbalance.

Seizures, usually in the form of generalized convulsions and often multiple, occur in the oliguric phase. Focal seizures may occur but are not usually consistently from the same site, unless they relate to an associated structural lesion. Patients may feel weak and demonstrate multifocal myoclonus that is so prominent that the muscles appear to be fasciculating. Action myoclonus has been described. Tetany may also be found. Focal signs such as hemiparesis are not rare but subside with dialysis and may switch sides with recurrent episodes. Cranial nerve function is usually intact, although the fundi may reflect arterial hypertension.

The electroencephalogram reflects the level of consciousness: Slowing of frequencies occurs in parallel with the severity of the encephalopathy. Generalized epileptiform discharges occur in about 25% of children with acute uremia, but these are rare in adults.

The main differential diagnosis is accelerated hypertension with hypertensive encephalopathy. The latter is usually associated with papilledema, which is rare and unexpected in uremic encephalopathy. Elevated cerebrospinal fluid (CSF) protein is more characteristic of hypertensive than uremic encephalopathy.

Other conditions that may cause both encephalopathy and systemic acidosis include reactions to exogenous toxins such as methanol, ethylene glycol, salicylates, and paraldehyde. Diabetic ketoacidosis, anoxia, sepsis with circulatory failure, and lactic acidosis should not pose diagnostic difficulty.

Penicillin intoxication (caused by huge doses) may cause an encephalopathy with seizures as well as acute renal failure. In children, lead intoxication enters the differential diagnosis. Papilledema and other evidence of raised intracranial pressure are commonly present in childhood lead intoxication with impaired consciousness. There may be a "lead line" in the gingivae and radiologic bony abnormalities.

The first step is to determine the category and specific cause of ARF, especially to detect and treat reversible causes. Pre- and postrenal causes, precipitants (myoglobin, hemoglobin, urate crystals), and nephrotoxic drugs should be sought first.

Fluid intake should be adjusted in keeping with the cause of ARF but usually must be restricted, depending on urinary output. Steps should be taken to reduce catabolism by increasing carbohydrate intake. Serum potassium must be closely monitored, as life-threatening hyperkalemia is a constant risk. Complications such as congestive heart failure, acute hypertension, fluid and electrolyte imbalance, and infections should be looked for, prevented, and managed promptly when they occur.

Not all patients require dialysis; some can be managed conservatively with correction of the underlying cause and careful observation. Absolute indications for dialysis include development of central nervous system complications, resistant hypertension, fluid overload, severe acidosis, and uremic pericarditis. Symptomatic treatment with antiepileptic drugs is often necessary. Phenytoin has a number of advantages: it is easy to administer parenterally or enterally and loading doses can be given. Because uremic toxins displace phenytoin from plasma proteins, management is facilitated by the measurement of the free (unbound) portion.

## Chronic Uremic Encephalopathy

The first symptoms of uremia include lethargy, slowness in thinking, general malaise, sleep disturbance, headache, and decreased libido. Personality changes include apathy, flatness of affect, depression, or irritability. Restlessness and impaired concentration, attention, and memory are common. Occasionally, patients become frankly delirious. Symptoms are improved to varying degrees by hemodialysis or peritoneal dialysis, depending on their adequacy and frequency, but are completely reversed by successful renal transplantation.

Convulsive seizures are still occasionally encountered in chronic renal failure. If they are not a result of acute, severe metabolic derangement, they should raise the possibility of a complication such as a stroke, cerebral neoplasm or abscess, progressive dialysis encephalopathy, or drug-related reaction.

Persistent focal signs are rare in uremic encephalopathy and should prompt the search for a structural lesion. Diffuse motor phenomena such as postural tremor, asterixis, and multifocal myoclonus are not uncommon in uremia. Tremor is found in mild renal failure, even when treated by dialysis. Asterixis and multifocal myoclonus reflect a more severe or advanced metabolic disturbance.

Routine EEGs show mild, intermittent slowing in the theta frequency range (greater than 4-Hz but less than 8-Hz waves), which is more prominent in the anterior head (Figure 11.2). Arousal from sleep is often abnormal, showing rhythmic delta in adults. Spontaneous epileptiform activity is uncommon but may appear in a generalized fashion during photic stimulation. Triphasic waves or intermittent rhythmic delta are usually features of more advanced uremia that is sufficient to require hospitalization (Figure 11.3). Improvement in the EEG, quantitative EEG, and middle-latency evoked responses parallels clinical improvement following enhanced dialysis therapy or renal transplantation (Figure 11.4).

The differential diagnoses of uremic encephalopathy include drug intoxication (especially when renal excretion is a major determinant of the drug or its active metabolites, as with amantadine hydrochloride, opiates, and beta blockers); degenerative conditions such as Alzheimer's disease (usually associated with gradual decline in memory and then other intellectual functions in a steadily progressive

**PROJECTED THETA**

AWAKE                                                    63 yrs

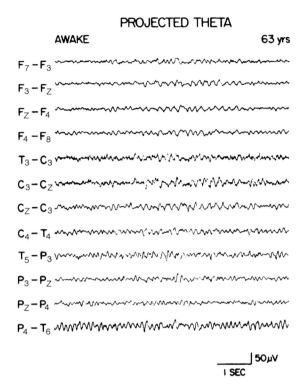

*Figure 11.2*   Recordings from a 63-year-old man with chronic renal failure. Intermittent 4- to 5-Hz low-voltage waves are accentuated in the anterior and mid head (top eight channels). (Reprinted with permission from CF Bolton, GB Young. Neurological Complications of Renal Disease. Boston: Butterworth, 1990.)

manner—confusion and fluctuation in mental status are not early features, as they often are in metabolic encephalopathies such as uremia); complications of dialysis, including subdural hematomas and progressive dialysis encephalopathy (see next section); depressive illness; and conditions that may affect both the kidneys and the brain, such as lead intoxication and certain collagen vascular diseases.

Management includes adequate clearance of uremic neurotoxins, for example, by increasing the frequency of dialysis treatments from twice to three times weekly.

## Neurologic Complications of Dialysis

### *Progressive Dialysis Encephalopathy*

Progressive dialysis encephalopathy (PDE), which is found in patients on long-term dialysis, has been shown to relate to aluminum intoxication of the brain. The encephalopathy may be associated with symptomatic aluminum poisoning of

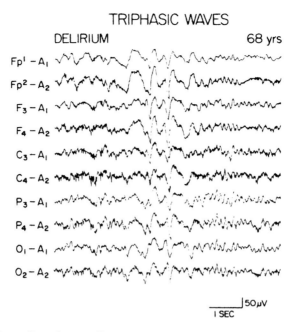

*Figure 11.3*   Recordings from a 68-year-old woman with chronic renal failure during a transient delirium. A burst of triphasic waves is seen in the middle of the tracing. (Reprinted with permission from CF Bolton, GB Young. Neurological Complications of Renal Disease. Boston: Butterworth, 1990.)

other organ systems, for example, vitamin D–resistant osteomalacia with a tendency for fractures, proximal myopathy in the lower limbs, and a severe, refractory, non–iron-deficiency, hypochromic, microcytic anemia.

The main manifestations of PDE include (1) a prominent speech disturbance, usually consisting of a nonfluent aphasia and dysarthria; (2) involuntary motor phenomena (myoclonus, tremor, asterixis, and seizures); (3) gait disturbance (ataxia or apraxia—wide based or small stepped); and (4) general mental decline or dementia. The symptoms and signs fluctuate considerably early in the course of the illness and are more progressive later in the course. The tempo varies markedly among patients.

The differential diagnoses include chronic uremic encephalopathy, drug intoxication, subdural hematoma, degenerative conditions, and Creutzfeldt-Jakob disease.

The EEG can help establish the diagnosis. Characteristically, there are generalized bursts of slow-frequency waves, triphasic waves, or irregular spike-and-wave. The EEG findings appear out of proportion to the uremia, and, unlike with uremic encephalopathy, the condition is not helped by increasing the frequency of dialysis treatments. Serum or bone aluminum concentrations and the desferrioxamine infusion tests give estimates of the body burden of aluminum and offer support of the diagnosis. Patients in the early stages of PDE often respond to

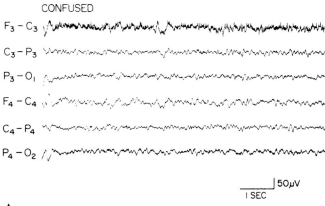

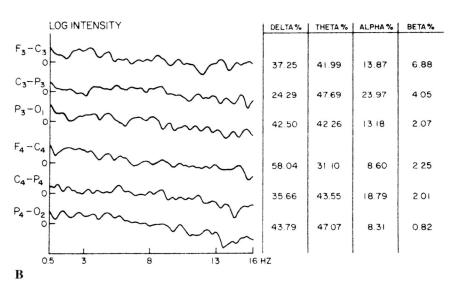

*Figure 11.4* Recordings from a 65-year-old woman with chronic renal failure treated with peritoneal dialysis. **(A)** shows the standard, "raw" electroencephalogram (EEG) showing excessive slowing. **(B)** shows excessive amounts of theta waves (>4 Hz but <8 Hz) and delta waves (≤4 Hz) in the quantitative EEG.

JAN. 17/85

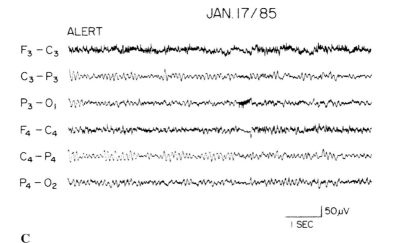

C

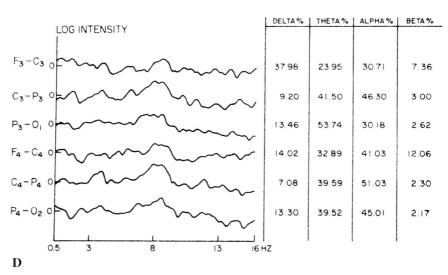

D

*Figure 11.4* (continued) (**C**) and (**D**) show a considerable improvement several months later. This improvement followed an increase in dialysis frequency from two to three times weekly. (Reprinted with permission from CF Bolton, GB Young. Neurological Complications of Renal Disease. Boston: Butterworth, 1990.)

administered benzodiazepines with prompt but temporary resolution of signs for several hours.

Management depends first of all on prevention. Epidemics related to high aluminum content in the tap water or dialysate have largely been eliminated, but it pays to remain vigilant. Aluminum-containing antacids, used to bind phosphate in the gut, are a source of aluminum exposure for some. Citrate increases aluminum absorption from the gastrointestinal tract. These substances are best replaced by calcium carbonate. Secondary treatment in the early phases includes elimination of aluminum exposure and the use of desferrioxamine. Benzodiazepines have only a transient beneficial effect.

## Subdural Hematoma

Chronic subdural hematomas, probably related to the intrinsic coagulopathy of uremia and the iatrogenic anticoagulation, occur in 3% of patients on hemodialysis. There may or may not be a history of trauma. Any adult age group may be affected.

The patient often complains of headache. When the condition is brought to medical attention, the level of consciousness is often diminished. Focal signs such as lateralized motor weakness are often present but may be hard to detect if the patient is obtunded or poorly cooperative or if bilateral subdural collections are present. Gait disturbance is especially common: for example, features of apraxia, ataxia, or hemiparesis may be found. Patients' signs and symptoms may fluctuate considerably.

Subdural hematomas are best confirmed by neuroimaging with CT or MRI scans. The treatment is almost always surgical, with drainage or evacuation of the clot.

## Dialysis Dysequilibrium

The full-blown condition of dialysis dysequilibrium rarely presents in office practice, but some patients exhibit transient symptoms of a less severe nature. This condition occurs mainly in individuals with chronic renal failure who have just started on hemodialysis. The condition relates to osmotic shifts of water that cause edema of the brain, especially of the cerebral cortex. It is associated with metabolic acidosis of the brain and cerebrospinal fluid.

Symptoms and signs include headache, anorexia, nausea, vomiting, dizziness, blurring of vision, and muscle cramps in milder cases; more severely affected patients may experience myoclonus, tremors, seizures, and coma. The EEG may show generalized, excessive rhythmic slowing. The incidence is higher in children, hypertensives, and those with pre-existing brain disease (e.g., trauma or recent stroke).

The syndrome should be recognized and differentiated from PDE, dementing illness, and threatened stroke. Dialysis dysequilibrium can be prevented by using hemofiltration (no osmotic gradients) rather than dialysis. Slower hemodialysis or substitution of hemodialysis for long-term ambulatory peritoneal dialysis will also avoid the syndrome. Alternatively, the osmolality of the dialysate can be increased by the addition of mannitol, glycerol, or glucose. The substitution of bicarbonate for acetate in the dialysate has also been recommended.

## Hemodialysis Headache

Hemodialysis headache, which affects about 60% of patients on hemodialysis, begins within a few hours of dialysis, usually as a throbbing bifrontal or generalized headache, often with nausea or vomiting. Antimigraine treatment is often effective.

## Other Complications

Vitamin deficiencies are now uncommon, because supplements of water-soluble vitamins are provided to replace those lost from the body in dialysis. It is wise, however, to be on guard for the possibility of thiamine deficiency (which may cause a Wernicke's encephalopathy or a polyneuropathy) and biotin deficiency (which may also produce a neuropathy with or without an encephalopathy characterized by myoclonic jerks, asterixis, and amnesia).

## Neurologic Complications of Renal Transplantation

Primary central nervous system lymphoma and opportunistic infections of the brain or meninges are now much less frequent than before the advent of cyclosporine A. Cyclosporine A is the main immunosuppressant used in transplant patients. This drug has better success and fewer severe adverse effects than earlier immunosuppressive agents. Cyclosporine A does, however, have a number of neurologic side effects. These include postural tremors (22% of cases), seizures (up to 5%, often associated with hypomagnesemia), and less commonly cerebellar intention tremors or ataxia, burning feet, myoclonus, hallucinations, encephalopathy, polyneuropathy, or spinal cord dysfunction (rare). Lymphoma and infections still occur, however, and present special problems (Table 11.3).

The mortality and morbidity among post-transplant patients result from a variety of conditions that continue to complicate the post-transplant state and reduced survival to 45% at 10 years.

In assessing the post transplant patient, one may establish the diagnosis by the typical symptoms and signs of the primary disease, for example, a typical skin lesion in herpes zoster. In many instances the history and physical findings give no clue as to the nature of the condition. In these cases, however, hospital admission and comprehensive investigations are indicated.

Central nervous system involvement is common and presents a difficult differential diagnosis (see Table 11.3). If the organ transplant is recent, a medication-related effect such as complication of cyclosporine treatment or the phenomenon of rejection encephalopathy should be considered. Then, infection should be thoroughly investigated. Blood, urine, and, if indicated, other specimens should be cultured for viruses, bacteria, and fungi. Serologic studies should also be done for specific changes in antibody titer, including that for human immunosuppressive virus. For example, the diagnosis of cytomegalovirus is established by a fourfold or greater seroconversion in cytomegalovirus antibody titers. All types of infections—viral, bacterial, or fungal—if left unchecked produce systemic symptoms, not as a result of direct invasion of organisms but as a septic syndrome and multiorgan failure. The nervous system effects may be septic encephalopathy or critical-illness polyneuropathy.

The EEG and CT scan or MRI are of great value (see Table 11.3). The finding of a mass lesion on CT scan contraindicates performing a subsequent lumbar puncture. Lumbar puncture is also contraindicated if there is any bleeding tendency, that is, low platelet levels, anticoagulant treatment, or aspergillosis. CSF should be tested as for any suspected central nervous system infection. Polymerase chain reaction of the CSF, if available, may provide the earliest diagno-

*Table 11.3*   Differential diagnosis of nervous system complications following organ transplantation

| Condition/ organism | Time after transplant | Neurologic manifestations | Cerebrospinal fluid | Computed tomographic head scan | Treatment |
|---|---|---|---|---|---|
| Cyclosporin complications | 0–3 mos | Tremor, ataxia, seizures, confusion, coma, paraplegia | Normal, or mild increase in protein and lymphocytic reaction | Normal, or white-matter edema | Stop cyclosporin, give parenteral magnesium |
| Septic encephalopathy | 0–3 mos | Diffuse encephalopathy, mild or severe | Normal, or mildly increased protein | Normal | Treat sepsis and multiple organ failure |
| Critical-illness poly-neuropathy | 0–3 mos | Failed weaning from ventilator, axonal polyneuropathy | Normal, or mildly increased protein | Normal | Treat sepsis and multiple organ failure |
| Rejection encephalo-pathy | 1–3 mos | Headache, confusion, and convulsions | Increased pressure | Normal or edema | Give steroids, manage hypertension and fluid balance |
| Cerebrovascular disease | Any time | Sudden onset of focal cerebral deficit | Normal, or signs of sub-arachnoid hemorrhage | Relatively specific for subdural hematoma, infarction, or hemorrhage | Conservative |
| Viruses | | | | | |
| Cytomegalovirus | 1–4 mos | None | Normal | Normal | Prophylaxis only |
| Epstein-Barr | 2–6 mos | None, or B cell lym-phoma (rare) | Normal | Normal, or B cell lymphoma (rare) | Prophylaxis only |
| Herpes simplex | Any time | Encephalitis (rare) | Increased white blood cells (WBC), red blood cells, and protein; normal or decreased glucose | Areas of decreased density, occasional small hemorrhages in frontal and temporal lobes | Acyclovir |
| Varicella-zoster | Any time | Encephalitis (rare) | Increased WBC and protein, normal glucose | ? | Acyclovir |

*Table 11.3* (continued)

| Condition/ organism | Time after transplant | Neurologic manifestations | Cerebrospinal fluid | Computed tomographic head scan | Treatment |
|---|---|---|---|---|---|
| Human immunodeficiency virus | Any time | Encephalopathy, myelopathy, peripheral neuropathy | Variable | Variable, depending on type of infection or malignancy | None |
| JC virus | Any time | Progressive multifocal leukoencephalopathy | Normal | Areas of decreased density with no enhancement | None |
| Bacteria | | | | | |
| Listeria monocytogenes | 1–3 mos (?) | Acute meningitis | Increased WBC (mainly neutrophils and protein, decreased glucose) | Normal, or generalized edema | Penicillin and tobramycin |
| Mycobacteria | Any time | Subacute and chronic meningitis or focal signs | Increased WBC (mainly lymphocytes) and protein, decreased glucose | Normal, or hydro-cephalus | Isoniazid, rifampin |
| Fungi | | | | | |
| Cryptococci | 1–8 mos | Mild, chronic meningitis | Increased WBC and protein, decreased glucose | Normal, or hydro-cephalus | Amphotericin B |
| Coccidioides organisms | 1–8 mos | Chronic meningitis | Increased WBC and protein, decreased glucose | Normal, or hydro-cephalus | Amphotericin B |

Source: Adapted with permission from CF Bolton, GB Young. Neurological Complications of Renal Disease. Boston: Butterworth, 1990.

sis. In many instances, a precise diagnosis of central nervous system infection is not possible, and empirical therapy should be started.

After these measures, the diagnosis may still be in doubt. For example, all microbiologic studies may initially have been negative and no malignant cells may have been found in the cerebrospinal fluid. A CT scan may show single or multiple lesions of a nonspecific nature. In this case, brain biopsy may be necessary. The neuropathologist and microbiologist should be notified in advance of this procedure and should be prepared to study the tissue comprehensively.

Treatment will depend upon the underlying condition (see Table 11.3).

## Stroke

Uremic patients have an increased incidence of stroke, compared to the general population. While patients are on dialysis, there is an increased risk of intracranial hemorrhage. Following transplantation, the principal type of stroke is ischemic. Risk factors include lipid abnormalities, coincident diabetes mellitus, hypertension, and secondary polycythemia.

Hemorrhagic strokes occur in the usual sites for hypertensive hemorrhages: basal ganglia, thalamus, cerebellum, and brain stem. Subarachnoid hemorrhages are also increased, however. Ischemic strokes can relate either to large-vessel occlusion or small-vessel damage (lacunar strokes). The latter may fit into syndromes—for example, pure motor hemiplegia, pure sensory stroke, ataxic hemiparesis—or may be multiple, with added deficits producing a mixed picture or pseudobulbar palsy. Sometimes the strokes relate to associated diseases, for example, systemic lupus erythematosus with Libman-Sacks endocarditis and embolism or diabetes mellitus.

## Peripheral Nervous System

### Uremic Polyneuropathy

In the early stages of chronic renal failure, during conservative management, uremic polyneuropathy is usually not clinically evident, although mild abnormalities may be detected with electrophysiologic studies or very mild clinical signs may be evident. It is only when end-stage renal failure has been reached, when the creatinine clearance is less than 5 ml per minute, that significant polyneuropathy occurs. Then, 60% of patients will have some evidence of uremic polyneuropathy. The commonest early symptoms are restless legs syndrome, cramps, numbness and tingling, and uncomfortable sensations, but these may be relatively nonspecific and may occasionally occur in the absence of clinical or electrophysiologic evidence of uremic neuropathy. They may be related to transient neural membrane dysfunction brought about by changes in water and electrolytes. The earliest clear-cut clinical signs are impaired vibratory perception in the toes and reduced ankle jerks. Rarely, the neuropathy is severe, with distal wasting and weakness, absent deep tendon reflexes, severe distal sensory loss in all modalities, and an inability to walk.

On occasion, uremic polyneuropathy seems to advance rapidly over a matter of weeks and may be predominantly of a motor variety. It is likely that this type of neuropathy is associated with underlying sepsis that occurs at the site of shunts or fistulas or follows intercurrent operation. The neuropathy is more properly called *critical-illness polyneuropathy*. It reverses satisfactorily once the sepsis is brought fully under control.

The autonomic nervous system is commonly involved in a mild form that is detected only by testing of the cardiac P-R interval; the normal variation in this interval is lost or diminished. Overt clinical evidence of autonomic nervous system dysfunction is uncommon, however. Any manifestations of autonomic neuropathy stabilize during chronic hemodialysis and improve following successful renal transplantation.

In uremic polyneuropathy, electrophysiologic studies show a primary axonal degeneration of motor and sensory fibers. There may be a secondary segmental demyelination. Hence, conduction velocities may be moderately reduced and distal latencies prolonged. Compound muscle-action-potential amplitudes and sensory-action-potential amplitudes are the earliest to be involved, along with prolongation of H- or F-wave latencies. These electrophysiologic abnormalities may be present in up to 80% of patients on chronic hemodialysis, whether children or adults. Because of the discomfort, needle electromyography need not be performed except in polyneuropathies that are moderate or severe. We have observed that abnormal spontaneous activity, positive sharp waves and fibrillation potentials, may be strangely absent when there is clinical and histologic evidence of denervation of muscle. We have speculated that uremic toxins may, in some way, inhibit the production of this abnormal spontaneous activity.

Clinical and electrophysiologic assessment of the peripheral nervous system in patients on chronic hemodialysis is a valuable method of determining how well controlled the uremic syndrome is by the particular dialysis techniques. Thus, if the polyneuropathy appears to have worsened (because it should normally stabilize during chronic hemodialysis), efforts should be made to optimize the hemodialysis. The nephrologist may do this in a variety of ways (e.g., increase the weekly frequency, change the type of dialyzer). Improvement in the neuropathy may not occur, however, for a number of months or may not occur at all. Hence, if the uremic neuropathy continues to worsen, the patient should be strongly considered for renal transplantation. When this is done, one can expect prompt and progressive improvement in the uremic polyneuropathy, even in severe cases.

Peritoneal dialysis does not appear to be any more effective than long-term hemodialysis in controlling uremic polyneuropathy.

## Uremic Mononeuropathy

A variety of mononeuropathies may occur during chronic hemodialysis, because uremic toxins render nerves susceptible to damage from focal compression or ischemia.

### Carpal Tunnel Syndrome

Carpal tunnel syndrome may occur in 31% of patients on long-term hemodialysis. It causes symptoms remarkably similar to those experienced by patients

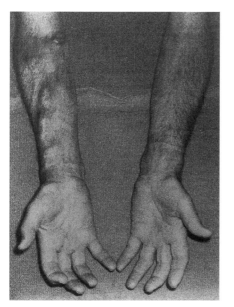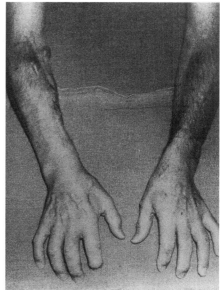

*Figure 11.5*  The upper limbs of a patient who had beta$_2$-microglobulin amyloidosis. It caused bilateral carpal tunnel syndrome (note proximal thenar wasting) and a right ulnar neuropathy (note wasting of interosseus muscles). Tissue biopsied at the time of carpal tunnel surgery revealed infiltration of blood vessels by amyloid. The pain may have been a result of an arthropathy (note thickening and flexion contraction of interphalangeal joints) and periodic nerve ischemia. Repeated surgery for carpal tunnel syndrome provided only transient relief. (The Brescia-Cimino forearm fistula caused the dilated veins of the right forearm.) (Reprinted with permission from CF Bolton, GB Young. Neurological Complications of Renal Disease. Boston: Butterworth, 1990.)

who are not in chronic renal failure. Thus, periodic numbness and tingling throughout the median nerve distribution and aching pain radiating proximally occur commonly and are characteristically worsened by acts such as reading a newspaper, repeatedly grasping objects, and so forth. These symptoms may seriously disturb the patient's sleep. However, a distinctive feature is that, in patients in long-term hemodialysis who have this syndrome, the symptoms are worse during each hemodialysis procedure. Moreover, the carpal tunnel syndrome is more likely to occur in the arm that contains the Brescia-Cimino fistula (Figure 11.5). Physical signs of median nerve compression, such as wasting of the thenar eminence, are late signs, and hence electrophysiologic studies are usually necessary to establish the diagnosis. Abnormalities in sensory conduction are the first to appear.

In most cases, the carpal tunnel syndrome is of uncertain cause or is clearly secondary to the forearm Brescia-Cimino fistula. Less commonly, however, patients develop amyloidosis (see Figure 11.5) after they have been on hemodialysis for longer than 10 years. This condition produces generalized arthropathy, in addition to carpal tunnel syndrome. This type of amyloidosis is seen only in chronic renal failure and is a result of the accumulation of beta microglobulin, a substance that is normally present in the body in very small amounts but that accumulates in end-stage renal failure. When carpal tunnel syndrome appears, appropriate stains for this type of amyloid must be performed in order to establish the diagnosis. Avoidance of the use of cuprophan membranes for long-term hemodialysis may eliminate this serious complication.

Conservative management, such as splinting the wrists, is usually not effective in treating carpal tunnel syndrome, but sectioning of the flexor retinaculum is usually quite effective. If it appears that the Brescia-Cimino fistula is a significant contributing factor, it may ultimately be necessary to band or ligate the fistula or perform angioplasty.

## Mononeuropathies Associated with Arteriovenous Fistula or Shunts

The Brescia-Cimino fistula commonly used for access during long-term hemodialysis occasionally produces periodic aching and burning in the hand. This condition is really an arterial steal syndrome, caused by periodic ischemia to the tissues. The symptoms often worsen during each hemodialysis procedure. It is common after graft placement but soon resolves spontaneously. If it becomes chronic, however, digital photoplethysmography, pulse oximetry, and angiography should be performed. Transcatheter balloon angioplasty or embolization may be effective in selected cases; ligation of the distal radial artery is the method of choice in some patients. The condition may be successfully treated with either banding or ligation of the fistula.

In some instances, true carpal tunnel syndrome develops as a result of vascular congestion and ischemia in the region of the carpal tunnel. In rare circumstances, a shunt placed more proximally in the upper arm may induce a sudden, severe ischemic neuropathy affecting the median, ulnar, and radial nerves. These neuropathic complications are most prevalent in diabetics. This occurrence is an emergency situation that requires immediate clinical and electrophysiologic documentation of the neuropathy, and investigation and management of tissue ischemia as described above. Even then, the neuropathy may not improve.

## Eighth-Nerve Dysfunction

In chronic renal failure, either because of the presence of uremic toxins or the use of antibiotics or diuretics, both cochlear and vestibular divisions may be affected. Improvement may occur either through hemodialysis or through successful renal transplantation.

## Compartment Syndromes

Because of the tendency to excessive bleeding in chronic renal failure, and particularly if anticoagulant drugs are being used, compartment syndrome may develop suddenly. A typical site is the psoas muscle. There may be sudden, severe pain and motor and sensory loss within the distribution of the femoral nerve. CT scanning may demonstrate the acute hemorrhage and surgical decompression may be beneficial.

### Combined Diabetic and Uremic Polyneuropathy

More diabetic patients are being accepted into dialysis and transplant programs, and thus the problem of combined diabetic and uremic polyneuropathy is being seen with increasing frequency. In both types of polyneuropathy, there is a symmetric motor and sensory involvement, with reduced deep tendon reflexes, ataxia, and distal loss of sensation. However, diabetic polyneuropathy is more likely to induce compressive palsies, such as tardy ulnar palsy or carpal tunnel syndrome, and autonomic disturbances and multifocal denervation of muscle are more common. Also, in diabetic polyneuropathy, conduction velocities tend to be lower and attempts at collateral reinnervation are usually more successful than in uremic polyneuropathy.

Each polyneuropathy also acts differently in response to organ transplantation. As already noted, uremic polyneuropathy improves promptly with successful kidney transplantation. On the other hand, pancreatic transplantation causes minimal improvement in diabetic polyneuropathy.

Bolton and colleagues observed four patients who had subacute, predominantly motor polyneuropathy associated with diabetes mellitus and end-stage renal disease. Electrophysiologic studies and muscle biopsy indicated a primary axonal degeneration of nerve with secondary segmental demyelination, and mild-to-moderate acute and chronic denervation of muscle. A relative absence of denervation potentials on needle electromyography was an unusual feature, possibly resulting from uremic toxins' inhibiting the generation of such potentials. Three patients improved with a switch from conventional to high-flux hemodialysis. Bolton and colleagues speculated that this may have been a result of enhanced removal of advanced glycosylation end products. Advanced glycosylation end products result from enzymatic reactions, termed Maillard reactions, that occur between glucose and proteins, and promote cytokine and growth factor release, matrix protein synthesis, increased vascular permeability, and procoagulant activity through interactions with vascular endothelium. They have been implicated in the complications of diabetes mellitus and aging: namely, cataracts, atherosclerosis, and renal disease. They may also be implicated in combined diabetic and uremic polyneuropathy.

### Disturbances of Muscle in Uremia

Defects in neuromuscular transmission are quite uncommon and, when present, are caused by certain antibiotic drugs or high levels of magnesium. Such defects can readily be demonstrated in the electromyographic laboratory by repetitive nerve stimulation techniques.

Severe disturbances of water or electrolytes may induce significant muscle weakness. Attacks of hyperkalemic periodic paralysis may occur in uremic patients and, in contrast to familial varieties, the serum potassium remains abnormal between attacks.

Tetany is a rare manifestation of chronic uremia and is caused by lowered serum levels of calcium or magnesium or to respiratory alkalosis. Hypocalcemia occurs in renal failure as a result of the kidney's inability to synthesize 1,25-dihydroxyvitamin $D_3$. It may also be caused by poor mobilization of calcium salts from bone. The rarity of tetany in renal failure is likely a result of the corrective action of the associated acidosis. Thus, it only becomes manifest if patients are treated with large amounts of alkali. Tetany is manifest as numbness and tingling in the extremities, light-headedness, and carpopedal spasm or laryngospasm. Percussion of a peripheral nerve may induce contraction of the muscle it supplies (Chvostek's sign). During electrophysiologic studies, needle electromyography may reveal spontaneous repetitive discharges that appear as double, triple, or multiple discharges; these discharges have the typical appearance of motor unit potentials. Tetany is successfully treated by correction of hypocalcemia and alkalosis.

In rare circumstances when high-dose steroids are used to treat certain forms of primary renal disease, a steroid myopathy may be induced. This myopathy is usually relatively mild and is characterized by normal levels of creatine phosphokinase and normal electrophysiologic studies, including needle electromyography of muscle. Muscle biopsy may be normal or may reveal a type 2 fiber atrophy.

When bone is significantly affected by hyperparathyroidism or aluminum accumulation, the result may be pain and, sometimes, severe wasting of muscle, particularly in proximal muscles (see Figure 11.1). As in steroid myopathy, however, electrophysiologic and morphologic studies of muscle are often normal or biopsy may reveal type 2 fiber atrophy, a nonspecific finding. These features are also present in patients who have muscle wasting as a result of the cachexia of renal failure.

Myoglobinuria may be a cause of acute and severe renal failure requiring hemodialysis. The muscles may be weak, swollen, and painful, but are occasionally surprisingly normal on examination. The creatinine phosphokinase is invariably considerably elevated. With successful treatment, muscle strength usually promptly returns to normal.

## SUGGESTED READING

Alfrey AC, LeGendre GR, Kaehny WD. The dialysis encephalopathy syndrome: possible aluminum intoxication. N Engl J Med 1976;294:184–188.
Asbury AK, Victor M, Adams RD. Uremic polyneuropathy. Arch Neurol 1963;8:413–428.
Baker LRI, Brown AL, Byrne J, et al. Head scan appearances and cognitive function in renal failure. Clin Nephrol 1989;32:242–248.
Bolton CF, Driedger AA, Lindsay RM. Ischemic neuropathy in uremic patients due to arteriovenous fistulas. J Neurol Neurosurg Psychiatry 1979;42:810–814.
Bolton CF, Young GB. Neurological Complications of Renal Disease. Boston: Butterworth, 1990.
Bolton CF, Young GB, Zochodne DW. The neurological complications of sepsis. Ann Neurol 1993;33:94–100.
Bosch BA, Schlebush L. Neurophysiological deficits associated with uraemic encephalopathy. S Afr Med J 1991;79:560–562.
Bruyn GW, De Wolff FA. Plumbism. In PJ Vinken, GW Bruyn (eds), Handbook of Clinical Neurology. Amsterdam: Elsevier, 1994;431–442.
Cadilhac J, Ribstein M. The EEG in metabolic disorders. World Neurol 1961;2:296–308.

Cassaretto AA, Marchiuro JC, Bagdade JD. Hyperlipidemia following renal transplant. Trans Am Soc Artif Intern Organs 1973;19:154.

Chadwick D, French AT. Uraemic myoclonus: an example of reticular reflex myoclonus? J Neurol Neurosurg Psychiatry 1979;42:52–55.

Chaptal J, Passouant P, Puech P. Sur la forme hypertensive des glomérulonéphrites de l'enfant. Arch Fr Pediatr 1954;11:192–196.

Conger JD, Schrier RW. Acute Renal Failure: Pathogenesis, Diagnosis, and Management. In RW Schrier (ed), Renal and Electrolyte Disorders. Boston: Little, Brown, 1985.

Fassbinder W, Challah S, Brynger H. The long-term renal allograft recipient. Transplant Proc 1987;19: 3754–3757.

Folstein MF, Folstein SE, McHugh PR. Mini-Mental State: a practical guide for grading the cognitive state of patients for the clinician. J Psychiatr Res 1975;12:189–198.

Gowers WR. A Manual of Diseases of the Nervous System. Philadelphia: Blackiston, 1888;535–536.

Higgins MR, Grace M, Dossetor JB. Survival of patients treated for end-stage renal disease by dialysis and transplantation. Can Med Assoc J 1977;117:880–883.

Hou SH. Hospital-acquired renal insufficiency: a prospective study. Am J Med 1983;74:243–247.

Ingelfinger JR, Grupe WE, Levey RH. Post-transplant hypertension in the absence of rejection or recurrent disease. Clin Nephrol 1981;15:235–239.

Jablecki CK. Myopathies. In WF Brown, CF Bolton (eds), Clinical Electromyography. Boston: Butterworth–Heinemann, 1987;385.

Knezevic W, Mastaglia FL. Neuropathy associated with Brescia-Cimino arteriovenous fistulas. Arch Neurol 1984;41:1184–1186.

Locke S, Merrill JP, Tyler HR. Neurologic complications of acute uremia. Arch Intern Med 1961;108:519–530.

Mahoney JF, Sheil AGR, Etheridge SB, et al. Delayed complications of renal transplantation and their prevention. Med J Aust 1982;2:426–429.

Nielsen VK. Pathophysiological Aspects of Uraemic Neuropathy. In N Canal, G Pozza (eds), Peripheral Neuropathies. New York: Elsevier/North Holland, 1978;197.

O'Hare JA, Callaghan NM, Murnaghan DJ. Dialysis encephalopathy: clinical, electro-encephalographic and interventional aspects. Medicine 1983;62:129–141.

Okada J, Yoshikawa K, Matsuo H, et al. Reversible MRI and CT findings in uremic encephalopathy. Neuroradiology 1961;33:524–526.

Onoyama K, Kumagai H, Miischima T, et al. Incidence of strokes and its prognosis in patients on maintenance hemodialysis. Jpn Heart J 1986;27:685-691.

Penn AS. Myoglobinuria. In AG Engel, BQ Banker (eds), Myology. New York: McGraw-Hill, 1986.

Plum F, Posner JB. The Diagnosis of Stupor and Coma (3rd ed). Philadelphia: Davis, 1980.

Rotter W, Roettger P. Comparative pathologic-anatomic study of cases of chronic global renal insufficiency with and without preceding hemodialysis. Clin Nephrol 1973;1:257–265.

Shields RW, Root KE, Wilbourn AJ. Compartment syndromes and compression neuropathies in coma. Neurology 1986;36:1370–1374.

Swift TR. Disorders of neuromuscular transmission other than myasthenia gravis. Muscle Nerve 1984;4:334–353.

Tegner R, Lindholm B. Vibratory perception threshold compared with nerve conduction velocity in the evaluation of uraemic neuropathy. Acta Neurol Scand 1985;71:284–289.

Tyler HR. Neurologic disorders in renal failure. Am J Med 1968;44:734–748.

Valji K, Hye RJ, Roberts AC, et al. Hand ischemia in patients with hemodialysis access grafts: angiographic diagnosis and treatment. Radiology 1995;196:697–701.

Vallance P, Leone A, Calver A, et al. Accumulation of an endogenous inhibitor of nitric acid synthetase in chronic renal failure. Lancet 1992;339:572–575.

Wilson SAK. Neurology. London: Edward Arnold, 1940;1097.

Wyrtzes L, Markley HG, Fisher M, Alfred AJ. Brachial neuropathy after brachial artery-antecubital vein shunts for chronic hemodialysis. Neurology 1987;37:1398–1400.

Zochodne DW, Bolton CF, Wells GA, et al. Polyneuropathy associated with critical illness: a complication of sepsis and multiple organ failure. Brain 1987;110:819–842.

# 12
# Hematology
## Martin A. Samuels

## ANEMIA

Anemia is present when the concentration of hemoglobin in the peripheral blood is below the normal range for the patient's age and sex (i.e., 14±2 g/dl for women, 16±2 g/dl for men, and 12±2 g/dl for children). When anemia is present, the red blood cell population is usually reduced. The normal red blood cell count is $4.8±0.6 \times 10^6$ per $mm^3$ for women and $5.4±0.9 \times 10^6$ per $mm^3$ for men. The hematocrit indicates the proportion of red blood cells in the blood. Greater than 40% for men and 37% for women is considered normal. The major red blood cell indices, which may be helpful in the differential diagnosis of anemia, are the mean corpuscular volume (MCV), which is the average red blood cell size (normal is $87±5 \ \mu m^3$); the mean corpuscular hemoglobin (MCH), which is the amount of hemoglobin per cell (normal is 29±2 pg of hemoglobin per cell); and the mean corpuscular hemoglobin concentration (MCHC), which is the average concentration of hemoglobin per cell (normal is 34±2%).

These erythrocyte indices may be useful, but it should be emphasized that they are averages. Complete evaluation requires microscopic examination of the peripheral blood smear, which reveals evidence of red blood cell size (macrocytosis, microcytosis) and shape as well as evidence of the degree of maturity of the red blood cells (i.e., presence of reticulocytes or nucleated cells), the intensity of hemoglobin staining (hypochromia, normochromia, or hyperchromia), or the presence of macrocytes, target cells, spherocytes, schistocytes, or other abnormally shaped cells. In some situations, automated analysis of erythrocyte indices may reveal normal range results, but direct observation of the peripheral blood smear shows evidence of a dimorphic anemia (e.g., iron deficiency anemia plus megaloblastic anemia) in which some cells are clearly microcytic and hypochromic and others are macrocytic. This circumstance accounts for the normal indices, which reflect an automated average of the two abnormalities. No analysis of anemia is complete without a direct observation of the peripheral blood smear by an experienced observer. A normal peripheral blood smear is

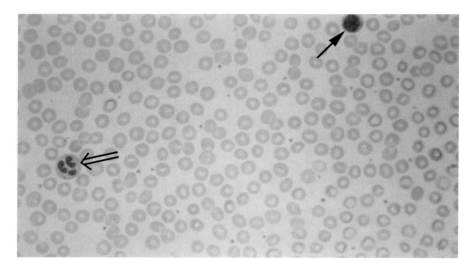

*Figure 12.1*    Normal blood smear. Note the normal size and morphology of the red blood cells. They are slightly smaller than the neighboring lymphocyte (*single arrow*) and have a paler center resulting from their biconcave shape. Note also the normal polymorphonuclear leukocyte (*double arrow*) with its three-lobed nucleus.

shown in Figure 12.1. Note the normal size of the red blood cells by comparing them to a neighboring lymphocyte. Also note the morphology of a normal polymorphonuclear leukocyte and the normal paler center of the red blood cells resulting from their biconcave shape (see Figure 12.1). In some circumstances, full evaluation of an anemia will require an examination of the bone marrow. Further details on the analysis of anemia are beyond the scope of this chapter but are readily available elsewhere.

## Nonspecific Neurologic Effects of Anemia

There are very few neurologic effects of anemia per se. Headache and light-headedness may occur in severe anemias, but these symptoms usually appear only when the hemoglobin concentration is reduced by at least one-half. In slowly developing anemias, many patients may have little or no neurologic symptoms with hemoglobin concentrations as low as one-tenth the normal level. The most easily examinable part of the nervous system that reflects the effect of anemia itself is the eye. The retina and optic nerve head and their vascular supply are easily observed with the ophthalmoscope and probably reflect similar changes in the rest of the brain. The reddish color of the fundus results when the light reflected from the ophthalmoscope by the choroidal blood is altered to a pink color by the pigment content of the retinal epithelium. As the hemoglobin concentration falls, the reddish color of the fundus pales. The optic disc also becomes paler, and the color contrast normally seen between arteries and veins is reduced.

Aside from pallor of the optic fundus, the most common ocular lesion in anemia is retinal hemorrhage, which is usually small and spindle shaped and occasionally associated with a cotton-wool exudate. The presence of hemorrhage correlates with the degree of anemia. It is very unusual to see a retinal hemorrhage when the hemoglobin concentration is greater than 50% of normal. It is believed that blood escapes from the capillaries by diapedesis and that the exudates are composed of fibrin. Both the hemorrhages and the exudates seen in anemia are transient. In severe anemia (i.e., hemoglobin concentration below 6 g/dl) a minor degree of edema of the optic disc and adjoining retina may be observed. This finding is not surprising, because the oxygenation of the optic nerve head depends not only on local blood flow but also on the oxygen-carrying capacity of the blood. The retinal vessels appear to be of different caliber than normal in anemic patients. The arteries are widened, and the usual width relationship between arteries and veins of 2 to 3 approaches 1 to 1.

There have been rare reports of patients who presented with focal cerebral symptoms with moderately severe chronic anemia (i.e., hemoglobin less than 10 g/dl) resulting from blood loss, which resolved upon transfusion. Whether the symptoms reflected an unmasking of underlying, previously asymptomatic, occlusive vascular disease is not clear, but it is certain that focal cerebral symptomatology is a very rare manifestation of anemia per se. Aside from these few general features, anemia itself has little neurologic expression. The following sections review the specific neurologic effects of particular anemias: namely, iron deficiency anemia, megaloblastic anemias (vitamin $B_{12}$ and folate deficiency), and hemoglobinopathies (sickle cell anemia and thalassemia).

## Iron Deficiency Anemia

Iron deficiency from chronic blood loss remains the most common form of anemia. Iron deficiency in the absence of anemia (sideropenia) may decrease the deformability of red blood cells and lead to ischemia in the distribution of small cerebral vessels. This mechanism is particularly important in the context of polycythemia (either primary or secondary) in which there are increased numbers of red blood cells, each one of which may be iron deficient. Both the polycythemia and the relative sideropenia lead to increased blood viscosity with associated neurologic symptoms and signs (see the section on hyperviscosity below). Iron deficiency causes a microcytic, hypochromic anemia (Figure 12.2).

Iron deficiency (usually but not always with anemia) is associated with obsessive-compulsive behaviors that fall into two categories: compulsive eating (pica) and compulsive moving of the limbs, usually the legs (restless legs). Common pica behaviors include the eating of starch, paint chips, clay (terra sigillata), earth (geophagia), and ice (pagophagia). The relationship between the iron deficiency and pica is unknown. Clearly it does not represent replacement of iron, because ice eating—the most common pica behavior—usually does nothing to help in this regard, and many clays contain substances that actually chelate iron, thereby worsening the problem. It seems more likely that pica represents some form of compulsive behavior akin to a tic.

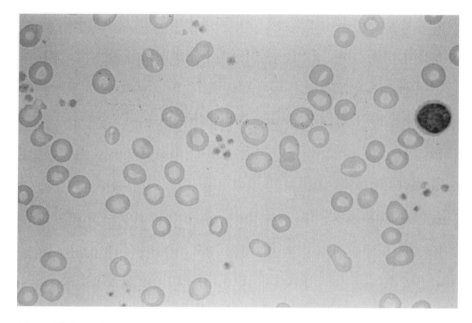

*Figure 12.2*  Peripheral blood smear in a patient with iron deficiency anemia. Note that the red blood cells are much smaller than the neighboring lymphocyte (microcytosis) and have larger, paler centers (hypochromia).

The restless legs syndrome is a very common cause of insomnia. It consists of an unpleasant creeping sensation that occurs deep in the legs (and occasionally in the arms) when the person is at rest. The person feels compelled to move the legs to avoid the unpleasant feeling. Most sufferers are women, who pace the floors at night and complain of insomnia. Polysomnographic studies often reveal nocturnal myoclonus (periodic movements of sleep). It is likely that restless legs, nocturnal myoclonus, and akathisia represent various fragments of a single disorder, sometimes called the Ekbom syndrome. Many such patients are iron deficient, in which case the symptoms respond to iron replacement. The rest are treated, usually very successfully, with clonazepam or another benzodiazepine at bedtime. Some patients who fail to respond to a benzodiazepine will derive benefit from L-dopa, clonidine, or clomipramine hydrochloride. Patients diagnosed as having the restless legs syndrome should undergo a careful anemia evaluation, including microscopic study of the blood smear, measurements of serum iron and total iron-binding capacity, and several stool occult blood tests.

## Megaloblastic Anemias

The term *megaloblastic anemia* refers to a characteristic pattern of morphologic abnormality in the blood and bone marrow that probably arises from impaired

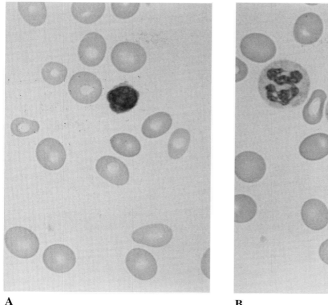
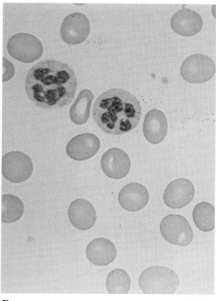

**A**        **B**

*Figure 12.3*  Peripheral blood smear from a patient with megaloblastic anemia. (**A**) Note that the red blood cells are larger than the neighboring lymphocyte (macrocytosis). (**B**) Note also that the polymorphonuclear leukocytes contain nuclei with five or more segments (hypersegmentation).

DNA synthesis. Clinically, this is usually the result of a deficiency of one of two factors, vitamin $B_{12}$ or folic acid, both of which are essential to the formation of the deoxyribosyl precursors of DNA. This deficiency results in abnormal development of erythroblasts in the marrow such that there is intramedullary hemolysis resulting in anemia. The peripheral blood contains macrocytic erythrocytes. The disordered DNA metabolism also affects the maturation of granulocytes, which results in the presence of hypersegmented polymorphonuclear leukocytes in the peripheral blood (Figure 12.3).

This disordered DNA metabolism is clearly not confined to the blood cells, because giant epithelial cells are found in many organs, including the mouth, stomach, and skin. The neurologic effects of the megaloblastic anemias are probably a result of a primary metabolic derangement in neural tissue and are clearly not directly related to the anemia per se. Because the blood-forming organs are particularly sensitive to the effects of $B_{12}$ or folate deficiency, it is unusual to find the neurologic effects in patients in whom no disorders of the blood are seen. Anemia is, however, only one and probably a relatively late sign of $B_{12}$ or folate deficiency, so it is possible to find a clear example of the neurologic effects of $B_{12}$ or folate deficiency without anemia. It is distinctly rare, on the other hand, to find no hematologic signs of $B_{12}$ or folate deficiency in a patient with proven neurologic effects of these vitamin deficiencies. Some patients of this kind have been reported, but the degree of completeness of the hematologic evaluation or the precise nature of the neurologic lesions is often questioned in analyzing these rare case reports. Some of these cases may represent other forms of degenerative spinal cord disease in which the lateral and posterior columns are primarily affected that are totally unassociated with vitamin $B_{12}$ deficiency. Because reliable methods of measuring serum vitamin $B_{12}$ levels have become available only relatively recently, cases reported prior to the availability of these methods in which no hematologic manifestations of $B_{12}$ or folate deficiency were noted must be viewed with a degree of skepticism.

## Vitamin $B_{12}$ Deficiency

Vitamin $B_{12}$ deficiency may be the result of a number of causes, which are summarized as follows:

1. Defective diet (low in animal or bacterial products)
2. Defective absorption
   a. Deficiency of intrinsic factor
      (1) Pernicious anemia
      (2) Gastrectomy
   b. Intestinal disease
      (1) Malabsorption (sprue; resection, bypass, or disease of terminal ileum)
      (2) Blind loop syndrome
      (3) Fish tapeworm infestation
3. Deranged metabolism or increased requirement (thyrotoxicosis, pregnancy, neoplasia)

Of these, the most prevalent form of $B_{12}$ deficiency, at least in North America, is pernicious anemia (or Addison's anemia, Biermer's anemia, primary anemia). It arises from failure of the gastric fundus to secrete adequate amounts of intrinsic factor to insure intestinal absorption of vitamin $B_{12}$. This failure of secretion of the mucoprotein intrinsic factor is a result of atrophy of the fundic glandular mucosa, a process that is usually immune mediated, but may be familial or result from gastric neoplasia. Assessment of histamine fast achlorhydria is a reliable method of diagnosing pernicious anemia, but it has now often been supplanted by measurements of anti-intrinsic factor and anti–parietal-cell antibodies. Patients with autoimmune pernicious anemia often have clinical and laboratory evidence of other conditions characterized by autoimmunity, such as vitiligo and thyroiditis. Serum $B_{12}$ levels have occasionally been measured erroneously to be normal in documented cases, so it is now routine to assess intracellular function by directly measuring serum homocysteine and methylmalonic acid. Cobalamin (vitamin $B_{12}$ or extrinsic factor) exists in two forms, methylcobalamin and adenosylcobalamin, each of which acts as an important cofactor in reactions vital to cellular function. The methylcobalamin system acts to transfer methyl groups from methyltetrahydrofolate to homocysteine, thereby creating tetrahydrofolate, which is required for DNA synthesis, and methionine (Figure 12.4). Failure of this system results in impaired DNA synthesis and accumulation of homocysteine. Nitrous oxide, an inhibitor of methyl transferase, causes the syndrome of subacute combined degeneration of the nervous system. This fact argues that DNA synthesis failure can cause neurologic disease, even though neurons are post-

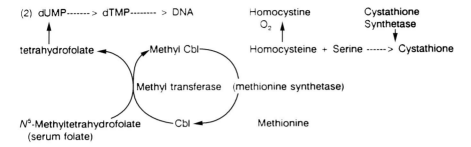

*Figure 12.4* Methylcobalamin-mediated methyl transferase system, which converts serum folate ($N^5$-methyltetrahydrofolate) to tetrahydrofolate by transferring a methyl group to homocysteine, thereby producing methionine as a consequence.

mitotic and therefore are themselves resistant to such a toxin. It is likely that this toxicity acts on oligodendrocytes, resulting in the demyelinating lesion that is characteristic of subacute combined degeneration.

The adenosyl cobalamin system acts to metabolize propionic acid by converting methylmalonyl coenzyme A to succinyl coenzyme A, which then enters the Krebs cycle (Figure 12.5). Failure of this system results in an accumulation of methyl-malonic acid, which is toxic to the nervous system by promoting the formation of long-chain fatty acids with odd numbers of carbon atoms. Normal long-chain fatty acids, which contain even numbers of carbon atoms, are formed using malonic acid. Therefore, when methylmalonic acid replaces malonic acid, an extra methyl group leads to odd numbers of carbon atoms and an unstable myelin.

Thus, serum homocysteine and methylmalonic acid levels are elevated when there is intracellular failure of the two cobalamin-related chemical reactions. This fact makes measurement of the levels of these two substances the most sensitive test for vitamin $B_{12}$ deficiency.

Because vitamin $B_{12}$ is stored in various tissues in large amounts, the appearance of cobalamin deficiency after the cessation of $B_{12}$ absorption or intake is delayed by at least 3 years. Despite the fact that pernicious anemia is the most common cause of $B_{12}$ deficiency, it seems clear that vitamin $B_{12}$ deficiency resulting from any of the above-listed causes may result in the identical clinical picture. The three neurologic manifestations of vitamin $B_{12}$ deficiency are subacute combined degeneration of the spinal cord, mental changes, and optic neuropathy.

*Subacute combined degeneration of the spinal cord* (or subacute combined sclerosis, posterolateral sclerosis) is the term used to designate the spinal cord disease resulting from cobalamin deficiency. The patients tend to complain of generalized weakness and paresthesias, which begin distally and progress proximally. As these symptoms progress, stiffness and weakness in the limbs develop. Loss of vibration sense is the most profound sign, often joined later in the course by loss of joint position sense as well. Romberg's sign is positive, and the gait is unsteady and awkward. Weakness and spasticity are usually worse in the legs than in the arms and may progress to a spastic paraplegia if untreated. Babinski's signs are present, but the deep tendon reflexes are variable. They may be grossly increased

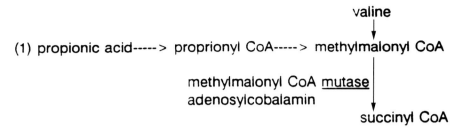

valine

(1) propionic acid-----> proprionyl CoA-----> methylmalonyl CoA

methylmalonyl CoA <u>mutase</u>
adenosylcobalamin

succinyl CoA

*Figure 12.5*   Role of adenosyl cobalamin in converting the potentially toxic methylmalonyl coenzyme A (CoA) to succinyl CoA.

with clonus, absent, or show any intermediate degree of activity. Occasionally, a sensory level may be found on the trunk that implicates the spinothalamic tracts. This finding should always be viewed with the greatest skepticism and lead one to exhaustively exclude other causes of spinal cord disease. All of the findings of pure vitamin $B_{12}$ deficiency may be attributable to myelopathy alone, and there is no convincing evidence that $B_{12}$ deficiency itself causes a neuropathy. In practice, however, the frequent concomitant existence of folate and other vitamin deficiencies makes it difficult to be sure of this point. Many patients with vitamin $B_{12}$ deficiency have distal symmetric impairment of cutaneous sensation, absent deep tendon reflexes, and even slowed nerve conduction velocities, findings that suggest a neuropathic component. These findings are probably a result of concomitant folate deficiency, but the outside chance that vitamin $B_{12}$ deficiency itself may cause a peripheral neuropathy cannot be rigorously excluded. Pathologically, the lesion in the nervous system is a degeneration of white matter in the spinal cord and occasionally the brain. The myelin sheaths and axis cylinders are both involved, the former more profoundly than the latter. These changes begin in the posterior columns of the lower cervical and upper thoracic segments and spread from there up and down and also laterally in the cord to involve the lateral columns. Microscopic study shows early changes consisting of swelling and destruction of myelin sheath with subsequent axonal destruction. Later, a cribriform appearance develops. Eventually, white matter is lost and is replaced by gliosis. The focal lesions have a rough but not absolute symmetry, and they extend caudally and rostrally so that ultimately the entire area of the dorsal columns is involved. In the meantime, the lesions have begun in the lateral columns and extend into the other long tracts. The gray matter is spared. Similar changes can be seen in the cerebral hemispheres and optic nerves. The myelin of peripheral nerves may also be involved, but axons have not been shown to be unequivocally affected.

*Mental changes* are frequent in patients with vitamin $B_{12}$ deficiency. In most cases these changes reflect abnormalities in level of consciousness, with inattention, confusion, somnolence, apathy, and delirium being the cardinal features. True dementia, defined as intellectual impairment in the absence of a disorder of level of consciousness, is certainly a relatively rare manifestation of pure vitamin $B_{12}$ deficiency. Pure mental change as the only manifestation of vitamin $B_{12}$ deficiency is exquisitely uncommon. Case reports of true dementia and pure mental change as manifestations of vitamin $B_{12}$ deficiency are contaminated with concomitant causes of dementia and disordered mental status.

*Optic neuropathy* is the third and last major neurologic complication of vitamin $B_{12}$ deficiency. It is characterized by bilateral involvement of the optic nerves, resulting in loss of central visual acuity and depressed sensitivity in the centrocecal area of the field of vision that is greater for color than for white. Optic neuropathy is the rarest of the three neurologic manifestations of vitamin $B_{12}$ deficiency, but it may be the only or the presenting manifestation of the syndrome. It may be found to be subclinically present in many more cases than previously believed if one uses a very sensitive measurement of optic nerve function such as visual evoked responses. This syndrome is clinically similar to a number of other bilateral optic neuropathy syndromes, including so called tobacco-alcohol amblyopia, diabetic optic neuritis, Leber's hereditary optic atrophy, and tropical ataxic neuropathy. Some believe that the cause of all of these syndromes, including vitamin $B_{12}$–deficiency optic neuropathy, is linked to an abnormality in cyanide metabolism resulting from a shortage of sulfur-donating amino acids. An epidemic of optic neuropathy and myelopathy in Cuba is thought to have been caused by multiple B-vitamin deficiencies caused by malnutrition combined with intake of alcohol and cyanide from cigar smoking and cassava consumption. The epidemic was terminated by vitamin supplementation.

Folic Acid (Folate) Deficiency

Folate deficiency accounts for nearly all of the cases of megaloblastic anemia that are not caused by vitamin $B_{12}$ deficiency. The causes of folate deficiency may be summarized as follows:

1. Defective diet (low in vegetables and liver)
2. Defective absorption
    a. Intestinal malabsorption (sprue; steatorrhea, massive diverticulosis, short circuits of gastrointestinal tract)
    b. Blind loop syndrome
3. Deranged metabolism
    a. Increased requirement (hemolytic anemia, pregnancy, neoplasia)
    b. Impaired utilization (liver disease, administration of folic acid antagonists or anticonvulsants)

Unlike with vitamin $B_{12}$, the bodily stores of folic acid are quite limited. A folate deficiency syndrome may commence within several months of dietary deprivation; for this reason, it is a much more common problem among the malnourished than is vitamin $B_{12}$ deficiency. Folate, once absorbed through the entire small intestine, is reduced by specific liver enzymes to tetrahydrofolic acid, a compound that plays a major role in the metabolism of one-carbon fragments by its synthesis and transfer of methyl groups. Via this mechanism, folate is vital for the conversion of deoxyuridine to thymidine, a precursor needed for DNA synthesis. Thus, tetrahydrofolate derivations are closely linked to vitamin $B_{12}$–dependent reactions, and the hematologic alterations in vitamin $B_{12}$ and folate deficiency are indistinguishable. Deficiencies of the two vitamins have very similar effects, and a deficiency of one may lead to faulty utilization of the other.

For example, patients with vitamin $B_{12}$ deficiency may have an initially elevated serum folate that plummets rapidly when vitamin $B_{12}$ is administered. Concomitant treatment with folate is thus required to prevent a folate deficiency state that was previously masked by the vitamin $B_{12}$ deficiency from becoming clinically significant. Many patients with vitamin $B_{12}$ deficiency have concomitant folate deficiency; however, the vast majority of those with the overwhelmingly more common folate deficiency state will have no vitamin $B_{12}$ deficiency. Folic acid deficiency is almost never pure. Because it accompanies malnutrition, it is nearly always associated with multiple vitamin deficiencies. The most common neurologic manifestation of this state is a polyneuropathy.

The symptomatology of nutritional polyneuropathy includes distal paresthesias, burning, and weakness. On examination, there is a distal loss of reflexes and sensation. The essential pathologic change is an axonal degeneration with a dying back of the axons according to length. Some minor degrees of segmental demyelination may also occur, usually a result of entrapment of metabolically weakened nerves. The common entrapment neuropathies (e.g., carpal tunnel syndrome, meralgia paresthetica, peroneal palsy, ulnar palsy) are all more frequent in patients with an underlying metabolic axonopathy such as that caused by vitamin deficiency. In circumstances in which the major vitamin deficiency is likely to be folic acid deficiency (i.e., when folate antagonists have been given), a mild polyneuropathy of the type described above occurs. There is no evidence that pure folate deficiency has any other neurologic manifestations.

## Hemoglobinopathies and Thalassemia

In normal people, variations in the concentrations of the three normal varieties of hemoglobin (A, $A_2$, and F) are known to take place with aging. Disorders in which the presence of a structurally abnormal hemoglobin is considered to play a primary pathologic role are referred to as hemoglobinopathies. Disturbances involving alterations in the percentages of normal forms of hemoglobin are designated by individual terms, such as *thalassemia*. Hemoglobin consists of four coiled polypeptide chains. The four chains are of two varieties, so that two of each type are present. There are four normal polypeptide sequences, designated alpha, beta, gamma, and delta. Hemoglobin A consists of two alpha and two beta chains, designated $\alpha_2\beta_2$. $HbA_2$ consists of $\alpha_2\delta_2$ and HbF consists of $\alpha_2\gamma_2$. Several mechanisms that result in abnormal hemoglobin are known. Many examples of abnormal hemoglobins have been defined in which a single amino acid substitution has occurred in one of the two pairs of polypeptide chains. Other abnormal hemoglobins result from crossing over of the adjacent structural genes for the beta, gamma, and delta polypeptides. Hemoglobins consisting of a single variety of polypeptide rather than the normal two have been described, and abnormalities resulting in the switch from fetal to adult hemoglobin are known. Finally, abnormalities in the mechanism controlling the rate of release or synthesis of various polypeptide chains are thought to result in the thalassemia group of disorders. Most of the abnormal hemoglobins cause no hematologic difficulty. However, some diseases are directly attributable to changes in hemoglobin structure that lead to a variety of steric changes in the molecule. Sickle hemoglobin forms insoluble polymers when deoxygenated. The HbM variants lead to excessive lev-

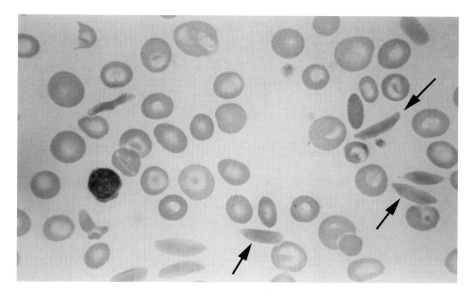

*Figure 12.6*   Peripheral blood smear from a patient with sickle cell anemia. Sickled red blood cells are marked with arrows.

els of methemoglobin. HgM combines irreversibly with oxygen, whereas other types such as HbQ are easily denatured and precipitate within the erythrocytes to form Heinz bodies.

A person homozygous for a structural mutation involving one of the polypeptide chains of HbA produces only a single abnormal adult variety of hemoglobin. Three examples of such a disease are HbS, HbC, and HbE. Of these, the most important is HbS, which causes sickle cell anemia. HbC and HbE diseases are generally mild and have no known neurologic complications.

## Sickle Cell Anemia (HbS disease)

Most of the manifestations of sickle cell anemia are related to the characteristic property of HbS to crystallize under conditions of reduced oxygen tension. Because of this property, sickled erythrocytes become trapped in terminal arterioles and capillaries; the result is more hypoxia, increased sickling, thrombosis, and infarction. Figure 12.6 is a peripheral blood smear from a patient with sickle cell anemia. Tissues that normally contain blood at low oxygen tensions, such as renal medulla and pulmonary arterioles, are at greatest risk, but sickling may occur in other organs, including the relatively well-oxygenated brain and spinal cord. The hemolysis results largely from the fact that the sickled erythrocytes are mechanically rigid, less flexible, and more fragile than normal cells.

The neurologic complications of sickle cell anemia may be divided into four categories: painful crises, vascular disease, infection, and fat embolism.

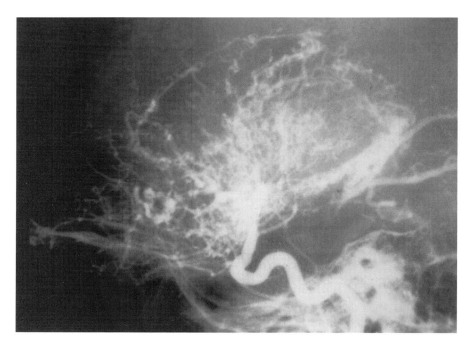

*Figure 12.7*    Cerebral angiogram of a patient with sickle cell anemia. Progressive stenosis of the supraclinoid portion of the internal carotid artery has resulted in the development of a fragile array of collateral vessels, which are subject to rupture leading to intracerebral hemorrhage. This angiographic pattern known as *moyamoya* (meaning "puff of smoke") is seen in Japanese patients without hemoglobinopathies but is most common in North America in patients with sickle cell anemia.

Painful crises are among the most common clinical problems in the management of patients with sickle cell anemia. The abdominal and bone pain so common in this disease is probably ischemic pain related to the sickling phenomenon as described above. The treatment consists of hydration, bed rest, and analgesia.

Vascular disease is the more serious neurologic aspect of this disorder and probably contributes in a major way to the decreased life expectancy of patients with sickle cell anemia. The incidence of overt strokes is about 20% among patients with sickle cell anemia, obviously a massive increase over that among other patients of similar age. Most of the strokes are caused by small-vessel occlusions, which often result in seizures at the onset of the stroke. In some cases, progressive small-vessel occlusions with recurrent development of collaterals can lead to a bizarre angiographic picture similar to that seen in moyamoya disease (Figure 12.7). Hemorrhages may occur as a result of rupture of these fragile collateral vessels, leading to intracerebral, subarachnoid, spinal, and retinal hemorrhagic strokes in patients with sickle cell disease. The progressive stenosis of the supraclinoid internal carotid artery that leads to the development of the moyamoya pattern may be detected noninvasively using transcranial Doppler ultrasonography. Strokes may be preventable if cerebral bypass surgery or prophylactic transfusions are used. Among children under the age of 15 years, sickle cell anemia is present in 7% of patients with strokes; it is thus an important cause of stroke in childhood. Spinal cord infarction is also seen much more commonly in patients with sickle cell anemia than in the general population. Massive intracranial hemorrhage has been said to be a rare but real complication of sickle cell anemia. Most of the literature, however, comes from the era before computed tomography (CT), and it is not clear whether the incidence of intracranial hemorrhage is higher in patients with sickle cell anemia than in a matched control population. Large-vessel occlusions have also been reported to occur in patients with sickle cell anemia. The supraclinoid carotid has been the most common site. The mechanism for large-vessel disease in this circumstance is unclear. Some believe that a hyperdynamic circulation leads to endothelial damage. Others hold that chronic stasis leads to diminished blood volume and thrombosis. Still others have postulated that sickled erythrocytes occlude the vasa vasorum of large vessel; this occlusion then causes ischemic damage to the vessel wall and leads to thrombosis.

Sepsis is the most common cause of death in patients with sickle cell anemia. Bacterial infection is the reason for as many as one-half of all hospitalizations in these patients. Of all the infections, meningitis is particularly important, accounting for 20% of the deaths from sepsis. Meningitis has been reported in some older children and adults, but most of the patients are under 3 years of age. *Streptococcus pneumoniae* is an unusually common organism in these patients and accounts for about three-fourths of the cases of meningitis, most of which are in patients under 3 years of age. For other children in this age group with meningitis, *Haemophilus influenzae* type B tends to be the leading cause of infection. In patients under 3 years with sickle cell anemia, meningitis has a peculiarly malignant course, often leading to death within a few hours. Recurrent meningitis seems also to be unusually common in these patients. The unusual susceptibility of patients with sickle cell anemia to infection is not totally understood, but the factors believed to be most important include their functional asplenia and an opsonizing defect that causes leukocyte malfunction.

Fat embolism occurs in sickle cell anemia patients with higher than expected frequency, and the brain is involved in greater than 80% of the patients in whom it is examined. Bone pain, fever, and changes in mental status are the major presenting features. Treatment is controversial, but most advocate systemic anticoagulation and exchange transfusion.

## Heterozygous Hemoglobin States and Complex Hemoglobin Combinations

Only the presence of some amount of HbS leads to the risk of a neurologic problem. Sickle cell trait is occasionally associated with neurologic complications, especially when patients at risk are exposed to an extremely low oxygen tension (e.g., high-altitude flying, anesthesia). The HbSC-, HbSD-, HbSF-, and HbS-thalassemia syndromes are all situations in which there is a risk of neurologic complications similar to those mentioned above for homozygous HbS disease. There are fewer neurologic problems, however, in these combined hemoglobin disorders than in the pure sickle cell disease.

Thalassemia

The genetic defect underlying thalassemia involves rates of synthesis of the individual polypeptide chains. Two major varieties of thalassemia exist: one involving defective alpha chain synthesis, the other involving beta chain synthesis. The more common beta-thalassemia may occur in the heterozygous or homozygous form to produce the syndromes of thalassemia trait or Cooley's anemia (thalassemia major) respectively. Heterozygosity for alpha-thalassemia results in a very mild condition and may require an associated hemoglobin abnormality for clinical expression (thalassemia minor). Homozygous alpha-thalassemia is thought to be incompatible with normal fetal development.

The neurologic dysfunction seen in the thalassemias may be divided into three distinct categories: meningitis following splenectomy (discussed above in the section on sickle cell anemia), spinal cord compression resulting from extramedullary hematopoiesis, and a mixed group of neuromuscular disorders.

The susceptibility to infection seen in thalassemia corresponds to that seen in sickle cell anemia, but is confined to those patients who have undergone splenectomy for control of their hemolysis.

Approximately one-third of patients with myelopathy caused by extramedullary hematopoiesis have thalassemia as their underlying disease. When extramedullary hematopoiesis exists in the presence of a hemolytic anemia, it is believed to be produced as a compensatory mechanism by totipotential cells in various locations. The usual location for extramedullary hematopoiesis is various parts of the reticuloendothelial system, particularly the liver, spleen, and lymph nodes. The spinal epidural space, however, and rarely the intracranial subdural space, may be involved, with consequent compression of the spinal cord or brain. Figure 12.8 is a magnetic resonance image (MRI) taken from a patient with thalassemia major who developed diplopia caused by bilateral abducens palsies. A mass of extramedullary hematopoiesis is seen on the clivus. Nearly all spinal cases have involved the thoracic spinal segments posteriorly, usually over multiple levels, and treatment with surgical decompression or radiotherapy has lead to dramatic and sometimes prolonged remissions of myelopathic symptoms and signs.

In addition to the complications of infection and extramedullary hematopoiesis, a large number of other less well defined syndromes may exist in thalassemia. Logethetis and colleagues (1972) reported on 138 patients with thalassemia major from their own experience. Twenty percent had transient episodes of dizziness, blurred vision, and fainting, which improved on transfusion. Two strokes occurred. One had convulsions followed by an acute transient hemiparesis 4 days following splenectomy, and the other had headaches and visual blurring followed by a right hemiparesis 2 days after a transfusion. Major motor seizures were observed in 7%. Forty-nine percent had absent or diminished deep tendon reflexes. Muscular abnormalities were prominent in 23%, muscle cramps in 4%, and muscle wasting in 32%. Nineteen percent had a myopathic syndrome; eleven of these had a myopathic electrophysiologic study. The pathophysiologic mechanism for this myopathic syndrome is totally unexplained.

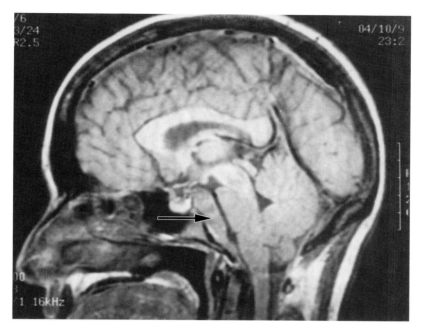

*Figure 12.8* Mass on the clivus (*arrow*) caused by extramedullary hematopoiesis in a patient with thalassemia major. The patient presented with diplopia caused by bilateral abducens palsies.

## MYELOPROLIFERATIVE DISORDERS

The myeloproliferative disorders include polycythemia vera, myelofibrosis with myeloid metaplasia, chronic myelogenous leukemia, and essential thrombocythemia. The proliferation in all of these diseases originates in the bone marrow or in the liver or spleen, where extramedullary blood formation may occur. The growth is self-perpetuating and involves all cell lines, although in each syndrome one line may predominate. This proliferation may be confined to a single cell form or may involve several different strains of cells simultaneously or at separate times. Because overlap syndromes occur so frequently, precise diagnosis in a given patient is often difficult and perhaps fruitless.

The neurologic manifestations of these conditions depend primarily on the tendency to thrombosis, hyperviscosity, or the effects of extramedullary hematopoiesis.

Strokes are the most common neurologic complication seen in polycythemia vera and occur in 15–32% of the patients. As many as 15% of patients with polycythemia vera die of a stroke, five times that of an age-matched control population. Headache, which occurs in nearly half the patients, and dizziness and vertigo, which occur in approximately one-third of the patients, are the most frequent neurologic symptoms.

Several cases of sudden unilateral or bilateral chorea have been described. The pathogenesis of these cases is presumed to be vascular, but the precise location of the lesions has been variable in different case reports. Most often they involve the subthalamic nuclei, cerebral cortex, and corpus striatum bilaterally in various combinations.

Extramedullary hematopoiesis is a common manifestation of the myeloproliferative disorders (see Figure 12.8). Complications resulting from extramedullary hematopoiesis are rare. A few cases of intracranial dura matter involvement by extramedullary hematopoiesis have been recorded, but all were asymptomatic and only found incidentally at autopsy or by imaging techniques. Approximately one-half of the cases of extramedullary hematopoiesis are associated with a myeloproliferative disorder; in the rest it is secondary to various hemolytic anemias, the most frequent of which is thalassemia (see the section of this chapter on hemoglobinopathies and thalassemia).

Polycythemia may rarely be caused by an erythropoietin-secreting cerebellar hemangioblastoma.

## HEMORRHAGIC DIATHESIS

### Hemophilia

Hemophilia may be defined as an inherited hemorrhagic diathesis characterized by impairment of the first stage of coagulation, the production of thromboplastin from the interaction of platelets and three or more plasma factors. Among the factors necessary for thromboplastin formation are antihemophiliac globin (AHG, or factor VIII), plasma thromboplastin component (PTC or factor IX or Christmas factor), and plasma thromboplastin antecedent (PTA or factor XI). Factor VIII deficiency is responsible for about 80% of cases of hemophilia, factor IX deficiency for about 15%, and factor XI deficiency for about 5%. Factor VIII and factor IX deficiencies are X-linked recessive disorders and therefore are seen almost exclusively in men. Factor XI deficiency is inherited as an autosomal dominant trait and is thus seen equally in men and women; it is found primarily in those of Ashkenazi Jewish descent. It is possible to determine specifically the deficient factor in the patient's plasma and, except in hemophiliac patients who have circulating antibodies to specific factors, produce normal hemostasis by factor replacement. One may classify the hemorrhagic diathesis as mild (7–15% of normal factor levels), moderate (1–6% of normal levels), and severe (<1% of normal levels). Neurologic complications of hemophilia may be divided into those affecting the peripheral nervous system and those affecting the central nervous system.

Peripheral Nervous System Complications of Hemophilia

The major problem with respect to the peripheral nervous system results from intramuscular hemorrhages, which may expand muscle tissue or extend into fascial planes and compress peripheral nerves. Such compression most commonly

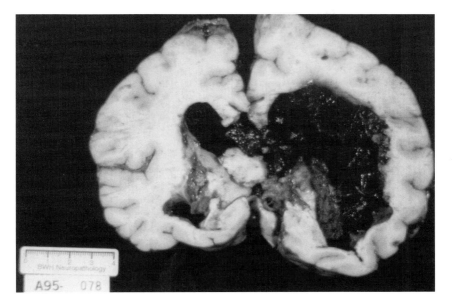

*Figure 12.9*   Intracerebral and intraventricular hemorrhage in a hemophiliac patient with acquired immunodeficiency syndrome.

occurs with the femoral or ulnar nerves, but cases involving the sciatic, peroneal, median, and even facial nerves have been reported. Actual intraneural hemorrhages have been postulated but never proved. Most patients with peripheral nerve compressions may be managed with factor replacement alone, but some may require fasciotomy as well.

## Central Nervous System Complications of Hemophilia

Intracranial hemorrhage is becoming increasingly common in patients with hemophilia, possibly because of the more active lives permitted by vigorous replacement therapy for intra-articular hemorrhages. Intracranial hemorrhage is an important cause of death in hemophiliac patients, possibly the largest hemophilia-related mortality factor other than acquired immunodeficiency syndrome (AIDS) (Figure 12.9). Bleeding may be intracerebral, subarachnoid, subdural, and epidural. Before 1960, the mortality rate from intracranial bleeding was 70%. It is now about 30%. In mild cases (7–15% of normal factor levels), intracranial bleeding occurs only after significant trauma. In patients with moderate cases (1–6% of normal levels), only minor trauma is required, and, in severe cases (<1% of normal levels), no trauma at all. The best method for accurate diagnosis of intracranial hemorrhage in this setting is the CT scan or MRI.

Subarachnoid hemorrhage may be treated successfully with factor replacement alone, although a ventricular catheter may be required to treat hydrocephalus. Subdural and epidural hemorrhages usually do not respond to factor replacement alone and ordinarily require surgical therapy. Surgical evacuation of the hematoma may be safely accomplished after factor replacement. Intracerebral hemorrhages are the most difficult to treat. Some patients have been successfully managed with medical therapy alone or with medical therapy plus a ventricular cannula for measurement and control of intracranial pressure. If the hematoma is accessible, however, surgical resection may lead to higher rates of recovery. General guidelines for the management of head trauma in hemophiliac patients are as follows. In patients with mild head trauma and a normal neurologic examination, one would suggest factor infusion to a measured postinfusion level of 70% of normal. In patients with more severe head trauma or abnormal neurologic examination, an emergency CT scan should be obtained. If it is normal, then 48 hours of 30–70% factor levels should be maintained by factor infusion. If the CT scan shows a hemorrhage, then factor infusions should continue for 7–10 days after the bleeding has stopped or 14 days after the neurosurgical procedure, whichever is longer.

## Thrombocytopenia and Other Purpuras

Thrombocytopenia is usually an acquired reduction in the number of platelets caused by either diminished production or increased peripheral destruction. Thrombocytopenia resulting from diminished production is seen from drug effects on the bone marrow, myelophthisic phenomena, and ineffective thrombopoiesis. Thrombocytopenia caused by increased peripheral destruction of platelets may be a result of mechanical factors such as a prosthetic device or vasculitis, disseminated intravascular coagulation, or thrombotic thrombocytopenic purpura. Thrombocytopenia not of mechanical origin but caused by peripheral destruction of platelets has been called immune thrombocytopenic purpura. Immune thrombocytopenic purpura may be subdivided into the secondary forms caused by drugs, virus, lymphoproliferative disorders, and collagen vascular diseases, and primary or idiopathic thrombocytopenic purpura. Splenomegaly, while it does not shorten platelet life span, increases the size of the sequestered platelet pool and causes thrombocytopenia.

The neurologic complications of thrombocytopenia revolve around intracranial bleeding, the severity and frequency of which are dependent on the severity of the thrombocytopenia rather than the underlying diseases. There are a few exceptions to this rule in which the underlying disease affects the neurologic picture apart from the thrombocytopenia itself. Those are lupus erythematosus, thrombotic thrombocytopenic purpura (see next section in this chapter), and leukemia, in which the leukemic infiltrates in the brain add to the tendency for intracranial hemorrhage.

The incidence of intracranial bleeding in thrombocytopenia is substantial; figures range from as high as 26% in older work to around 1.5% in more recent surveys. This wide variation is partly a result of improvement in treatment, but also reflects the definition of cases said to have intracranial hemorrhage. The more recent surveys generally refer only to true intracerebral hemorrhage and exclude cases in which hemorrhagic spinal fluid is found in the absence of signs of an intraparenchymal hemorrhage. The CT scan has made this an easy differential point; only large intracerebral hemorrhages would be seen by this technique, whereas episodes of "brain purpura" with hemorrhagic spinal fluid would not likely yield a positive CT scan. It has been frequently stated that intracerebral hemorrhage is the most common cause of death directly attributable to thrombocytopenia.

Intracranial bleeding in thrombocytopenia can be in the form of multiple small punctate or petechial hemorrhages caused by capillary bleeding. This brain purpura consists of small, ring-shaped hemorrhages in both the gray and white matter of the brain. It has been suggested that the basic pathophysiology of hemorrhage in thrombocytopenia is capillary bleeding, which may become confluent with continued bleeding in severe cases, leading to frank intracerebral hemorrhages. This intracerebral source of bleeding probably explains the sparsity of subdural, subarachnoid, and epidural hematomas seen in the thrombocytopenias compared with the frequency of intracerebral hemorrhages. Peripheral nerve involvement with hemorrhage and spinal cord hemorrhage are both rare in the thrombocytopenias. The symptom complex associated with brain purpura is not known. It is probable that most of these petechiae are asymptomatic.

Treatment depends on the etiology of the thrombocytopenia. Platelet transfusions are useful in situations in which decreased production is the difficulty. When increased platelet destruction or splenic sequestration is an important factor, therapy may require splenectomy, administration of corticosteroids, intravenous immunoglobulin (IVIg) administration, and platelet transfusions. In the presence of central nervous system bleeding, corticosteroid and IVIg administration and platelet transfusions may be performed. Emergency splenectomy has been advocated when intracerebral hemorrhage is suspected in a patient with immune thrombocytopenia, even before a full evaluation of the intracerebral hemorrhage is carried out. This is accompanied by corticosteroid and platelet administration, followed by neurosurgical evacuation of the hemorrhage if technically possible. The efficacy of IVIg, which can transiently raise the platelet count in patients with idiopathic thrombocytopenic purpura, may alter this practice.

## Thrombotic Thrombocytopenic Purpura

Thrombotic thrombocytopenic purpura (Moschcowitz's disease) is usually considered a triad of thrombocytopenic purpura, hemolytic anemia, and neurologic manifestations. Fever and evidence of renal disease are also almost invariably present. The diagnosis requires histologic demonstration of the characteristic pathologic lesion, which consists of widespread hyaline occlusion of terminal arterioles and capillaries (Figure 12.10). This can be accomplished using many tissues, the most accessible of which are lymph node, bone marrow, skin, and spleen. The blood smear often shows a microangiopathic hemolytic anemia (Figure 12.11). The most important pathologic changes in the nervous system are a striking increase in the cellularity of the walls of arterioles and capillaries, and platelet thrombi associated with multiple small foci of parenchymal necrosis and petechial hemorrhages. These changes are identical to those seen in other organs and thus are considered part of a systemic disease. Gray matter is affected to a greater extent than white matter (Figure 12.12). The neurologic manifestations of the disease reflect the widespread gray-matter involvement. The most common are headache; mental change, including altered states of consciousness, agitation, confusion, and

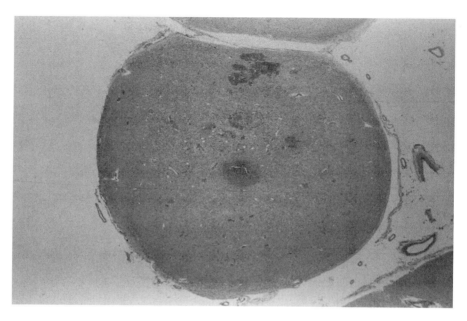

*Figure 12.10*   Typical lesion of thrombotic thrombocytopenic purpura characterized by hyaline occlusion of small vessels in multiple organs, including the brain.

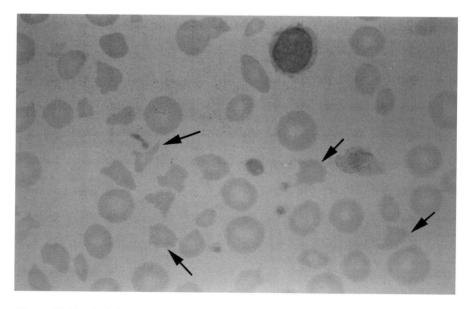

*Figure 12.11*   Peripheral blood smear from a patient with thrombotic thrombocytopenic purpura. It shows a microangiopathic pattern with many damaged erythrocytes (schistocytes), some of which are marked with arrows.

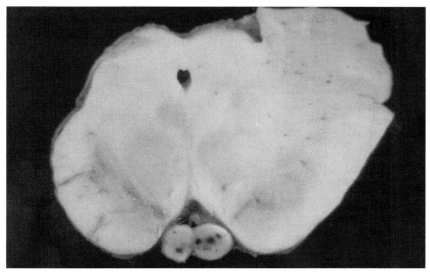

A

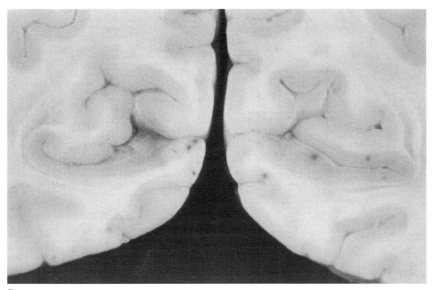

B

*Figure 12.12* **(A)** Typical lesions of thrombotic thrombocytopenic purpura seen in the mamillary bodies. **(B)** Typical lesions of thrombotic thrombocytopenic purpura seen in the primary visual cortex.

delirium; hemiparesis; aphasia; syncope; visual changes; dysarthria; seizures; coma; cranial nerve palsies; paresthesias; and vertigo.

The pathogenesis of thrombotic thrombocytopenic purpura remains obscure. Many possible causes, including exposure to toxins, drug sensitivity, bacterial infections, autoimmune reactions, collagen disease, abnormality of serum lipids, intravascular thrombosis, and hemolysis as related to intravascular thrombosis, have been postulated. At present, most arguments favor an immunologically mediated phenomenon. The disorder has occurred in association with an immune response (triggered by vaccination or infection) and in the course of certain autoimmune diseases such as systemic lupus erythematosus. Subnormal levels of serum complement and immunoglobulins in the vascular lesions, elevated levels of platelet-bound immunoglobulins, and the presence in serum of complement-dependent activity cytotoxic for endothelial cells have been reported. Hemolytic uremic syndrome, a childhood disorder similar in many respects to thrombotic thrombocytopenic purpura, may be triggered by immune complexes. The same can be said for the HELLP (hemolytic anemia, elevated liver function tests, low platelets) syndrome seen in peripartum patients. Exchange transfusion has been reported to dramatically reverse the syndrome. It has also been noted that remission can be induced with fresh frozen plasma but not albumin. If there were an unusual class of immune complex active against vascular tissue, and perhaps platelets, that provoked thrombotic thrombocytopenic purpura, then the effectiveness of exchange transfusions would be explained. Furthermore, normal plasma might promote clearing of these presumptive immune complexes if, fortuitously, it contained an antibody with high affinity for their antigenic component. These postulated immune complexes have not yet been identified, however. Other treatments for thrombotic thrombocytopenic purpura have included heparin, antiplatelet agents, corticosteroids, dextran, and splenectomy, all aimed at various parts of the syndrome. The prognosis is poor, and mortality in most cases is about 70%, though better results have been reported in groups receiving exchange transfusions with whole blood or plasmapheresis.

## Hereditary Hemorrhagic Telangiectasia

Hereditary hemorrhagic telangiectasia (Osler-Weber-Rendu disease) is a disease with an autosomal dominant mode of inheritance that involves several systems. The neurologic manifestations may be produced by vascular malformations of the central nervous system or by complications of pulmonary arteriovenous malformations.

Pulmonary arteriovenous malformations are the most common large visceral vascular anomalies in hereditary hemorrhagic telangiectasia. Several mechanisms may cause the development of neurogenic symptoms: erythrocytosis may induce cerebral thrombosis; cerebral air embolism may follow hemoptysis; thrombosis may develop in the pulmonary malformation, with subsequent cerebral embolism; and the right-to-left extracardiac shunt that allows bacteria and septic microemboli to bypass the pulmonary filter predisposes to the development of brain abscess. Multiple and solitary abscesses have been described as occurring anywhere in the brain.

In addition, the brain, spinal cord, or meninges may be the site of telangiectasias or larger vascular malformation. Seizures, headaches, progressive neurologic deficits, and spontaneous subarachnoid or intracerebral hemorrhage are the typical clinical presentations.

## Henoch-Schönlein Purpura

Henoch-Schönlein (allergic or anaphylactoid) purpura is characterized by serosanguinous effusions into the subcutaneous submucous and subserous tissues. The pathogenesis of the disorder is obscure, but much indirect evidence suggests an allergic etiology. The disorder is most common in children and young adults. The skin lesions are variable in appearance, but the purpura is usually associated with one of the manifestations of allergy such as erythema or urticaria. Effusions into joints or viscera may produce various localized symptoms such as joint pain or abdominal pain. Involvement of the nervous system is rare, but cerebral hemorrhages and peripheral nerve involvement have been reported. Treatment is largely symptomatic. Corticosteroids have been used but with questionable success.

## Disseminated Intravascular Coagulation

Disseminated intravascular coagulation (DIC) is a relatively common acquired hemorrhagic thrombotic syndrome that occurs as a result of the presence of thrombin in the systemic circulation. The syndrome follows other disease states such as viral infections, bacterial infections, obstetric and surgical complications, neoplasms, fat embolism, diabetic ketoacidosis, and head injury. DIC causes thrombosis and bleeding at multiple sites, including the nervous system. The essential neuropathologic changes are multiple infarctions, petechial hemorrhages, and occasionally small subdural and subarachnoid hemorrhages. Fibrin thrombi are found in the cerebral vessels. The clinical syndrome depends on the particular pathology but may include seizures, mental changes, and focal findings. Most patients with DIC show xanthochromic cerebrospinal fluid and angiographic abnormalities consistent with multiple small-vessel occlusions. Subacute or chronic DIC, particularly in patients with thrombotic complications, has been treated effectively with heparin. However, no specific treatment apart from removal of the underlying cause (e.g., evacuation of the uterus in cases of abruptio placentae) is useful in acute DIC.

## Anticoagulant Therapy

Hypoprothrombinemia is a common cause of clinical bleeding. The rare causes include congenital (vitamin K–resistant) and idiopathic (vitamin K–responsive) hypoprothrombinemia, a hemorrhagic disease of the newborn as yet unable to provide its own vitamin K; diseases that interfere with vitamin K absorption (e.g., sprue, steatorrhea, surgical resection); disorders that interfere with bile access to the vitamin K in the gut (biliary obstruction); liver diseases that interfere with prothrombin production; and salicylate therapy. By far the most important and frequent cause of hypoprothrombinemia, however, is anticoagulant drugs. The neurologic complications of anticoagulant drug usage are related to the presence of hypoprothrombinemia. Any other cause of hypoprothrombinemia as listed above can result in the same spectrum of disorders. In addition, the following discussion includes the neurologic complications of heparin therapy, a drug that inactivates thrombin, inhibits the conversion of prothrombin to thrombin, and prevents the agglutination of platelets. Its complication spectrum is similar to that of the agents that lower the prothrombin content of the blood by acting as a metabolic antagonist to vitamin K (e.g., coumarin and related agents).

In patients on anticoagulants, nervous system hemorrhage may occur in numerous locations, including intracerebral, subarachnoid, subdural, cranial epidural, spinal epidural, and spinal intramedullary. In addition, roots, plexus, and peripheral nerves may also be compressed by bleeding of this type. Before the advent of CT scanning, lumbar punctures were used to diagnose nervous system bleeding of this type. Lumbar puncture itself, however, may be dangerous in the presence of a hemorrhagic diathesis and has led to epidural and cauda equinal compression syndromes. When CT scanning is not available, every effort should be made to correct the coagulation defect before the lumbar puncture is performed, although this process should not be permitted to delay a lumbar puncture too long if an infection is suspected.

## PLASMA CELL DYSCRASIAS

Paraproteinemias may be seen in many conditions, including connective tissue diseases, multiple types of malignancies, and even in the absence of any known underlying disease. The most important group of disorders associated with the production of abnormal proteins is the plasma cell dyscrasias.

The plasma cell dyscrasias are a group of disorders characterized by the uncontrolled proliferation of cells normally involved in antibody synthesis. This is usually accompanied by the synthesis of a homogeneous immunoglobulin or one of its constituent polypeptide chains. These disorders are often classified according to the type of protein that is produced. Thus, they fall into three major categories: (1) multiple myeloma—IgG, IgA, IgD, and IgE; (2) macroglobulinemia—IgM; and (3) heavy-chain diseases—gamma, alpha, and mu.

### Multiple Myeloma

Multiple myeloma is the most common plasma cell dyscrasia and is characterized by infiltration of the bone marrow with neoplastic plasma cells. Characteristic "punched-out" bony lesions, often involving the skull and associated with hypercalcemia, may be found, but the disease may certainly be present without any bony lesions. The disease may be present in a subclinical form for many years before the development of symptomatology. The most characteristic components are (1) frequent and recurrent bacterial infections due to impaired normal antibody synthesis; (2) chronic renal dysfunction caused by several factors, including tubular damage secondary to the reabsorption of large amounts of Bence Jones proteins (light chains) filtered by the glomeruli, secondary amyloid renal

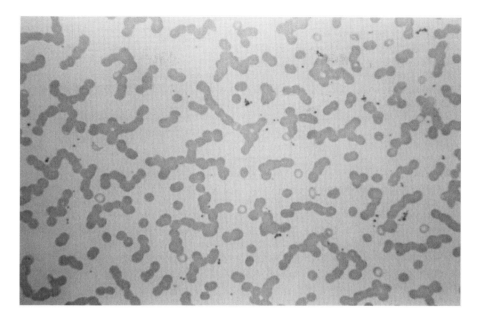

*Figure 12.13* Peripheral blood smear from a patient with multiple myeloma. The abnormal paraprotein has coated the usually charged red cell surfaces, so that there is clumping of the erythrocytes like stacks of coins (rouleaux).

disease, hypercalcemic renal damage, recurrent pyelonephritis, and hyperuricemia; and (3) damage to other organs, such as the spinal cord and nerve roots by pathologically fractured vertebrae or local development of plasmacytomas. In approximately 5–10% of patients with multiple myeloma, symptoms are induced by the presence of the abnormal proteins, the characteristics of which are described below. The peripheral blood smear may show abnormal clumping of erythrocytes in a stack of coinlike rows (rouleaux), a result of the fact that the normally charged surfaces that cause red cells to repel each other are coated with the paraprotein (Figure 12.13).

## Macroglobulinemia

Macroglobulinemia is defined by the presence of an excessive amount of IgM gamma globulin in the serum. It includes a spectrum of disorders ranging from an apparently benign monoclonal gammopathy to progressive malignant lymphoma. Clinically the disease is generally seen in the elderly and resembles a malignant lymphoma. Weakness, weight loss, adenopathy, and hepatosplenomegaly form the characteristic clinical picture. Bone lesions are rare. Like myeloma, anemia is occasionally seen as a complication. Neurologic complications are primarily related to the viscosity of the large abnormal protein or the development of malignant lymphoma.

## Heavy-Chain Diseases

Heavy-chain diseases are defined by the finding of characteristic immunoglobulin heavy-chain fragments in the serum or urine. Three of the five possible types of heavy-chain disease have been recognized. Gamma heavy-chain disease resembles a lymphoma more than a myeloma. Alpha heavy-chain disease is the most common heavy-chain disease and is the almost invariable accompaniment of a malignant lymphoma of the intestine with malabsorption. Mu heavy-chain disease is the rarest of these disorders and has been seen in association with chronic lymphocytic leukemia.

Neurologic manifestations of the paraproteinemias may be divided into the following categories: hyperviscosity syndrome, cryoglobulinemia, cold agglutinin disease, amyloidosis, hemorrhagic diathesis, polyneuropathy, mononeuropathy, paraneoplastic syndromes (e.g., progressive multifocal leukoencephalopathy, cerebellar degeneration), encephalopathy (Bing-Neel syndrome), and infections (fungal, bacterial).

*Hyperviscosity syndrome* refers to the symptom and sign complex of abnormal levels of consciousness (inattention, drowsiness, stupor, coma, delirium), fundoscopic changes characterized by venous engorgement ("sausage veins"), retinal hemorrhages and exudates, blurred vision, and headache. The term *coma paraproteinemia* refers to the encephalopathy of the hyperviscosity syndrome. The syndrome requires that the relative viscosity of the blood as measured by a viscosimeter be greater than 3.0 (normal is less than 2.0). This increase in viscosity may be caused by an increased red blood cell mass (as in polycythemia), but more often it is caused by the presence of large amounts of an abnormal protein, usually a macroglobulin. When abnormal proteins are the cause, treatment consists of plasmapheresis, which usually provides dramatic relief of the symptoms and signs. When indicated, treatment must then be directed toward the underlying disease (e.g., plasma cell dyscrasia, polycythemia).

*Cryoglobulinemia* refers to the presence in the serum of proteins that precipitate in the cold and redissolve on warming. These proteins are most often associated with myeloma and macroglobulinemia but may be seen as part of a connective tissue disease or as an isolated finding in the absence of any known underlying cause. Approximately one-third of the cryoglobulins are myeloma IgG proteins (type I), one-third are IgM macroglobulins (type II), and one-third are a mixture of IgM and IgG molecules (type III). Many cryoglobulins may actually be antibodies against gamma globulins. The mechanism of the cryoprecipitation is not known, and there is not a direct relationship between the amount of cryoglobulin or the temperature at which precipitation occurs and the symptom complex. The neurologic syndrome associated with cryoglobulinemia is most common in the type III form, which is the type most often related to an underlying connective tissue disease. These patients often show purpura and a progressive renal lesion that is suggestive of an antigen-antibody (immune) complex nephritis. The most frequent neurologic syndrome is a sensorimotor polyneuropathy, the precise pathology of which is not understood. It may represent a form of mononeuropathy multiplex caused by disease of the vasa nervorum or an axonal polyneuropathy. There is no clear explanation for the latter possibility. Central nervous system syndromes are poorly described but may represent episodes of brain purpura associated with the bleeding diathesis.

Cold agglutinins are an unusual group of macroglobulins that induce red cell agglutination and hemolysis on exposure to cold. Although the phenomenon may be seen transiently in certain infections such as mononucleosis, it rarely causes clinically relevant hemolysis in conditions other than lymphomas and macroglobulinemia. These proteins contain only kappa light chains and are generally directed against the I antigen of erythrocytes. These proteins may also interact with clotting factors or coat platelets, thus interfering with the blood coagulation mechanism. This interference may lead to central nervous system bleeding and the retinal hemorrhages so commonly seen in the para-proteinemia states.

Polyneuropathies have been described in cases of paraproteinemias, particularly in myeloma and macroglobulinemia. Most often there is a sensory polyneuropathy manifested by cramps, paresthesias, and acral sensory loss. Cranial nerve palsies and an acute demyelinating polyneuropathy (Guillain-Barré–like illness) have been encountered; however, the number of such cases is so few that it is difficult to ascribe the polyneuropathy to any particular characteristic of the para-proteinemia state. Some cases may represent paraneoplastic syndromes, while others may be the result of more common concomitant causes of peripheral nerve dysfunction, such as vitamin deficiency.

Paraneoplastic syndromes of many types—including polymyositis, cerebellar degeneration, polyneuropathy, and progressive multifocal leukoencephalopathy—have been recorded in patients with various paraproteinemias. The cause of progressive multifocal leukoencephalopathy is known to be a viral infection. The etiologies of the other syndromes in this group remain cryptic, though an immune-mediated mechanism is most likely.

*Bing-Neel syndrome* is loosely defined as the central nervous system syndrome seen in macroglobulinemia and was actually described prior to Waldenström's naming of the disease in 1944. Central nervous system involvement occurs in about 5–15% of the patients with macroglobulinemia; however, it is clear that many of the manifestations of the syndrome are a result of the effects of hyperviscosity. This aspect of the Bing-Neel syndrome is reviewed above in the discussion on hyperviscosity syndrome. In addition, however, some patients show a multifocal disease with a rapid downhill course that is uniformly fatal and unresponsive to plasmapheresis. The spinal fluid in these patients is abnormal, with some pleocytosis and elevated protein. The pathology consists of infiltration of lymphocytes and plasma cells, particularly around veins. Sometimes the pathologic appearance is that of a histiocytic lymphoma (formerly called reticulum cell sarcoma or microglioma) of the brain.

Infections are common in patients with paraproteinemias, probably because of the paucity of normal immunoglobulins associated with the overproduction of the abnormal proteins. Because the defect is mainly in the sphere of humoral immunity, the patients are most susceptible to bacterial and fungal infections, which may affect the nervous system. The most important of these include fungal and tubercular meningitis and bacterial meningitis.

POEMS syndrome (for polyneuropathy, organomegaly, endocrinopathy, monoclonal gammopathy, skin changes) is a multisystem syndrome seen in patients with osteosclerotic myeloma. The mechanism is unknown, but it is likely that it is an immune-mediated paraneoplastic syndrome. The polyneuropathy is a subacute or chronic painful polyneuropathy. There is usually hepatosplenomegaly, sexual impotence, and various skin lesions. The M component in the serum is produced by an osteosclerotic myeloma; when it is treated, there is improvement in all components of the syndrome.

## HYPERCOAGULABLE STATES

Patients are considered to have hypercoagulable states if they have laboratory-revealed abnormalities or clinical conditions that are associated with an increased risk of thrombosis (prethrombotic states) or if they have recurrent thrombosis without recognizable predisposing factors (thrombosis proneness). The hypercoagulable states are subdivided into two categories: those in which a clearly identified, specific abnormality in hemostasis can be found (primary hypercoagulable states), and those accompanying various diverse clinical conditions that have been associated with an increased risk of thrombosis (secondary hypercoagulable states). In both circumstances, it is becoming increasingly clear that cerebral thrombosis (venous and arterial) and embolism are important manifestations.

### Primary Hypercoagulable States

The primary hypercoagulable states are a result of failure of one of the three physiologic anticoagulant mechanisms (e.g., antithrombin III, protein C, and the fibrinolytic system) and include antithrombin III deficiency, protein C deficiency, protein S deficiency, fibrinolytic disorders, dysfibrinogenemia, factor XII deficiency, prekallikrein deficiency, and the antiphospholipid antibody syndrome.

Antithrombin III Deficiency

Antithrombin III deficiency may be either inherited as an autosomal dominant trait or acquired as a result of urinary excretion of the protein in patients with the nephrotic syndrome or in patients with severe disease of the liver, where much of the protein is produced. Venous thrombosis is more common than arterial thrombosis. Treatment consists of intravenous administration of heparin.

Protein C Deficiency

Protein C deficiency is inherited as an autosomal dominant trait, and occasionally is acquired by patients with severe liver disease or disseminated intravascular coagulation. Protein S acts as a cofactor for the anticoagulant effects of protein C and can be deficient as a result of inheritance of the trait or in severe liver disease or DIC. The treatment of people with protein C or protein S deficiency who suffer recurrent thrombosis is long-term warfarin therapy.

## Fibrinolytic Abnormalities

Various fibrinolytic abnormalities can lead to defective digestion of fibrin. Some patients with hypercoagulable states have been found to have defective release of plasminogen activator from endothelial cells in the vessel walls. There may also be circulating inhibitors of plasminogen activators. Neurologists and neurosurgeons have ceased using epsilon aminocaproic acid (Amicar) to prevent rebleeding in subarachnoid hemorrhage patients because of the hypercoagulable state that is produced by this drug's inhibition of circulating plasminogen activator. Genetically produced tissue plasminogen activator may have a role in treating such patients, but the risk of hemorrhage may outweigh the potential benefits.

## Dysfibrinogenemia

In a few patients with hypercoagulable states there is formation of a functionally abnormal fibrinogen molecule, which creates gels that are extremely rigid and resistant to removal by the fibrinolytic system. These dysfibrinogenemias are probably very rare causes of the hypercoagulable state.

## Factor XII and Prekallikrein Deficiency

Patients with autosomal recessively inherited deficiencies of factor XII (Hageman factor) or other factors involved in contact activation of the coagulation cascade (e.g., prekallikrein and high-molecular-weight kininogen) have prolonged partial thromboplastin times but paradoxically have an increased tendency to thrombosis, probably because these factors promote blood fluidity by helping to activate the fibrinolytic system and generate vasodilator kinins.

## Antiphospholipid Antibody Syndrome

Two major antiphospholipid syndromes are known: the lupus anticoagulant and the anticardiolipin antibody syndromes. The so-called lupus anticoagulant is actually an antibody to phospholipids that interferes with the formation of the prothrombin activator (a complex of calcium ions, factor Xa, factor V), and a source of phospholipid (usually the platelet membrane in the coagulation cascade). This IgG or IgM antiphospholipid antibody often, but not always, causes prolongation of phospholipid-dependent coagulation tests, such as the activated partial thromboplastin time (PTT). This antibody is present in approximately 25% of patients with systemic lupus erythematosus (Figure 12.14); it may cross-react with cardiolipin, the antigen commonly used in a blood-screening test for syphilis, thus producing a biologic false positive. Despite the prolonged PTT, this antiphospholipid antibody is actually a procoagulant caused by several mechanisms, including increased platelet adhesiveness, interference with the production of the vasodilator and antiplatelet aggregator prostacyclin by the endothelial cell, and decreased production of plasminogen activator. The lupus anticoagulant

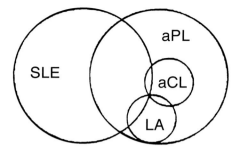

*Figure 12.14*   Venn diagram showing the approximate relationship among lupus patients (SLE), antiphospholipid antibodies (aPL), anticardiolipin antibodies (aCL), and the lupus anticoagulant (LA).

can only be diagnosed using a three-step functional test: (1) screening test such as a PTT, (2) mixing test to determine that the factor which prolongs the PTT is in the serum, and (3) phospholipid loading test such as platelet addition or octagonal phase to determine that the plasma factor which prolongs the PTT is an antiphospholipid antibody. It cannot be quantified using an enzyme-linked immunosorbent assay. In addition to patients with systemic lupus erythematosus, other people at risk for the anticardiolipin antibody syndrome include patients on neuroleptic drugs, patients with neoplasms, and patients with other autoimmune disorders. Some people with the syndrome have no apparent underlying disorders. Those without underlying disease are said to have the primary anticardiolipin antibody syndrome.

The primary anticardiolipin antibody syndrome is characterized by recurrent episodes of venous or arterial thrombosis, thrombocytopenia, and in pregnant women, recurrent mid-pregnancy spontaneous abortions. Migraine, mitral valve prolapse, and livedo reticularis are also over-represented in these patients. Echocardiography frequently reveals the presence of vegetations on the mitral valve, which presumably represent foci of Libman-Sacks endocarditis. The nervous system is commonly affected, with large- and small-vessel arterial occlusions, venous occlusions, and emboli that probably arise from nonbacterial thrombotic endocarditis, which in turn results from the hypercoagulable state. Many of the neurologic syndromes seen in systemic lupus erythematosus patients can be conceptualized as being a result of either thrombosis in situ or emboli from nonbacterial thrombotic endocarditis (known as *Libman-Sacks endocarditis* in systemic lupus erythematosus patients). Treatment of patients who have the antiphospholipid antibody and who suffer recurrent thrombosis is long-term warfarin therapy. The precise dosage of warfarin is unknown, but it is likely that fairly intense anticoagulation is required (i.e., international normalized ratio of 3.0–3.5).

## Secondary Hypercoagulable States

The secondary hypercoagulable states may be divided into three major groups based on the presumed predominant pathophysiologic mechanism: (1) abnormalities of coagulation and fibrinolysis, such as occur with malignancy, pregnancy, use of oral contraceptives, infusion of prothrombin complex concentrates, and nephrotic syndrome; (2) abnormalities of platelets, such as occurs with

myeloproliferative disorders, paroxysmal nocturnal hemoglobinuria, hyperlipidemia, diabetes mellitus, and heparin-induced thrombocytopenia; and (3) abnormalities of blood vessels or rheology, such as in conditions promoting venous
stasis (e.g., immobilization, obesity, advanced age, postoperative state), artificial
surfaces, vasculitis and chronic occlusive arterial disease, homocystinuria, hyperviscosity (e.g., polycythemia, leukemia, sickle cell disease, leukoagglutination,
increased serum viscosity), and thrombotic thrombocytopenia purpura.

## Hypercoagulable States Related to Underlying Malignancy

The relationship between increased tendency for thrombosis and malignancy has
been known ever since Armand Trousseau described the syndrome that bears his
name. Migratory thrombophlebitis, pulmonary emboli, and transient or permanent
focal neurologic deficits are known as a paraneoplastic syndrome, and usually
occur in patients with mucin-secreting adenocarcinomas. Some of the neurologic
deficits are a result of thrombosis in situ of cerebral vessels. Others are a result of
emboli that arise from nonbacterial thrombotic endocarditis, which itself is caused
by the paraneoplastic hypercoagulable state. Most data support the concept that
this hypercoagulable state is caused by a general activation of the clotting system,
which results in chronic DIC. This DIC may be initiated by the tumor's production of a procoagulant, such as a cysteine protease that has been found in malignant cells and is known to activate factor X.

## Hypercoagulable States Related to Pregnancy

Pregnancy increases the risk of thrombosis, probably as a consequence of the
chronic low-grade DIC that develops normally in pregnancy, presumably in
preparation for the hemostatic challenge of placental separation. Cerebral venous
thrombosis is the major neurologic complication of this hypercoagulable state;
it is seen primarily in the postpartum period. It takes two major clinical forms:
venous sinus occlusion and cortical vein occlusion. Though these two clinical
forms often fuse as the illness progresses, venous sinus thrombosis usually presents with increased intracranial pressure, whereas cortical vein thrombosis usually begins with partial seizures that are often very resistant to anticonvulsant
therapy. As in any venous occlusions, the resulting infarctions, if any, are hemorrhagic, and, as such, are usually easily visible by imaging techniques. MRI has
proved particularly useful in demonstrating the characteristic triangular thrombosis (inverted delta sign) in the superior sagittal sinus even when hemorrhagic
infarction is not present. Treatment for the hypercoagulable state of pregnancy is
reserved for patients with demonstrated thrombosis and consists of administering heparin, because warfarin crosses the placenta and is possibly teratogenic.

## Hypercoagulable States Related to Oral Contraceptive Use

Use of oral contraceptives significantly increases the risk of thrombosis in a way
similar to that which occurs in late pregnancy; however, unlike in pregnancy, the
fibrinolytic response is not inappropriately blunted. Epidemiologic studies have

suggested that the use of oral contraceptives raises the risk of stroke in young women, particularly in those with a history of migraine.

## Hypercoagulable States Related to Prothrombin Complex Infusion

Prothrombin complex concentrates contain the vitamin K–dependent clotting factors II, VII, IX, and X and are used to treat patients with deficiencies of these factors. Transfusion with these concentrates is associated with an increased risk of thrombosis and DIC, including stroke, particularly in patients with underlying liver disease. The thrombogenicity of these concentrates may be a result of the presence of small quantities of activated clotting factors that cannot be adequately cleared by the patient's diseased liver.

## Hypercoagulable States Related to Nephrotic Syndrome

In patients with nephrotic syndrome, there is an increased risk of stroke; it is probably related in large part to an acquired antithrombin III deficiency caused by urinary loss of the protein.

## Hypercoagulable States Related to Platelet Abnormalities

Abnormalities in platelet function probably partially underlie the thrombotic tendency seen in patients with myeloproliferative disorders, thrombocytosis, paroxysmal nocturnal hemoglobinuria, hyperlipidemia, and heparin-induced thrombocytopenia.

## Hypercoagulable States Related to Abnormalities of Blood Vessels or Rheology

Many abnormalities in blood vessels and rheology may promote coagulation and thus produce cerebral thrombosis. Of particular importance from a neurologic perspective are artificial surfaces, such as are found when patients are placed on extracorporeal circulation; vasculitic conditions, such as giant cell arteritis of the brain and Behçet's disease; homocystinemia; and hyperviscosity of any cause.

## SUGGESTED READING

Adams RD, Kubik CS. Subacute degeneration of the brain in pernicious anemia. N Engl J Med 1944;231:1–9.
Beck WS. Neuropsychiatric consequences of cobalamin deficiency. Adv Intern Med 1991;36:33–56.
Bing J, Neel AV. Two cases of hyperglobulinemia with affection of the central nervous system on a toxic-infectious basis. Acta Med Scand 1936;88:492–506.

Charache S, Adams RJ. Neurologic Complications Associated with Disorders of Red Blood Cells. In CG Goetz, CM Tanner, MJ Aminoff (eds), Systemic Diseases (pt 1). Handbook of Clinical Neurology, Vol. 63. Amsterdam: Elsevier, 1993;249–269.

Grotta JC, Manner C, Pettigrew LC, Yatsu FM. Red blood cell disorders and stroke. Stroke 1986;17: 811–817.

Healton EB, Savage DG, Brust JCM, et al. Neurologic aspects of cobalamin deficiency. Medicine 1991;70:229–245.

Kinsella LJ, Green R. "Anesthesia paresthetica": nitrous oxide-induced cobalamin deficiency. Neurology 1995;45:1608–1610.

Logethetis J, Constantoulakis M, Economidau J, et al. Thalassemia major: a survey of 138 cases with emphasis on neurologic and muscular aspects. Neurology 1972;22:294–304.

Moschcowitz E. An acute febrile pleiochromic anemia with hyaline thrombosis of the terminal arterioles and capillaries: an undescribed disease. Arch Intern Med 1975;35:89–95.

Nachman RL, Silverstein R. Hypercoagulable states. Ann Intern Med 1993;119:819–827.

Samuels MA. Neurologic aspects of hematologic disease. Curr Neurol 1992;12:215–240.

Samuels MA. Neurologic Manifestations of Hematologic Diseases. In A Asbury, G McKhann, I McDonald (eds), Diseases of the Nervous System (2nd ed). Philadelphia: Saunders, 1992;1510–1521.

Samuels MA, Schiller AL. Case records of the Massachusetts General Hospital (Case 23-1981). N Engl J Med 1981;304:1411–1421.

Samuels MA, Thalinger K. Cerebrovascular manifestations of selected hematologic diseases. Semin Neurol 1991;11:411–418.

Schafer AI. The hypercoagulable states. Ann Intern Med 1985;102:814–828.

Silverstein MN. Intracranial bleeding in hemophilia. Arch Neurol 1960;3:1415–1420.

Toh B-H, VanDriel IR, Gleeson PA. Mechanisms of disease: pernicious anemia. N Engl J Med 1997;337: 1441–1448.

Trousseau A. Phelegmasia alba dolens. Clin Med Hotel Dieu de Paris 1865;3:94–100.

# 13
# Neurologic Problems in Oncology
## Lisa M. DeAngelis and S. Clifford Schold, Jr.

Neurologic symptoms are among the most common reasons for consultations on hospitalized patients with cancer and are second only to routine chemotherapy as a reason for hospital admission of cancer patients. Because many neurologic complications of cancer and its treatment occur late in the course of disease or are delayed effects, neurologic syndromes have become more frequent as cancer patients survive longer. A number of conditions can cause neurologic symptoms in cancer patients (Table 13.1). Complications related to metastatic cancer and chemotherapy or radiotherapy are the most common causes; however, infections, cerebrovascular disease, and metabolic disturbances—as well as neurologic disease unrelated to cancer, such as Parkinson's disease or multiple sclerosis—occur in these patients. Consequently, the diagnosis of the neurologic disorder is often complex. Specific types of cancer produce particular neurologic problems; thus, knowing the biology of each cancer can aid the neurologic consultant. To assist with these issues, we have divided this chapter into two sections. The first section describes the common neurologic symptoms and signs in cancer patients; the second section details the common neurologic conditions associated with specific cancers.

## PRESENTING SYMPTOMS AND SIGNS

### Back and Neck Pain

Back and neck pain are the most common reasons for neurologic consultation in hospitalized cancer patients. Table 13.2 shows common causes of back pain in cancer patients. In a large series examining both inpatient and outpatient neurologic consultations in a dedicated cancer hospital, epidural spinal metastasis was found to account for one-third of all cases of back pain in cancer patients, and isolated vertebral body metastasis was found to account for an additional one-third. Only 12%

*Table 13.1*   Conditions causing neurologic symptoms in cancer patients

Nervous system metastases
Damage from chemotherapy or radiation
Vascular disorders
Infections
Metabolic disorders
Nutritional disorders
Paraneoplastic syndromes

*Table 13.2*   Common causes of back pain in cancer patients

Metastasis
    Epidural space
    Bone
    Leptomeninges
    Nerve plexus
    Paravertebral space
Degenerative spine disease
Epidural abscess
Vertebral compression fracture (tumor, osteoporosis)
Referred pain from intrathoracic or intra-abdominal process

had a nonmetastatic cause, primarily degenerative disease, whereas the remainder had other metastatic causes such as leptomeningeal, paravertebral, or plexus tumor. Back pain usually heralds a serious process in a cancer patient.

Back pain in cancer patients is usually subacute and progressive. Acute back pain in this population is most commonly caused by a vertebral compression fracture related to either bony metastatic disease or osteoporosis. Distinguishing benign from malignant causes of back pain can be difficult, but several clinical features are helpful. Spinal metastasis usually involves the thoracic spine, which is an uncommon site of pain from herniated intervertebral disc or other degenerative disorders. Back pain that intensifies on lying down is often a result of metastatic disease, whereas pain from degenerative disease typically improves with lying down. Cancer patients with a history of degenerative disease often describe this difference when they develop back pain from metastasis; however, there are occasional patients whose spine metastasis produces symptoms that exactly recapitulate prior back pain from disk disease. Point tenderness over a single spinous process increases the suspicion that tumor is present. Most important, back pain from metastatic cancer usually occurs in the setting of known metastatic disease from tumors that commonly spread to bone.

Several pitfalls may lead the clinician astray. Significant epidural tumor may cause only pain; the absence of other neurologic symptoms or signs is not an assurance that spinal cord compression is absent. Radicular pain may accompany back pain and does not differentiate metastatic disease from a nonmetastatic process; however, when produced by metastasis, radicular pain often indicates epidural extension of tumor or leptomeningeal metastasis. Occasionally, pain from spinal epidural tumor presents as referred pain without pain in the back or neck. Finally, radicular pain from herpes zoster (which occurs more often in certain forms of cancer) may precede the rash and suggests metastatic disease when none is present.

Any constant or progressive back or neck pain in a cancer patient warrants prompt evaluation because of possible epidural metastasis, the most neurologically threatening cause of back pain. Epidural spinal cord metastasis can produce either a myelopathy or a cauda equina syndrome. Whereas epidural tumor may grow slowly and cause only insidious pain for months, abrupt decompensation may cause a sudden and often permanent disabling myelopathy. Early diagnosis to avoid myelopathy is critical, because the patient's neurologic condition at diagnosis is the most important determinant of neurologic function after treatment. Patients with paraplegia or severe paraparesis at diagnosis have a slim chance of recovering meaningful function even after definitive treatment has been administered, whereas patients who are ambulatory at the time of diagnosis usually maintain ambulation following treatment. Spinal magnetic resonance imaging (MRI), or myelography in patients unable to undergo MRI, is the definitive diagnostic test. A non–contrast-enhanced MRI scan is often sufficient to visualize epidural metastasis. Although plain films and radionuclide bone scan may be performed before MRI and are often abnormal in the presence of tumor, these tests cannot exclude epidural metastasis. MRI is more sensitive for the detection of bone metastasis and can be positive when the bone scan is negative. Although expensive, MRI as the initial diagnostic test in cancer patients with back pain is probably more cost effective than a more conservative approach. The initial spinal MRI yields the correct diagnosis—including the diagnoses of epidural tumor, paravertebral metastasis, bone metastasis, and degenerative disease—in more than 80% of cancer patients with back pain. Patients in whom a diagnosis of epidural metastasis is made should subsequently have their complete spine imaged (if such imaging was not done in the initial study) because of the 5–10% incidence of multiple sites of epidural tumor. The 20% of patients for whom a definitive diagnosis is not made from the initial MRI may require repeat MRI with gadolinium to visualize leptomeningeal metastasis or the rare intramedullary metastasis. Occasionally tumor plexopathy, retroperitoneal adenopathy or a pancreatic mass, or a posterior mediastinal or intrathoracic tumor presents as back pain. These require additional imaging procedures.

The treatment of back pain is determined by the specific diagnosis, but there are a few general guidelines. Initially the patient's back pain may be so severe as to require immediate relief before a satisfactory imaging study can be obtained. In patients with severe back pain for whom there is high suspicion of epidural metastasis (e.g., patients with known bone metastases, radicular pain, or signs that suggest spinal cord or root compression), high-dose corticosteroids should be administered intravenously before the MRI is obtained. In patients with lymphomas, corticosteroids can cause substantial tumor shrinkage and thereby produce a false-negative study, but that risk is acceptable in the face of rapidly progressing neurologic dysfunction. The immediate and marked response to high-dose steroids is so characteristic of epidural tumor as to be almost diagnostic. In some patients steroids must be combined with opioids to produce adequate pain relief, but often steroids alone are sufficient. Patients who have

*Table 13.3*   Common causes of headache in cancer patients

Nonstructural causes
   Tension headache
   Migraine
   Headache associated with fever, anemia, or systemic illness
   Drug-related headache (e.g., caused by all-*trans*-retinoic acid)
   Procedure-related headache (e.g., post–lumbar puncture)
Structural causes
   Metastasis: brain, leptomeninges, skull base, upper cervical spine
   Intracranial hemorrhage
   Central nervous system infection
   Venous sinus occlusion

epidural metastasis confirmed on neuroimaging studies but who have not yet received corticosteroids should receive parenteral high-dose steroids as soon as possible. An intravenous dose of 100 mg of dexamethasone has been shown in retrospective studies to be associated with excellent pain control; it is unknown if such high doses of steroids produce better neurologic outcome than more conventional doses or if different steroid preparations would have equivalent efficacy. If epidural tumor is found, definitive treatment may include radiotherapy, surgery, or possibly chemotherapy or hormonal manipulation, depending upon the tumor type and the specific clinical situation.

## Headache

Headache accounts for approximately 15% of all neurologic consultations in cancer patients. Although most headaches have a benign cause even in patients known to have cancer, the possibility of intracranial hemorrhage, abscess, or metastasis usually prompts consultation. Table 13.3 shows common causes of headache in cancer patients. Clinically, most headaches in these patients are generalized and nonspecific. Some patients have typical migraine with hemicranial throbbing pain, with or without visual scotomata. Localized headache is relatively uncommon, even in patients with focal disease. However, a focal, nonmigrainous headache is more likely to be associated with localized intracranial disease. Neither type of headache is particularly associated with structural intracranial disease except when accompanied by other symptoms or signs of increased intracranial pressure or focal neurologic signs. Often, headaches occur within the context of another acute systemic illness, such as infection with fever, and do not necessarily indicate structural disease of the nervous system. A less-common systemic cause of headache is severe anemia (hemoglobin $\leq 5.0$ g/dl), which can cause raised intracranial pressure and papilledema. Intracranial structural disease accounts for only about 40% of headaches in the cancer population and is usually accompanied by lateralizing signs. The principal cause is metastatic tumor—usually intracerebral, but sometimes to the leptomeninges, skull base, or cervical spine. Intracranial hemorrhage is a relatively uncommon cause of headache in the cancer patient. Hemorrhage may cause the abrupt onset of severe

*Table 13.4*   Common causes of altered mental status in cancer patients

Metabolic encephalopathy
Toxic encephalopathy (e.g., from opioids, ifosfamide)
Intracranial metastasis (brain, leptomeninges)
Intracranial hemorrhage
Postoperative delirium
Cerebrovascular disease
Central nervous system infection
Psychiatric disorder

headache with alteration of consciousness, but it can also cause a persistent generalized headache indistinguishable from headache associated with benign conditions; this is a result of the common occurrence of small hemorrhages or subacute oozing of blood into a brain metastasis. Other causes of headache in the cancer patient include treatment with all-*trans*-retinoic acid (usually for acute promyelocytic leukemia), which can produce a pseudotumor cerebri syndrome; venous thrombosis (either spontaneous or associated with asparaginase therapy for acute lymphocytic leukemia); jugular vein occlusion from head and neck cancer or an indwelling central line; and post–lumbar-puncture headache, which also rarely is present after bone marrow harvest for transplantation.

Even though headache in the cancer patient is usually benign, cranial imaging is warranted in most cancer patients with a recent onset of headache. If the headache is accompanied by neurologic signs, particularly if they are lateralizing, imaging is mandatory. MRI identifies most structural causes of headache. MRI venography to visualize venous sinuses and lumbar puncture to document leptomeningeal metastasis may also be necessary. Nonstructural causes of headache usually respond to mild analgesics or correction of the underlying contributory illness. If brain metastases are found on MRI, administration of a corticosteroid, usually 16 mg per day of dexamethasone or its equivalent, often produces rapid relief of headache and amelioration of neurologic symptoms and signs. Corticosteroids reduce edema that surrounds metastatic brain lesions and thereby improve the patient's condition. Definitive treatment of brain metastases may include whole-brain radiotherapy, surgery, stereotactic radiosurgery, or, less commonly, chemotherapy.

## Altered Mental Status

Altered mental status is second only to pain as a cause for neurologic consultation in hospitalized cancer patients. It accounted for 17% of all neurologic consults in the Memorial Sloan-Kettering Cancer Center series. The term *altered mental status* includes all degrees of impairment of cognitive function, from mild confusion to language deficits to coma, and its causes are multiple (Table 13.4). Structural disease, usually intracerebral or leptomeningeal metastases, account for a minority of cases, although structural disease is more likely when the cognitive abnormalities are accompanied by lateralizing signs.

In approximately 60% of cancer patients with altered mental status, the cause is metabolic. Fever and infection, hypoxia and ischemia, organ failure (particularly of the liver or kidney), hypercalcemia, and abnormalities of sodium and glucose are the most common causes of metabolic encephalopathy. Sedative drugs, even at doses that do not ordinarily affect cognition, may contribute to the mental status abnormalities in the presence of one of these metabolic derangements. In fact, the majority of cancer patients with a metabolic encephalopathy have multiple metabolic abnormalities, and it is the cumulative effect, rather than a single cause, that is responsible.

Disseminated intravascular coagulation may also cause an encephalopathy with or without focal neurologic signs, and it can be present in a compensated but symptomatic state even when the platelet count and prothrombin time are normal. Demonstration of fibrin degradation products or, specifically, D-dimer, establishes the diagnosis. Heparin is the appropriate treatment.

An encephalopathy also occurs as a toxic response to some chemotherapeutic drugs, particularly ifosfamide, interferons, and cyclosporine. High doses of nitrosoureas have also produced encephalopathy.

Postoperative delirium and so-called intensive care unit (ICU) psychosis are also seen with some frequency in hospitalized cancer patients. Septic encephalopathy or metabolic disturbances may contribute to confusion in these settings; however, in some patients no identifiable factor is found other than recent surgery, usually surgery lasting many hours, or a prolonged stay in the ICU.

Altered mental status may accompany paraneoplastic neurologic conditions, particularly so-called limbic encephalitis. A chronic and relatively mild dementia can occur in other paraneoplastic conditions.

Other rare, but potentially reversible, causes of encephalopathy in the cancer patient include Wernicke's syndrome, pellagra in the carcinoid syndrome, acute radiation encephalopathy, and acute uremia associated with the tumor lysis syndrome. Again, multiple factors may contribute.

In addition, patients with a clear metabolic cause of confusion may have coexisting structural disease. Consequently, most patients with altered mental status should undergo neuroimaging, preferably with an enhanced MRI, as well as a full metabolic evaluation. A lumbar puncture is indicated if leptomeningeal tumor or infection is suspected. Electroencephalography (EEG) may be warranted if there is any suspicion of nonconvulsive status epilepticus. Despite the fact that many cancer patients with altered mental status have ultimately incurable conditions that produce their encephalopathy, the majority achieve meaningful neurologic improvement if the underlying metabolic disorder is corrected or the structural brain disease is effectively treated.

## Seizures

Seizures account for about 5% of neurologic consultations in hospitalized cancer patients. Occasionally the diagnosis of a seizure itself is difficult, but in most cases there is no doubt that an epileptic event has occurred. In cancer patients, seizures are often the first indication of structural brain disease, which is usually metastasis, but infection, stroke, or even a new primary brain tumor may be responsible (Table 13.5). Venous sinus thrombosis, specifically sagittal sinus

*Table 13.5*   Common causes of seizures in cancer patients

Intracranial metastasis: brain, leptomeninges, dura
Cerebral infarction
Central nervous system infection
Venous sinus thrombosis
Primary epilepsy
Hyponatremia
Hypoglycemia

thrombosis, is not uncommon in certain types of cancer, and it often presents with seizures. Tumor infiltration of the sinus, a hypercoagulable state, and dehydration are the most common predisposing factors for sinus thrombosis.

All cancer patients with a new seizure should have a cranial MRI with gadolinium and a metabolic screen. Some require MRI venography and lumbar puncture, depending on the circumstances. EEG is rarely helpful for either diagnosis or treatment decisions if it is clear that a seizure has occurred. Treatment of seizures in the cancer population does not differ from their treatment in the general population. Seizures associated with specific metabolic derangements (e.g., hyponatremia) usually do not require treatment with anticonvulsants if the metabolic abnormality can be corrected.

Some specific concerns regarding the use of anticonvulsants in cancer patients include (1) the potential myelosuppressive effects of carbamazepine, which may accentuate chemotherapy-induced myelosuppression (this is more of a theoretic concern than a frequent practical issue; however, it is seen in the occasional patient); (2) the enhanced potential for a Stevens-Johnson reaction from phenytoin when used in a patient who is receiving concurrent corticosteroid and cranial radiotherapy; such reaction has also been described with carbamazepine; (3) in patients with major organ failure, blood levels of phenytoin, phenobarbital, valproic acid, and carbamazepine must be followed closely; free levels, if available, may be particularly helpful with phenytoin; (4) specific drug interactions are also common in the cancer population. Concurrent use of corticosteroids with anticonvulsants, particularly phenytoin, can enhance drug metabolism and decrease the serum level, especially as the steroid dosage is increased. Alternatively, the addition of phenytoin to the drug regimen of a patient on a stable dosage of a corticosteroid can increase steroid metabolism and sometimes result in symptoms of steroid withdrawal. Another common drug regimen is the use of sucralfate as a gastrointestinal protective agent in a patient maintained on corticosteroids. Sucralfate inhibits absorption of oral phenytoin, reducing its serum level and therefore its efficacy, despite a stable phenytoin dosage.

## Focal Neurologic Signs

Lateralizing signs such as hemiparesis, aphasia, or a visual field defect in a cancer patient indicate structural brain disease. Common causes of lateralizing neurologic signs in cancer patients are given in Table 13.6. The tempo of symptom

*Table 13.6*    Common causes of lateralizing neurologic signs in cancer patients

---

Cranial
    Metastasis: brain, dura, leptomeninges
    Stroke: hemorrhage, infarction, nonbacterial thrombotic endocarditis, venous sinus
        thrombosis
    Infection
    Radionecrosis
Spinal
    Metastasis: epidural space, intramedullary, leptomeninges
    Radiation myelopathy
    Infection: epidural abscess, herpes zoster myelitis
    Infarction
Peripheral
    Plexopathy: tumor, radiation
    Entrapment neuropathy

---

onset often suggests the underlying cause. An abrupt onset may indicate hemorrhage into an underlying lesion. The most common forms of brain metastasis that bleed are melanoma, choriocarcinoma, and lung, renal, and thyroid carcinomas. Stroke in cancer patients may have the usual atherosclerotic causes associated with standard risk factors, or it may be the result of a hypercoagulable state associated with systemic cancer. Hypercoagulability is usually a manifestation of nonbacterial thrombotic endocarditis. Rarely, stroke is caused by herpes zoster vasculitis, which usually occurs after the rash has cleared. Sometimes, the acute appearance of focal neurologic signs is caused by a postictal paralysis (Todd's paralysis) from a new seizure, with the ictal event either missed or unobserved; generally, seizures that leave residual, albeit temporary, focal signs are associated with underlying structural brain lesions. A more subacute and progressive development of lateralizing signs often indicates a growing brain metastasis or, less likely, focal infection or even the development of a primary brain tumor as a second malignancy. MRI is the diagnostic method of choice for cancer patients with localizing signs or symptoms. If the patient has had a stroke, further workup depends on the clinical situation; it may include MRI angiography, carotid ultrasonography, and echocardiography, including a transesophageal study, particularly if nonbacterial thrombotic endocarditis is suspected. Treatment is dictated by the specific diagnosis.

Myelopathy usually points to epidural tumor or infection that compresses the cord, an intramedullary metastasis, a meningioma or neurofibroma, or late radiation damage to the cord. Most patients with myelopathy have a classic spinal cord presentation with a sensory level deficit, leg weakness, or sphincter disturbance. A Brown-Séquard syndrome suggests radiation myelopathy, but it can occur as a manifestation of epidural cord compression. Occasionally patients present with ataxia as the sole manifestation of thoracic cord compression. This condition is a result of disruption of the spinocerebellar tracts and can be confused with cerebellar disease.

Unilateral limb pain or weakness is another relatively common reason for requesting a neurologic evaluation. Limb pain or weakness may be the first symptom of an epidural metastasis, particularly in patients who also have back pain, because radiculopathy is a frequent manifestation of epidural tumor. Radicular pain is often the first and may be the only manifestation of cutaneous herpes zoster, which often occurs in patients who are receiving long-term corticosteroid administration or who have lymphoma or leukemia. Limb pain or weakness is usually the first sign of plexopathy, either brachial or lumbosacral. Tumor plexopathy is typically painful and associated with sensory symptoms. Radiation plexopathy is usually painless, associated with lymphedema of the affected limb, and slowly progressive. When a brachial plexopathy is associated with Horner's syndrome, there is a high likelihood of an associated cervical epidural lesion, which has usually extended directly from the paravertebral space. Radiculopathy is also a frequent initial symptom of leptomeningeal metastasis; often multiple noncontiguous roots are involved, suggesting a multilevel process. Although neurologic examination can often distinguish among these conditions, proper imaging is essential. Selection of the initial imaging study depends on the clinical impression. Epidural metastasis can be identified with a noncontrast spinal MRI, whereas leptomeningeal metastasis requires either a gadolinium-enhanced MRI to identify intradural nodules or a lumbar puncture to demonstrate tumor cells in the cerebrospinal fluid. A computed tomographic (CT) scan or MRI of the brachial or lumbosacral plexus identifies most tumors in these areas. Radiation plexopathy is often a diagnosis made by excluding the presence of tumor and verifying that the clinically affected areas were within the radiation fields. Radiation plexopathy is characterized by myokymia on electrophysiologic studies in about 60% of patients; myokymia is not seen in tumor plexopathy. Rarely, imaging and electrophysiologic tests are inadequate to discriminate between tumor and radiation plexopathy, and a surgical exploration of the plexus is necessary for pathologic confirmation.

Peripheral neuropathy occurs frequently in cancer patients. The most common cause is chemotherapy-induced neuropathy from cisplatin, the vinca alkaloids (usually vincristine sulfate), or the taxanes (principally paclitaxel). The neuropathy from these drugs is widely recognized by oncologists, and neurologic consultation is rarely requested; however, when the neuropathy is severe or unusual (e.g., a cranial neuropathy from vincristine) consultation is more likely to be sought. Often, a critical question is whether additional drug can be given safely. When vincristine has produced a prominent motor neuropathy, typically foot drop, the drug should be withheld or the neuropathy will progress and become irreversible. Neuropathy is rarely dose-limiting with the taxanes, and the neuropathy in some patients can improve or stabilize even when the drug continues. The neuropathy from cisplatin is usually delayed, and the full extent of damage, usually to large sensory fibers, may not be apparent until after the course of treatment has been completed. If the patient develops a prominent sensory ataxia before completion of the prescribed course of therapy, the drug should be withheld, because the neuropathy will progress with additional doses, and the patient may be left with a severe, permanent disability.

Cachexia may contribute to neuropathy in patients with extensive disease, but it rarely disables the patient. Paraneoplastic disease is a rare cause of peripheral neuropathy and most commonly produces a painful sensory neuropathy. Non–cancer-related causes of neuropathy, particularly alcohol neuropathy (especially in head and neck cancer patients) and diabetic neuropathy, are also seen in the cancer population.

In most cancer patients with peripheral neuropathy, the history and examination establish the diagnosis and etiology. Occasionally patients require evaluation with a gadolinium-enhanced spinal MRI scan or lumbar puncture to exclude leptomeningeal metastases, which can mimic peripheral neuropathy. Electrophysiologic studies are usually not necessary to establish a diagnosis, and even less commonly is a nerve or muscle biopsy needed. These are often reserved for the patient in whom the diagnosis is difficult because the problem is hard to localize or has multiple causes, or when looking for rare complications of leukemia or lymphoma such as peripheral nerve infiltration by tumor.

Entrapment neuropathies are also seen with regularity in cancer patients. Peroneal nerve palsy is observed in cachectic patients who have been bedridden for an extended period of time; it is often confused with an $L_5$ radiculopathy, which has a more serious significance. Stretch injuries, particularly of the brachial plexus, can be seen after prolonged surgical procedures. Femoral neuropathy may be a complication of intra-abdominal or intrapelvic operations or may be caused by a retroperitoneal hematoma in a patient who is receiving anticoagulation therapy or who has thrombocytopenia. Usually the neurologic examination suffices to make the diagnosis of nerve compression. Occasionally, imaging is needed to exclude a more serious problem or to identify the cause; for example, pelvic CT scan may be required to visualize a hematoma.

It is important to remember that cancer patients may also develop neurologic disease that is unrelated to their tumor or its treatment. This is particularly true for patients who are in remission or have been cured of their neoplasm. Attacks of multiple sclerosis, vascular disease, and episodes of Guillain-Barré syndrome are but a few of the more common noncancer causes of focal neurologic signs in cancer patients.

## Multifocal Signs

Multifocal signs pointing to involvement of the nervous system at different levels are a hallmark of leptomeningeal metastasis. This condition may coexist with brain metastasis or occur as the only site of tumor spread. Leptomeningeal metastasis can produce cranial neuropathies (most commonly of cranial nerves III, VI, and VII), hydrocephalus with headache or confusion, seizures, and radiculopathies. Often the patient presents with a combination of these neurologic abnormalities.

Multifocal epidural metastasis is present in about 5% of patients with a single site of documented epidural involvement. This condition can produce confusing signs on neurologic examination and is a justification for imaging of the entire spine in any patient with known epidural tumor.

Apparent multifocality may appear in cancer patients who have more than one neurologic problem. The coexistence of multiple diagnoses is common and is seen primarily in patients with late-stage cancer. A lymphoma patient with leg weakness may have vincristine neuropathy and leptomeningeal metastasis. A patient with brain metastases on long-term steroid therapy may develop limb pain due to cutaneous herpes zoster, leptomeningeal metastasis, or a plexopathy. A patient with epidural spinal cord compression who develops increasing leg weakness may have a steroid myopathy or progressive cord compression. These are a few examples to illustrate the common issues confronting the con-

*Table 13.7*   Common neurologic syndromes by specific tumor type

| Tumor type | Brain metastasis | Leptomeningeal metastasis | Epidural spinal cord metastasis | Treatment effect | Paraneoplastic syndromes |
|---|---|---|---|---|---|
| Non–small-cell lung | +++ | ++ | ++ | ++ | + |
| Small-cell lung | +++ | +++ | ++ | ++ | +++ |
| Breast | ++ | +++ | ++ | ++ | + |
| Colon | + | + | + | + | 0 |
| Prostate | 0 | 0 | +++ | + | 0 |
| Pancreas | 0 | 0 | + | 0 | ++ |
| Genitourinary | ++ | + | ++ | + | ++ |
| Melanoma | +++ | +++ | ++ | + | 0 |
| Leukemias | 0 | +++ | 0 | ++ | 0 |
| Lymphomas/ Hodgkin's disease | 0 | ++ | ++ | +++ | + |
| Myeloma | 0 | + | +++ | + | + |

+++ = frequent; ++ = occasional; + = infrequent; 0 = rare.

sulting neurologist. The potential multiplicity of diagnoses makes a thorough neurologic examination and appropriate imaging essential to clarifying the nature of neurologic illness in the cancer patient.

# NEUROLOGIC SYNDROMES IN SPECIFIC FORMS OF CANCER

The most common neurologic complications of cancer are produced by metastases to the nervous system or its surrounding structures, but indirect complications and complications of cancer therapy also occur frequently. The incidence of neurologic complications of cancer and cancer therapy varies significantly with the type of cancer afflicting the patient, so the appropriate differential diagnosis and the weight given to various diagnostic possibilities depends on a knowledge of these patterns. The next sections describe neurologic complications of systemic cancer organized by specific neoplasm (Table 13.7).

## Non–Small-Cell Lung Cancer

This group of primary lung cancers includes squamous cell carcinomas, adenocarcinomas, and undifferentiated tumors. The most common neurologic effects of these tumors are direct metastases to the brain or epidural space of the spinal cord. Non–small-cell lung cancer is the most frequent cause of brain metastasis. These tumors also produce leptomeningeal metastasis. They rarely produce paraneoplastic neurologic syndromes; however, nonbacterial thrombotic endocarditis may be associated with widespread systemic tumor, and hypercalcemia may be associated with bone metastases. Radiation damage or tumor infiltration of the brachial plexus occasionally occurs if the tumor is situated in the upper lobe or has spread to the supraclavicular lymph nodes. Potentially neurotoxic chemotherapeutic agents used in these patients include cisplatin, vincristine, and paclitaxel, all of which can produce a dose-related neuropathy.

## Small-Cell Lung Cancer

Small-cell lung cancer is a form of primary lung cancer that frequently produces brain, epidural spinal cord, and leptomeningeal metastases. It is also the tumor most commonly associated with paraneoplastic syndromes, such as the Lambert-Eaton myasthenic syndrome, subacute sensory neuropathy, and subacute cerebellar degeneration. It can produce hypercalcemia and hyponatremia that can lead to metabolic encephalopathy or seizures. As in non–small-cell lung cancer, cisplatin, vincristine, and paclitaxel are often used in patients with small-cell lung cancer, and each can produce a polyneuropathy.

## Breast Cancer

Breast cancer can metastasize to the brain, the epidural space of the spinal cord, and the leptomeninges. Frequently more than one neurologic site is affected in the same patient. Patients with breast cancer are also susceptible to tumor invasion of the brachial plexus, radiation damage to the brachial plexus, and some paraneoplastic neurologic syndromes. Among the chemotherapeutic agents commonly used to treat breast cancer, perhaps the one that most often produces neurologic toxicity is cisplatin. Paclitaxel, which is increasingly used in the breast cancer population, can also produce a toxic neuropathy. A new vinca alkaloid, vindesine sulfate, is being used in the treatment of disseminated breast cancer. By itself, it causes a mild peripheral neuropathy, but the neuropathy can be severe in patients previously treated with paclitaxel. Tamoxifen citrate can cause diminished vision from retinal toxicity.

## Colon Cancer

Although colon cancer is one of the most common forms of cancer, it does not usually metastasize to the brain, the leptomeninges, or the epidural spinal space. Brain metastasis is the most frequent site of metastasis to the nervous system. Colon cancer metastasis has a predilection for the posterior fossa, particularly the cerebellum. A more clinically significant problem for the neurologist evaluating the patient with colon cancer is tumor infiltration of the lumbosacral plexus or radiation damage to these plexuses. Other treatment-related neurologic toxicities in patients with colon cancer include a cerebellar syndrome from fluorouracil (which is rare at the drug dosages currently in use) and an encephalopathy from levamisole hydrochloride in combination with fluorouracil. Because colon cancer so commonly metastasizes to liver, metabolic encephalopathy from drugs that undergo hepatic metabolism is relatively frequent in this population.

## Prostate Cancer

The most common neurologic complication of prostate cancer is epidural spinal cord compression, which reflects the tendency of this tumor to metastasize to bone. Metastasis to brain or leptomeninges is rare; however, prostate cancer does occasionally spread to the dura, producing intracranial, though not intra-cerebral, metastases. Local spread of the primary tumor in the pelvis can produce a sacral plexopathy, and the lumbar and sacral plexuses are also susceptible to radiation injury if they were within the treatment field. Paraneoplastic neurologic effects do not occur in prostate cancer.

## Pancreatic Cancer

Like colon cancer, pancreatic cancer is relatively common but usually does not affect the nervous system. It has a greater tendency to spread locally in the abdom-inal cavity, causing back and abdominal pain, than to metastasize throughout the body. Central nervous system ischemia or infarction can occur because of the ten-dency for pancreatic cancer to produce a hypercoagulable state leading to non-bacterial thrombotic endocarditis or disseminated intravascular coagulation.

## Melanoma

As many as 80% of patients who die from metastatic melanoma have a nervous system metastasis at autopsy. Most often, it is brain metastasis, which is fre-quently multiple and sometimes hemorrhagic. Leptomeningeal metastasis from melanoma is also relatively common and may coexist with brain metastases. Epidural spinal cord compression is much less common, because melanoma does not have a great predilection to metastasize to bone. Paraneoplastic neuro-logic syndromes very rarely occur in patients with melanoma. Treatment-related neurologic complications are relatively few in these patients, but interferon-α can produce an encephalopathy.

## Genitourinary Cancer

Carcinoma of the kidney often metastasizes to brain, frequently causing hemor-rhagic lesions. Epidural spinal cord compression is relatively common, but lep-tomeningeal and plexus metastases are rare. As in melanoma, renal cancer may have a relatively long latency period from the original diagnosis and treatment of the primary tumor to the development of metastases. This pattern certainly is not always the case, but it occurs more often than in most other lethal cancers, in which a 5-year disease-free survival represents a cure. Because renal carcinoma is particularly radioresistant, surgery is often the initial treatment for nervous sys-tem metastasis, if feasible.

Testicular tumors used to metastasize frequently to the brain, but the introduc-tion of more effective treatment at diagnosis (namely, cisplatin and its derivatives) has dramatically reduced the incidence of neurologic complications. Cisplatin neuropathy and radiation damage to the lumbar or sacral plexus are now probably a more common cause of neurologic problems than are metastases. Ovarian cancer rarely leads to nervous system metastases. However, cisplatin and paclitaxel neuropathy are seen frequently in these patients, particularly when the two agents have been used sequentially. Cervical and endometrial cancers usually produce neurologic effects by local infiltration of nerves, but both can produce brain metastases. Choriocarcinoma has a high incidence of brain metastasis that is usually hemorrhagic. Bladder cancer is usually locally invasive and produces neurologic problems by infiltrating the nerve plexuses in the pelvis. It can disseminate, however, and produce brain metastases. It also occasionally produces leptomeningeal metastases. Neither kidney, testicular, nor bladder cancer commonly produces paraneoplastic neurologic complications, although they have been reported. Ovarian cancer and occasionally endometrial cancer are associated with selected paraneoplastic conditions, particularly subacute cerebellar degeneration.

## Leukemias

Acute forms of leukemia have a pronounced tendency to involve the leptomeninges. This occurs so commonly in acute lymphocytic leukemia that prophylactic treatment to the meninges (either radiation or intrathecal chemotherapy) is used at the time of initial therapy. The incidence of meningeal invasion by the acute granulocytic leukemias varies with the cell type of the neoplasm, and prophylactic therapy is administered accordingly. Leptomeningeal metastasis is considerably less common in the chronic leukemias. Unlike lung and breast cancer, the leukemias rarely produce intraparenchymal mass lesions (so-called chloromas). Occasionally, leukemic cells invade peripheral nerves, producing a mononeuritis multiplex. Hyperviscosity syndromes from marked leukocytosis can also lead to transient or permanent neurologic dysfunction. Treatment-related neurologic syndromes in patients with leukemia include radiation or methotrexate leukoencephalopathy, vincristine neuropathy, asparaginase-induced sagittal sinus thrombosis, and an acute cerebellar syndrome from high-dose cytosine arabinoside. Of course, treatment of acute leukemia usually produces severe bone marrow suppression, and patients are susceptible to intracranial hemorrhage and to central nervous system infections during the periods of thrombocytopenia and neutropenia.

## Lymphomas and Hodgkin's Disease

Most early-stage non-Hodgkin's lymphomas and Hodgkin's disease are curable with primary therapy and do not affect the nervous system. Late-stage or disseminated lymphomas commonly spread to the leptomeninges, but they rarely spread to the parenchyma of the central nervous system. Curiously, Hodgkin's disease rarely produces leptomeningeal metastases, even when the tumor is widespread. Both lymphomas and Hodgkin's disease can produce epidural spinal cord compression, and unlike most solid tumors, they may do so by growth through the neural foramina and not by metastasis to the vertebral bodies. Consequently, radionuclide bone scans and other imaging studies that are directed primarily at bone may not detect epidural tumor. Lymphomas are not commonly associated with paraneoplastic neurologic conditions. Hodgkin's disease is rarely associated with an atypical form of subacute cerebellar degeneration, and a rare form of anterior horn cell disease occurs with increased frequency in these patients. Hodgkin's disease is associated with depressed cell-mediated immunity, and opportunistic infections of the nervous system are seen with increased frequency. Both lymphomas and Hodgkin's disease are treated with radiation and often with vincristine as a component of their combination chemotherapy, so patients are susceptible to the neurologic effects of these agents. Cutaneous herpes zoster is a common complication of the lymphomas and Hodgkin's disease, and it is often followed by postherpetic neuralgia.

## Multiple Myeloma

Myeloma can produce neurologic effects by forming an epidural spinal cord mass or, rarely, spreading to the leptomeninges. It is also associated with a paraneoplastic polyneuropathy, particularly in the osteosclerotic form of myeloma.

## Miscellaneous Tumors

Bone, soft tissue, and other sarcomas can produce neurologic effects either by local infiltration of nerves and plexuses or by metastasis to the brain or epidural space of the spinal cord. Carcinoid tumors can metastasize to the brain. Salivary gland, parotid, paranasal sinus, and other head and neck tumors can infiltrate adjacent cranial nerves and, rarely, form leptomeningeal metastases by direct invasion. Nasopharyngeal cancer also tends to invade locally and can produce leptomeningeal tumor by this route. Other forms of head and neck tumors generally do not affect the nervous system except by local infiltration or by therapy-related damage to nerves (from surgery, radiation, cisplatin chemotherapy). Although stomach cancer was one of the first cancers recognized to be associated with leptomeningeal metastases, it is now a much less common tumor than in the early part of the twentieth century. Consequently, neurologic complications from stomach cancer are less common than they once were.

## CONCLUDING REMARKS

Hospitalized cancer patients are susceptible to a wide variety of neurologic problems. The diagnostic complexity is reduced somewhat if one recognizes that certain syndromes are more commonly associated with certain forms of cancer. Yet, there is no doubt that more than one form of neurologic complication often occurs in the same cancer patient, which, of course, increases the diagnostic challenge. Finally, the guidelines described in this chapter are statistical generalizations. In practice, neurologic complications in an individual patient with cancer may not follow these broad guidelines. Thus, the clinician must be sensitive to unique situations, particularly as new forms of therapy are introduced and patients survive for longer periods with their disease.

## SUGGESTED READING

Byrne TN, Waxman SG. Spinal Cord Compression: Diagnosis and Principles of Management. Philadelphia: Davis, 1990.

Clouston PD, DeAngelis LM, Posner JB. The spectrum of neurological disease in patients with systemic cancer. Ann Neurol 1992;31:268–273.

DeAngelis LM. Management of brain metastases. Cancer Invest 1994;12:156–165.

Delattre JY, Krol G, Thaler H, et al. Distribution of brain metastases. Arch Neurol 1988;45:741–744.

Freilich RJ, Krol G, DeAngelis LM. Neuroimaging and cerebrospinal fluid cytology in the diagnosis of leptomeningeal metastasis. Ann Neurol 1995;38:51–57.

Gilbert RW, Kim JH, Posner JB. Epidural spinal cord compression from metastatic tumor: diagnosis and treatment. Ann Neurol 1978;3:40–51.

Jordan JE, Donaldson SS, Enzmann DR. Cost effectiveness and outcome assessment of magnetic resonance imaging in diagnosing cord compression. Cancer 1995;75:2579–2586.

Nussbaum ES, Djalilian HR, Chok H, Hall WA. Brain metastases: histology, multiplicity, surgery, and survival. Cancer 1996;78:1781–1788.

Posner JB. Neurologic Complications of Cancer. Philadelphia: Davis, 1995.

Rodichok LD, Harper GR, Ruckdeschel JC, et al. Early diagnosis of spinal epidural metastases. Am J Med 1981;70:1181–1188.

van Oosterhout AGM, van de Pol M, ten Velde GPM, Twijnstra A. Neurologic disorders in 203 consecutive patients with small cell lung cancer. Cancer 1996;77:1434–1441.

Wasserstrom WR, Glass P, Posner JB. Diagnosis and treatment of leptomeningeal metastases from solid tumors: experience with 90 patients. Cancer 1981;49:759–772.

# 14
# Cardiology

Raymond Tak Fai Cheung and Vladimir Hachinski

Neurologic consultations from cardiology are the most common among all consultations from the various medical specialties for several reasons. The coincidental occurrence of neurologic disease in cardiac patients is frequent, especially in older patients. Atherosclerosis, hypertension, hyperlipidemia, diabetes mellitus, obesity, cigarette smoking, alcohol abuse, and family history of vascular diseases are risk factors for both coronary artery and cerebrovascular diseases. In addition, the presence of either coronary artery disease or cerebrovascular disease signals an increased chance that the other is also present. Cardiac conditions and invasive cardiologic procedures may result in neurologic complications, and cardioembolism is a major cause of ischemic stroke. Less commonly, multisystem diseases have both neurologic and cardiac features, and recognition of these features assists in achieving the correct clinical diagnosis. Sometimes, neurologic conditions with prominent cardiac features masquerade as cardiac diseases.

A cardiologist typically consults neurology service for one of the following reasons. First, a patient has new neurologic symptoms or signs to suggest a neurologic complication of the cardiologic condition or treatment. Yet it is possible the neurologic condition may pre-exist unrecognized or may be a coincidental event. Second, the patient has a known or suspected neurologic diagnosis that may or may not interfere with treatment of the cardiologic condition. Third, the cardiovascular diagnosis has the potential of causing neurologic complications. The responding neurologist should confirm the existence of a neurologic problem, make the correct diagnosis, assess the risk for any potential neurologic complication, advise on investigations, estimate the prognosis, and formulate the management plan.

A detailed description of every possible neurologic diagnosis encountered in neurologic consultations from cardiology is beyond the scope of this chapter. Neurologic consultation problems from cardiothoracic surgery and pediatric cardiology and cardiac surgery are covered in Chapters 19 and 30, respectively. Major neurologic symptoms, such as altered mental status, behavior disturbances, seizures, and weakness, and special issues such as stroke, drugs, toxins, and electrolyte disorders are the topics of chapters in Part I. The emphasis in this chapter is on analyzing the possible relationship between cardiac problems and neurologic diagnoses and on recognizing the circumstances under which neurologic problems arise. Thus, common scenarios are outlined, and neurologic complications of major cardiac conditions are highlighted. The neurologic and cardiac causes of syncope, which is a common symptom for referral, are also described. Included is an elaboration on neurogenic or cerebrogenic cardiovascular disturbances, and finally, some guidelines are given for approaching neurologic consultations originating from cardiology.

## COMMON NEUROLOGIC CONSULTATIONS

### Scenarios from the Intensive Care Unit or Coronary Care Unit

In one scenario, a patient is admitted into an intensive care unit because of post-cardiac arrest and does not wake up despite being hemodynamically stable after successful cardiopulmonary resuscitation. Recurrent focal or generalized seizures may occur, and bedside neurologic assessment may reveal some focal motor deficits or brain stem signs. The differential diagnoses include diffuse ischemic hypoxic encephalopathy, bilateral hemispheric infarctions, brain stem infarction, status epilepticus, and metabolic or toxic encephalopathy. The cardiac arrest, however, may be the consequence of a primary neurologic condition such as stroke, seizure, head trauma, or rapidly enlarging brain tumor (a result of hemorrhage that causes herniation and brain stem compression).

In another scenario, a patient under coronary care has a neurologic complication after a myocardial infarction, diagnostic coronary angiography, or therapeutic percutaneous transluminal coronary angioplasty with or without stenting. Presence of focal neurologic deficits may indicate a transient ischemic attack or stroke, cranial nerve palsy, limb plexopathy, peripheral neuropathy, myelopathy, or myopathy. On the other hand, focal or generalized seizures may be the prominent feature. Finally, the patient could have neurobehavioral and cognitive symptoms, including confusion, delirium, altered consciousness, aggressive behavior, hallucinations, delusions, depression, mania, memory loss, and impaired higher cognitive functions. The diagnoses are usually straightforward according to the symptoms, signs, results of investigations, and clinical circumstances. The possible pathogenic mechanisms may include cardioembolism, artery-to-artery embolism, foreign-body or air embolism, systemic hypotension (resulting from arrhythmia, heart failure, or major hemorrhage with or without significant extracranial or intracranial arterial stenosis of cerebral artery), intracranial hemorrhage (resulting from systemic anticoagulation or thrombolysis), direct local or regional complication of the cardiologic procedure, contrast encephalopathy, neurotoxic effects of polypharmacy, intensive care psychosis, and others. A potential trap exists when focal neurologic symptoms and signs of sudden onset are accompanied by some evidence of myocardial ischemia, or arrhythmia. The differential diagnoses are cardioembolic stroke and acute stroke with neurogenic cardiac abnormalities, and thus the management may be different.

## Scenarios from the Cardiology Ward

Patients admitted for treatment or investigation of other cardiologic diagnoses such as congestive heart failure, infective endocarditis, valvular heart disease, and cardiomyopathy can develop transient or persistent focal neurologic deficits, seizures, or episodic loss of consciousness. Alternatively, they may have asymptomatic or symptomatic carotid bruits. Similarly, when an invasive cardiologic procedure or cardiovascular surgery is planned for a patient who has carotid stenosis or a history of stroke, a neurologist's opinion is usually sought. Patients admitted into the cardiology ward may also have chronic neurologic conditions such as Parkinson's disease and multiple sclerosis, in which case advice is sought regarding adjustment in medication because of concomitant use of cardiac drugs.

## Analysis Based on the Patterns of Neurologic Manifestations

These scenarios illustrate some general points. First, the most common reason for a neurologic consultation originating from an intensive care unit or coronary care unit is a suspected neurologic complication in one of three common clinical settings—postcardiac resuscitation, acute myocardial infarction, and invasive cardiologic procedures. Any one or any combination of the following common patterns of neurologic manifestations can occur: focal neurologic deficits, seizures, altered or depressed state of consciousness, and behavioral disturbances or cognitive impairment. In contrast, suspected neurologic complications, asymptomatic or symptomatic carotid stenosis, and a history of transient ischemic attacks, stroke, or other neurologic diagnoses are the main reasons for consultations from a cardiologic ward. In addition, the clinical settings include patients with a wide variety of stable or unstable cardiac conditions and patients who have undergone invasive cardiologic procedures. Nevertheless, the patterns of neurologic manifestations are almost the same, with two exceptions: (1) the patient may be neurologically asymptomatic at the time of consultation (e.g., asymptomatic carotid stenosis); and (2) the consultation may be for a chronic neurologic condition or other specific diagnosis.

Second, one practical approach to neurologic consultations from cardiology is to recognize the patterns of neurologic manifestations, work out the differential diagnoses, establish the underlying etiologies, and formulate the plan of management (Table 14.1). Alternatively, we can focus on the clinical setting and alert ourselves to the neurologic problems that are commonly associated with the particular setting for one reason or another (please refer to the section Highlights of Some Important Neurocardiac Conditions).

Third, the possible neurologic conditions encountered in hospital consultations from cardiology are unlimited within the scope of clinical neurology, but some are more common under certain circumstances. There are six possible relationships between neurologic conditions and cardiac diseases: (1) coincidental neurologic and cardiac problems, (2) neurologic complications of cardiac diseases, (3) neurologic complications of cardiac and related drugs, (4) neurologic complications of invasive cardiologic procedures, (5) multisystem diseases with neurologic and cardiac features, and (6) neurologic diagnoses presenting with cardiac features.

*Table 14.1*   Major patterns of neurologic manifestations seen in consultations from cardiology[a]

| Major patterns | Differential diagnoses | Main etiologies | Management of diagnosis |
|---|---|---|---|
| Focal deficit | Transient ischemic attack, ischemic stroke | Atherothrombotic, cardioembolic, lacunar, prothrombotic, other arteriopathy | Ix: CT or MRI, carotid USG, MRA, angiography, ECG, echocardiography, routine blood tests, screen hyperlipidemia[b] and hypercoagulability<br>Tx: Thrombolysis, anticoagulation, carotid surgery, treat and prevent complications, control risk factors, rehabilitation |
| | Hemorrhagic stroke | Intracerebral hemorrhage, subarachnoid hemorrhage, subdural hematoma, extradural hematoma | Ix: CT or MRI, routine blood tests, coagulation screen, angiography<br>Tx: Stop anticoagulation, treat coagulopathy, surgical decompression, $Ca^{2+}$ antagonist for SAH, aneurysmal surgery, treat and prevent complications, control hypertension, rehabilitation |
| | Cranial nerve palsy | Iatrogenic, stroke | Ix: CT or MRI, more Ix if result of stroke<br>Tx: Conservative, more Tx if due to stroke |
| | Myelopathy | Aortic dissection, extrinsic compression | Ix: Plain radiographs, MRI, myelogram, CT myelogram, CSF, SER, MRA, angiogram<br>Tx: According to the underlying cause, steroid, decompression |
| | Plexopathy | Iatrogenic | Ix: NCS, EMG, SER, MRI, coagulation screen<br>Tx: Conservative, physiotherapy |
| | Peripheral neuropathy | Iatrogenic, previously unrecognized | Ix: NCS, EMG, routine blood test, ESR, FBS, heavy metal screen, toxic screen, review drug history, screen for vitamin deficiency, autoimmune screen, CSF, nerve biopsy<br>Tx: According to the underlying cause |
| | Myopathy | Metabolic, drug related | Ix: ESR, muscle enzymes, autoimmune and endocrine screen, review drug history, EMG, NCS, muscle biopsy<br>Tx: According to the underlying cause |
| Seizure | Focal seizure | Stroke, trauma, tumor, abscess, epilepsy | Ix: EEG, CT or MRI, CSF, electrolytes, BSL, pH, arterial blood gases, muscle enzymes, toxic screen, review drug history, brain biopsy<br>Tx: According to the underlying cause, anticonvulsants, airway protection |

| Major patterns | Differential diagnoses | Main etiologies | Management of diagnosis |
|---|---|---|---|
| | Generalized seizure | Stroke, encephalopathy, epilepsy | Ix and Tx: Same as for focal seizure |
| | Status epilepticus | Encephalopathy, stroke, raised ICP, epilepsy | Ix: Same as for focal seizure, monitor ICP, EEG, and vital signs<br>Tx: ICU admission, $O_2$, IV diazepam, correct metabolic disturbances, IV phenytoin or phenobarbital sodium, consider IV steroid, anesthetization, muscular paralysis, and artificial ventilation for refractory cases |
| | Epilepsy | Coincidental | Ix and Tx: Same as for focal seizure |
| Altered consciousness | Coma | Massive stroke, brain stem stroke, encephalopathy, status epilepticus, sedatives, raised ICP | Ix: CT or MRI, EEG, CSF, BAER, monitor ICP, routine blood tests, BSL, pH, arterial blood gases, electrolytes, toxic screen, review drug history, brain biopsy<br>Tx: According to the underlying cause |
| | Depressed consciousness or confusion | Stroke, encephalopathy, postictal, sedatives, raised ICP | Ix and Tx: Same as for coma |
| | Syncope | See subsection on syncope and Table 14.11 | See subsection on syncope |
| Behavioral disturbances | Dementia, amnesia, delirium, psychosis, neurosis, depression | Stroke, encephalopathy, drug induced, previously unrecognized problem | Ix: Mental state examination, neuropsychological tests, toxic and metabolic screen, EEG, review drug history, other Ix according to the suspected cause<br>Tx: According to the cause and diagnosis |
| Others | Carotid stenosis | Atherosclerosis | See subsection on coincidental carotid stenosis, Tables 14.7 and 14.8 |
| | Specific diagnosis | Vary with diagnosis | Ix and Tx: According to the underlying diagnosis |
| | Headache | Migraine, tension, stroke, raised ICP | Ix and Tx: According to the suspected diagnosis |
| | Dizziness | Vertigo, nonspecific | Ix and Tx: According to the diagnosis |

Ix = investigation; CT = computed tomographic scan; MRI = magnetic resonance imaging; USG = ultrasonography; MRA = magnetic resonance angiography; ECG = electrocardiogram; Tx = treatment; $Ca^{2+}$ = calcium; CSF = cerebrospinal fluid; SER = somatosensory evoked response; NCS = nerve conduction study; EMG = electromyography; ESR = erythrocyte sedimentation rate; FBS = fasting blood sugar; EEG = electroencephalogram; BSL = blood sugar level; ICP = intracerebral pressure; $O_2$ = oxygen; IV = intravenous; BAER = brain stem auditory evoked response.
[a]The lists of differential diagnoses, etiologies, investigations, and treatment are meant for quick reference only, as the lists do not include every possibility.
[b]Lipids may be artificially low after a myocardial infarction.

## POSSIBLE RELATIONSHIPS BETWEEN NEUROLOGIC AND CARDIAC PROBLEMS

### Coincidental Neurologic and Cardiac Problems

In adult cardiology wards, the single most common cardiac condition is coronary artery disease with or without complications. Affected patients are middle-aged or older. Thus, unrelated neurologic conditions that are commonly seen in middle-aged and older people may be encountered in cardiology inpatients. These unrelated neurologic diagnoses occur with their usual frequencies. Common neurologic problems are headache and facial pain, syncopes (see the subsection Syncopes), seizures and epilepsy, carotid stenosis (see the subsection Coincidental Carotid Stenosis), transient ischemic attacks and stroke, Parkinson's disease and other extrapyramidal disorders, multiple sclerosis, and dementia. The reasons for referral include a change in severity of the neurologic conditions, a need for advice on medications because of potentially adverse interactions with cardiac drugs, and diagnosis of some previously unrecognized neurologic condition. Except in the last case, the diagnoses are usually apparent from history and clinical examination, and investigations are hardly required.

Coronary artery and cerebrovascular diseases share similar vascular risk factors, and coronary artery disease is associated with extracranial and intracranial atherosclerosis as well as cardioembolism. In addition, atherothromboembolism is a major pathogenic mechanism in both conditions. Thus, patients with coronary artery disease have increased risk for stroke, and transient ischemic attacks and stroke are strong predictors of cardiac death. When stroke occurs in close temporal relation to an acute cardiac condition or a recent invasive cardiologic procedure, however, the possibility that the stroke is a complication should be considered.

### Neurologic Complications of Cardiac Diseases

Neurologic problems may complicate cardiac diseases such as acute myocardial infarction, congestive heart failure, infective endocarditis, valvular heart disease, congenital heart disease, cor pulmonale, aortic aneurysm, acute severe hypertension, postural hypotension, and cardiomyopathy. Although the relative risk of individual neurologic complication varies among these cardiac diseases, the spectrum of neurologic complications is similar. Thus, cardioembolism or systemic hypotension (causing cerebral hypoperfusion) produces stroke, transient ischemic attacks, or vascular cognitive impairment. Septic emboli (from infective endocarditis or cyanotic congenital heart disease) result in suppurative intracranial infections. Underlying pulmonary causes of cor pulmonale impair cerebral metabolism through hypoxia or hypercapnia. The latter also disturbs the cerebral vasoreactivity and so impairs cerebrovascular autoregulation, which may be exceeded by extreme fluctuations in arterial blood pressure.

### Neurologic Complications of Cardiac or Related Drugs

Commonly used drugs in cardiology can produce neurologic complications through overdosage, side effects, or adverse drug interactions. For example, excessive anticoagulation with heparin or warfarin sodium (Coumadin) increases the risk of systemic and intracranial hemorrhage. Paradoxically, heparin may cause arterial thrombosis through heparin-platelet interactions or reduction of antithrombin III level. Use of sedatives in cardiologic procedures such as transesophageal echocardiography and cardiac catheterization may result in confusion or altered state of consciousness. High dose of contrast, especially in patients with impaired renal functions, can lead to toxic encephalopathy. Adverse drug interactions may arise from therapeutic or prophylactic use of antibiotics (such as chloramphenicol and aminoglycosides) for infective endocarditis. Chloramphenicol inhibits hepatic enzymes and so could lead to accumulation of warfarin, carbamazepine, phenytoin, or diazepam. Aminoglycosides, antiarrhythmic drugs (such as procainamide hydrochloride, quinidine bisulfate, and lignocaine), narcotics, sedatives, and potassium-wasting diuretics can worsen the muscular weakness in myasthenia gravis or precipitate a myasthenic crisis. Patients on monoamine-reuptake–inhibiting antidepressants (such as imipramine and amitriptyline hydrochloride) manifest enhanced cardiovascular responses to noradrenaline and adrenaline. Conversely, users of monoamine oxidase inhibitors have excessive sensitivity to sympathomimetics or narcotics, which cause acute hypertensive crisis and central nervous system excitation, respectively. Parkinsonian drugs like levodopa and bromocriptine mesylate increase the hypotensive effects of many antihypertensive medications.

## Neurologic Complications of Invasive Cardiologic Procedures

Traditional Invasive Cardiologic Procedures

Historically, diagnostic cardiac catheterization and coronary angiography were the only invasive cardiologic procedures that could result in complications (Table 14.2). Fortunately, central nervous system complications of cardiac catheterization are uncommon (0.1–1.0%) and have become rarer with improvement in the techniques, setup, catheters, guide wires, and radiologic contrast medium.

Transesophageal Echocardiography

The advent of transesophageal echocardiography and new (diagnostic and therapeutic) cardiac catheterization procedures creates new situations in which neurologic and non-neurologic complications may arise. In general, echocardiography permits a safe, accurate, and thorough functional and anatomic evaluation of the heart and related structures. Unlike surface or transthoracic echocardiography, transesophageal echocardiography uses a transducer mounted on the tip of a flexible endoscope to visualize the cardiac and aortic structures through the esophagus. Thus, this technique overcomes the inadequate imaging of transthoracic echocardiography caused by pulmonary disease, obesity, and prosthetic valves, and allows satisfactory visualization of the left atrium, left atrial appendage, interatrial septum, and aorta. As a semi-invasive procedure, transesophageal echocardiography can be performed safely as an outpatient, inpatient,

*Table 14.2*   Major or common complications of traditional diagnostic cardiac catheterization or coronary angiography

| Types | Major or common complications |
|---|---|
| Cardiac | Arrhythmias, myocardial ischemia and infarction, cardiac arrest |
| Neurological | Focal neurologic deficits (transient ischemic attack or stroke), encephalopathy, seizures |
| | Mechanisms for transient ischemic attack or stroke: embolism (air, platelet, clot, foreign body; more common in the vertebrobasilar territory), cerebral hypoperfusion |
| | Mechanisms for encephalopathy and seizures: systemic hypotension, arrhythmias, contrast toxicity, dehydration, oversedation, excessive blood loss |
| Systemic | Hypotension, embolism, sepsis, internal hemorrhage, allergic to contrast |
| Local | Sepsis, trauma, external hemorrhage |

or intraoperative investigation. Neurologic complication is mainly related to the concomitant use of mild sedation.

## New Invasive Cardiologic Procedures

New diagnostic or therapeutic cardiac catheterization procedures are summarized in Table 14.3. The spectrum of neurologic complications is the same as in diagnostic cardiac catheterization, but the frequency of various complications may be higher because of the complexity and length of the procedures, multiple exchanges of guide wires, repeated entries of larger catheters, temporary obstruction of circulation (causing hypotension), extended duration of anticoagulation, and use of a larger volume of contrast material.

## Multisystem Diseases with Neurologic and Cardiac Features

Patients with multisystem diseases may have both neurologic and cardiac features and present to the cardiology service or require cardiologic treatment because of prominent cardiac features. For example, uremia causes hypertension, arrhythmias, pericarditis, peripheral neuropathy, seizures, and encephalopathy. Pernicious anemia produces peripheral neuropathy, combined degeneration of cord, optic neuritis, encephalopathy, dementia, and heart failure. Encephalopathy, seizures, meningism, psychiatric disturbances, focal neurologic deficits, mononeuritis multiplex, peripheral neuropathy, endocarditis, aortic or mitral valvular lesions, pericarditis, and cardiac failure are features of systemic lupus erythematosus. Thyrotoxicosis or hypothyroidism can lead to encephalopathy, dementia, psychiatric disturbances, arrhythmias, hypertension, and heart failure. In acute rheumatic fever, Sydenham's chorea, tachycardia, electrocardiographic changes, pericarditis, myocarditis, and endocarditis may occur. Both cardiovascular syphilis (causing aortitis, aortic regurgitation, aortic aneurysm, or angina) and neurosyphilis (producing

*Table 14.3* New diagnostic or therapeutic cardiac catheterization procedures

| Type | Name of procedure |
| --- | --- |
| Diagnostic | Percutaneous transcatheter endomyocardial biopsy |
| | Cardiac electrophysiologic studies |
| Therapeutic | Percutaneous transluminal coronary angioplasty |
| | Percutaneous transluminal coronary stenting |
| | Percutaneous balloon or blade atrial septostomy |
| | Percutaneous balloon valvuloplasty for stenosis of pulmonic, mitral, or aortic valve |
| | Percutaneous balloon dilation for coarctation of the aorta |
| | Percutaneous transcatheter electrical ablation of accessory pathway or atrioventricular node |
| | Percutaneous transcatheter closure of congenital defects (such as patent ductus arteriosus, atrial septal defect, and ventricular septal defect) |

meningovascular syphilis, tabes dorsalis, or general paralysis of the insane) are late complications of untreated or inadequately treated infection caused by *Treponema pallidum*. Severe thiamine or vitamin B$_1$ deficiency in chronic alcoholics causes beri-beri, which is characterized by peripheral neuropathy, Wernicke's encephalopathy, Korsakoff's psychosis, anemia, and heart failure. Encephalopathy and heart failure are features of hemochromatosis. In carcinoid syndrome, excessive production and release of serotonin is associated with cerebral metastasis, valvular stenosis, and cor pulmonale. Patients with fibromuscular dysplasia or Takayasu's syndrome have hypertension and cerebrovascular ischemia. Severe electrolyte disturbances could produce encephalopathy, seizures, tetany, muscle cramp, nonspecific weakness, paresthesias, and arrhythmias.

## Neurologic Diagnoses Presenting with Cardiac Features

Although neurologic diseases presenting acutely with prominent cardiac features are uncommon, these are important clinically, as affected patients should be under the joint care of both neurologists and cardiologists. Theoretically, presence of the neurologic features and recognition of the temporal relationship between the neurologic and cardiac features would lead to the correct diagnosis. In clinical practice, confusion often exists as to whether the cardiac abnormalities are the causes or the consequences of the neurologic events. The differentiation has, however, very important implications for the subsequent management.

Various neurologic diseases (including stroke of all types, head injury, brain tumor, seizures and epilepsy, meningitis, hydrocephalus, increased intracranial pressure, multiple sclerosis, and spinal cord lesions), neurosurgical manipulation, psychiatric diseases, and strong emotional stresses can lead to disturbances in autonomic activity; cardiac arrhythmias; repolarization changes on electrocardiography; electrical, enzymatic, or pathologic evidence of myocardial damage; and disturbances of arterial blood pressure regulation. Similar alterations in autonomic activity may produce fatal cardiac arrhythmias and cause sudden death syndrome.

Autonomic neuropathy or failure may be a marked feature in neurologic conditions such as Shy-Drager syndrome, Parkinson's disease, and Guillain-Barré syndrome. Mild autonomic disturbances are reported in about 65% of patients with Guillain-Barré syndrome; these disturbances include arrhythmias, hypertension, hypotension, labile blood pressure, vasovagal spells, nonspecific electrocardiographic changes, changes in sweating, urinary retention, and paralytic ileus. Both neuromuscular features and cardiomyopathy are features of muscular dystrophies, myotonias, and hereditary ataxias.

## HIGHLIGHTS OF SOME IMPORTANT NEUROCARDIAC CONDITIONS

### Cardiogenic Embolism and Stroke

The Diagnostic Problem

One in five ischemic strokes is probably a result of cardioembolism. Nevertheless, varying degrees of uncertainty exist in the clinical diagnosis of cardioembolic stroke, because the mere existence of a potential cardiac source of embolism in a patient with cerebral ischemia is insufficient to make such a diagnosis. Other possible causes of stroke, such as carotid stenosis and prothrombotic states, are present in about 25% of stroke patients who have a cardioembolic source. Table 14.4 illustrates the clinical features and diagnostic criteria of cardioembolic stroke. Table 14.5 summarizes the commonly accepted causes of cardiogenic embolism and the consensus long-term treatment strategies. These different conditions have varying risk of causing strokes, and the chance of detecting such conditions depends on thoroughness of the evaluation.

Chronic Antithrombotic Therapy

Long-term treatment depends on the specific cardioembolic source (relating to the risk of embolism), associated conditions (such as carotid stenosis), risk of hemorrhagic complications, and purpose of therapy (i.e., primary or secondary prevention). In general, long-term anticoagulation should be considered on an individual basis in high-risk conditions unless otherwise contraindicated, and aspirin may be a useful alternative in some situations (see Table 14.5).

Anticoagulation in Acute Cardioembolic Stroke

Optimum therapy in the acute phase of cardioembolic stroke remains uncertain. The potential usefulness of early anticoagulation to prevent recurrent embolism should be balanced against the risk of causing secondary intracerebral hemorrhage. Spontaneous hemorrhagic transformation revealed on computed tomographic (CT) scan of the head occurs in up to 40% of cardioembolic strokes and most often develops within 2–4 days. A delay of 48 hours for small- to moderate-sized infarcts or 7–10 days for large infarcts before starting anticoagulation

*Table 14.4*   Clinicoradiologic features and diagnostic criteria of cardioembolic stroke

Clinical features suggesting cardioembolic stroke
    Nonprogressive onset
    Isolated hemianopia
    Wernicke's aphasia
    Ideomotor apraxia
    Paucity of vascular risk factors
Topographic features suggesting cardioembolic stroke
    Posterior division of the middle cerebral artery
    Anterior cerebral artery
    Cerebellar arteries
    Multiple territories
Neuroradiologic features suggesting cardioembolic stroke
    Superficial cortical location in the above territories
    Multifocal infarcts
    Hemorrhagic transformation
Clinical diagnosis of probable cardioembolic stroke requires all of the following:
    Presence of a cardioembolic source
    Nonlacunar stroke
    Absence of significant carotid stenosis, other causes of stroke, and major vascular risk
        factors (such as hypertension and diabetes mellitus)
Clinical diagnosis of definite cardioembolic stroke requires all of the following:
    Presence of a cardioembolic source
    Angiography showing one of the following:
        Embolic occlusion without significant atherosclerosis
        Normal findings in a nonlacunar stroke
        Normal findings in a lacunar stroke without hypertension and diabetes mellitus

is prudent, and neuroimaging should be repeated to exclude spontaneous hemorrhagic transformation prior to anticoagulation.

## Coronary Artery Disease and Myocardial Infarction

### Mechanisms Responsible for Neurologic Complications

Transient ischemic attacks and stroke complicate acute myocardial infarction. The common mechanism for ischemic stroke is cerebral embolization, and intracranial hemorrhage can be caused by systemic anticoagulation or thrombolysis. Occasionally, hemodynamic causes of cerebral hypoperfusion (secondary to arrhythmias, cardiac arrest, or left ventricular failure) are responsible for cerebral damage in the watershed territories.

### Incidence, Timing, and Risk Factors

In general, the incidence of in-hospital stroke after acute myocardial infarction is about 1–2%. Approximately one-third of the stroke complications occur simul-

*Table 14.5*   Commonly accepted causes of cardiogenic embolism and the consensus long-term treatment strategies

| Types | Causes | Consensus treatment |
|---|---|---|
| Valvular heart disease | Rheumatic heart disease,[a] especially mitral stenosis | Anticoagulation unless contraindicated |
| | Prosthetic valves,[a] especially mechanical | Anticoagulation unless contraindicated |
| | Infective endocarditis[b] | Antibiotics, ?anticoagulation |
| | Calcific aortic stenosis[a] | ?Aspirin |
| | Mitral annulus calcification[a] | Variable |
| | Nonbacterial thrombotic endocarditis | Aspirin, ?anticoagulation |
| | Mitral valve prolapse[a] | ?Aspirin |
| | Inflammatory valvulitis, e.g., Libman-Sacks endocarditis, Behçet's disease, syphilitic aortic regurgitation | According to underlying cause |
| Coronary artery disease | Acute myocardial infarction with or without mural thrombus[c] | Aspirin if without thrombus, anticoagulation if with mural thrombus |
| | Left ventricular aneurysm,[c] left ventricular dyskinesia | According to the manifestation |
| Arrhythmias associated with atrial thrombi | Atrial fibrillation[d] | Anticoagulation or aspirin according to risk profiles[e] |
| | Sick sinus syndrome | ? |
| Nonischemic cardiomyopathy | Dilating[f] | Anticoagulation unless contraindicated |
| | Hypertrophic[f] | Beta blocker, surgery |
| Prothrombotic states | Antiphospholipid antibodies syndrome | ? |
| Intracardiac tumors | Primary, e.g., atrial myxoma | Surgery |
| | Metastatic (rare) | Palliative, ?surgery |
| Paradoxical emboli | Atrial septal defects[g] | ? |
| | Patent foramen ovale[h] | ? |
| | Ventricular septal defects[g] | ? |
| | Pulmonary arteriovenous fistulas | ? |
| Others | Atrial septal aneurysms | ? |
| | Invasive cardiologic procedures[h] | Prevention |

? = controversial or unknown.

[a]See subsection on valvular heart disease.

[b]See subsection on infective endocarditis, and Tables 14.9 and 14.10.

[c]See subsection on coronary artery disease and myocardial infarction.

[d]See subsection on nonvalvular atrial fibrillation.

[e]See Table 14.6.

[f]See subsection on cardiomyopathy.

[g]See subsection on congenital heart disease.

[h]See subsection on neurologic complications of invasive cardiologic procedures and Table 14.2.

taneously with acute myocardial infarction, and more than 90% occur within the first 2 weeks. These stroke complications are clinically important, as they worsen the prognosis. Risk factors for the occurrence of stroke complicating myocardial infarction include large infarct size (as reflected by a greater rise in the cardiac enzyme levels), apical or anterior infarction (as compared with inferior myocardial infarction), low cardiac output state or left ventricular failure, presence of atrial fibrillation or flutter, older age, and previous history of stroke.

## Mural Thrombus

Many of these risk factors are associated with the presence of mural thrombus. Nevertheless, systematic echocardiographic studies reveal a high incidence of mural thrombus in patients with acute myocardial infarction (40–67%) and in those with healed or older infarction (approximately 25%). Thus, clinically evident cerebral embolism occurs in a small proportion of patients harboring mural thrombi. Pedunculated or mobile mural thrombi appear to have a higher propensity for systemic embolism. Systemic anticoagulation does not improve the overall mortality nor reduce the incidence of mural thrombus after myocardial infarction, but it lessens the risk of systemic embolism. While large, randomized, placebo-controlled clinical trials are awaited to define the role of anticoagulation in acute myocardial infarction, anticoagulation therapy for patients with postinfarction left ventricular thrombus is prudent in the absence of contraindication, and aspirin is a useful alternative.

## Left Ventricular Aneurysm

Postinfarction left ventricular aneurysm, a localized cavitary protrusion of the left ventricular free wall, complicates 7–10% of cases of acute myocardial infarction, especially apical-septal myocardial infarction. Patients with left ventricular aneurysm are at risk of congestive heart failure, ventricular arrhythmias, and systemic embolism. Despite the high incidence of an associated mural thrombus, the overall risk of clinically evident cerebral embolism in left ventricular aneurysm remains low (about 3%).

## Thrombolysis and Neurologic Complications

Current standard management of acute myocardial infarction includes thrombolytic therapy. Although thrombolysis reduces the mortality from acute myocardial infarction, it carries a 1–2% risk of intracerebral hemorrhage; half of these hemorrhages are fatal. Pooled data from placebo-controlled thrombolysis trials and comparative trials of thrombolytic agents indicate no overall increase in stroke risk but a change in the subtypes of stroke. Because patients with recent or previous strokes were excluded from these trials, the risk of stroke found in these thrombolytic studies was an underestimate. Nevertheless, thrombolytic therapy increases the risk of stroke on the day of and day after thrombolysis; these are mostly hemorrhagic strokes or intracerebral hemorrhages and are often fatal or disabling. Thrombolysis-related hemorrhagic strokes are usually lobar but occasionally occur in the thalamus and cerebellum; sometimes hemorrhages are multiple. Conversely, thrombolysis salvages ischemic myocardium, lessens wall motion abnormalities, and achieves direct lysis of intracardiac thrombus, and thus reduces the incidence of ischemic stroke. Use of tissue plasminogen activator or anisoylated plasminogen streptokinase activator complex is associated with a higher risk of stroke than use of streptokinase, because of an increased risk of intracerebral hemorrhage. Adding aspirin appears to reduce the risk of stroke after acute myocardial infarction, whereas heparin anticoagulation is not useful.

## Nonvalvular Atrial Fibrillation

### Prevalence, Pathogenesis, and Clinical Importance

Three percent of the population over age 65 have atrial fibrillation, and the prevalence increases sharply with rising age. Decline in the frequency of rheumatic heart disease has made nonvalvular atrial fibrillation the single most common cause of this cardiac arrhythmia (accounting for about 80–90% of all cases). Atrial fibrillation increases the risk of stroke mainly by systemic embolization of stasis-induced thrombi that form in the left atrium or left atrial appendage. Nevertheless, the associated cardiac abnormalities, coexistent cardiovascular diseases, and intrinsic cerebrovascular diseases may account for 25–33% of the strokes associated with atrial fibrillation. Owing to its frequent occurrence, nonvalvular atrial fibrillation probably accounts for 45% of all cardioembolic stroke. In addition, silent cerebral infarcts revealed on CT of the head are present in about 25% of patients with nonvalvular atrial fibrillation and are often multiple or bilateral.

### Optimum Long-Term Management for Primary Prevention

Despite the absence of proof from well-designed randomized clinical trials, systemic anticoagulation with warfarin sodium is the accepted standard treatment for patients with both valvular heart disease and atrial fibrillation; the risk of stroke is 17 times that for comparable control subjects. Conversely, randomized trials have revealed the risk of stroke (about 5% per year or six times that of control subjects) in patients with nonvalvular atrial fibrillation and have proved the safety and benefit of long-term anticoagulation with warfarin sodium. As determined by meta-analysis, the overall relative risk reduction for stroke among patients treated with warfarin sodium as compared with placebo is 64%, and the corresponding benefit of aspirin is 22%.

Despite close monitoring, low-intensity anticoagulation (with international normalized ratios between 2 and 3) carries an extra risk of severe bleeding of about 1%, including an annual incidence of 0.3% for intracerebral hemorrhage. Older patients (more than 75 years) have a higher risk of stroke but are more sensitive to toxicity from oral anticoagulation. Paroxysmal atrial fibrillation or concomitant asymptomatic carotid stenosis does not increase the risk of thromboembolism or stroke. Thus, high-risk patients with atrial fibrillation (Table 14.6) should be given anticoagulation therapy with warfarin sodium if there is no contraindication. An international normalized ratio of 2–3 is safe and effective for those aged 75 years or

*Table 14.6*  Factors associated with a higher risk of thromboembolic stroke in nonvalvular atrial fibrillation

| Types | Factors |
|---|---|
| Clinical | Older than 65 yrs |
| | Hypertension |
| | Diabetes mellitus |
| | Recent heart failure |
| | Previous history of stroke |
| | Transient ischemic attack |
| Echocardiographic | Enlarged left atrium |
| | Left ventricular dysfunctions |

younger, whereas a ratio of 2 seems to be logical for those older than 75 years. Low-risk patients with atrial fibrillation and those with contraindications for warfarin sodium should be given aspirin at 325 mg per day to prevent stroke.

## Secondary Prevention of Stroke

In the absence of contraindication, anticoagulation is indicated for secondary prevention of stroke in patients with atrial fibrillation to reduce the risk of recurrence (10% per year). Oral anticoagulation should be delayed for a few days to a week or more for a sizable infarction to reduce the risk of hemorrhagic transformation of the bland infarct. Other causes of stroke should also be investigated, however; for example, elective carotid endarterectomy should be performed for ipsilateral severe carotid stenosis before chronic anticoagulation. Significant carotid stenosis is present in about 12% of elderly patients with atrial fibrillation.

## Coincidental Carotid Stenosis

### Coronary Artery Disease, Carotid Stenosis, and Atherosclerosis

As many as 40% of patients with carotid disease have asymptomatic coronary artery disease, and patients with asymptomatic carotid bruit have increased risk of myocardial infarction. Pathologically, carotid stenosis is secondary to atherosclerosis in the great majority of cases. Fibromuscular dysplasia and other rare conditions cause carotid stenosis very occasionally. Carotid stenosis causes amaurosis fugax, retinal stroke, hemispheric transient ischemic attack, and ischemic stroke on the ipsilateral side by two main mechanisms: thromboembolic and hemodynamic.

### Medical Management

The best medical treatment of all vascular risk factors together with aspirin (or ticlopidine hydrochloride in cases of aspirin intolerance or failure) should be offered to all patients with carotid stenosis. A high-quality and reliable ultrasonographic

*Table 14.7*   Factors associated with a higher risk of thromboembolic stroke
in carotid stenosis

---

Cerebrovascular ischemic symptoms
Severe degree of stenosis
Plaque ulceration
Contralateral stenosis or occlusion
Inadequate collateral circulation
Large number of vascular risk factors
Cerebral infarction on neuroimaging

---

assessment of the presence, location, and severity of the stenosis is essential, and the nature of the plaque should be determined, if possible.

## Carotid Endarterectomy

Despite improvement in the perioperative risk and the angiographic technique, elective carotid endarterectomy in good surgical centers carries a significant perioperative risk of stroke and death (2–6%). Thus, the risk of stroke without endarterectomy (Table 14.7), the chance of nonstroke death, the risk of angiography, and the perioperative mortality and morbidity should be carefully considered before recommending elective carotid endarterectomy. In general, patients with transient ischemic attacks related to severe carotid stenosis have a 12–13% rate of stroke in the first year and a cumulative rate of 30–35% in 5 years, whereas those presenting with strokes have a 5–9% annual rate of recurrence and a 5-year rate of 25–45%. After successful carotid endarterectomy, patients who presented with transient ischemic attacks continue to have a 1–2% annual risk of ipsilateral hemispheric stroke, whereas a presenting history of stroke carries a 2–3% per year rate of subsequent ipsilateral stroke. The risk of stroke in asymptomatic carotid disease is low: an annual rate below 2% if the linear stenosis is 60% or less, and an annual stroke rate of 2% or more when the stenosis is more than 60%. Current guidelines for carotid endarterectomy for symptomatic or asymptomatic stenosis are summarized in Table 14.8.

## Combined Coronary and Carotid Surgery

The optimal strategy for managing patients with combined coronary artery and carotid disease remains unresolved. Meta-analysis of the available reports indicates that combined carotid and coronary surgery carries the same perioperative stroke rate as when carotid endarterectomy precedes coronary artery bypass grafting and that the stroke rate is highest if carotid surgery follows coronary surgery. Nevertheless, the risk of myocardial infarction or death is greater when carotid surgery precedes coronary artery bypass grafting. Thus, a prospective randomized trial is needed to resolve the controversy.

*Table 14.8*   Current guidelines for carotid endarterectomy for symptomatic or asymptomatic stenosis[a]

| Types | Indications for carotid endarterectomy |
|---|---|
| Symptomatic | Proven: Good-risk patients with 70–99% stenosis plus <6% perioperative morbidity and mortality rate |
| | Not proven: <70% stenosis plus 6% surgical risk; surgical risk approaches 10% plus any degree of stenosis |
| | Acceptable: <70% stenosis in an ongoing prospective contemporary randomized trial plus <6% surgical risk; 50–69% stenosis without the option of referral to a randomized trial plus <6% surgical risk |
| Asymptomatic | Proven: None |
| | Acceptable: ≥75% stenosis plus <3% surgical risk[b] |
| | Not proven: ≥3% surgical risk plus any degree of stenosis |

[a]Degree of stenosis is measured according to the method used in the North American Symptomatic Carotid Endarterectomy Trial.
[b]The Asymptomatic Carotid Atherosclerosis Study (ACAS) reported a statistically significant 53% relative risk reduction in favor of carotid endarterectomy in asymptomatic persons with linear stenosis of 60% or more. Nevertheless, the absolute risk reduction is only 5.9% over 5 years, and the positive results are critically dependent on a remarkably low perioperative rate of 2.3%. In addition, women were not found to benefit from the surgery, and no information was available to indicate any higher risk subgroup in which carotid endarterectomy for asymptomatic stenosis may be more appropriate. More important, no difference in the risk of disabling stroke was present between the surgical and medical arms of the ACAS.

# Valvular Heart Disease

The major neurologic complications of valvular heart disease are cerebral embolization, dizziness, and syncope. Cerebral embolization is preventable with antithrombotic therapy at the expense of a slightly increased risk of major bleeding, including intracranial hemorrhage. The incidence of arterial thromboembolism varies according to the underlying cause, involved valve or valves, degree of left atrial enlargement, presence of atrial fibrillation, and age of the patient.

## Aortic Valve Disease

In general, isolated aortic valve disease is not rheumatic in origin but calcific. The risk for systemic embolization is very low in aortic valve disease (stenosis with or without regurgitation), unless it is accompanied by infective endocarditis, mitral valve disease, or atrial fibrillation; thus, systemic anticoagulation is not indicated. Exercise-related symptoms such as dizziness, syncope, arrhythmias, angina, dyspnea, and sudden death are not uncommon in moderate to severe aortic stenosis.

## Mitral Valve Disease

Despite the reduction in incidence of rheumatic heart disease, mitral valve disease (stenosis with or without regurgitation) remains the most common type of valvular disease causing arterial thromboembolism. Thrombus formation in the left atrium is related to stasis of blood, low cardiac output, degree of left atrial enlargement, and presence of atrial fibrillation; age is also a risk factor for embolization. Isolated mitral regurgitation has a lower risk of thromboembolism than mitral stenosis. Systemic anticoagulation is the accepted treatment despite the lack of scientific evidence.

Mitral Valve Prolapse

Some 5–10% of the population have mitral valve prolapse, which is associated with transient ischemic attacks, cerebral and cerebellar infarction, intracerebral and subarachnoid hemorrhage, seizures, and retinal stroke. Nevertheless, the risk of embolism is low, and prophylactic antithrombotic therapy for primary prevention of stroke is not indicated. On the other hand, when mitral valve prolapse is discovered in patients with cerebrovascular ischemic symptoms, investigations should be arranged to rule out other causes. Long-term aspirin therapy may be used in patients with mitral valve prolapse and repeated episodes of otherwise unexplained cerebral ischemic events.

Mitral Annular Calcification

Mitral annular calcification occurs more commonly in elderly females and is associated with mitral valve disease, calcific aortic stenosis, arrhythmias, infective endocarditis, and embolic stroke. Presence of mitral annular calcification appears to be an independent risk factor for stroke. The types of emboli include fibrin clots and calcific particles. Thus, anticoagulation is indicated for true thromboembolism or an associated condition like mitral valve disease or atrial fibrillation. Mitral valve replacement may be useful when anticoagulation fails or when calcific emboli are responsible for cerebrovascular ischemic symptoms.

Prosthetic Valve Disease

Successful valve replacement improves the symptoms and quality of life and prolongs the survival when the native valves are severely diseased. Artificial valves are either mechanical or tissue prostheses. Thromboembolism is a major complication of all prosthetic valves except the aortic homograft. Lifelong anticoagulation therapy is indicated for all patients with mechanical valves but remains controversial for patients with tissue valves. It is a popular practice to provide anticoagulation therapy to all bioprosthetic valve patients for 6–8 weeks initially; long-term anticoagulation therapy is reserved for those at high risk of thromboembolism as a result of other factors.

**Infective Endocarditis**

There have been changes in the epidemiology of infective endocarditis (such as increasing age of the patients, reduced prevalence of rheumatic heart disease, and

*Table 14.9*   Neurologic complications of infective endocarditis

| Complications | Mean incidence (%) |
|---|---|
| Cerebral embolization | 13.4 |
| Intracranial hemorrhage (intracerebral hemorrhage + subarachnoid hemorrhage) | 3.6 |
| Mycotic aneurysm[a] | 1.5 |
| Meningitis | 7 |
| Brain abscess | 1.9 |
| Encephalopathy | 6.4 |
| Seizure (focal + generalized) | 3.5 |
| Severe headache | 3.7 |
| Others[b] | 1.0 |

[a]Symptoms and signs attributed to expansion, leakage, or rupture.

[b]Uncommon complications include visual disturbances (from retinal emboli or cranial nerve involvement), psychiatric abnormalities, extrapyramidal features, spinal cord involvement, and peripheral nerve involvement.

rising frequency of intravenous drug abuse), its diagnosis (use of echocardiography), and its treatment (with antimicrobials and valve replacement surgery); nevertheless, there has been no alteration in the incidence of neurologic complications, which occur in about 30% (range: 20–40%) of the affected patients (Table 14.9).

## Neurologic Complications

About 16–23% of patients with infective endocarditis present with neurologic manifestations, but neurologic complications can occur later, usually within the first 2 weeks of initiation of antimicrobial therapy. Less commonly, cerebral embolization occurs months or a few years following an apparently successful course of treatment, and complications of intracranial mycotic aneurysms can develop years later. Presence of neurologic complications is associated with a worse prognosis. Table 14.10 summarizes factors that increase the risk of neurologic complications in infective endocarditis.

Cerebral embolization, the most common complication, very often affects the middle cerebral artery territories and manifests as contralateral motor or sensory deficits, aphasia, cortical sensory loss, hemianopia, and apraxia. Basal ganglia involvement produces parkinsonism or chorea, whereas brain stem damage results in dysphagia, nausea, vomiting, vertigo, dysarthria, ataxia, nystagmus, or diplopia. Occasionally, multiple microemboli cause seizures, fluctuating neurologic signs, disturbed consciousness, delirium, or psychosis. Intracranial hemorrhage is related to mycotic aneurysm, hemorrhagic transformation of cerebral infarction, and use of anticoagulants. In contrast to congenital cerebral aneurysms, which are located at the circle of Willis, intracranial mycotic aneurysms are characteristically found at the bifurcation of small secondary or tertiary branches. The middle cerebral artery is affected four times as often as in the anterior or posterior cerebral artery. Cranial nerve palsy, headache, nuchal rigidity, homonymous hemianopia, and cerebral embolization may be caused by an enlarging or leaking mycotic aneurysm. Confirmation by angiography and

*Table 14.10*    Factors associated with a higher risk of developing neurologic complications in infective endocarditis

---

Left-sided infective endocarditis

Mitral valve involvement

Presence of congestive heart failure

Infections caused by more virulent organisms (such as *Staphylococcus aureus*, *Streptococcus pneumoniae*, enterobacteriaceae, and anaerobes)

Presence of large vegetations (as a result of *Haemophilus* species, nutritionally variant streptococci, group B beta-hemolytic streptococci, fungi, and mixed microorganisms)

Intravenous drug abuse with left-sided infective endocarditis

---

Note: Systemic embolization from right-sided infective endocarditis is rare but may occur because of a patent foramen ovale or a pulmonary arteriovenous fistula or as a result of septic thrombi from pulmonary veins. Similarly, intravenous drug abusers with pure right-sided infections do not have a high risk of neurologic complications. In contrast to some previous reports, more recent reviews show that prosthetic valve endocarditis does not have increased risk for neurologic complications.

definitive treatment by surgical excision may prevent the life-threatening complications of rupture: subarachnoid or intracerebral hemorrhage. Pathogenic mechanisms for encephalopathy and seizures include abscesses, emboli, hypoxia, metabolic derangement, bacterial toxins, immunologic factors, and drug toxicity.

## Optimum Management

A full course of antimicrobial therapy remains the cornerstone of management. Initiation of antimicrobial treatment is associated temporally with a marked reduction in incidence of embolization. Neurosurgery is reserved for the complications of mycotic aneurysms, aneurysms that persist despite antimicrobial therapy, or drainage of large intracranial abscesses. The use of anticoagulation therapy in infective endocarditis is controversial. Anticoagulation in native valve infection does not prevent embolization but increases the risk of intracranial hemorrhage. On the other hand, carefully controlled anticoagulation should be maintained in prosthetic valve endocarditis. When central nervous system complications arise, anticoagulation should be temporarily stopped and investigations arranged to exclude intracranial hemorrhage.

## Cardiomyopathy

Dilated or congestive cardiomyopathy carries a significant risk of systemic and cerebral embolism, and systemic anticoagulation is advised unless otherwise contraindicated. Hypertrophic cardiomyopathy is associated with atrial fibrillation, systemic embolism, and exercise-induced syncope. Cardiomyopathy, congestive heart failure, and other cardiac abnormalities are common features of hereditary muscular dystrophies with or without myotonias.

## Congenital Heart Disease

Stroke, cerebral abscess, and mental retardation or developmental delay are neurologic complications of congenital heart disease. The advent of surgical repair and palliative procedures has improved the prognosis and prolonged the survival of patients with congenital heart disease. Thus, spontaneously occurring neurologic complications have become less common, whereas complications from invasive cardiologic procedures and surgery have increased in frequency. Infective endocarditis remains a potential risk in all types of congenital heart disease, especially in the presence of prosthetic materials or artificial valves. Serious bradyarrhythmias or tachyarrhythmias may cause dizziness, syncope, and seizures.

### Cyanotic Congenital Heart Disease

Fallot's tetralogy and transposition of the great arteries are the common types of cyanotic congenital heart disease in which the right-to-left shunt is associated with severe hypoxemia and a variety of hematologic abnormalities. The latter includes polycythemia, hyperviscosity, and consumptive coagulopathy (causing thrombocytopenia, hypofibrinogenemia, and deficiency in clotting factors). Thus, there is increased risk for thrombotic cerebral infarction, embolic stroke (from peripheral venous thrombosis and paradoxical embolism), cerebral venous sinus thrombosis, cerebral abscess, and intracerebral hemorrhage. Sometimes, a prolonged hypercyanotic spell may cause syncope, seizure, hypoxic brain damage, or even death.

### Acyanotic Congenital Heart Disease

Common types of acyanotic congenital heart disease encountered in adults include atrial septal defect, ventricular septal defect, and coarctation of the aorta. The slightly increased risk of embolic stroke in cases of congenital septal defect is probably a result of paradoxical embolization during a Valsalva maneuver. Patients with atrial septal defects have an increased risk of developing chronic atrial fibrillation. Coarctation of aorta is associated with intracranial arterial aneurysms, congenital cerebral arteriovenous fistulas, and systemic hypertension, and so there is an increased risk for stroke. Rarely, dilated collateral arteries within the spinal canal may compress the spinal cord and cause paraplegia.

## Syncope

Syncope is a common complaint. Although cardiac and arrhythmic causes predominate, neurologic or other disorders can also produce syncopes (Table 14.11). Evaluation of syncope begins with history-taking and physical examination. The history may reveal features of vertebrobasilar transient ischemic attacks, seizures, subclavian steal syndrome, cardioneurogenic syncope, or an underlying cardiac disorder. The physical examination should be focused on the neurologic and cardiovascular systems. Twelve-lead electrocardiography and serum electrolyte test-

*Table 14.11*   Major causes of syncope

Cardiac arrhythmias
    Cardioneurogenic syncope (also known as vasovagal, vasoreactive, or reflex syncope)
    Bradycardias resulting from sinus node dysfunction, atrioventricular node disorder, or
       His-Purkinje disease
    Tachyarrhythmias caused by supraventricular or ventricular tachycardia, or ventricular
       fibrillation
Mechanical cardiac disorders
    Valvular stenosis (including aortic, mitral, or pulmonary valves)
    Prosthetic valve obstruction
    Obstructive cardiomyopathy
    Left atrial myxoma
    Aortic dissection
    Pulmonary embolus
    Pulmonary hypertension
Neurologic diseases
    Vertebrobasilar transient ischemic attacks
    Subclavian steal syndrome
    Normal pressure hydrocephalus
    Seizures
Metabolic conditions
    Hyperventilation
    Hypoxia
    Hypoglycemia
Psychiatric diagnoses
    Panic attacks
    Hysteria

ing are essential in the baseline assessment. Choice of subsequent investigations depends on the results of the initial evaluation. Thus, electroencephalography, neuroimaging, or angiography are indicated for neurologic causes. Tilt-table testing, which is useful in cardioneurogenic syncope, may be omitted if the history is classic, because treatment should be initiated anyway. Further cardiologic investigations, including echocardiography, treadmill exercise testing, Holter monitoring, and cardiac catheterization, are considered if cardiac causes are suspected or if the cause remains unclear; referral to a cardiologist should be arranged.

## Cardiovascular Consequences of Central Nervous System Disease

### Neural Control of Cardiovascular Functions

The brain controls cardiovascular functions through the autonomic nervous system and endocrine-humoral system, although the heart can function in an autonomous and isolated manner. This brain-heart control enables second-to-second regulation of cardiac activity and vasomotor tone in response to physical activities, threats, and stresses, and changes in emotional state. Apart from normal cardiovascular control, the central nervous system can alter cardiovascular functions and produce serious consequences under certain abnormal conditions.

## Mechanisms of Neurogenic Cardiovascular Disturbance

The peripheral mechanisms of neurogenic cardiovascular disturbance include an increase in the sympathetic nervous discharge, hypersecretion of adrenomedullary catecholamines, and a change in the parasympathetic nervous activity. The central mechanisms, however, are uncertain. Evidence from both experimental and clinical research has shifted the attention from the hypothalamus, brain stem cardiovascular centers, and spinal autonomic outflows to the cortical and subcortical regions such as the insular cortex and amygdala as possible sites of origin of neurogenic cardiovascular dysfunction.

## Causes and Types of Neurogenic Cardiovascular Disturbance

As mentioned before, neurologic conditions, neurosurgery, psychiatric diseases, and emotional stresses can produce various combinations of cardiovascular disturbances of different degrees of severity. Presence of these disturbances may either worsen the general condition or be associated with a poorer prognosis. Thus, the caring physician should be alerted of such possibilities, and patients who manifest neurogenic cardiovascular dysfunctions should be put under close monitoring, preferably in an intensive care setting. These neurogenic or cerebrogenic cardiovascular effects can be grouped into the following categories: (1) myocardial ischemia, (2) cardiac arrhythmias, (3) disturbances of blood pressure regulation, and (4) neurogenic pulmonary edema.

### Myocardial Ischemia

Acute neurologic conditions have long been known to cause myocardial ischemia in the absence of acute coronary events, as evidenced by electrocardiographic changes, elevation of cardiac enzymes, and myocardial pathologic changes. The reported electrocardiographic changes include prolonged QT intervals, depressed ST segments, flat or inverted T waves, U waves, tall peaked T waves, notched T waves, elevated ST segments, peaked P waves, Q waves, and increased QRS amplitudes. These changes usually evolve for several days and disappear within 2 weeks, except that QT prolongation or U waves may become permanent.

Elevation of cardiac enzymes has been observed in many but not all patients with neurogenic electrocardiographic changes. This elevation cannot be explained by contamination from skeletal muscle enzymes, because the cardiospecific isoenzyme creatine kinase myocardial band (CK-MB) is often increased in patients with neurogenic electrocardiographic changes but is undetectable in those without such changes. In addition, a significant correlation has been found between the elevation of CK-MB and the presence of electrocardiographic changes and cardiac arrhythmias in acute stroke patients. Unlike in myocardial infarction, CK-MB levels rise slowly after stroke and peak on around day 4.

Postmortem examination of the heart reveals focal myocytolysis, myofibrillar degeneration, subendocardial congestion or hemorrhages, lipofuscin pigment deposition in myofibrils, and histiocytic infiltration. These pathologic changes are unrelated to coronary artery disease but may be experimentally reproduced either by increasing the sympathetic nervous activity or by infusing catecholamines.

## Cardiac Arrhythmias

Cardiac arrhythmias are particularly common in subarachnoid hemorrhage and seizures, but they can also occur in other neurologic conditions and with neurosurgical procedures. The types of arrhythmia include bradycardia, supraventricular tachycardias, atrial flutter, atrial fibrillation, ectopic ventricular beats, multifocal ventricular tachycardias, torsades de pointes, ventricular flutter, and ventricular fibrillation.

Evidence suggests that asymmetric innervation of the heart by the autonomic nervous system or imbalance between the sympathetic and parasympathetic components are important pathogenic mechanisms of neurogenic cardiac arrhythmias. In general, the predominant innervation of the sinoatrial and atrioventricular nodes comes from the parasympathetic nervous system, whereas the ventricular muscle is affected more by the sympathetic nervous system. The right vagus nerve has more effect on the sinoatrial node, whereas the left vagus nerve has more influence on the atrioventricular node. The left stellate ganglion or the left-sided sympathetic activity is much more arrhythmogenic than the right cardiac sympathetic innervation. Although these neurogenic cardiac arrhythmias are usually transient, severe hypotension, cardiogenic embolism, secondary brain damage, and sudden unexpected death can be the consequences.

## Disturbances of Blood Pressure Regulation

Various conditions of the central nervous system can produce acute hypertension, profound hypotension, or orthostatic hypotension. Acute hypertension secondary to sympathoadrenal hyperactivity has been found in patients who have ischemic, degenerative, or neoplastic lesions of the hypothalamus, medulla oblongata, or posterior fossa. The classic Cushing response of hypertension, bradycardia, and apnea can be caused by different kinds of damage within the posterior fossa or by raised intracranial pressure. The immediate mechanism appears to involve ischemia or distortion of the dorsal medulla along the floor of the fourth ventricle. Acute hypertension is a common finding in seizures, epilepsy, and stroke.

Hypotension associated with spinal shock is well recognized. Rarely, destructive lesions involving the rostral ventrolateral medulla (the medullary sympathetic center) or its outflow pathways result in profound hypotension resembling spinal shock. Nevertheless, arrhythmia-induced hypotension is more common.

Despite postural changes, arterial blood pressure is well maintained because of the baroreceptor reflex. The latter can be impaired by interruption of the central pathways, as occurs, for example, in Shy-Drager syndrome.

*Neurogenic Pulmonary Edema*

The mechanisms of neurogenic pulmonary edema are transiently increased pulmonary intravascular pressure and more prolonged pulmonary capillary leakage. The second mechanism results in a protein-rich fluid, which is not found in cardiogenic pulmonary edema. Neurogenic pulmonary edema has been observed in cases of subarachnoid hemorrhage, generalized seizures, head injury, increased intracranial pressure, focal lesions or surgical manipulation of the hypothalamus or brain stem, and bulbar poliomyelitis.

## APPROACH TO NEUROLOGIC CONSULTATIONS FROM CARDIOLOGY

The evaluation begins with the history, physical examination, results of investigations that are already available, and the clinical circumstances. In most cases, a neurologic diagnosis or a short list of differential diagnoses is apparent from the history and physical examination. The results of investigations that are already available and the clinical circumstances are helpful in the analysis of the possible relationship between the neurologic condition and the cardiac disease. This analysis is crucial because it permits the inclusion of all potential diagnoses, provides guidance in the selection of appropriate investigations, suggests the correct diagnosis while awaiting confirmation, and directs the definitive therapy.

Diagnosing a coincidental neurologic disease should be straightforward, and the appropriate investigation should be arranged. Management depends mainly on the neurologic diagnosis. Sometimes, the coexisting cardiac condition influences the choice of management.

When the neurologic condition is a complication of the underlying cardiac disease, the management should include appropriate investigations and treatment of both the cardiac and neurologic conditions, long-term prophylactic therapy, and consideration of immediate treatment to prevent early recurrence. The risk and benefit of any prophylactic measure should be carefully considered on an individual basis. In general, results from prospective randomized trials provide the best reference in the decision-making process.

Polypharmacy is common in hospital inpatients, especially in the elderly. The list of medications should be under constant review, and any unnecessary medication should be discontinued. Otherwise, the management of medication-related neurologic complications is conservative and supportive. In addition, efforts and attention should be directed to the prevention of these complications. Very occasionally, specific antidotes or detoxification measures are used.

Neurologic complications of invasive cardiologic procedures are highly situation-specific, and the risk of spontaneous recurrence is low. The management is mainly supportive, with appropriate investigations to define the extent of neurologic damage. As most of these complications are potentially preventable, appropriate precautions, prophylactic measures, and meticulous techniques should be ensured in the cardiac catheterization laboratory.

In multisystem disease with both neurologic and cardiac features, appropriate investigations should be arranged early to confirm the diagnosis so that the correct management may be initiated. Not uncommonly, both the neurologic and cardiac manifestations require their own specific treatments.

Advances in both clinical and basic research on neurogenic cardiovascular disturbances are beginning to unravel the central and peripheral pathogenic mechanisms, anatomic substrates, and neurotransmitter and neuropeptide changes, as well as the real magnitude of this important clinical problem. At this stage, the possibility of a neurologic disease with secondary cardiovascular features should always be considered. Management, jointly provided by a neurologist and a cardiologist, should include close monitoring plus appropriate investigations and treatment of both the neurologic and cardiovascular features. As the neurologic condition becomes stabilized, the cardiovascular complications usually disappear. Thus, long-term cardiovascular treatment is rarely required.

## SUGGESTED READING

Barnett HJM, Meldrum HE, Eliasziw M. The dilemma of surgical treatment for patients with asymptomatic carotid disease. Ann Intern Med 1995;123:723–725.

Dalos NP, Borel C, Hanley DF. Cardiovascular autonomic dysfunction in Guillain-Barré syndrome: therapeutic implications of Swan-Ganz monitoring. Arch Neurol 1988;45:115–117.

Davis PH, Hachinski VC. The cardiac factor in stroke. Curr Opin Neurol Neurosurg 1992;5:39–43.

Executive Committee for the Asymptomatic Carotid Atherosclerosis Study. Endarterectomy for asymptomatic carotid artery stenosis. JAMA 1995;273:1421–1428.

Fogoros RN. Cardiac arrhythmias—syncope and stroke. Neurol Clin 1993;11:375–389.

Furlan AJ, Sila CA, Chimowitz MI, Jones SC. Neurologic complications related to cardiac surgery. Neurol Clin 1992;10:145–166.

Hachinski VC. The clinical problem of brain and heart. Stroke 1993;24[suppl I]:I-1–I-2.

Hart RG. Cardiogenic embolism to the brain. Lancet 1992;339:589–594.

Hart RG, Halperin JL. Atrial fibrillation and stroke—revisiting the dilemmas. Stroke 1994;25:1337–1341.

Hess DC, D'Cruz IA, Adams RJ, Nichols FT III. Coronary artery disease, myocardial infarction, and brain embolism. Neurol Clin 1993;11:399–417.

Moore WS, Barnett HJM, Beebe HG, et al. Guidelines for carotid endarterectomy—a multidisciplinary consensus statement from the Ad Hoc Committee, American Heart Association. Stroke 1995;26:188–201.

Oppenheimer SM, Cechetto DF, Hachinski VC. Cerebrogenic cardiac arrhythmias: cerebral electrocardiographic influences and their role in sudden death. Arch Neurol 1990;47:513–519.

Oppenheimer SM, Hachinski VC. The cardiac consequences of stroke. Neurol Clin 1992;10:167–176.

Park SC, Neches WH. The neurologic complications of congenital heart disease. Neurol Clin 1993;11:441–462.

Samuels MA. Neurally induced cardiac damage. Neurol Clin 1993;11:273–291.

Talman WT. Cardiovascular regulation and lesion of the central nervous system. Ann Neurol 1985;18:1–12.

Tunkel AR, Kaye D. Neurologic complications of infective endocarditis. Neurol Clin 1993;11:419–440.

Usher BW. Cardiac valvular disease and stroke. Neurol Clin 1993;11:391–398.

# 15
# Rheumatic Diseases

Patricia M. Moore

The rheumatic diseases are characterized by inflammation and autoimmune tissue injury that usually affects connective tissues, blood vessels, joints, and muscles. The pattern and extent of disease as well as specific serologic, histologic, and, sometimes, radiographic features render individual diseases distinctive. Typically, these disorders are multisystemic, but occasionally a single organ may be involved. Neurologic abnormalities, prominent in some disorders, occasionally herald the disease. Some of the rheumatic diseases occur frequently. Rheumatoid arthritis has an incidence in the United States of 1 in 100 persons. Other disorders such as some of the vasculitides are distinctly unusual. In Table 15.1, the disorders are classified into three groups: the vasculitides, the connective tissue diseases, and the chronic inflammatory disorders.

The neurologist encounters patients with these diseases in several settings. In some cases, a neurologic abnormality is an early problem, and the physician must help decide if there is an underlying connective tissue disease or vasculitis. In other cases, the patient has an established diagnosis and a new neurologic event that may indicate (1) undertreated disease, (2) a complication of treatment or infection, or (3) an initially inaccurate diagnosis requiring revision.

Because the causes of systemic inflammation and its consequences on the nervous system are broad and many of the underlying diseases may be difficult to diagnose early, this chapter provides some broad outlines to the approach, describes some of these diseases, and suggests potential pitfalls in interpreting neurodiagnostic studies.

Almost by definition, patients with rheumatic disease have immunologic abnormalities. Immune derangements may result from the underlying disease or from the therapies used to treat the disease. This fact has practical importance because these patients are quite susceptible to infections and, indeed, have a high rate of infections with a variety of organisms. Thus, the first advice for the neurologic consultant is to *be vigilant for infections* and to recognize the limitations of studies (such as a sin-

*Table 15.1*    Rheumatic disorders

Vasculitides
    Hypersensitivity vasculitis
    Polyarteritis nodosa
    Churg-Strauss angiitis
    Wegener's granulomatosis
    Lymphomatoid granulomatosis
    Temporal arteritis
    Takayasu's arteritis
    Isolated angiitis of the central nervous system
    Behçet's disease
Connective tissue diseases
    Systemic lupus erythematosus
    Sjögren's syndrome
    Rheumatoid arthritis
    Progressive systemic sclerosis
    Polymyositis/dermatomyositis
Chronic, undifferentiated inflammatory disorders
    Cryoglobulinemia
    Undifferentiated tissue disease

gle spinal fluid analysis in an immunosuppressed patient) in the diagnosis. The next point is to *be cautious in the interpretation of blood studies*. A serologic study such as the antinuclear antibody (ANA) titer is not specific for any disease; it may indicate chronic inflammation from many sources. When possible, identify and treat the source of inflammation. The third precept is to *initiate therapy with glucocorticoids or immunosuppressants only with a clear therapeutic goal, a framework for the duration of therapy, and knowledge of the side effects of medication.*

## CLINICAL CLASSIFICATION

### Idiopathic Vasculitides

The vasculitides are a group of disorders characterized by inflammation of the blood vessel wall with attendant tissue injury. Ischemia is the common denominator of tissue injury. Classification of vasculitic syndromes incorporates clinical, radiologic, and pathologic features. Identification of any underlying cause of vasculitis is central to the management, as this guides treatment [1–4].

Case 1

    A 47-year-old man in excellent health, except for a transient left median nerve mononeuropathy 6 months earlier, developed low-grade fevers and a 10-lb weight loss over 3 weeks. He described abdominal and right flank pain 2 days before admission. On the day of admission, he awakened with headache and dizziness and went to an acute care center. On general and neurologic examinations, the following were notable: (1) diaphoresis and skin pallor, (2) blood pressure of 170/110 mm Hg, (3) left VI cranial neuropathy, and (4) right common peroneal neuropathy.

Laboratory studies revealed an erythrocyte sedimentation rate of 45 mm per hour, ANA titer of 1:64, hepatitis B + antigenemia, and urinalysis with proteinuria and red blood cell casts. Further, renal angiography revealed multiple aneurysms. Sural nerve biopsy demonstrated inflammation and necrosis in the wall of several arterioles.

## Polyarteritis Nodosa

Polyarteritis nodosa (PAN), classically a systemic necrotizing vasculitis, affects small and medium-sized muscular arteries, especially bifurcations and branchings. Clinically, the disease affects the kidneys, musculoskeletal system, nervous system, gastrointestinal tract, skin, heart, and genitourinary system. Hypertension is present in more than half the patients. Laboratory findings may reflect systemic inflammation but are not diagnostic. Diagnosis depends on angiography and biopsy. Peripheral neuropathies, which may be the presenting manifestation of PAN, occur in 60% of patients. Six major patterns of neuropathy, mononeuropathy multiplex, extensive mononeuropathy multiplex, polyneuropathy, cutaneous neuropathy, brachial plexopathy, and radiculopathy may appear. Central nervous system (CNS) abnormalities, including encephalopathies, subarachnoid hemorrhage, seizures, strokes, and cranial neuropathies, develop in 40% of patients. These usually occur in the course of the disease [5–14].

## Churg-Strauss Syndrome

Churg-Strauss syndrome (CSS) was first described in 1951 in an autopsy study of 13 patients with asthma, eosinophilia, and a systemic illness. The disease is often heralded by rhinitis and then increasingly severe asthma. This prodrome may precede the onset of vasculitis by 2–20 years. Clinical and hematologic features distinguish it from PAN. Early features may include anemia, weight loss, heart failure, recurrent pneumonia, and bloody diarrhea. Pulmonary involvement is typical in CSS and rare in PAN. Similarly, the eosinophilia that is characteristic of CSS is not a feature of PAN. Cutaneous manifestations include palpable purpura, erythema, and subcutaneous nodules. The disease involves the peripheral nerves, and kidneys are involved in 60–65% of patients.

Histologically, medium-sized and small vessels are affected. Debate continues over the necessity for strict histologic criteria (necrotizing vasculitis, tissue infiltration by eosinophils, and extravascular granuloma) to establish a diagnosis. Studies of the potential mechanisms for vascular and tissue injury center on the eosinophil [15,16]. The two diagnostically essential lesions are angiitis and extravascular necrotizing granulomas, usually with eosinophilic infiltrates [17]. In any single biopsy specimen, however, the changes may appear very similar to those in PAN.

Neurologic abnormalities are similar to those in PAN, but the occurrence of encephalopathies early in the course of the disease is more frequent in CSS and probably reflects the small size of vessels involved [18]. CNS abnormalities include memory loss, confusion, seizures, subarachnoid hemorrhage, and chorea [19–21]. Visual abnormalities are a prominent part of the disease [22,23]. In the absence of histologic evidence of vasculitis in the brain, however, the frequency of cerebrovascular inflammatory disease remains conjectural. Peripheral neuropathies are a prominent manifestation of CSS. In 38% of cases in one series, peripheral neuropathies were the predominant clinical feature of the disease. Overall, 50–75% of patients have some manifestation of neuropathy. Peripheral neuropathies classically present as mononeuropathies multiplex, but polyneuropathies also occur [15–21,23–26].

Laboratory features reflect general systemic inflammation. Although the erythrocyte sedimentation rate is elevated, and ANAs may be present in low titer, no autoantibodies are diagnostic of the disease. Antineutrophil cytoplasmic antibodies (ANCAs) are not reliably present. Thus, the clinical features again provide the critical information for diagnosis. Characteristically, the triad of asthma, eosinophilia, and vasculitis in two extrapulmonary organs defines the disease. Neurologic abnormalities are similar to those in PAN with an increased incidence of encephalopathies, which may occur early in the course of the disease. Peripheral neuropathies are common. Adult-onset asthma, particularly in association with eosinophilia, should suggest the diagnosis.

## Hypersensitivity Vasculitis

Hypersensitivity vasculitis, the most frequently encountered of all the vasculitides, is a heterogeneous group of clinical syndromes characterized by inflammation of small vessels, most prominently the venules. The skin is the organ most affected. In many instances, the vessel inflammation can be identified as a response to a precipitating antigen such as a drug, foreign protein, or microbe. Several groups of hypersensitivity vasculitis, including serum sickness, Henoch-Schönlein purpura, and vasculitis with mixed cryoglobulinemia, have distinctive clinicopathologic characteristics. Involvement of the nervous system is variable. Neurologic abnormalities are frequent in serum sickness and include encephalopathy, seizures, stroke, brachial plexopathy, and peripheral neuropathies. In other subgroups of hypersensitive vasculitis, neurologic involvement is unusual. Occasional reports of subarachnoid hemorrhage and peripheral neuropathies exist [27–32].

## Case 2

A 54-year-old man presented with a history of 4 months of progressive hearing loss in his right ear. He described a chronic nonproductive cough. Two days before admission he developed acute onset of diplopia most prominent on gaze left. The day of admission he complained of acute flank pain and blood in his urine.

General physical examination revealed a thin, ill-appearing man with a blood pressure of 172/94 mm Hg and pulse of 92. His left eye was ecchymotic, and some blood was crusted around his nostril. His chest examination revealed bilateral rhonchi, but his heart had a regular rate and rhythm without murmurs, rubs, or gallops. Neurologic examination revealed a normal level of arousal, intact cognition, and an appropriate affect. He had left sixth-cranial-nerve, seventh-cranial-nerve, and right eighth-cranial-nerve palsies. Although his motor examination was normal, there was bilateral symmetric diminished sensation in his feet.

Laboratory studies included a chest radiograph revealing bilateral nodular infiltrates, urinalysis with red cell casts and 3+ proteinuria, and electrocardiogram (ECG) showing a sinus tachycardia. His sedimentation rate was 85 mm per hour, ANA titer was 1:640, and cytoplasmic ANCA (cANCA) was 1:2,560. Bronchoscopy with biopsy revealed a necrotizing vasculitis with prominent granuloma.

## Wegener's Granulomatosis

Wegener's granulomatosis is a systemic necrotizing vasculitis with a characteristic organ specificity. The involvement of the upper and lower respiratory tracts with granulomatous vasculitis, together with a necrotizing glomerulonephritis, is quite distinctive. Histologically, granulomata are prominent in the vasculitic lesions. The diagnosis is often suggested by cough, hemoptysis, or recurrent sinus abnormalities in a patient with systemic inflammation. Neurologic abnormalities, particularly cranial neuropathies, may be among the presenting manifestations of the disease. Ocular abnormalities, including proptosis and inflammation of the anterior structures of the eye, occur in just under half of the patients. Wegener's granulomatosis is unusual among the vasculitides in the strong association between the disease and an autoantibody, cANCA. Classic cANCA is strongly associated with Wegener's granulomatosis and microscopic polyarteritis, whereas the peripheral perinuclear ANCA (pANCA) is nonspecific for disease. Controversy still exists over whether these antibodies are serologic markers for disease activity, are pathogenic, or neither. In Wegener's granulomatosis, neurologic abnormalities develop from contiguous extension of granulomas from primary sites in the nasopharynx (cranial neuropathies, cavernous sinus compression, diabetes insipidus) and vasculitis (peripheral neuropathies, encephalopathies, stroke). Magnetic resonance imaging (MRI) has dramatically changed the approach to the neurologic abnormalities by enabling us to distinguish between granulomas and infarction, for example. Histology still remains essential for the diagnosis [33–38].

## Lymphomatoid Granulomatosis

Lymphomatoid granulomatosis is a rare disease affecting the lungs, skin, and nervous system. Histologic lesions are characterized by infiltration of vessels with atypical lymphocytes, plasmacytes, and histiocytes in an angiocentric angiodestructive pattern. Granulomas are plentiful. Both the central and peripheral nervous system may be affected. CNS dysfunction is reported in 20% of patients and peripheral nervous system dysfunction in 40%. The spectrum of neurologic abnormalities is wide and includes visual loss, nystagmus, cranial neuropathies, ataxia, aphasia, encephalopathies, and upper-motor-neuron changes [39–41].

## Giant Cell Arteritis

Two histologically similar but clinically distinct diseases are included under the term *giant cell arteritis*: temporal arteritis and Takayasu's arteritis.

### Case 3

A 62-year-old woman presented with headache of new onset and some discomfort chewing her food over the previous 2 weeks. Her only medical problem was mild diabetes, well controlled on oral agents for the past 8 years. She denied vision problems, hearing loss, or change in memory. Her brief, general physical examination was considered normal. Samples were drawn for laboratory studies, and she was given a return appointment for 2 weeks and referred for dental evaluation.

Two days later she appeared in the emergency room with acute loss of vision in her right eye. Her headaches remained unabated. Examination was as before except that the vision in her right eye had declined to light perception only. Review of the laboratory studies initiated several days before revealed normal results from blood chemistries but an elevated sedimentation rate of 78 mm per hour. A temporal artery biopsy was performed, which revealed an inflammatory infiltrate in the media with destruction of elastic tissue.

*Temporal arteritis* is a systemic panarteritis affecting mainly patients over the age of 50. Despite the widespread nature of the vasculitis, symptoms below the neck are unusual. Neurologically, headache, visual loss, ophthalmoplegia, and other cranial neuropathies predominate. Jaw claudication is often present. Although temporal arteritis is traditionally considered to be a disorder of the extracranial circulation, histologic and clinical evidence of posterior circulation disease exists. Encephalopathies, strokes, and peripheral neuropathies occur with somewhat increased frequency in these patients, although it is not certain that these are effects of inflammatory vascular disease. Because blindness occurs in temporal arteritis, it is important that physicians remain vigilant for the disease. Temporal arteritis is considered a neurologic emergency. Two factors underlie the importance of early, accurate diagnosis: elderly patients have an even higher complication rate from corticosteroids than do younger patients, and an overlap exists between temporal arteritis and polymyalgia rheumatica (which responds well to a lower dosage of corticosteroids). Both statements illustrate the importance of temporal artery biopsy to confirm the diagnosis so that the need for the higher dose of corticosteroids can be determined. Temporal artery biopsy usually reveals a granulomatous inflammation, which is typically found in the media but extends from the intima to the adventitia. A fairly nonspecific cellular infiltrate consists of lymphocytes, histiocytes, monocytes, giant cells, and occasional eosinophils. The sensitivity of biopsy varies from 65–97%. Although the pathophysiology of temporal arteritis is unclear, the pathologic distribution draws attention to the elastic lamina as an antigenic target. Histologically, the posterior circulation also reveals evidence of vascular inflammation, and this finding appears to explain the symptoms and signs referable to the posterior fossa. Encephalopathies develop in patients with temporal arteritis, but the histologic associations in this older population are not yet clear.

Diagnosis depends on keeping a high index of suspicion when encountering new-onset headaches or visual changes in persons over the age of 50. An elevated sedimentation rate is almost invariable. Liver function abnormalities are frequently encountered. Temporal artery angiography has not been as helpful as anticipated, but arteriography in other regions of the body is strongly recommended if symptoms suggest that a systemic vasculitis may be present [42–51].

*Takayasu's arteritis* is a large-vessel arteritis that affects the aortic arch and its branches by a process that is initially inflammatory and later occlusive. Although the disease was first described in young Asian women, it is now recognized worldwide. Takayasu's arteritis is often called the *pulseless disease*, and absence of at least one arterial pulse is identified in 98% of patients. Bruits are often heard. Typically, Takayasu's arteritis is recognized by signs of decreased blood flow to the limbs and viscera. Most of the neurologic abnormalities occur in the latter vaso-occlusive stage of the illness. Hypertension exacerbates the vascular disease. Neurologically, strokes, transient ischemic attacks, and syncope are prominent [52–54].

## Behçet's Disease

Behçet's disease, initially characterized by the triad of relapsing ocular lesions and recurrent oral and genital ulcers, is in fact a systemic disease. Many organs exhibit a small-vessel vasculitis. Thrombophlebitis, arthritis, and erythema nodosum occur frequently. The course is usually frustrating but benign, unless the nervous system is involved. Neurologic involvement increases the morbidity of the disease to a variable degree. Various series report neurologic abnormalities in 10–50% of patients; these include meningoencephalitis, brain stem abnormalities, and focal CNS changes. The diagnosis is strongly clinical. The varied abnormalities are nonspecific on neuroradiographic studies (MRI and computed tomographic [CT] scan) but occasionally initiate the search for the correct diagnosis. Cerebrospinal fluid analysis frequently reveals inflammation but has not yet shown itself to be a reliable guide for determining the efficacy of therapy [52,55–61].

Vasculitis is clinically restricted to the CNS.

## Case 4

A 53-year-old woman presented with a 1-year history of diminished memory and paresthesias in her left arm. Diagnostic evaluation included an MRI (normal results), sedimentation rate (normal results), ANA titer (no antibodies present), cerebrospinal fluid analysis (normal results), and an electroencephalogram (EEG) (showing mild diffuse slowing). Two weeks before her admission, she developed decreased vision in her left eye (acuity of 20/100), a generalized major motor seizure, and a mild spastic paraparesis. MRI revealed two areas of decreased attenuation in the white matter. Cerebral angiography showed multiple areas of segmental narrowing in the anterior and posterior circulations bilaterally. Leptomeningeal/wedge cortical biopsy revealed several arteries with a prominent mononuclear cell infiltrate in and around vessel walls. Cultures and tissue strains were negative for fungal and mycobacterial infection.

## Isolated Angiitis of the Central Nervous System

Isolated angiitis of the CNS is a recurrent inflammatory disease of the small and medium-sized blood vessels of the brain and spinal cord. Symptoms and signs are restricted to the nervous system and typically include headaches, encephalopathies, strokes, cranial neuropathies, and myelopathies. Notably, symptoms or laboratory evidence of systemic inflammation is absent. This disease illustrates the fact that, in a persistent vascular inflammatory disease, the sedimentation rate, ANA titer, and tests for rheumatoid factor and immune complexes may all have normal (or negative) results. Neurodiagnostic studies reflect the degree and locations of parenchymal abnormalities. EEG and CT scans may be abnormal but do not specifically suggest or exclude the diagnosis. Similarly, MRI often, but not invariably, reveals evidence of parenchymal lesions consistent with ischemic damage. Although magnetic resonance angiography is potentially useful, much of the disease occurs beyond its current resolution. Studies that yield the most complete information on abnormalities in the cerebral vasculature are angiography and biopsy. Angiography is the gold standard for diagnosing vasculitis to date, although the findings may be normal in up to 10–15% of patients with exclusively small-vessel vasculitis. Features that suggest the diagnosis of vasculitis are recurrent segmental narrowing, abrupt termination of blood vessels, and neovascularization. A notable caution is that there are no angiographic features that are specific for vasculitis, nor do they distinguish between primary and secondary vasculitides. Biopsy of tissue is important for determination of vascular inflammation and exclusion of alternate diagnoses such as neoplasia and infection, which are the two most common causes of similar clinical abnormalities in large series. Because the diagnostic evaluation is invasive and expensive, the prudent physician often inquires which clinical features are most suggestive of isolated angiitis of the CNS. In our experience, the features that most often alert the physician to a correct diagnosis of vasculitis are headaches, encephalopathy, and multifocal signs [60,62–67].

## Other

Several reports and series describe patients with neurologic abnormalities that cannot readily be classified into the above disease groups. Among these are a vasculitis restricted to the peripheral nervous system; a small-vessel vasculitis restricted to the CNS, skin, and muscle; and a vasculitis characterized by encephalopathy and deafness.

## Secondary Vasculitides

### Infections

The most prominent cause of CNS vascular inflammation is infection. A wide variety of CNS infections result in clinically critical inflammation. CNS infections reveal the clearest association between a specific etiology and vasculitis. Infectious agents inducing a vasculitis include bacteria, fungi, viruses, treponemes, mycobacteria, rickettsiae, and parasites. Multiple mechanisms can lead to vascular inflammation: direct infection of the vessel wall, immune complexes, or toxic products of bacteria. The infection may vary in tempo and severity. At times, an infection is so indolent (as with aspergillosis) that only a rigorous search for the cause of a vasculitis reveals the pathogen. Vasculitis secondary to fungal infections (indolent processes often unaccompanied by evidence of systemic inflammation) may be difficult to distinguish clinically from an idiopathic vasculitis. The need for histologic analysis and tissue culture before immunosuppression is thus emphasized. Viruses also induce vascular inflammation, which may be acute or delayed. A contralateral hemiplegia 3–8 weeks after herpes zoster ophthalmicus is well described; the direct cause may be vasculitis or thrombosis. Vascular inflammation is also notorious in treponemal infections, but the underlying agent can more easily be identified by serologic studies [68–74].

## Toxins

The earliest reports of toxin-associated vasculitis are probably those of sulfonamide-induced hypersensitivity vasculitides. Amphetamine abuse is associated with both a systemic necrotizing vasculitis and a vasculitis restricted to the CNS. Cocaine is a frequently encountered cause of stroke; the underlying mechanism is occasionally vasculitis [75–77].

## Neoplasia

Neoplasia may cause a vasculitis, typically by immune complex formation secondary to a large tumor load. Hodgkin's disease is associated with a CNS vasculitis; the mechanism is unknown. Accurate diagnosis is important, because the vasculitis resolves with treatment of the underlying disease [78,79].

## Connective Tissue Diseases

The connective tissue diseases are a group of multisystem diseases characterized by inflammation of joints, muscles, and skin. Although vascular inflammation may be a component of these diseases, they are clinically distinct from the vasculitides. There is a genetic predisposition to these diseases, because relatives of patients frequently have in vitro evidence of immunoregulatory abnormalities, if not clinical disease. Several of these diseases occur spontaneously in animals. Typically these disorders are multisystemic, but sporadically a single organ may be involved. Neurologic abnormalities, prominent in some disorders, occasionally herald the disease.

## Case 5

A 23-year-old woman with a history of trigeminal neuralgia at the age of 19 and monocular vision loss lasting 2 weeks at the age of 21 developed partial complex seizures. These were initially well controlled with carbamazepine.

Four months before admission she developed a confusional episode that lasted for 2 days, during which time she stayed at home in bed. Her family reported that she was uncharacteristically depressed after this episode. Her past medical history was entirely normal except for occasional joint and muscle aches after running. Family history was normal except that a sister had arthritis. The patient's general physical and neurologic examinations were normal with the following exceptions: She had (1) several small areas of hair loss, (2) abnormal short-term memory testing with two-thirds recall at 5 and 10 minutes, and (3) horizontal nystagmus with left lateral gaze. Laboratory testing revealed the following: ANA, 1:320; anti-DNA, 1:32; blood urea nitrogen, 19 mg/dl; creatinine, 1.0 mg/dl. The creatinine clearance was 76 ml per minute. A scalp biopsy revealed immunoglobulin deposition along the dermal epidermal junction.

## Systemic Lupus Erythematosus

Systemic lupus erythematosus (SLE) is a multisystem autoimmune disease that characteristically affects young women. Cutaneous, renal, hematologic, musculoskeletal, neurologic, cardiac, pulmonary, and gastrointestinal abnormalities are frequent. The course ranges from indolent to fulminant. Persistence of autoantibodies is a hallmark of SLE. Patients and animals with this disease show exaggerated responses to exogenous stimuli and spontaneous production of autoantibodies, some to unique antigens. Autoantibodies to nuclear components, including nucleic acids, proteins, and nucleoprotein complexes, are prominent. The particular pattern of autoantibody formation may be an important diagnostic feature. Immune complex deposition with subsequent inflammation is the principal pathogenesis of the renal and cutaneous disease. Anemia, leukopenia, thrombocytopenia, and some coagulopathies probably result from direct antibody-mediated effects.

The frequent and protean neurologic abnormalities are broadly grouped in Table 15.2. The neurologic abnormalities result from multiple pathogenic mechanisms. Notably for the clinician, some develop from acute immunologic mechanisms and are treatable; others are the result of chronic injury, and therapy may produce more complications than benefit. A list of immunopathogenic mechanisms in neuro-SLE is shown in Table 15.3. Critically important to the consultant is the fact that perhaps half of the neurologic abnormalities in these patients

*Table 15.2*   Neurologic manifestations of systemic lupus erythematosus

Seizures
Encephalopathies
Psychiatric symptoms
Movement disorders
Cranial neuropathies
Focal motor/sensory symptoms
Ataxia
Myelopathies
Peripheral neuropathies

*Table 15.3*  Mechanisms of the neurologic abnormalities of systemic lupus erythematosus

---

Neurologic abnormalities result from the following mechanisms:
  Primary: Immune-mediated direct effects
          1. Immune complex
          2. Autoantibodies
          Immune-mediated indirect effects
          1. Vasculopathy
          2. Coagulopathy
          3. Cardiac emboli
  Secondary: Infectious, metabolic, toxic

---

are secondary complications (of infections, medications, metabolic abnormalities) rather than primarily immunologic features of SLE. When the SLE itself does affect the nervous system, contributions from autoantibodies reactive with neuronal tissue, ischemia from coagulopathies, and behavioral changes from activation of the hypothalamic-pituitary-adrenal axis all appear likely.

Vascular disease occurs from emboli, coagulopathies, and degenerative processes in the vessel wall. Histologic evidence of vasculitis is rare. The cause of the vasculopathy is not clear. Despite the absence of inflammation in the vessel wall, an immune-mediated process is the likely mechanism. Studies of the coronary vascular system in autoimmune mice of varying genetic backgrounds provide clues to the pathogeneses. The consequent histologic feature of circulating immune complex deposition depends on the titer and the chronicity of the circulating complexes as well as genetic features of the host. Predisposed animals with low levels of immune complexes developed a degenerative process without a cellular infiltrate [16,80–90].

Mixed connective tissue disease, initially described on the basis of high titers of antibodies to ribonucleoprotein (RNP), clinically appears to be a mild variant of SLE. The clinical features of generalized systemic inflammation, scleroderma, and polymyositis associated with Raynaud's phenomenon suggest the disease. Titers of greater than 1:4,000 anti–U1 RNP are typical. Neurologic manifestations occur in over half the patients and include aseptic meningitis, psychosis, febrile headaches, peripheral neuropathies, trigeminal neuropathy, and seizures.

## Sjögren's Syndrome

Sjögren's syndrome is a chronic autoimmune inflammatory disease characterized by diminished lacrimal and salivary secretion resulting in keratoconjunctivitis sicca and xerostomia. It is usually a relatively benign disease manifested primarily by exocrine gland impairment caused by the presence of destructive mononuclear infiltrates in the lacrimal and salivary glands. In a number of patients, however, visceral involvement occurs, and a wide spectrum of extraglandular manifestations may arise as a result of lymphoid infiltration of lung, kidney, skin, thyroid gland, stomach, liver, and muscle. There is a strong association between Sjögren's syndrome and anti-Ro (SSA) antibodies, although anti-La (SSB) antibodies also occur. The importance of these autoantibodies in the pathogene-

*Table 15.4*   Manifestations of Sjögren's syndrome

Lymphocyte-mediated destruction of exocrine tissue
Visceral involvement (variable)
Cell-mediated and antibody-mediated tissue damage
High levels of anti-La (SSB) antibodies (frequent)
Neurologic abnormalities (10–32% of patients)
   Trigeminal neuropathy
   Sensory neuropathy
   Seizures, myelopathies, subarachnoid hemorrhage

sis of the disease is not established. Diagnosis of Sjögren's rests on clinical features, lip biopsy demonstrating lymphocyte infiltration, and, usually, the presence of circulating autoantibodies.

Neurologic manifestations (Table 15.4) are more frequent in the peripheral than the central nervous system. Cranial neuropathies, particularly trigeminal neuropathy, are common and may occur in up to 40% of patients. Both central and peripheral nervous system abnormalities occur, although the histology is not convincingly vasculitis. In one series of nerve biopsies, however, 8 of 11 patients had findings consistent with or highly suggestive of vasculitis; other patients had a perivascular inflammatory response. An alternative, distinctive neuropathy in Sjögren's is not vasculitis but a dorsal root ganglionitis. These patients present with a sensory neuropathy and ataxia, usually associated with autonomic insufficiency [91–98].

## Rheumatoid Arthritis

Rheumatoid arthritis consists of progressive erosive inflammation of the joints. Activation of a cellular immune response in the genetically susceptible host generates the early stages. Ensuing proliferation of polyclonal B cells results in proliferative synovitis. Cytokines drive the proliferation of synovial cells, which invade and destroy articular cartilage. Because the damage to the joints is widespread, secondary injury to the nervous system occurs. Cervical spine abnormalities are seen in up to 25% of patients. Potentially devastating is the dissolution of the transverse ligament, which allows forward displacement of the skull and atlas. Physicians must be vigilant for this condition to prevent a high cervical myelopathy in these patients. Peripheral neuropathies develop from several mechanisms. Compression from swollen tissue and subcutaneous nodules typically result in the chronic, progressive neuropathies. Another pathogenic mechanism of neuropathy is ischemia. Vascular occlusions both from vasculitis and from obliterative vasculopathy cause neuropathies, which are usually more acute in onset than the compressive neuropathies. CNS abnormalities are less common and are caused by subcutaneous nodules or the systemic vasculitis that is a complication in a small percentage of rheumatoid arthritis cases [99–104].

## Progressive Systemic Sclerosis (Systemic Scleroderma)

Progressive systemic sclerosis (systemic scleroderma) involves the cardinal features of (1) proliferative intimal arterial lesions, (2) obliterative microvascular defects, and (3) atrophy and fibrosis of the involved organs. The disease is largely a cell-mediated (by T lymphocytes and mast cells) immune process. Some distinctive autoantibodies may be markers of the disease. Neurologic abnormalities are unusual; in one large series they occurred in less than 1% of patients. When clinical neurologic disease does occur, it is usually a consequence of accelerated hypertension, uremia, or pulmonary insufficiency. Rarely, a vasculitis may complicate scleroderma, and this vasculitis may involve the CNS [102,105–107].

## Immunopathogenic Mechanisms

The immunopathogenic mechanisms of the connective tissue diseases are complex and remain poorly defined. Typically, autoantibodies, immune complexes, cytokines, and some form of vascular inflammation or degeneration are present. Autoantibody formation is a normal, transient phenomenon in both humans and animals. In some diseases, circulating autoantibodies are persistent. These autoantibodies may be nonspecific manifestations of inflammation, markers for a specific disease, or, occasionally, pathogenic. Autoantibody-mediated disease develops through several mechanisms. Antibodies can bind to their cognate antigen, altering cell function or causing cell death. The antibodies to the acetylcholine receptor in myasthenia gravis and to a skin antigen in pemphigus illustrate the range of pathogenic antibodies that can exist. In SLE, autoantibody-mediated abnormalities are most clearly delineated in the hematologic changes. In many connective tissue diseases, the lack of association of the target antigens and clinical features indicate that the mechanism of disease is at least one step removed from direct binding of antibody to the antigen. The pathogenicity of autoantibodies directed against intracellular antigens is a result of immune complex formation. Thus, antibodies to autoantigens such as DNA and Sm produce renal and cutaneous vascular damage largely by immune-complex-recruited inflammation [108–110].

Cytokines play a prominent role in the pathogenesis of joint inflammation and destruction in rheumatoid arthritis and may be similarly important in the organ damage of the other diseases. Excessive cytokine production occurs in several diseases, including SLE and Sjögren's disease. The potential role of cytokines as a cause of neurologic abnormalities is suggested by the documented behavioral changes and sleep disturbances caused by interleukin-1 (IL-1) administration in animals. IL-2 administration in humans is associated with neurologic changes. IL-6 is also implicated in behavioral and cognitive abnormalities [111,112].

Vasculitis is characterized by the accumulation of cells in the vessel wall. Tissue injury in the inflammatory vascular diseases (vasculitides) results largely from ischemia. At least three separate components of the inflammation contribute to the ischemia: direct effects of inflammation, altered vasomotor reactivity, and hypercoagulation.

Vascular inflammation itself has three currently identifiable immunopathogenic mechanisms: (1) T lymphocyte–endothelial interactions, (2) immune complex deposition, and (3) certain autoantibodies. Endothelial cells are in an immunologically unique position: they direct traffic of lymphocytes by expression of cell surface (homing) molecules, they function as antigen-presenting cells, express major histocompatability antigens, Fc receptors, and complement receptors; and they secrete cytokines, which recruit an inflammatory response. Cytokines, released by the endothelium, are a major group of molecules that govern the chemotaxis and adherence of leukocytes through adhesion molecules, changes in permeability of the vessel wall, and molecular and cellular transport across the endothelial barrier [113–116].

Adhesion molecules are the second major group of inducible molecules prominent in inflammation. These signals on the vascular endothelium evolve during the course of inflammation and display tissue diversity. The selectin family of adhesion molecules tethers the leukocyte to the vessel wall and allows it to roll in the direction of flow. The expression of integrins on the leukocyte and their ligands, cell adhesion molecules such as intercellular adhesion molecule–1 on endothelial cells, and lymphocyte-function-associated antigen–1 on the lymphocyte provide a firmer adhesion. Finally, another group of molecules, the chemoattractants, direct transendothelial migration of leukocytes into the tissue [117].

Vascular smooth muscle and perivascular cells may also signal and initiate inflammation, but information about these cells is scantier. Overall, this reaction mediated by *leukocytes and endothelial cells* is a physiologic process that is a central part of the body's vigilance against infection; it may also result in vascular disease.

Another inflammatory process resulting in vasculitis is *immune complex deposition*. Immune complexes are a normal, transient phenomenon. They are efficiently cleared from the circulation by several mechanisms. When the body's ability to clear complexes is overwhelmed or the complexes are numerous or persistent, antigen-antibody complexes of certain sizes and valences may deposit in the blood vessels. Deposition of circulating immune complexes or in situ formation of immune complexes (with filtered or planted antigen) both occur. The immune complexes, trapped along the basement membrane, activate complement components. Complement-derived chemotactic factors (C3a, C5a, C567) cause accumulation of the polymorphonuclear leukocytes. These cells release lysosomal enzymes such as collagenase and elastase that cause subsequent damage and necrosis of the vessel wall. Thrombosis, occlusion, and hemorrhage ensue. Lesions usually heal with prominent scarring.

Antibodies alone do not usually cause vascular inflammation. Under special conditions, *autoantibodies that are not usually pathogenic*, such as antiendothelial antibodies, may cause disease. In Kawasaki's disease, antiendothelial antibodies become cytotoxic when the high levels of circulating interleukins induce neoantigens on endothelial cells. Another large group of antibodies, antiphospholipid antibodies, at least in vitro bind to endothelial cells and theoretically could result in vascular inflammation. The presence of antiphospholipid antibodies, associated or unassociated with clinical SLE, have been linked to thrombotic vascular occlusions. This family of antibodies shares reactivity with negatively charged phosphodiester moieties. Potential targets of antiphospholipid antibodies are the endothelial cell, prostacyclin, protein C, protein C-S complex, and platelets. Both acute effects on coagulation and chronic effects on the vessel wall are plausible. Whether these antibodies are pathogenic remains controversial, and a direct pathogenic role of antiphospholipid antibodies in stroke is not established.

Finally, another group of antibodies is strongly associated with an interesting subgroup of vasculitides. These antibodies, the ANCAs, react with two molecules, myeloperoxidase (pANCA) and proteinase 3 (cANCA) in neutrophils. The cANCAs occur in patients with Wegener's granulomatosis and microscopic polyarteritis and are fairly specific for these diseases. Although their pathophysiologic relevance is not established, in vitro they activate cytokine-primed neutrophils; the result is an oxidative burst and degranulation that could damage the endothelium [118–120].

The common denominator of these immunopathogenic mechanisms is the accrual of cells in the vessel wall with obstruction of the lumen and, often, necrosis of the vessel wall. Clinical features may not only present acutely, with the inflammation, but may also be delayed by years when the ischemia results from scarring and narrowing of blood vessels. This fact emphasizes the importance of prompt diagnosis and therapy.

The inflammatory process influences other physiologic processes important to normal blood flow. Inflammation-associated changes in *vasomotor reactivity* are particularly important in the CNS, which normally exerts tight autoregulation of blood flow. Clinically, these changes in vasomotor reactivity are important and limit our ability to correlate angiographic changes with vessel wall induration. Endothelial cells, known regulators of blood flow through their action on vascular smooth muscle, mediate these changes through vasodilators and vasoconstrictors. Local synthesis of these vasoconstrictor and vasodilating factors may be altered by inflammation and may contribute to regional variations in blood flow. Endothelium-dependent relaxation is provided mainly by two pathways: the prostaglandin pathway and the nitric oxide pathway. Factors that initiate vasoconstriction include superoxidase anions, thromboxane (from platelets), and endothelin-1 [121–123].

Another prominent effect of inflammation is that exerted on the *coagulation* system. The coagulation system is a highly regulated cascade of surface-associated enzymes and cofactors that results in the generation of thrombin. The interactions of the coagulant and anticoagulant proteins and the fibrinolytic system occur at the cell surface. Acquired hypercoagulable states occur with abnormalities of coagulation proteins, abnormalities of platelet function, or endothelial cell dysfunction. Inflammation alters the normally anticoagulant properties of the endothelium to create a net procoagulant effect. Antibodies and cytokines appear to induce many of these changes. IL-1 and other cytokines also induce the production of thromboplastin, prostacyclin, and platelet-activating factors from endothelial cells; the result is altered vascular permeability and thrombosis. IL-2 prominently induces increased vascular permeability. Platelet-activating factor appears to be another important proinflammatory mediator [124].

Not all immune interactions with the vessel wall result in flagrant, histologically demonstrable inflammation. More subtle but equally damaging to the blood vessel wall are the effects of chronic inflammation. The pathophysiologic mechanisms are not delineated in humans, but in animals low levels of immune complexes circulating over a long period in a genetically susceptible host result in mural degeneration of some medium-sized arteries. Similarly, in other models of chronic inflammation, serum amyloid A protein and acute-phase reactants associated with high-density lipoproteins displace apoprotein A. Thus the ability to shuttle free fatty acids across the wall is diminished, and as a result they are deposited in the vessel wall. Concurrent features in human disease, such as the presence of hypertension or corticosteroid therapy, may accelerate this process and result in early atherosclerotic disease.

Clinically, the most frequently recognized immune-associated vasculopathies of the nervous system are seen in connective tissue diseases, particularly SLE. Whether this vasculopathy is related to chronic inflammation, the presence of antibodies reactive with the blood vessel wall, or inappropriate activation of adhesion molecules is not known.

## GUIDES TO NEUROLOGIC CONSULTATION ON PATIENTS WITH RHEUMATIC DISEASES

1. Diagnostic considerations when neurologic abnormalities are present and an underlying diagnosis is not established include the following: Does this patient with a peripheral neuropathy (or seizures, encephalopathy) have SLE, polyarteritis nodosa, or Sjögren's syndrome?

When neurologic abnormalities occur and an underlying connective tissue disease or vasculitis is a possible cause, the clinician must use a combination of clinical features and laboratory studies for accurate diagnosis (Table 15.5). Often the clinical features strongly suggest a particular disease. Examples include hemoptysis, cranial neuropathies, and mononeuropathy multiplex in Wegener's granulomatosis; trigeminal neuropathy and sicca complex in Sjögren's disease; butterfly rash, encephalopathy, pleuritic pain, and proteinuria in SLE. Histologic studies would confirm the diagnosis in each of the above. Sometimes a clinical presentation is consistent with several diseases; for example, fever, malaise, azotemia, and seizures could be caused by polyarteritis, SLE, or chronic infection. An ANA titer would likely be elevated in all three conditions and would not

*Table 15.5*   Clinical approach to neurologic abnormalities in rheumatic disorders

Evaluation
  Delineate neurologic abnormalities: central or peripheral nervous system; white or grey matter; mixed
  Determine evidence of systemic disease: renal, cutaneous, cardiac, hepatic, ocular
  Document immunologic clefts: autoantibodies, immune complexes, cellular infiltrates
  Discover any underlying conditions: infections, neoplasias, toxins
Management
  Evaluate immunopathogenic mechanisms
  Remove any underlying causes
  Determine extent of tissue damage
  Make as accurate a diagnosis as possible
  Determine least toxic and most effective treatment
  Plan dose, duration, and goals of therapy

be diagnostically useful. An abnormal angiogram would help diagnose PAN and render SLE and infection less likely. Similarly, high titers of anti-DNA and anti-Sm would diagnose SLE and exclude PAN and infection. Histologic studies of tissue would confirm either diagnosis, and culture and histologic studies might be necessary to diagnose an infection such as tuberculosis. Cerebrospinal fluid analysis is a critical study, although it may or may not reveal evidence of inflammation. Oligoclonal bands are present in up to one-half of the patients with neuropsychiatric SLE or Sjögren's syndrome.

Thus, the clinician must make appropriate use of serologic and histologic studies, realizing that in several of these diseases there may be no serologic markers of a progressive disease. Histology is central to the diagnosis in most of the vasculitides and is important in SLE and Sjögren's disease. Serologic studies (for autoantibodies) may be diagnostic or may at least narrow the diagnostic possibilities when there are high titers of anti-DNA, anti-Sm, anti-Ro, anti-La, and ANCA. Angiography is useful in the medium- and large-vessel vasculitides. Among the valuable information provided by angiography is the distribution of the disease and serial evaluations to show healing or progression.

Sometimes, particularly early in the course of the disease, mild clinical symptoms and marginal laboratory abnormalities make diagnosis difficult. Then, it is prudent to withhold a specific diagnosis until distinctive features have evolved.

2. Diagnostic considerations when neurologic abnormalities occur in the setting of previously diagnosed disease include the following: Are this patient's seizures (or encephalopathy, cranial neuropathy) part of the primary disease, secondary to other end-organ disease, or a complication of therapy?

The neurologist is also asked to evaluate patients with an identified connective tissue disease or vasculitis and new neurologic symptoms. In this situation, the new features usually result from inexorable disease progression or inadequate therapy, or are a complication of the treatment regimen. Occasionally the initial diagnosis was incorrect, and the clinician must re-evaluate the data for diagnosis.

Among the most important clinical concerns in this group of patients are complications of therapy, largely because these are either avoidable or treatable. Because many of these patients are immunosuppressed—either because of their disease or, more likely, because of their treatment—infections occur and contribute prominently to morbidity and mortality. The diagnosis of infection may be overlooked because symptoms (malaise, fever, headache) and signs are attributed to the underlying disease. Specifically, the usually indolent CNS fungal infections are underdiagnosed. A high clinical index of suspicion, repeated cerebrospinal fluid analyses, and occasionally brain biopsy are important. Other complications of therapy include the side effects of medications. Corticosteroids are frequent causes of psychopathy, visual changes, and myopathy, as well as certain types of memory abnormalities. Antihypertensive medications may cause headaches and cognitive changes.

3. Therapy includes the following: When clinical conditions require pharmacotherapy, the physician chooses among the current options of anti-inflammatory and immunosuppressive treatments. Several reviews of these are available, and the choice of agent is usually dictated by the efficacy of the medications in the lowest effective dose according to recent series. Therapies emerging in the treatment of rheumatoid arthritis hold promise for use in other connective tissue diseases [125–135].

# REFERENCES

1. Hunder GG, Arend WP, Bloch DA, et al. The American College of Rheumatology 1990 criteria for the classification of vasculitis. Introduction. Arthritis Rheum 1990;33:1065–1067.
2. Moore PM. Neurological manifestation of vasculitis: update on immunopathogenic mechanisms and clinical features. Ann Neurol 1995;37(suppl):S131–S141.
3. Alpern RJ. Southwestern Internal Medicine Conference: vasculitis—it's time to reclassify [review]. Am J Med Sci 1995;309:235–248.
4. Watts RA, Carruthers DM, Scott DG. Epidemiology of systemic vasculitis: changing incidence or definition? Semin Arthritis Rheum 1995;25:28–34.
5. Moore PM, Calabrese LH. Neurology manifestations of systemic vasculitides [review]. Semin Neurol 1994;14:300–306.
6. Lightfoot RW Jr, Michel BA, Bloch DA, et al. The American College of Rheumatology 1990: criteria for the classification of polyarteritis nodosa. Arthritis Rheum 1990;33:1088–1093.
7. Guillevin L, Le Thi Huong Du, Godeau P, et al. Clinical findings and prognosis of polyarteritis nodosa and Churg Strauss angiitis: a study in 165 patients. Br J Rheumatol 1988;27:258–264.
8. Montanaro A. Vasculitis in older patients: presentations and significance. Geriatrics 1988;43:75–86.
9. Akova YA, Jabbur NS, Foster CS. Ocular presentation of polyarteritis nodosa. Ophthalmology 1993;100:1775–1781.
10. Topaloglu R, Besbas N, Saatci U, et al. Cranial nerve involvement in childhood polyarteritis nodosa. Clin Neurol Neurosurg 1992;94:11–13.
11. Kirkali P, Topaloglu R, Kansu T, Baddaloglu A. Third nerve palsy and internuclear ophthalmoplegia in periarteritis nodosa. J Pediatr Ophthalmol Strabismus 1991;1:45–46.
12. Said G, Lacrois-Ciaudo C, Fujimura H. The peripheral neuropathy of necrotizing arteritis: a clinicopathologic study. Ann Neurol 1988;23:461–465.
13. Genereau T, Lortholary O, Leclerq P, et al. Treatment of systemic vasculitis with cyclophosphamide and steroids: daily oral low-dose cyclophosphamide administration after failure of a pulse intravenous high-dose regimen in four patients. Br J Rheumatol 1994;33:959–962.
14. Liou HH, Yip PK, Liu HM. Allergic granulomatosis and angiitis (Churg-Strauss syndrome) presenting as prominent neurology lesions and optic neuritis. J Rheumatol 1994;21:2380–2384.
15. Tai PC, Holt ME, Denny P, et al. Deposition of eosinophil cationic protein in granulomas in allergic granulomatosis and vasculitis: the Churg-Strauss syndrome. BMJ 1984;289:400–402.
16. West SG, Emlen W, Wener MK, Kotzin BL. Neuropsychiatric lupus erythematosus: a 10-year prospective study on the value of diagnostic tests. Am J Med 1995;99:153–163.
17. Masi AT, Hunder GG, Lie JT, et al. The American College of Rheumatology 1990 criteria for the classification of Churg-Strauss syndrome (allergic granulomatosis and angiitis). Arthritis Rheum 1990;33:1094–1100.
18. Lichtig C, Ludatscher R, Eisenberg E, Bental E. Small blood vessel disease in allergic granulomatous angiitis (Churg-Strauss syndrome). J Clin Pathol 1989;42:1001–1002.
19. Sehgal M, Swanson J, DeRemee R, Colby T. Neurologic manifestations of Churg-Strauss syndrome. Mayo Clin Proc 1995;70:337–341.
20. Chang Y, Karga S, Goates J, Horoupian D. Intraventricular and subarachnoid hemorrhage resulting from necrotizing vasculitis of the choroid plexus in a patient with Churg-Strauss syndrome. Clin Neuropathol 1993;12:84–87.
21. Kok J, Bosseray A, Brion J, Micoud M. Chorea in a child with Churg Strauss syndrome. Stroke 1993;24:1263–1264.
22. Weinstein JM, Chui H, Lane S, et al. Churg Strauss syndrome (allergic granulomatous angiitis): neuro-ophthalmologic manifestations. Arch Ophthalmol 1983;101:1217–1220.
23. Acheson JF, Cockerell OC, Bentley CR, Sanders MD. Churg Strauss vasculitis presenting with severe visual loss due to bilateral sequential optic neuropathy. Br J Ophthalmol 1993;77:118–119.
24. Liou H, Yip P, Chang Y, Liu H. Allergic granulomatosis and angiitis (Churg-Strauss syndrome) presenting as prominent neurologic lesions and optic neuritis. J Rheumatol 1994;21:2380–2384.
25. O'Donovan CA, Keogan M, Staunton H, et al. Peripheral neuropathy in Churg-Strauss syndrome associated with IgA-C3 deposits. Ann Neurol 1992;32:411.
26. Dixon FJ. The pathogenesis of murine systemic lupus erythematosus. Am J Pathol 1979;97:10–16.
27. Calabrese LH, Michel BA, Bloch DA, et al. The American College of Rheumatology 1990 criteria for the classification of hypersensitivity vasculitis. Arthritis Rheum 1990;33:1108–1113.
28. Lie JT. Illustrated histopathologic classification criteria for selected vasculitis syndrome. Arthritis Rheum 1990;33:1074–1087.

29. Smoller BR, McNutt NS, Contreras F. The natural history of vasculitis. Arch Dermatol 1990;126:84–89.
30. Hodge SJ, Callen JP, Ekenstam E. Cutaneous leukocytoclastic vasculitis: correlation of histopathological changes with clinical severity and course. J Cutan Pathol 1987;14:279–284.
31. Gibson LE, Su WP. Cutaneous vasculitis [review]. Rheum Dis Clin North Am 1995;21:1097–1113.
32. Calabrese LH, Clough JD. Hypersensitivity vasculitis group (HVG): a case oriented review of a continuing clinical spectrum. Cleve Clin Q 1982;49:17–42.
33. Nishino H, Rubino FA, DeRemee RA, et al. Neurological involvement in Wegener's granulomatosis: an analysis of 324 consecutive patients at the Mayo Clinic. Ann Neurol 1993;33:4–9.
34. Hoffman GS, Kerr GS, Leavitt RY, et al. Wegener granulomatosis: an analysis of 158 patients. Ann Intern Med 1992;116:488–498.
35. Miller K, Miller K. Wegener's granulomatosis presenting as a primary seizure disorder with brain lesions demonstrated by magnetic resonance imaging. Chest 1993;103:316–318.
36. Bullen CL, Liesegang TJ, McDonald TJ, DeRemee RA. Ocular complications of Wegener's granulomatosis. Am J Ophthalmol 1989;90:279–290.
37. Stern GM, Hoffbrand AV, Urich H. The peripheral nerves and skeletal muscles in Wegener's granulomatosis: a clinico-pathological study of four cases. Brain 1989;58:151–164.
38. van der Woude FJ, Rasmussen N, Lobatto S, et al. Autoantibodies against neutrophils and monocytes: tool for diagnosis and marker of disease activity in Wegener's granulomatosis. Lancet 1985;1(8426):425–429.
39. Schmidt BJ, Meagher-Villemure K, Carpio JD. Lymphomatoid granulomatosis with isolated involvement of the brain. Ann Neurol 1984;15:478–481.
40. Jenkins TR, Zaloznik AJ. Lymphomatoid granulomatosis. a case for aggressive therapy. Cancer 1989;64:1362–1365.
41. Simard H, LeBlanc P. Radiotherapy: an effective treatment of cerebral involvement by lymphomatoid granulomatosis. Chest 1993;103:650–651.
42. Hunder GG, Lie JT, Goronzy JJ, Weyand CM. Pathogenesis of giant cell arteritis. Arthritis Rheum 1993;36:757–761.
43. Mehler MF, Rainowich L. The clinical neuro-ophthalmologic spectrum of temporal arteritis. Am J Med 1988;85:839–844.
44. Moreira F, Defreitas MRG, Caldas MLR. Giant cell arteritis and peripheral neuropathy: a report of 2 cases and review of the literature. J Rheumatol 1987;14:129–134.
45. Selma JK, Raine CS, Cross AH. Anti-tumor necrosis factor therapy abrogates autoimmune demyelination. Ann Neurol 1991;30:694–700.
46. Caselli RJ, Hunder GG, Whisnant JP. Neurologic disease in biopsy-proven giant cell (temporal) arteritis. Neurology 1988;38:352–359.
47. Bengtsson BA, Malmvall B-E. Prognosis of giant cell arteritis including temporal arteritis and polymyalgia rheumatica: a follow-up study on ninety patients treated with corticosteroids. Acta Med Scand 1981;209:1–14.
48. Allison MC, Gallagher PJ. Temporal artery biopsy and corticosteroid treatment. Ann Rheum Dis 1984;43:416–417.
49. Golbus J, McCune WJ. Giant cell arteritis and peripheral neuropathy: a report of 2 cases and review of the literature. J Rheumatol 1987;14:129–134.
50. Stevens RJ, Hughes RA. The aetiopathogenesis of giant cell arteritis [review]. Br J Rheumatol 1995;34:960–965.
51. Mertens JC, Willemsen G, Van Saase JL, et al. Polymyalgia rheumatica and temporal arteritis: a retrospective study of 111 patients. Clin Rheumatol 1995;14:650–655.
52. Edwards KK, Lindsley HB, Lai C, Van Veldhuizen PJ. Takayasu arteritis presenting as retinal and vertebrobasilar ischemia. J Rheumatol 1989;16:1000–1002.
53. Vinijchaikul K. Primary arteritis of the aorta and its main branches (Takayasu's arteriopathy): a clinicopathologic autopsy study of eight cases. Am J Med 1967;43:15–27.
54. Weyand CM, Goronzy JJ. Molecular approaches toward pathologic mechanisms in giant cell arteritis and Takayasu's arteritis [review]. Curr Opin Rheumatol 1995;7:30–36.
55. O'Duffy JD. Behçet's syndrome. N Engl J Med 1990;322:326–328.
56. Rubinstien LJ, Urich H. Meningo-encephalitis of Behçet's disease: case report with pathological findings. Brain 1986;86:151–160.
57. Serdaroglu P, Yazici H, Ozdemir C, et al. Neurologic involvement in Behçet's syndrome. A prospective study. Arch Neurol 1989;46:265–269.
58. Kuroiwa Y, Toghi H, Kanayama H. Neuro-Behçet's disease with alternating hemiparesis. Neuroradiology 1986;28:284–285.
59. Ben-itzhak J, Keren J, Simon J. Intracranial venous thrombosis in Behçet's syndrome. Neuroradiology 1985;27:450–451.

60. Hurst RW, Grossman RI. Neuroradiology of central nervous system vasculitis [review]. Semin Neurol 1994;14:320–340.
61. Parisi JE, Moore PM. The role of biopsy in vasculitis of the central nervous system. Semin Neurol 1994;14:341–348.
62. Moore PM. Vasculitis of the central nervous system. Semin Neurol 1994;14:307–312.
63. Alhalabi M, Moore PM. Serial angiography in isolated angiitis of the central nervous system. Neurology 1994;44:1221–1226.
64. Moore PM. Diagnosis and management of isolated angiitis of the central nervous system. Neurology 1989;39:167–173.
65. Calabrese LH, Gragg LA, Furlan AJ. Benign angiopathy: a distinct subset of angiographically defined primary angiitis of the central nervous system. J Rheumatol 1993;20:2046–2050.
66. Calabrese LH, Mallek JA. Primary angiitis of the central nervous system: report of 8 new cases, review of the literature, and proposal for diagnostic criteria. Medicine 1988;67:20–39.
67. Garner BF, Burns P, Bunning RD, Laureno R. Acute blood pressure elevation can mimic arteriographic appearance of cerebral vasculitis (a postpartum case with relative hypertension). J Rheumatol 1990;17:93–97.
68. Giang DW. Central nervous system vasculitis secondary to infections, toxins, and neoplasms. Semin Neurol 1994;14:313–319.
69. Williams PL, Johnson R, Pappagianis D. Vasculitic and encephalitic complications associated with *Coccidioides immitis* infection of the central nervous system in humans: report of 10 cases and review. Clin Infect Dis 1992;14:673–682.
70. Meurers B, Kohlepp W, Gold R, et al. Histopathologic findings of the central and peripheral nervous system in neuroborreliosis: a report of three cases. J Neurol 1990;237:113–116.
71. Wheat LJ, Batteiger BE, Sathapatayavongs B. Histoplasma capsulatum infections of the central nervous systema: a clinical review. Medicine 1990;69:244–260.
72. de la Torre FE, Gorraez MT. Toxoplasma-induced occlusive hypertrophic arteritis as the cause of discrete coagulative necrosis in the CNS. Hum Pathol 1989;20:604.
73. Nurick S, Blackwood W, Mair WGP. Giant cell granulomatous angiitis of the central nervous system. Brain 1982;95:133–142.
74. Walsh TJ, Hier DB, Caplan LR. Aspergillosis of the central nervous system: clinicopathological analysis of 17 patients. Ann Neurol 1985;18:574–582.
75. Halpern M, Citron BP. Necrotizing angiitis associated with drug abuse. Am J Roentgenol Radiat Ther Nucl Med 1971;111:166–176.
76. Krendel DA, Ditter SM, Frankel MR, Ross WK. Biopsy-proven cerebral vasculitis associated with cocaine abuse. Neurology 1990;40:1092–1094.
77. Stafford CR, Bodgoff BM, Green L, Spector HB. Mononeuropathy multiplex as a complication of amphetamine angiitis. Neurology 1975;25:570–572.
78. Roux S, Grossin M, De Brandt M, et al. Angiotropic large cell lymphoma with mononeuritis multiplex mimicking systemic vasculitis. J Neurol Neurosurg Psychiatry 1995;58:363–366.
79. Greer JM, Longley S, Edwards NL, et al. Vasculitis associated with malignancy: experience with 13 patients and literature review. Medicine 1988;67:220–230.
80. Hay EM, Huddy A, Black D, et al. A prospective study of psychiatric disorder and cognitive function in systemic lupus erythematosus. Ann Rheum Dis 1994;53:298–303.
81. Hopkinson NP, Gardner-Medwin J. Antiphospholipid antibodies (aPL) in systemic lupus erythematosus: are they specific tools for the diagnosis of aPL syndrome? Ann Rheum Dis 1994;53:619–620.
82. McNicholl JM, Glynn D, Mongey A, et al. A prospective study of neurophysiologic, neurologic and immunologic abnormalities in systemic lupus erythematosus. J Rheumatol 1994;21:1061–1066.
83. Mills JA. Systemic lupus erythematosus. N Engl J Med 1994;330:1871–1879.
84. Vogelweid CM, Wright DC, Johnson JC, et al. Evaluation of memory, learning ability, and clinical neurologic function in pathogen-free mice with systemic lupus erythematosus. Arthritis Rheum 1994;37:889–897.
85. Cervera R, Khamashta MA, Font J, et al. Systemic lupus erythematosus: clinical and immunologic patterns of disease expression in a cohort of 1,000 patients. Medicine 1993;72:113–123.
86. Fisk JD, Eastwood B, Sherwood G, Hanly JG. Patterns of cognitive impairment in patients with systemic lupus erythematosus. Br J Rheumatol 1993;458–462.
87. Lewis S, Goldman R, Cronstein B. Acute syphilitic meningitis in a patient with systemic lupus erythematosus. J Rheumatol 1993;20:870–871.
88. Beneivelli W, Vitali C, Isenberg DA, et al. Disease activity in systemic lupus erythematosus: report of the consensus study group of the European Workshop for Rheumatology Research, III: develop-

ment of a computerized clinical chart and its application to the comparison of different indices of disease activity. Clin Exp Rheumatol 1992;10:549–554.

89. Hanly JG, Walsh NMG, Sangalang V. Brain pathology in systemic lupus erythematosus. J Rheumatol 1992;19:732–741.

90. Lammens M, Robberecht W, Waer M, et al. Purulent meningitis due to aspergillosis in a patient with systemic lupus erythematosus. Clin Neurol Neurosurg 1992;94:39–43.

91. Alexander EL, Arnett FC, Provost TT, Stevens MB. Sjögren's syndrome: association of anti-Ro (SS-A) antibodies with vasculitis, hematological abnormalities, and serologic hyperreactivity. Ann Intern Med 1983;98:155–159.

92. Malinow K, Yannakakis GD, Glusman SM. Subacute sensory neuronopathy secondary to dorsal root ganglionitis in primary Sjögren's syndrome. Ann Neurol 1986;20:535–537.

93. Oxholm P, Asmussen K. Classification of disease manifestations in primary Sjögren's syndrome: present status and a new proposal [review]. Clin Rheumatol 1997;14:3–7.

94. Fox RI. Sjögren's syndrome [review]. Curr Opin Rheumatol 1995;7:409–416.

95. Price EJ, Venables PJ. The etiopathogenesis of Sjögren's syndrome [review]. Semin Arthritis Rheum 1995;25:117–133.

96. Hietaharju A, Yli-Kerttula U, Hakkinen V, Frey H. Nervous system manifestations in Sjögren's syndrome. Acta Neurol Scand 1990;81:144–152.

97. Vrethem M, Ernerudh J, Lindstrom F, Skogh T. Immunoglobulins within the central nervous system in primary Sjögren's syndrome. J Neurol Sci 1990;100:186–192.

98. Molina H, Provost TT, Alexander EL. Peripheral inflammatory vascular disease in Sjögren's syndrome: association with nervous system complications. Arthritis Rheum 1985;28:1341–1347.

99. Harris ED Jr. Rheumatoid arthritis. N Engl J Med 1990;322:1277–1289.

100. Scott DGI, Bacon PA, Tribe CR. Systemic rheumatoid vasculitis: a clinical and laboratory study of 50 cases. Medicine 1981;60:288–297.

101. Arend WP, Dayer JM. Cytokines and cytokine inhibitors or antagonists in rheumatoid arthritis. Arthritis Rheum 1990;33:305–315.

102. Hietaharju A, Jantti V, Korpela M, Frey H. Nervous system involvement in systemic lupus erythematosus, Sjögren syndrome and scleroderma. Acta Med Scand 1993;88:299–308.

103. Beck DO, Corbett JJ. Seizures due to central nervous system rheumatoid meningovasculitis. Neurology 1983;35:1058–1061.

104. Conn DL, McDuffie FC, Dyck PJ. Immunopathologic study of sural nerves in rheumatoid arthritis. Arthritis Rheum 1972;15:135–143.

105. Clements PJ. Measuring disease activity and severity in scleroderma. Curr Opin Rheumatol 1995;7:517–521.

106. Saitoh H, Tomkiel J, Cooke CA, et al. CENP-C, an autoantigen in scleroderma, is a component of the human inner kinetochore plate. Cell 1992;70:115–125.

107. Farrell DA, Medsger TA Jr. Trigeminal neuropathy in progressive systemic sclerosis. Am J Med Sci 1982;73:57–62.

108. von Muhlen CA, Tan EM. Autoantibodies in the diagnosis of systemic rheumatic diseases [review]. Semin Arthritis Rheum 1995;24:323–358.

109. Abu-Shakra M, Smythe H, Lewtas J, et al. Outcome of polyarteritis nodosa and Churg-Strauss syndrome: an analysis of twenty-five patients. Arthritis Rheum 1994;37:1798–1803.

110. Rahman MAA, Isenberg DA. Autoantibodies in systemic lupus erythematosus. Curr Opin Rheumatol 1994;6:468–473.

111. Kekow J, Szymkowiak CH, Sticherling M, et al. Pro- and anti-inflammatory cytokines in primary systemic vasculitis. Adv Exp Med Biol 1993;336:341–344.

112. Braquet P, Hosford D, Braquet M, et al. Role of cytokines and platelet-activating factor in microvascular immune injury. Int Arch Allergy Appl Immunol 1989;88:88–100.

113. Savage COS, Cooke SP. The role of the endothelium in systemic vasculitis. J Autoimmun 1993;6:237–249.

114. Osborn L. Leukocyte adhesion to endothelium in inflammation. Cell 1990;62:3–6.

115. Cines DB, Tomaski A, Tannenbaum S. Immune endothelial-cell injury in heparin-associated thrombocytopenia. N Engl J Med 1987;316:581–589.

116. Henson PM, Johnston RB Jr. Tissue injury in inflammation: oxidants, proteinases, and cationic proteins. J Clin Invest 1987;79:669–674.

117. Argenbright LW, Barton RW. Interactions of leukocyte integrins with intercellular adhesion molecule 1 in the production of inflammatory vascular injury in vivo. J Clin Invest 1992;89:259–272.

118. Gross WL, Schmitt WH, Csernok E. ANCA and associated diseases: immunodiagnostic and pathogenetic aspects. Clin Exp Immunol 1993;91:1–12.

119. Kallenberg CGM. Autoantibodies in vasculitis: current perspectives. Clin Exp Rheumatol 1993;11:355–360.
120. Falk RJ, Jennette JC. Anti-neutrophil cytoplasmic autoantibodies with specificity for myeloperoxidase in patients with systemic vasculitis and idiopathic necrotizing and crescentic glomerulonephritis. N Engl J Med 1988;318:1651–1657.
121. Hallenbeck JM, Dutka AJ. Background review and current concepts of reperfusion injury. Arch Neurol 1990;47:1245–1254.
122. Vanhoutte PM, Shimokawa H. Endothelium-derived relaxing factor and coronary spasm. Circulation 1989;80:1–9.
123. Shiozawa S, Kuroki Y, Kim M, et al. Interferon alpha lupus psychosis in lupus psychosis [abstract]. Arthritis Rheum 1992;35:417–422.
124. Johnson RJ. Platelets in inflammatory glomerular injury. Semin Nephrol 1991;11:276–284.
125. Valente RM, Conn DL. Current therapies for systemic vasculitis. Semin Neurol 1994;14:380–386.
126. Lockwood CM. Approaches to specific immunotherapy for systemic vasculitis. Semin Neurol 1994;14:387–392.
127. Bacon PA. Therapy of vasculitis. J Rheumatol 1994;21:788–790.
128. Campion EW. Desperate diseases and plasmapheresis. N Engl J Med 1992;326:1425–1427.
129. Conn DL, Tompkins RB, Nichols WL. Glucocorticoids in the management of vasculitis—a double edge sword? J Rheumatol 1988;15:1181–1183.
130. Sharkey J, Appel NM, DeSouza EB. Alterations in local cerebral glucose utilization following central administration of corticotropin-releasing factor in rats. Synapse 1989;4:80–87.
131. Maini RN. A perspective on anti-cytokine and anti-T cell-directed therapies in rheumatoid arthritis [review]. Clin Exp Rheumatol 1995;13:S35–S40.
132. Dickler HB, Albright JF. Immunosuppression in the treatment of disease. J Allergy Clin Immunol 1994;93:669–676.
133. Kalden JR. Biologic agents in the therapy of inflammatory rheumatic diseases, including therapeutic antibodies, cytokines, and cytokine antagonists [review]. Curr Opin Rheumatol 1994;6:281–286.
134. Boumpas DT, Yamada H, Patronas NJ, et al. Pulse cyclophosphamide for severe neuropsychiatric lupus. Q J Med 1991;81:975–984.
135. Wolkowitz OM, Reus VI, Weingartner H, et al. Cognitive effects of corticosteroids. Am J Psychiatry 1990;147:1297–1303.

# 16
# Vascular Medicine and Surgery

Dawn M. Pearson and Frances Jensen

This chapter describes neurologic disorders frequently encountered in patients hospitalized for a primary vascular disease. The vast majority of these patients have complications of atherosclerotic vascular disease secondary to hypertension, hypercholesterolemia, or diabetes. Less frequent causes for admission include arteritis, venous thrombotic disease, and congenital vascular syndromes. Although a great many patients hospitalized on a vascular medicine or surgery service have associated coronary artery disease and complications of cardiac ischemia, specific neurologic complications of cardiac disease are covered in Chapter 14.

In the present chapter we focus in detail on stroke syndromes, because in our experience stroke is the most common diagnosis considered at the time of neurologic consultation to the vascular service. Stroke or transient cerebral ischemic attack can present as a coincidental new event during hospitalization for an unrelated vascular problem or can occur as a direct complication of a vascular surgical procedure such as carotid endarterectomy, surgery involving the aortic arch, and thrombectomy with undiagnosed source for paradoxical embolus. Ischemic stroke is by far the most commonly encountered problem, but hemorrhagic stroke is seen in this population in the setting of anticoagulant therapy, hypertension, and angiopathy, and less frequently as a perioperative complication. Encephalopathy is a very frequent cause for neurologic consultation on the vascular service, either in the setting of hypertension or arteritis, or as perioperative complication. The chapter closes with descriptions of other entities that may present on neurologic consultation, such as frequently encountered peripheral neuropathies that occur in patients with diabetes and autoimmune diseases.

## CEREBROVASCULAR DISEASE

Sudden focal neurologic deficits resulting from cerebrovascular disease can be broadly classified into several categories. The most common form is atherothrom-

*Table 16.1*   Classification of stroke

Atherothrombotic brain infarction
    Large-vessel thrombosis
    Lacunar disease
    Transient monocular blindness
Cerebral embolism
    Artery-artery
    Cardiogenic
Transient ischemic attack
Hemorrhage
    Subarachnoid
    Intracerebral
    Hypertensive
    Amyloid angiopathic
Other
    Coagulopathies
    Vasculopathies
    Migraine
    Dissection
    Venous occlusive disease

botic stroke, which includes lacunar disease in addition to large-vessel disease (Table 16.1). Transient ischemic attacks (TIAs) occur almost as frequently, followed by cerebral embolism. Hemorrhagic disease accounts for the majority of the remainder of cases, including intracerebral hemorrhage (ICH) and subarachnoid hemorrhage (SAH).

## Risk Factors for Stroke and Transient Ischemic Attack

Many of the risk factors for stroke are the same as those for atherosclerotic vascular disease. According to the Framingham Study, the most prominent risk factor is *hypertension* [1]. The relative risk of stroke in hypertensive persons is 3.1 in men and 2.9 in women compared with normotensive controls. Borderline hypertension has a relative risk of 1.5 compared with normotensive controls. The relative contribution of systolic versus diastolic pressure remains controversial. Isolated systolic hypertension significantly increases stroke risk [2,3]. Stroke risk is directly related to systolic pressure for any given diastolic value. The role of diastolic pressure is less clear, and there is no evidence that diastolic pressure has a primary role [4,5]. *Coronary artery disease* and *myocardial infarction* (MI) increase stroke risk as a result of arterial embolism from a cardiac source. Anterior wall MIs carry a higher risk for thrombus formation and subsequent cardioembolic stroke other than transmural MIs [6]. Both symptomatic and silent MI carry an increased risk of stroke. A major risk factor for cerebral embolism is *atrial fibrillation* (AF), either isolated or associated with valvular disease. Chronic AF is associated with a 5.6-fold increased incidence of stroke; risk increases with age, and AF is the cause of 36% of all strokes by the ninth decade [7]. In contrast, if AF is accompanied by rheumatic heart disease, the relative risk rises to 17 times that of the control population [8]. *Diabetes mellitus* is another major risk factor and increases the risk of stroke 1.8–4.0 times [9,10]. Diabetes also contributes to the progression of other diseases that represent independent risks, such as atherosclerosis and coronary artery disease. *Cigarette smoking* has been demonstrated to be an independent factor in both ischemic and hemorrhagic stroke. Smoking increases the risk to 1.56 in men and 1.86 in women compared with nonsmokers. The risk is directly related to the number of cigarettes smoked per day; patients who smoke 40 cigarettes per day have approximately twice the risk of stroke of those who smoke 10 cigarettes per day [11]. The relationship between *elevated serum lipids* and stroke is less clear than that for coronary artery disease. In fact, cholesterol, lipid, and triglyceride levels have not been directly related to an increase in ischemic stroke. However, a low serum cholesterol has been related to intracerebral hemorrhage, especially when diastolic blood pressure is elevated [12]. Other risk factors for stroke include *obesity*, *elevated hematocrit*, *elevated fibrinogen*, and *homocystenemia*. *Oral contraceptive* use raises stroke risk, and this risk is further increased by concomitant cigarette smoking [13]. The risk of stroke also increases with use of oral contraceptives containing high levels of estrogen. Stroke can occur as a complication of systemic disease, including *autoimmune diseases* such as systemic lupus erythematosus and antiphospholipid antibody syndrome, temporal arteritis, polyarteritis, and Wegener's granulomatosis. *Coagulopathies* such as thrombotic thrombocytopenic purpura, antithrombin III deficiency, and protein S and protein C deficiencies are rarer causes of stroke and must especially be considered in younger patients. Other causes of stroke in the young include *paradoxical cardiac emboli* from a right-left shunt, complicated *migraine*, ischemic or hemorrhagic stroke associated with use of a *sympathomimetic* such as cocaine, and ruptured *arteriovenous malformations*.

The differential diagnosis of stroke and TIA encompasses all entities that may cause acute onset of a focal neurologic deficit or alteration of consciousness. These include syncope, seizure, classic migraine, brain tumor, metabolic encephalopathy, vestibular vertigo, drug intoxication, and conversion reaction. The symptom complexes that constitute the major forms of cerebrovascular disease are detailed in the following sections.

## Stroke Syndromes

Transient Ischemic Attacks

*Clinical presentation*

TIAs are defined as episodes of neurologic deficit lasting less than 24 hours. The vast majority of TIAs last less than 30–60 minutes and usually less than 10 minutes. TIAs can occur in all vascular territories. When transient ischemia occurs in the retinal arteries as a complication of carotid artery disease, vision is temporarily obscured, and the phenomenon is termed *transient monocular blindness* or *amaurosis fugax*. The classic description is one of a shade descending monocularly, but often the patient simply describes the condition as "blurred," "foggy," or "hazy" vision. Symptoms such as bright lights or flashes can also occur as a manifestation of transient retinal ischemia. Although hemispheric strokes are not common after *transient monocular blindness,* this entity should be evaluated as thoroughly as is a TIA. TIAs carry a relative risk of subsequent stroke of 5% per year and 35% over 5 years [1]. However, the risk of coronary heart disease remains greater than the risk of stroke in this population.

## Etiology

TIAs can occur in thrombotic, lacunar, and embolic disease, although TIAs are usually associated with thrombotic disease. Embolic TIAs have been reported to be of longer duration than those that are thrombotic [14].

## Ischemic Stroke

### Carotid Disease

**Clinical presentation.**   Stenosis of the extracranial common and internal carotid arteries is a major cause of both hemispheric TIAs and strokes. Atherosclerosis of the carotid artery can affect territory within its middle cerebral artery (MCA) and anterior cerebral artery (ACA) divisions. The posterior cerebral artery (PCA) distribution is usually spared, because it is supplied primarily by the vertebrobasilar circulation. The major mechanisms of ischemic injury are reduced distal flow secondary to a proximal stenosis and artery-to-artery embolization from a proximal atherosclerotic plaque (Figure 16.1). Clinical deficits occurring as a result of distal artery insufficiency are often less severe than those occurring as a result of embolism. Clinical syndromes relate to disruption of function subserved by tissue within a given vascular territory.

1. *Symptomatic intracranial disease.* In ACA occlusion, medial frontoparietal ischemia causes weakness and sensory deficits in the contralateral lower extremities; other frontal lobe symptoms, such as incontinence and abulia, can also occur. With MCA occlusion, the more lateral aspects of the frontoparietal and temporal lobes can be affected. Deficits relate to the function these regions subserve, including strength and sensation in the contralateral face and upper extremities, and language (dominant hemisphere). In nondominant hemisphere ischemia, a severe neglect syndrome can result from parietal ischemia, in addition to contralateral weakness and sensory loss. Vision loss in the contralateral hemifield can occur as a result of ischemia to the radiating visual fibers that course through the parietal temporal region to the occipital lobes.

2. *Symptomatic extracranial carotid disease.* Distal insufficiency can occur with high-grade proximal carotid artery stenosis, with or without superimposed systemic hypotension. Carotid plaques can also generate artery-artery emboli or acutely worsen and cause complete carotid occlusion. Carotid bruits are present only in a portion of patients with significant stenosis. In the case of severe systemic hypotension, watershed infarcts occur in the end-circulation border zones of the MCA and ACA. Furthermore, symptomatic carotid stenosis is associated

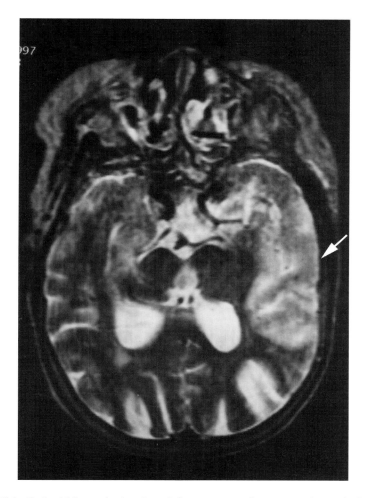

*Figure 16.1* Left middle cerebral territory infarct on magnetic resonance image in the setting of left internal carotid artery stenosis. (Courtesy of Mahesh R. Patel, M.D., Beth Israel Deaconess Medical Center, Boston.)

with a risk of future stroke of 2–15% per year, depending on the percentage of stenosis and the clinical presentation [15].

3. *Asymptomatic carotid stenosis.* Because of the accuracy and availability of carotid duplex technology, the documentation of internal carotid artery stenosis has been increasing. Asymptomatic bruit in the neck is a relatively common finding that occurs in 4–5% of persons between the ages of 45 and 80 years [16,17]. The frequency of this finding is even higher in patients with known peripheral vascular disease [18]. As with TIAs, the presence of a carotid bruit has been reported to present anywhere from a 1% to a 15% risk of stroke over a 2-

to 7-year period [19–21]. Asymptomatic carotid artery occlusion has been reported to carry a stroke risk of 2–5% per year, but these figures include strokes in all vascular territories, so that the risk is general rather than specific to the stenotic carotid artery [22–25].

**Etiology.**   Atherosclerotic lesions occur most commonly at the origin of the internal carotid artery in the neck. Common intracranial sites include the carotid siphon and the stems of the MCA and ACA. In whites, the extracranial circulation is affected more than intracranial sites, but in other races (blacks and Asians), intracranial MCA disease is more common than extracranial disease [26].

Premature atherosclerosis resulting from homocysteinemia is a cause of stroke in younger individuals. Homocystenemia is increasingly recognized as a risk factor for stroke. Homocystenemia can result from accumulation of homocysteine in plasma and urine, as in inherited deficiencies of metabolic enzymes, or from acquired nutritional deficiencies of vitamins $B_6$, $B_{12}$, or folate [27]. Elevated homocysteine levels have been shown to be related to increased stroke risk [28] and increased carotid wall intimal thickness. Elevated homocysteine levels can be detected in plasma and 24-hour urine samples.

Carotid dissection is another major cause of acute stroke, especially in younger patients (Table 16.2). Carotid dissection occurs as a result of traumatic or spontaneous tearing of the arterial wall, with subsequent hematoma formation and partial or total occlusion of the vascular lumen. Spontaneous dissection has been reported in younger patients [29] and can be associated with fibromuscular dysplasia. Fibromuscular dysplasia affects primarily the extracranial carotid and vertebrobasilar arteries, but can also affect intracranial vessels [30,31]. It is bilateral in most cases [32] and can also be associated with dysplasia of the renal arteries. A characteristic pattern resembling strings interrupted by beading can be seen on the angiogram as the renal wall narrows and dilates [33].

*Table 16.2*   Causes of stroke in young adults

Ischemic
    Cardiogenic embolism (including paradoxical from patent foramen ovale or atrial septal defect)
    Arterial dissection
    Migraine stroke
    Reversible cerebral angiopathies (toxic, eclamptic)
    Coagulopathy (autoimmune, paraneoplastic, sickle cell, thrombocytotic)
    Atherosclerosis (accounts for less than 20%)
    Cerebral venous thrombosis (pregnancy)
    Fibromuscular dysplasia
    Metabolic disorders (homocysteinuria; myopathy, encephalopathy, lactic acidosis, and stroke-like episodes [MELAS] syndrome)
Hemorrhagic
Arteriovenous malformation
Hypertension
Sympathomimetic agents
Anticoagulant therapy

*Lacunar Stroke*

**Clinical presentation.** Lacunes are small areas of infarction in the distribution of penetrating arteries in the brain. The risk of small-vessel disease increases with age, hypertension, diabetes, smoking, hypercoagulable state, and hyperlipidemia. Common locations of lacunes are the subcortical white matter, basal ganglia, thalamus, and brain stem [34]. Strokes in these locations result in specific syndromes of subtotal deficits (Table 16.3). Brain imaging reveals punctate hypodense lesions on computed tomographic (CT) scan or areas of increased T2 signal on magnetic resonance imaging (MRI). Frequently, patients have multiple lacunar lesions that have occurred over a protracted period. The cumulative effect of multiple lacunes is the so-called lacunar state. The course of this syndrome is one of stuttering, stepwise deterioration. The multilacune state is distinctly different from Binswanger's disease, which involves diffuse white-matter damage, termed *leukoariosis* [35]. In the latter syndrome, there is progressive rarefaction of the subcortical white matter, and CT or MRI reveals large confluent areas of damage around the ventricles, with ventricular enlargement due to atrophy. The incidence of the syndrome increases with age and hypertension. Symptoms are of insidious, gradual onset, and subcortical dementia in association with gait disorder and incontinence may be present in more severely affected individuals.

**Etiology.** The small-vessel occlusion in lacunar disease has been attributed to microatheromatous deposits [34,36]. Lipohyalinosis, fibrinoid necrosis, and microemboli are less common causes for lacunes. The exact pathophysiology of the disease is unknown, but may relate to the chronic effects of hypertension, because arterioles are seen to be thickened in areas of white-matter pallor [37].

*Vertebrobasilar Disease*

**Clinical presentation.** Symptoms of vertebrobasilar disease vary dramatically with small changes in the location of the ischemia, because much of the territory is the brain stem. The two vertebral arteries supply the cerebellum, medulla, and caudal pons before joining together to form the basilar artery. The two most common sites of infarction in the vertebral circulation are the

*Table 16.3* Common lacunar syndromes in vertebrobasilar disease

| Syndrome | Location |
|---|---|
| Dysarthria–clumsy hand | Contralateral pons |
| Pure motor hemiplegia | Contralateral cerebral peduncle, pons, or medulla |
| Pure hemisensory deficit | Contralateral ventral thalamus |
| Ataxic hemiparesis | Contralateral pons or ventral thalamus |
| Contralateral motor and sensory deficit | Ventral thalamus and adjacent internal capsule |
| Lateral medullary syndrome | |

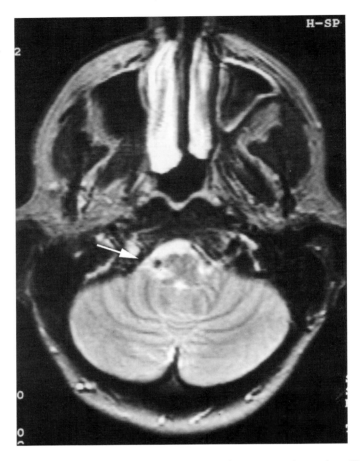

*Figure 16.2*    Right lateral medullary infarct on magnetic resonance image in a 51-year-old woman with Wallenberg's syndrome. (Courtesy of Mahesh R. Patel, M.D., Beth Israel Deaconess Medical Center, Boston.)

cerebellum and lateral medulla. Cerebellar infarction can result in ipsilateral limb ataxia and dysmetria. Occlusion of the posterior inferior cerebellar artery results in the lateral medullary syndrome (Wallenberg's syndrome), which is a distinct constellation of symptoms occurring from medullary ischemia, including vertigo, nystagmus, ataxia, ipsilateral Horner's syndrome, facial numbness and mild weakness, contralateral pain and temperature loss, and hoarseness and dysarthria caused by ipsilateral weakness of the vocal cords and palate (see Table 16.3; Figure 16.2). Basilar artery occlusion can result in subtotal deficits caused by partial ischemia to the pons and medulla, but complete occlusion of the basilar in this region causes a "locked-in" syndrome. Occlusion of the top of the basilar causes ischemia in the thalamus and decreases

*Table 16.4*   Most common causes of cardiogenic embolism (according to the Cerebral Embolism Task Force*)

| Cause | Percentage of all emboli |
|---|---|
| Nonvalvular atrial fibrillation | 45 |
| Acute myocardial infarction | 15 |
| Ventricular aneurysm | 10 |
| Rheumatic heart disease | 10 |
| Prosthetic valve | 10 |
| Other (i.e., paradoxical, myxoma, cardiomyopathy) | 10 |

*See refs. 39 and 40.

flow to both posterior cerebral arteries; the result is vision loss resulting from occipital lobe ischemia.

Lacunes (discussed above) occur commonly in the vertebrobasilar circulation, as there is an abundance of small, penetrating vessels in the brain stem and thalamus. Stereotypical syndromes have been described, including pure motor hemiplegia, pure sensory stroke, dysarthria–clumsy hand syndrome, ataxic hemiparesis, and sensorimotor stroke (see Table 16.3).

**Etiology.**   Like the carotid system, the vertebrobasilar circulation can be affected by atherosclerosis, lacunes, embolic occlusion, vasculopathy, and dissection. Extracranial vertebral artery disease is more common in whites than in other races and is more common in men than in women [26].

## Stroke Caused by Emboli of Cardiac or Ascending Aorta Origin

**Clinical presentation.**   Cardiovascular disease accounts for 15–20% of all ischemic strokes [38–40]. Embolic occlusion occurs most frequently at sites of arterial branching. The most common site is the MCA, with emboli less frequently going to the ACA or the vertebrobasilar system. Complications of cardiac-source emboli include hemorrhage transformation and distal migration of the embolic fragments. Hemorrhage occurs secondarily in some cases; the hemorrhage is usually within 72 hours of the onset of embolic stroke.

**Etiology.**   The most common cardiac conditions associated with embolism have been described by the Cerebral Embolism Task Force [39,40]. These include AF, acute MI, left ventricular aneurysm, atrial myxoma, and other left-sided sources as discussed above (Table 16.4). Paradoxical emboli originating from a right-left shunt can occur with patent foramen ovale, atrial septal defect, or, rarely, pulmonary arteriovenous fistula [41,42]. Septic emboli may arise from an infected valve, and in the past often occurred as a superinfection of valves damaged by rheumatic heart disease. However, as rheumatic heart disease declines, subacute bacterial endocarditis is encountered in individuals with prosthetic valves [43] and those with a history of intravenous drug abuse

*Table 16.5*  Stroke in inflammatory and autoimmune disease

Large-vessel involvement
    Temporal arteritis
    Takayasu's arteritis
Small-vessel or intracranial vessel involvement
    Polyarteritis nodosa
    Wegener's granulomatosis
    Systemic lupus erythematosus
        Cardiogenic embolism (with or without Libman-Sacks endocarditis)
        Thrombotic thrombocytopenic purpura
        Prothrombotic state associated with antiphospholipid antibody
    Bacterial and viral meningoencephalitis
    Behçet's disease

but otherwise normal valves. The organism associated with the highest rate of septic embolization is *Staphylococcus aureus*. Mycotic aneurysms and secondary hemorrhages are uncommon.

Aortic atherosclerotic disease is an increasingly recognized source of cerebral emboli. A likely association exists between complicated plaque with mobile components in the aorta and brain infarcts. Aortic arch atherosclerotic plaques provide a source of atherothrombotic or cholesterol embolism. Transesophageal echocardiography is able to detect plaques in the aortic arch [44].

## Stroke Caused by Inflammatory and Autoimmune Disease

**Clinical presentation.**  Strokes caused by hypercoagulable states can mimic the presentation of large- or small-vessel strokes; they should always be considered in the differential diagnosis, especially when the more common risk factors are not present or when the stroke is in a young person (see Table 16.2). The differential diagnosis can be considered after determining whether the presentation and imaging findings indicate large-vessel disease or small-vessel disease (Table 16.5).

**Etiology: large-vessel pattern.**  Temporal arteritis (giant cell arteritis) affects extracranial vessels [45] and rarely involves the intracranial vasculature. The incidence of the disease is greater in women and increases with age. Systemic involvement results in the syndrome of polymyalgia rheumatica, which often precedes the neurologic symptoms [46]. Headache is largely attributable to inflammation of the temporal arteries. The erythrocyte sedimentation rate (ESR) is often markedly elevated, but a normal value does not preclude the diagnosis of temporal arteritis. The ophthalmic artery becomes involved; this involvement leads to vision loss resulting from ischemic optic neuropathy and retinal artery occlusion. Vision loss is reported in up to 50% of cases; in most cases the loss is monocular [46]. Stroke resulting from giant cell arteritis is more common in the vertebrobasilar system than in the carotid territory [47]. Biopsy of the temporal artery reveals a granulomatous, giant cell arteritis. Takayasu's arteritis has a predilection for involvement of the aortic arch vessels but also can affect the extracranial carotid and vertebral circulation. [48]. Takayasu's arteritis typically occurs in young women and is more common in Asians. Symptoms include general malaise and fever; strokes and TIAs occur as a result of proximal vessel occlusion or embolic events. Subclavian steal syndrome can occur if the subclavian artery is occluded. The symptoms are accompanied by a high ESR, and angiography reveals stenosis of large vessels. The pathologic process is a granulomatous angiitis.

**Etiology: intracranial and small-vessel pattern.**   Several arteritic conditions involve intracranial vessels rather than the proximal carotid or vertebral arteries. Arteritis can accompany a bacterial meningitis, because vessels become occluded as they course through the meningeal covering of the brain. Isolated granulomatous angiitis affects small arterioles and veins and causes multifocal strokes [49,50]. Constitutional symptoms such as headache, fever, and malaise are common and are not correlated with the ESR, which is low or normal in some cases. Cerebrospinal fluid (CSF) analysis reveals a moderate pleocytosis but an elevated protein content (>100 dl). Angiography does not reliably demonstrate abnormalities but can show a "beading" pattern, and CT scans or MRI reveals multiple strokes and hemorrhage. Polyarteritis nodosa is another condition that affects small and medium-sized vessels in the brain. In polyarteritis, central nervous system involvement occurs usually when the systemic disease is well advanced [51,52]. Symptoms include headache, fever, seizures, and ischemic strokes; hemorrhagic strokes are less common. Serologic testing reveals an elevated antinuclear antibody (ANA) titer; the CSF analysis may show only moderate abnormalities. Arteritis can be documented by biopsy of an affected tissue, such as peripheral nerve. The vasculitis is necrotizing, and angiography may demonstrate aneurysmal dilation of the involved vessels.

Systemic lupus erythematosus (SLE) can be associated with stroke from a variety of mechanisms [53]. A vasculopathy affecting small and medium-sized intracranial vessels is present in some cases. This is not a vasculitis, but rather an inflammatory infiltrate in the perivascular space. More common causes of stroke in SLE are cardiac emboli from Libman-Sacks endocarditis or hyper-coagulability, or from associated thrombotic thrombocytopenic purpura (TTP) or antiphospholipid antibody syndrome [53,54]. Involvement of intracranial vessels in SLE can result in ischemic infarcts, hemorrhages, and, rarely, venous thrombosis. Wegener's granulomatosis causes a necrotizing vasculitis in medium-sized intracranial vessels as well as venous thrombophlebitis and thrombosis, and secondary intraparenchymal hemorrhages [55]. The intracranial disease occurs in the setting of glomerulonephritis and systemic vasculi-tis, particularly in the respiratory tract. Granuloma formation can occur systemically as well as intracranially. Laboratory testing reveals an elevated ANA level. Other less common inflammatory conditions causing stroke-like events are arterial narrowing following an episode of herpes zoster ophthalmi-cus, or inflammation associated with Sjögren's syndrome or rheumatoid arthri-tis. Behçet's disease is an inflammatory syndrome characterized by oral and genital ulcers, uveitis, and arthritis. The disease also causes an endarteritis in the brain and leptomeninges, and stroke-like events can occur in the setting of

*Table 16.6*   Hypercoagulable states

---

Systemic lupus erythematosus
   Antiphospholipid syndrome
   Thrombotic thrombocytopenic purpura
Antithrombin III deficiency
Protein S, protein C deficiencies
Puerperium
Malignancy (Trousseau's syndrome)
Polycythemia
Cryoglobulinemia
Sickle cell disease
Ulcerative colitis
Nephrotic syndrome

---

an aseptic meningitis. CSF evaluation reveals a moderate pleocytosis and increased protein, and MRI may reveal areas of increased signal intensity in the grey and white matter.

## Stroke Caused by Hypercoagulable States

Hypercoagulability can occur in some collagen vascular diseases as well as other hematologic conditions (Table 16.6). The two main conditions associated with SLE that can increase coagulability are the presence of antiphospholipids (lupus anticoagulant, anticardiolipin antibodies) and TTP. The antiphospholipid antibody syndrome can occur in patients with or without SLE [56]. Migraine-like headaches are a prominent symptom, and recurrent TIAs, strokes, and encephalopathy can occur. In women, the antiphospholipid antibody syndrome is associated with a high incidence of spontaneous abortion. Laboratory evaluation reveals the presence of antiphospholipid antibodies. CT scan or MRI shows primarily cortical infarct, and angiography may show stenosis in intracranial vessels as well as in the extracranial carotid and vertebrobasilar circulation. Patients have also been shown to have cardiac abnormalities on echocardiography, including valvular abnormalities and thrombi. Treatment begins with administration of antiplatelet agents, but cases with recurrent symptoms require administraion of corticosteroids, immunosuppressants, and anticoagulants. In TTP, microangiopathic changes consisting of arterial and capillary thrombi cause a range of symptoms, including headache, encephalopathy, seizures, and stroke-like events. Similar symptoms are observed in cryoglobulinemia, in which extra- and intracranial vessels may become occluded. Deficiencies of the anticoagulant proteins antithrombin III, protein S, and protein C occur as hereditary conditions and may also be acquired. Hypercoagulable states can be acquired as a result of intercurrent malignancy and infection and can occur in the perioperative period and in pregnancy. These conditions may also activate clotting factors such as factor V, factor VII, and factor VIII coagulant activity. Polycythemia and sickle cell disease both cause stroke by decreasing blood flow and should be included in the differential diagnosis of stroke etiology.

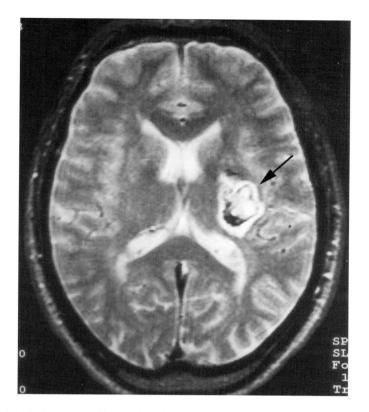

*Figure 16.3* Left putamenal hemorrhage in a 78-year-old man with hypertension. (Courtesy of Mahesh R. Patel, M.D., Beth Israel Deaconess Medical Center, Boston.)

## Hemorrhagic Stroke

### Clinical presentation and Etiology

Hemorrhage can occur in the brain parenchyma and subarachnoid, subdural, or epidural spaces. Intraparenchymal hemorrhage or ICH can occur secondarily, as a complication of an ischemic infarct, or as a primary event.

On a vascular service, the majority of ICHs are a result of either a hypertension hemorrhage or a hemorrhagic conversion of an ischemic infarct. When ICH is seen as a complication of severe hypertension, the location is typically in the basal ganglia (putamen), thalamus, deep hemisphere (lobe), or pons (Figure 16.3). The source of bleeding is believed to be the rupture of Charcot-Bouchard aneurysms related to chronic hypertension. Nonhypertensive causes of bleeding include cerebral amyloid angiopathy, which causes smaller hemorrhages, primarily located in the cortex and seen almost exclusively in elderly patients. Rupture of arteriovenous malformations (AVMs) can occur at any age and can at times result in large intraparenchymal hemorrhages, which are associated with high morbidity and mortality. ICH may occur in the setting of anticoagulant or thrombolytic therapy, sympathomimetic drug use, and alcohol abuse, and as a complication of a brain neoplasm.

Although SAH is uncommon in the patient population typically seen in a vascular service, it has an annual incidence of 4–10 per 100,000 and has a high mortality. SAH is caused by the rupture of saccular aneurysms of cerebral vessels. Most aneurysms are in the ACA and MCA distributions. Multiple aneurysm are seen in up to 30% of cases [57]. Before hemorrhage, patients may have premonitory headaches, which are thought to represent leaking from the unstable aneurysm (sentinel bleed). A sudden, severe headache heralds the SAH and is often accompanied by loss of consciousness. Stroke can occur in the distribution of the ruptured artery.

## Laboratory Diagnosis of Stroke

Table 16.7 lists components of the acute stroke workup. Expanded and more detailed diagnostic protocols are described for ischemic and hemorrhagic stroke (Table 16.8). Individual diagnostic procedures are detailed below.

Computed Tomography and Magnetic Resonance Imaging

Multiple modalities now exist for the localization of stroke and determination of its cause. Imaging of the infarct may be carried out by CT, MRI, and single photon emission CT. CT scans detect acute blood in the first 48 hours more easily than MRI. In addition, CT scan is the optimal technique for imaging blood over the brain convexities resulting from SAH and often makes it possible to avoid a diagnostic lumbar puncture. An ischemic infarct appears as a hypodense area on CT scan. Unless the infarct is very large, CT scans do not reliably show the lesion until 24–48 hours have passed. During

*Table 16.7*    Immediate diagnostic procedures after stroke onset

---

Vital signs
Neurologic examination: motor deficit, level of consciousness, with or without headache
Electrocardiogram, cardiac monitor
Chest x-ray (especially if impaired consciousness or swallowing)
Oxygen saturation
Complete blood count with differential, erythrocyte sedimentation rate, prothrombin time, partial thromboplastin time
Electrolytes, blood urea nitrogen, creatinine, glucose
Computed tomography (of head) to rule out bleed, subarachnoid hemorrhage, old strokes
Magnetic resonance imaging diffusion perfusion scan to detect early ischemic lesions within 30 mins after onset

---

*Table 16.8*  Expanded workup for differential diagnosis

Ischemic stroke
    Rule out hypercoagulable state or inflammatory process
        Complete blood count with differential, prothrombin time, partial thromboplastin
            time, erythrocyte sedimentation rate, serum protein electrophoresis
        Antinuclear antibody titer, antiphospholipid antibody, anticardiolipin antibody
        Protein S, protein C, antithrombin III, homocysteine levels
    Rule out cardiac source
        Echo (transesophageal echocardiogram if paradoxical embolus is suspected)
        Holter monitor
        Blood cultures if possibility exists of subacute bacterial endocarditis
    Rule out large-vessel disease
        Carotid noninvasive studies
        Magnetic resonance angiography if carotid stenosis on ultrasound >60% or equivocal
Hemorrhagic stroke
    Same workup as for ischemic stroke because often hemorrhagic conversion of ischemia
    Determine if patient has hypertensive history; if not, consider other causes, such as arte-
        riovenous malformation, amphetamine abuse
    Magnetic resonance angiography
    Angiography when indicated

the interval between 48 hours and 2 weeks, the infarct can actually become less discrete because of masking by intercurrent edema, which begins to peak at 72 hours. Later, the subacute or chronic infarct appears as a well-demarcated area of hypodensity. Both T1- and T2-weighted MRI imaging is available in most centers. MRI can reveal areas of infarction within the first 24 hours, earlier than CT scan. For lacunar stroke, brain imaging reveals punctate hypodense lesions on CT scan, or areas of increased T2 signal on MRI (Figure 16.4). MRI is the imaging method of choice, given its high resolution and the small size of lacunar and other small infarcts. Cardioembolic events typically result in distal vessel occlusion that leads to wedge-shaped lesions in superficial cortex. In addition, cardioemboli can produce multiple simultaneous infarcts, and it is not uncommon to see several lesions of the same age on the scan. Emboli from the heart or aorta tend to produce larger infarcts than those secondary to artery-artery emboli.

## Ultrasound Techniques

### Transcranial Doppler Ultrasonography

Intracranial blood flow can be documented noninvasively by duplex ultrasonography of the carotid and extracranial vertebral arteries, transcranial Doppler (TCD) ultrasonography of the intracranial vessels, and magnetic resonance angiography (MRA) for both intracranial and neck vessels. TCD ultrasonography can be useful in detecting reduced flow in large and medium-sized intracranial vessels.

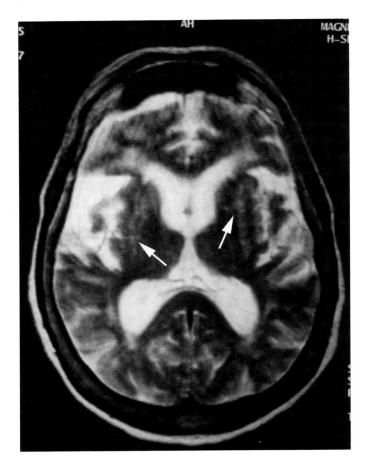

*Figure 16.4*   Small-vessel disease represented by small subcortical foci of increased T2 signal on magnetic resonance image in a 72-year-old woman with chronic hypertension and dementia. Cortical atrophy is also prominent.

## Carotid Duplex Ultrasonography

Carotid duplex ultrasonography is useful for assessment of the degree of extracranial stenosis as well as evaluation of plaque morphology. Duplex scanning can be more accurate than conventional angiography in detecting smaller plaque ulcerations or vessel wall irregularities. However, it has several limitations. Unusual vessel anatomy may not be detected. Calcification may obscure vascular anatomy. In addition, differentiation of complete occlusion and critical stenosis may be difficult. With the advances in MRA, carotid ultrasonography combined with MRA may be a less-invasive, adequate preoperative evaluation in some cases of carotid stenosis (Figure 16.5). A limitation of MRA is its use of an intravenous contrast agent that has been associated with minor renal effects in approximately 1% of patients [58].

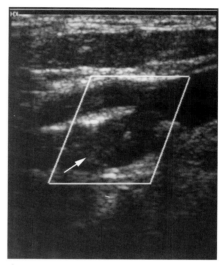

A

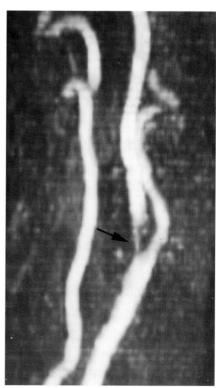

*Figure 16.5* **(A)** Carotid ultrasound image showing total occlusion of the left internal carotid artery. Thrombus can be seen within the vessel. (Courtesy of Colin McCardle, M.D., Beth Israel Deaconess Medical Center, Boston.) **(B)** Magnetic resonance angiogram showing 90–95% stenosis of the right internal carotid artery at its origin. (Courtesy of Mahesh R. Patel, M.D., Beth Israel Deaconess Medical Center, Boston.)

B

## Angiography

Angiography is still the test of choice if high resolution is required to visualize the local vessel lesions and small-caliber vascular structures. Unlike duplex ultrasonography, angiography can provide data about carotid anatomic variation and document the presence of intracranial stenosis as well as extracranial disease.

## Electrocardiography and Echocardiography

In cases of suspected cardioembolic stroke, cardiac arrhythmias are identified by electrocardiography and 24-hour monitoring. To isolate a source of cardiac emboli, echocardiography is appropriate for identifying valvular or wall abnormalities. For determining paradoxical emboli, transthoracic echocardiography with a bubble study is indicated. Transesophageal echocardiography (TEE) has even higher accuracy in detecting small right-to-left shunts. TEE also detects plaques in the aortic arch. The highest risk of stroke has been associated with plaques larger than 4 mm in the proximal arch. Plaque thickness and the presence of a mobile component can be best assessed with TEE.

## Serologic and Other Studies

A number of studies should be performed as a routine diagnostic screen in a patient with a new stoke. These include complete blood count with differential, prothrombin time, partial thromboplastin time (PTT), and blood glucose, cholesterol, and triglyceride levels. An expanded work-up to evaluate for hypercoagulability, autoimmune disease, and other occult causes includes ESR, serum protein electrophoresis, ANA titer, antiphospholipid antibody, anticardiolipin antibody, protein S level, protein C level, antithrombin III level, and serum and urine homocysteine levels. When temporal arteritis is being considered as a cause of stroke, temporal artery biopsy is indicated. Peripheral (sural) nerve biopsies can reveal arteritis in polyarteritis nodosa.

## Treatment of Stroke

### Treatment of Acute Ischemic Stroke

The management of acute ischemic stroke is changing rapidly with the advent of higher-resolution imaging as well as newer treatment modalities, including thrombolytic therapy. Acute treatment protocols are summarized in Table 16.9.

### Early Imaging and Diagnosis

Initial imaging and laboratory work required within the first hours following stroke are detailed in Table 16.9. Patients presenting with a new stroke should undergo immediate imaging to determine whether there is associated hemor-

*Table 16.9*   Treatment of ischemic stroke

Strict bedrest
Head of bed flat, except if congestive heart failure or paroxysmal nocturnal dyspnea
Isotonic fluids
Cardiac monitoring for at least first 24 hrs
Blood pressure maintained higher in hypertensives—do not overcorrect (do not treat systolic
    blood pressure <230 mm HG or diastolic <120 mm HG, slightly lower if on heparin)
Thrombolytic therapy, depending on history and presentation (initiate within first few hrs)
    CT scan with no acute infarction or hemorrhage, and subtotal clinical deficit
    t-PA for acute ischemic stroke
        0.9 mg/kg IV, 10% bolus, remainder over 60 mins
        No adjunctive anticoagulation or antiplatelet treatment for first 24 hrs
        Treatment within 90–180 mins after onset of symtoms
        Blood pressure maintained at systolic <180 mm HG and diastolic <100 mm HG
    t-PA exploratory subgroup study—increased intracranial hemorrhage
        >75 yrs
        Larger deficit, positive CT scan
        Prior aspirin use
Antiplatelet or anticoagulant therapy, depending on history and presentation
    For suspected cardioembolic source, large-vessel disease, hypercoagulable state, venous
        thrombosis, or arterial dissection, and if no operable carotid disease:
    Heparin without an initial bolus to avoid excess anticoagulation—start with a rate of
        1,000 U/hr for international normalized ratio of 2–3
    For large stroke visible on early CT, delay heparin by 48–72 hrs to decrease risk of
        hemorrhagic conversion
    Do not anticoagulate if subacute bacterial endocarditis suspected
    For lacunar stroke use aspirin, 325 mg qd, or ticlopidine hydrochloride (Ticlid), 250 mg bid
    Consider carotid endarterectomy if ipsilateral stenosis >70%
    Acute surgery if small, nonhemorrhagic subtotal stroke, with heparinization in interval
        before surgery
    Delayed surgery if large infarct visible on early CT or hemorrhagic stroke; delay
        heparinization for 48–72 hrs in interval before surgery

CT = computed tomography; t-PA = tissue-type plasminogen activator.

rhage. The CT scan is preferable for initial screening, because it can be obtained rapidly at most centers and readily visualizes acute blood. MRI sequences that can image acute hemorrhage are under development, but T1- and T2-weighted studies are inferior to CT scans for this purpose. If the patient has a mild to moderate subtotal stroke in a branch of a major intracranial artery, then acute anticoagulant therapy should be considered.

*Intravenous Tissue-Type Plasminogen Activator*

Intravenous clot lysis has become available with U.S. Food and Drug Administration–approved use of recombinant tissue-type plasminogen activator (t-PA) [59,60]. Use of t-PA, however, is only appropriate in a select patient population. Guidelines are referenced below. A major complication of t-PA treatment is the risk of subsequent intracranial hemorrhage, especially at the site of the infarction. Risk of hemorrhage has been shown to increase with patient age, previous aspirin use, and appearance of an infarct on the early CT. Intravenous t-PA should be administered only in hospital settings, where appropriate intensive care monitoring and neuroimaging are available to detect early clinical changes should a hemorrhage occur. One clinical study [60] indicated that administration of t-PA within 120 minutes of the onset of stroke significantly improved long-term functional outcome as evaluated at 3 months after stroke.

### Carotid Endarterectomy for Acute Stroke

Duplex ultrasonography and MRA should be performed to determine whether there is a stenosis greater than 70%. If a high-grade ipsilateral stenosis is seen, the patient should be considered for emergency carotid endarterectomy. The timing of carotid endarterectomy depends on the patient's clinical presentation. In patients presenting with a small nonhemorrhagic stroke and mild clinical deficit, immediate endarterectomy should be considered if a significant stenosis can be documented by duplex ultrasonography, MRA, or contrast angiography. However, in cases of infarcts complicated by hemorrhage or infarcts resulting from total or near-total intracranial branch occlusion, it is necessary to delay surgery until the acute lesion has resolved. In cases where no hemorrhage is demonstrated, anticoagulant therapy may be used to prevent recurrent strokes in the interim before surgery.

In patients with strokes or TIAs referable to the hemisphere or eye ipsilateral to a stenotic carotid artery, treatment is determined by the severity of the stenosis. The North American Symptom Carotid Endarterectomy Trial (NASCET) study revealed that endarterectomy significantly improved long-term outcome compared with medical therapy (aspirin) in patients with high-grade (70%) stenosis [61]. The European Cooperative study has also evaluated patients with moderate (30–69%) and low-grade (<30%) stenosis [62]. Although no benefit of surgical therapy has been demonstrated for patients in the low-grade group, the role of carotid endarterectomy in patients with moderate-grade (30–69%) stenosis is still under study. It is important to note that carotid endarterectomy may result in significant complications, including stroke secondary to emboli, local hypoperfusion, carotid occlusion, cranial nerve damage, and death. In the above studies demonstrating a benefit of endarterectomy over medical therapy, the risk of major stroke and death was low, in the range of 2.0–2.5%. Hence, the assessment of surgical mortality and mortality statistics is an integral part of determining management at a given institution.

### Carotid Endarterectomy in Patients with Asymptomatic Carotid Stenosis

In 1995, the Asymptomatic Carotid Atherosclerosis Study, a multicentered study including 39 sites in the United States and Canada, followed approximately 1,650 patients with greater than 60% carotid artery stenosis. All patients received aspirin and medical risk factor management. Those patients randomized to receive surgery underwent carotid endarterectomy. Primary outcome measures were cerebral infarction in the distribution of the study artery or any stroke or death occurring in the perioperative period. With median follow-up of 2.7 years, the projected aggregate risk over 5 years for ipsilateral stroke and perioperative stroke or death was estimated to be about 5% for surgical patients and 11% for medically treated patients. It was concluded that, for patients with greater than 60% carotid stenosis who are good surgical candidates, the 5-year risk of ipsilateral stroke will be reduced if carotid endarterectomy is performed with less than 3% perioperative morbidity and mortality and other stroke risk factors are modified. It should be noted that relative risk reduction in this study reached significance in men, not in women [63]. Hence, the decision to treat asymptomatic stenosis surgically is dependent on local surgical morbidity and mortality statistics as well as lesion severity. When a patient has an asymptomatic stenosis that is less than 60%, it is recommended that follow-up carotid studies using noninvasive methods be performed at least every 6–12 months to detect progression. Surgical therapy would be favored for rapidly progressing lesions at the time they reach greater than 60% stenosis.

## Anticoagulation and Antiplatelet Therapy for Acute Stroke

In nonsurgical patients, the decision to anticoagulate depends on the estimated size of the infarct as well as the cause of the condition. Patients with lacunar stroke do not benefit from anticoagulant therapy, and little evidence exists that antiplatelet therapy decreases the neurologic deficit or risk of recurrence, although it is accepted practice to treat patients with antiplatelet therapy if no contraindication exists. Early anticoagulation is also contraindicated in patients with a large stroke involving all territory within a major branch of the intracranial carotid. In these patients, appropriate measures to minimize edema should be taken, including fluid restriction and elevation of the head of the bed to 30 degrees. More aggressive measures such as mannitol administration may be used if edema progresses. Edema is maximal at 48–72 hours following stroke onset. Anticoagulation is deferred for at least 48 hours in the case of a large stroke, as this is the period of greatest risk for hemorrhagic transformation of the infarct. Likewise, in the case of a hemorrhagic infarct, anticoagulation is deferred for this period of time or longer, depending on the size of the hematoma.

Anticoagulant therapy can be indicated for patients suffering from subtotal strokes who show worsening of symptoms and who have been determined not to be candidates for endarterectomy. In these cases, it is generally advisable to begin heparin at 1,000 units per hour without an intravenous bolus to minimize risk of secondary hemorrhage. PTT levels should be checked within 4–6 hours of starting heparin, and the dose should be adjusted to produce PTT levels in the range of 60–80 seconds. Anticoagulant therapy is also indicated for patients who have suffered large strokes caused by significant carotid stenosis, but in whom surgery must be delayed because of the size of their infarcts. These patients should be treated as above, with a delay of at least 48–72 hours before initiation of anticoagulant therapy to prevent the risk of secondary hemorrhage.

A number of studies have evaluated risk reduction for stroke in patients with cardioembolic stroke. It is generally agreed that patients with valvular AF are candidates for anticoagulant therapy. In a study of patients with nonvalvular AF, the Stroke Prevention in Atrial Fibrillation trial randomly assigned patients to treatment with either aspirin or warfarin sodium [64]. The results suggest that warfarin sodium may be more useful in older patients. Similar findings were obtained from the Boston-area trial [65] and the Copenhagen study [66], with warfarin sodium statistically reducing the risk of stroke as well as the risk of death from other causes. The acceptable range for the international normalized ratio should be between 2 and 3.

Warfarin sodium and aspirin are both used in the prevention of stroke following MI. A meta-analysis combining several studies concluded that warfarin is superior [67]. However, aspirin still had a role in reducing the risk of complications from peripheral vascular disease other than stroke. Neither aspirin nor anticoagulant therapy is indicated in the case of emboli caused by subacute bacterial endocarditis, because of the high risk of recurrent embolization and secondary hemorrhage [43,68]. Repeat angiography performed after antibiotic therapy is useful in identifying residual aneurysms in patients such as those with prosthetic valves in whom long-term anticoagulation is indicated [43].

## Antiplatelet and Anticoagulant Therapy for Stroke Prevention

Prophylactic medical therapy for carotid disease in cases where operative therapy is not indicated consists largely of administration of antiplatelet agents or anticoagulants. Aspirin has been the mainstay of therapy and is usually the first-line agent used. Aspirin prevents platelet aggregation and has been shown in several large studies to reduce the risk of primary and secondary stroke related to carotid disease [69–75]. The dose used varied from 30 mg to 1,500 mg per day. Overall, the risk reduction in these studies ranged from 20% to 50% reduction for stroke and death. The optimal dose has been controversial, and 325 mg per day is used by most groups. The NASCET study is currently evaluating the relative risk reduction for secondary stroke in postendarterectomy patients taking 325 mg versus 1,300 mg of aspirin per day. Other agents that decrease platelet aggregation include dipyridamole (Persantine) [72], sulfinpyrazone [73,76], and suloctidil [77]. However, clinical trials and meta-analyses have shown no benefit of these agents either alone or in combination with aspirin [67]. In contrast, clinical trials have shown that ticlopidine hydrochloride, which inhibits ADP-dependent platelet activation and release, effectively prevents both primary and secondary stroke [78–81]. The usual dose of ticlopidine hydrochloride is 250 mg twice a day. Side effects of ticlopidine hydrochloride are more prominent than those of aspirin and can include diarrhea, rash, and neutropenia. The neutropenia has been reported in 1% of patients using ticlopidine hydrochloride but is reversed when the drug is discontinued.

Anticoagulant therapy is used in the treatment of secondary stroke prevention in appropriate nonsurgical candidates when aspirin and ticlopidine hydrochloride have failed. In addition, anticoagulation significantly reduces the risk of recurrent stroke in the setting of a known cardioembolic source. Heparin is generally reserved for acute induction of anticoagulation, usually in the management of a new ischemic stroke of any etiology or acute arterial occlusion. Heparin is also used for long-term anticoagulation when it is necessary during pregnancy, because warfarin sodium is teratogenic. Warfarin sodium is the anticoagulant of choice for outpatient prophylaxis in patients for whom antiplatelet therapy has been unsuccessful and who are not surgical candidates. The warfarin sodium dose should be managed to maintain a prothrombin time in the range of an international normalized ratio of 2 to 3 [82,83].

Finally, it is important to note that, for all atherothrombotic strokes, a mainstay of therapy is to reduce concurrent risk factors. Adequate treatment of hypertension, diabetes, hypercholesterolemia, hyperlipidemia, and hypercoagulable states, as well as discouragement of smoking and alcohol intake, are all important in the long-term management of patients at risk for a primary or secondary stroke. Management of intercurrent hypertension and diabetes is especially important in the setting of lacunar stroke, where there is little evidence that administration of antiplatelet agents and anticoagulants alter disease progression.

## Treatment of Stroke Caused by Autoimmune Disease

Immunosuppression is the mainstay of therapy for autoimmune causes of stroke such as temporal arteritis, Wegener's granulomatosis, and SLE. Therapies include administration of corticosteroids and cytotoxic agents such as cyclophosphamide. In Takayasu's arteritis, bypass surgery on major aortic branches may be required. Isolated granulomatous angiitis may improve with the above therapies, but progression of disease can be refractory to therapy.

## Treatment of Stroke Caused by Homocysteinemia

In the setting of homocysteinemia, administration of supplemental vitamins $B_6$, $B_{12}$, and folic acid may lower blood levels of homocysteine, but it has not been shown that this intervention reduces incidence of stroke [15].

## Treatment of Hemorrhagic Stroke

Treatment of hemorrhagic stroke is summarized in Table 16.10. ICH can frequently be a life-threatening event. If the patient has altered consciousness, then the airway should be protected, and the patient should be intubated if necessary. The main complication is increased intracranial pressure from an enlarging hematoma or from ensuing secondary edema. CT scan or MRI must be performed serially if herniation across the midline or infratentorially is suspected, and scans should be repeated with any significant clinical deterioration. Judicious fluid restriction and elevation of the head of the bed are minimal steps necessary in a mild hemorrhage without significant neurologic deficit. With larger hemorrhages, however, hyperventilation can be used as the first step in lowering intracranial pressure, followed by administration of mannitol if necessary. Underlying bleeding disorders should be promptly evaluated and treated. Hypertension should be corrected cautiously, because significant decreases in blood pressure when there is increased intracranial pressure may lower cerebral perfusion. Cerebral angiography is usually unrevealing in acute ICH, as involved cerebral vasculature is often obscured by the hematoma. Sur-

*Table 16.10*   Treatment of hemorrhagic stroke

Large infarct or intracerebral hemorrhage—reduce risk of herniation
Head of bed elevated >30 degrees
    Fluid restriction to two-thirds maintenance
    Cardiac monitor
    Blood pressure: avoid overcorrection, keep systolic blood pressure at 160–220 mm Hg
      and diastolic at 70–130 mm Hg
    Antiplatelet or anticoagulant therapy: avoid or discontinue for at least first 5–7 days
Herniation caused by large ischemic infarct or bleed
    Angiography if arteriovenous malformation suspected
    Intensive care unit transfer
    Diuretics
    Cardiac monitor
    Hyperventilation to keep $pCO_2$ around 25 mm Hg
    Neurosurgical decompression should be considered if cerebellar or nondominant
      hemisphere stroke
    Mannitol if diuretics and hyperventilation inadequate (20% solution, 1 g/kg over 15 mins)

gical therapy for ICH is performed only under certain circumstances. The decision to evacuate a hematoma usually is made if the bleed is easily accessible and if the procedure is lifesaving. A common indication for surgery is the occurrence of a cerebellar hemorrhage, where enlargement can cause compression of the brain stem and death.

AVMs may be diagnosed during a workup for a focal neurologic deficit or seizures, and the decision to resect them is made depending on their location and size. In addition to surgical resection, AVMs can also be reduced in size by stereotactic radiosurgery. In the case of very large AVMs, invasive neuroradiologic procedures such as embolization are performed before surgical resection in order to debulk the mass.

## Treatment of Subarachnoid Hemorrhage

The acute management of SAH is directed at controlling blood pressure, suppressing vasospasm, and preventing seizures, which may increase blood pressure and cause rebleeding. In addition, the patient must be monitored for the development of hyponatremia and syndrome of inappropriate secretion of antidiuretic hormone. Blood pressure can be reduced with agents such as sodium nitroprusside, and the calcium channel blocker nimodipine is used to prevent vasospasm and reduce the risk of secondary stroke. If vasospasm occurs, then blood pressure may be increased in order to maintain cerebral blood flow. Cerebral blood flow may be monitored with TCD ultrasonography. Anticonvulsants are given as a prophylactic against seizure activity. In most centers, patients undergo contrast angiography immediately, and, if an operable aneurysm is detected, surgical resection is performed as early as possible. Evidence indicates that early timing of surgery improves outcome.

*Table 16.11*  Common causes of encephalopathy

| Hypertensive | Increased blood pressure |
|---|---|
| | Infarct |
| | Hemorrhage |
| Postoperative | Infarct |
| | Hemorrhage |
| | Hypoxia |
| | Seizures |
| Metabolic or toxic | Medications |
| | Infection |
| | Hepatic dysfunction |
| | Uremia or renal dysfunction |
| | Electrolyte imbalance |
| | Alcohol withdrawal |

## ENCEPHALOPATHY

Encephalopathy is a common complication in the acute care setting and can be a manifestation of multiple underlying causes. *Encephalopathy* is a general term used to denote mental status changes that can range from increased drowsiness and lethargy to confusion and disorientation. In addition to mental status change, associated signs such as asterixis and myoclonus may also be present. Discussed here is acute or subacute change in mental state, which does not include the long-term cognitive decline seen with dementia. This section addresses the most common etiologies to be considered when consulting on a vascular patient with mental status change. The categories included are hypertensive encephalopathy, mental status change in the immediate postoperative setting, metabolic and toxic encephalopathy, and alcohol withdrawal. These are summarized in Table 16.11.

### Hypertensive Encephalopathy

Clinical Presentation

Hypertensive encephalopathy must be addressed when considering altered mental status in an inpatient on a vascular service. This condition is a neurologic syndrome consisting of headache, seizure, vision changes, and altered mental status in association with sustained elevated systemic blood pressure. Other neurologic signs such as cortical blindness, focal weakness, or aphasia may be present. The signs and symptoms can be rapidly progressive. If the syndrome is unrecognized or treatment delayed, it may be fatal. If the hypertension is treated, however, the neurologic changes are usually reversible. Other neurologic entities that can manifest similarly to hypertensive encephalopathy include stroke, intracranial hemorrhage, encephalitis, venous thrombosis, and tumor. Hypertensive encephalopathy has also been described in the context of bilateral carotid

endarterectomy and was thought to be related to dysfunction of carotid baroreceptor reflex sensitivity [84].

## Etiology

Pathophysiologically, the normal spectrum of autoregulation of cerebral blood
flow is exceeded in hypertensive encephalopathy. Studies suggest that abnormal
vasodilation caused by increased intraluminal pressure leads to vascular damage
and cerebral edema. The occipital lobes and watershed zones are the first areas
that demonstrate vasogenic edema. With persistent elevated pressures, though,
generalized cerebral edema can be seen.

## Laboratory Diagnosis

Neurodiagnostic testing can help sort out hypertensive encephalopathy from other
causes of mental status change in hypertensive patients. Establishing the presence
of an ischemic stroke in the brain becomes especially relevant when determining
treatment of elevated blood pressure. In hypertensive encephalopathy, both head CT
scans and head MRI can be normal or may show cerebral edema. Edema is characteristically in the occipital lobes and is seen as decreased attenuation on CT scan or
increased T2 signal on MRI. The occipital abnormalities are typically bilateral,
involving the subcortical white matter and often extending to the cortical surface
[85]. Electroencephalography (EEG) may show slowing of background activity,
which is particularly prominent in the posterior regions if cortical blindness is present. Lumbar puncture can reveal normal or elevated opening pressure. CSF protein
concentration may be as high as 150 mg/dl, and a few red cells can be seen. CSF
analysis is more helpful in ruling out other causes of encephalopathy, such as meningoencephalitis, than in establishing a diagnosis of hypertensive encephalopathy.

## Treatment

The goals of initial treatment for hypertensive encephalopathy are to decrease
blood pressure to within the range of cerebral autoregulation, to control seizures,
and to manage edema. The target blood pressure should be based in part on the
patient's baseline blood pressure and varies depending on whether the patient
was previously normotensive or chronically hypertensive. Overly aggressive
lowering of systemic blood pressure can be harmful, especially if ischemic
infarct is already present. No single antihypertensive agent is used in all scenarios. Relevant to this discussion is the concern that the agent chosen should
have minimal effect on cerebral vasculature. A medication such as nitroglycerin
that decreases peripheral vascular resistance also dilates cerebral vessels and
may worsen hypertensive encephalopathy. Labetalol hydrochloride, an alpha-
and beta-adrenergic blocking agent, is often preferred. Seizures may be adequately controlled with treatment of the hypertension. However, if they persist,
intravenous phenytoin may be required. If cerebral edema becomes widespread

and does not improve with lowering of blood pressure, the patient will most likely be comatose and may need intracranial monitoring and more aggressive therapy directed at vasogenic edema. Hyperventilation and corticosteroids can be effective. An osmotic diuretic, mannitol, potentially may worsen edema as it may cross the damaged blood-brain barrier [86].

## Postoperative Encephalopathy

### Clinical Presentation and Etiology

Several other causes of encephalopathy should be considered in the immediate postsurgical setting, expecially following vascular surgical procedures such as carotid endarterectomy. If a patient has difficulty waking up postanesthesia or is persistently confused postoperatively, cerebral ischemia and hypoxia may be factors.

Ischemic stroke can result when atherosclerotic emboli travel to distal arteries, most commonly within the anterior cerebral and middle cerebral territories. It is often easier to diagnose ischemic stroke if there are neurologic findings other than altered mental status, such as unilateral weakness. Embolic stroke following cardiovascular procedures is discussed in Chapter 14. Transient hypotension can lead to cerebral hypoperfusion; this in turn may cause arterial watershed zone infarcts, often bilaterally. These border zone areas, lying high over the cortical convexity, are most vulnerable when systemic arterial pressure is lowered. Infarction in these areas can result in cortical blindness, transcortical aphasias, and a proximal pattern of weakness bilaterally. Myoclonus may also be seen after hypoxic injury.

Nonconvulsive status (i.e., persistent electrical seizure activity not manifested with repetitive tonic-clonic movements) should also be considered in the patient who is difficult to arouse or agitated and confused postoperatively. Seizures often denote another underlying pathology, including severe hypertension, ischemia, hemorrhage, anoxia, or metabolic derangements. Infection and metabolic abnormalities are always possibilities in the differential diagnosis of postoperative encephalopathy and are discussed separately below.

### Diagnosis

Diagnostic tests that may be helpful in the setting of postoperative encephalopathy are a head image and an EEG. A CT scan is probably the head imaging method best tolerated by a surgical intensive care unit patient. Initially, it will demonstrate hemorrhage and possibly early changes resulting from ischemic stroke if the infarct is large. Otherwise, head CT scan best reveals ischemic damage between 24 and 48 hours of the stroke and may need to be repeated. In cases of global anoxic ischemic encephalopathy, cerebral edema may be evident on CT scan. EEG can help in ruling out continuous seizure activity as well as in confirming encephalopathy. CSF analysis is worth performing if the patient is febrile and there is no other clear source of infection.

Treatment

Treatment depends on the cause of the perioperative encephalopathy. While ischemic damage cannot be reversed entirely, it is important to maintain a steady blood pressure that supports cerebral perfusion and does not overwork the heart. The ideal systemic pressure will vary from patient to patient depending on the history of cardiovascular disease and the type of brain damage.

A patient with anoxic encephalopathy who is otherwise stable needs to be followed over time. It is difficult to determine prognosis in these situations, and absolute statements should be avoided. An amnesic syndrome similar to Korsakoff's may persist for weeks or remain permanently, presumably a result of hippocampal susceptibility to anoxic injury. Depression can also be a significant contributing factor in the long term. Behavioral neurologic evaluation and neuropsychologic testing can be helpful after discharge, both in determining cognitive problem areas and in providing strategies to compensate.

Infections or metabolic abnormalities should be treated accordingly. Seizure activity should be controlled with intravenous anticonvulsants while the cause is being determined.

## Metabolic and Toxic Encephalopathy

Clinical Presentation and Etiology

The spectrum of etiologies in metabolic and toxic encephalopathy ranges from medications to infection to metabolic derangements. Because the focus here is on the inpatient population, causative medications are usually those that have been introduced since the patient's admission. Common culprits contributing to encephalopathy are benzodiazepines and narcotic analgesics. Antiemetics such as metoclopramide hydrochloride (Reglan) and prochlorperazine edisylate (Compazine) and sedating medications such as antihistamines may also contribute. A careful review of the patient's medication regimen is always worthwhile when mental status change occurs.

When fever accompanies the encephalopathy, infection must be ruled out. If blood and urine cultures remain negative, and radiologic studies do not demonstrate a systemic source of fever (e.g., pneumonia, abscess), then a lumbar puncture for CSF evaluation should be considered. Associated signs and symptoms such as papilledema, headache, neck stiffness, vomiting, or seizures point more toward a diagnosis of meningitis or encephalitis.

Common metabolic abnormalities that may manifest with encephalopathy include renal or hepatic dysfunction; abnormal sodium, calcium, or magnesium metabolism; and hypoglycemia or hyperglycemia. Of course, often a combination of several factors is present. For example, a diabetic patient with chronic renal insufficiency may develop encephalopathy while an inpatient as a result of fluctuating blood sugars and rising blood urea nitrogen, independent of the reason for admission to hospital.

Heavy use or abuse of alcohol is common enough that alcohol withdrawal should always be considered in patients with acute mental status change. The timing and clinical signs can help with this diagnosis. In addition, if the diagnosis is suspected, treatment should be initiated. Confusion, disorientation, and agitation along with visual hallucinations commonly appear 12–72 hours after cessation of drinking. Tremors, nausea, anxiety, and increased sweating may begin within hours of the last intake of alcohol, however. This tremulous syndrome may herald full-blown delirium tremens. It is most helpful, although not always possible, to have an accurate alcohol history up front.

## Diagnosis

The need for diagnostic testing is dictated by the clinical setting. Relevant data is accumulated to confirm clinical suspicion based on the patient's presentation and underlying medical or surgical issues.

Head imaging helps define the presence of stroke or abscess but is not likely to differentiate one metabolic cause of encephalopathy from another. If a lumbar puncture is to be performed as part of an infection workup for acute mental status change and increased intracranial pressure is suspected, a head CT scan is indicated before the procedure to look for a space-occupying lesion or obstructive hydrocephalus. If bacterial meningitis or encephalitis is suspected, CSF evaluation should include CSF glucose and protein, red and white blood cell counts and differential, Gram's stain, cultures, and antibiotic sensitivities. Common pathogens in nosocomial meningitis in adults are *Escherichia coli* and *Klebsiella pneumoniae* [87].

Electrolyte and other metabolic disorders can be assessed with measurement of serum concentrations, for example, sodium level, liver chemistries, blood urea nitrogen level, and serum ammonia level.

## Treatment

Treatment is dictated by which factors are contributing to the encephalopathy. Sometimes simplifying a medication regimen is the only intervention needed. If central nervous system infection is suspected, antibiotic therapy should be started as soon as possible and should not be delayed while waiting for diagnostic studies. In the case of alcohol withdrawal, benzodiazepines can be helpful initially, along with nutritional support to correct thiamine, multivitamin, and magnesium deficiencies as needed.

## PERIPHERAL NEUROPATHY

Neurologic problems may also present within the peripheral nervous system in the acute care setting. This section discusses a few common entities that may be seen in vascular medicine and surgery patients with chronic illness such as diabetes and hypertension. Diabetes-related neuropathies and entrapment syndromes that may be encountered in acutely ill patients are mentioned.

The peripheral neuropathy most commonly seen in association with underlying diabetes is a distal symmetric polyneuropathy. Sensory loss is typically in a stocking-glove distribution. Small-fiber sensory neuropathy will present with deep burning pain and paresthesias, while large-fiber involvement may be painless with impairment of vibration and position sense. There may also be distal motor involvement in the lower extremities as well as autonomic system involvement.

Diabetic autonomic neuropathy can manifest with orthostatic hypotension, high resting heart rate, or pulse rate that is unresponsive to respiration. This condition is likely a contributing factor to the increased incidence of silent myocardial infarction in diabetic patients. Gastrointestinal motility problems, disorders of sweating, urinary retention, and impotence are also included in the spectrum of autonomic involvement.

Entrapment and compression neuropathies of the ulnar and peroneal nerves can be seen in patients who have been bedridden or relatively immobile. Diabetic patients also have an increased incidence of entrapment nerve syndromes [88]. Direct compression of the ulnar nerve is typically at the elbow in a patient who has undergone general anesthesia or has repeatedly leaned on the medial aspect of the elbow. Weakness is seen in the intrinsic hand muscles, the flexor carpi ulnaris and the flexor digitorum profundus of the fourth and fifth fingers. Sensory loss involves the fifth finger, part of the fourth finger, the hypothenar eminence, and part of the dorsum of the hand.

Common peroneal nerve compression is typically at the fibular head where the nerve is particularly vulnerable. Such compression is often seen as a result of repeated leg crossing or significant weight loss or in chronically ill patients. The condition may lead to weakness in the foot dorsiflexors and foot eversion, with sensory impairment over the lateral lower leg and dorsum of the foot. A foot drop may be seen if gait can be tested.

Femoral nerve involvement in the setting of retroperitoneal hematoma should also be considered here, especially in a patient population where anticoagulant therapy is common. Iliopsoas hematoma predominantly affects the femoral nerve but can also include obturator nerve and leads to weakness of hip flexors, knee extensors, and hip adductors, and decreased or absent patellar reflex. Groin pain may be significant and radiate into the thigh and leg, and paresthesias of the anteromedial thigh may be seen.

## REFERENCES

1. Wolf PA, D'Agostino RB, Belanger AJ, Kannel WB. Probability of stroke: a risk profile from the Framingham Study. Stroke 1991;22:312.
2. Colandrea MA, Friedman GD, Nichaman MZ. Systolic hypertension in the elderly: an epidemiologic assessment. Circulation 1970;41:239.
3. Kannel WB, Wolf PA, McGee DL. Systolic blood pressure, arterial rigidity, and risk of stroke: the Framingham Study. JAMA 1981;245:1225.
4. Fisher CM. The ascendancy of diastolic blood pressure over systolic. Lancet 1985;2:1349.
5. Rutan GH, McDonald RH, Kuller LH. A historical perspective of elevated systolic vs. diastolic blood pressure from an epidemiology and clinical trial viewpoint. J Clin Epidemiol 1989;42:663.
6. Stratton JR, Resnick AD. Increased embolic risk in patients with left ventricular thrombi. Circulation 1987;75:1004.
7. Wolf PA, Abbott RD, Kannel WB. Atrial fibrillation: a major contributor to stroke in the elderly: the Framingham Study. Arch Intern Med 1987;147:1561.

8. Wolf PA, Dawber TR, Thomas HE, Kannel WB. Epidemiologic assessment of chronic atrial fibrillation and risk of stroke: the Framingham Study. Neurology 1978;28:973.
9. Barrett-Connor E, Khaw K. Diabetes mellitus: an independent risk factor for stroke. Am J Epidemiol 1988;128:116.
10. Dorman JS, Laporte RE, Kuller LH, et al. The Pittsburgh insulin-dependent diabetes mellitus (IDDM) morbidity and mortality study. Mortality results. Diabetes 1984;33:271.
11. Shinton R, Beevers G. Meta-analysis of relation between cigarette smoking and stroke. BMJ 1989;298:789.
12. Iso H, Jacobs DR, Wentworth D. Serum cholesterol levels and six-year mortality from stroke in 350,977 men screened for the multiple risk factor intervention trial. N Engl J Med 1989; 320:904.
13. Collaborative Group for the Study of Stroke in Young Women. Oral contraception and stroke in young women: associated risk factors. JAMA 1975;231:718.
14. Pessin MS, Duncan GW, Mohr JP, Poskanzer DC. Clinical and angiographic features of carotid transient ischemic attacks. N Engl J Med 1977;296:358.
15. Sacco RL, Benjamin EJ, Broderick JP, et al. Risk factors. AHA conference proceedings. Stroke 1997;28:1507.
16. Heyman A, Wilkinson WE, Heyden S. Risk of stroke in asymptomatic persons with cervical arterial bruits. N Engl J Med 1980;302:838.
17. Wolf PA, Kannel WB, Sorlie P, McNamara P. Asymptomatic carotid bruit and the risk of stroke. JAMA 1981;245:1442.
18. Treiman RL, Foran RF, Shore EH, Levin PM. Carotid bruit. Arch Surg 1973;106:803.
19. Cooperman M, Martin EW, Evans WE. Significance of asymptomatic carotid bruits. Arch Surg 1978;113:1229.
20. Kagan A, Popper J, Rhoads GG. Epidemiologic Studies on Coronary Artery Disease and Stroke in Japanese Men Living in Japan, Hawaii, and California: Prevalence of Stroke. In P Scheinberg (ed), Cerebrovascular Diseases. New York: Raven, 1976;267.
21. Kartchner MM, McRae LP. Noninvasive evaluation and management of the "asymptomatic" carotid bruit. Surgery 1977;82:840.
22. Bernstein NM, Norris JW. Benign outcome of carotid occlusion. Neurology 1989;39:6.
23. Cote R, Barnett HJM, Taylor DW. Internal carotid occlusion: a prospective study. Stroke 1983;14:898.
24. Furlan AJ, Whisnant JP. Long-term prognosis after carotid artery occlusion. Neurology (Minneapolis) 1980;30:986.
25. Sacquegna T, DeCarolis P, Pazzaglia P. The clinical course and prognosis of carotid artery occlusion. J Neurol Neurosurg Psychiatry 1982;45:1037.
26. Caplan LR, Gorelick PB, Hier DB. Race, sex, and occlusive cerebrovascular disease: a review. Stroke 1986;17:648.
27. Mudd SH, Levy HL, Skovby F. Disorders of Transsulfuration. In CR Scriver et al. (eds), The Metabolic and Molecular Bases of Inherited Disease (7th ed). New York: McGraw-Hill, 1995.
28. Perry IJ, Refsum H, Morris RW, et al. Prospective study of serum total homocysteine concentration and risk of stroke in middle-aged British men. Lancet 1995;346:1395.
29. Fisher CM, Ojemann R, Roberson G. Spontaneous dissection of cervico-cerebral arteries. J Can Sci Neurol 1978;5:9.
30. Ringel S, Harrison S, Norenberg M. Fibromuscular dysplasia: multiple "spontaneous" dissecting aneurysms of the major cranial arteries. Ann Neurol 1977;1:301.
31. Stanley JC, Gewertz BL, Bove EL. Arterial fibrodysplasia: histopathologic character and current etiologic concepts. Arch Surg 1975;110:561.
32. Luscher TF, Stanson AW, Hauser OW. Arterial fibromuscular dysplasia. Mayo Clin Proc 1987;62:931.
33. Osborne AG, Anderson RE. Angiographic spectrum of cervical and intracranial fibromuscular dysplasia. Stroke 1977;8:617.
34. Fisher CM. Lacunar strokes and infarcts. Neurology 1982;32:871.
35. Hachinski VC, Potter P, Merksey H. Leukoariosis. Arch Neurol 1987;44:21.
36. Fisher CM. Capsular infarcts. Arch Neurology 1979;36:65.
37. Nichols FTI, Mohr JP. Binswanger's Subacute Arteriosclerotic Encephalopathy. In HJM Barnett, BM Stein, JP Mohr, FM Yatsu (eds), Stroke: Pathophysiology, Diagnosis and Management. New York: Churchill Livingstone, 1986;875.
38. Bogousslavsky J, Van Melle G, Regli F. The Lausanne Stroke Registry: analysis of 1000 consecutive patients with first stroke. Stroke 1988;19:1083.
39. Cerebral Embolism Task Force. Cardiogenic brain embolism. Arch Neurol 1986;43:727.

40. Cerebral Embolism Task Force. Cardiogenic brain embolism: the second report of the Cerebral Embolism Task Force. Arch Neurol 1989;46:727.
41. Jones HR Jr, Naggar CZ, Seljan MP, Downing LL. Cerebral emboli of paradoxical origin. Ann Neurol 1983;13:314.
42. Loscalzo J. Paradoxical embolism: clinical presentation, diagnostic strategies, and therapeutic options. Am Heart J 1986;112:141.
43. Davenport J, Hart RG. Prosthetic valve endocarditis 1976–1987: antibiotics, anticoagulation, and stroke. Stroke 1990;21:993.
44. Amarenco P, Cohen A, Tzourio C, et al. Atherosclerotic disease of the aortic arch and the risk of ischemic stroke. N Engl J Med 1994;331:1474.
45. Machado EDV, Michet CJ, Ballard DJ. Trends in incidence and clinical presentation of temporal arteritis in Olmsted County, Minnesota, 1950–1985. Arthritis Rheum 1988;31:745.
46. Huston KA, Hunder GG, Lie JT. Temporal arteritis: a 25-year epidemiologic, clinical and pathologic study. Ann Intern Med 1978;88:162.
47. Missen GA. Involvement of the vertebrocarotid arterial system in giant cell arteritis. J Pathol 1972;106:ii.
48. Hall S, Barr W, Lie JT. Takayasu arteritis: a study of 32 American patients. Medicine 1985;64:89.
49. Calabrese LH, Mallek JA. Primary angiitis of the central nervous system: report of 8 new cases, review of the literature, and proposal for diagnosis. Medicine (Baltimore) 1988;67:20.
50. Moore PM. Diagnosis and management of isolated angiitis of the nervous system. Neurology 1989;39:167.
51. Ford RG, Siekert RG. Central nervous system manifestations of polyarteritis nodosa. Neurology 1965;15:114.
52. Travers RL, Allison DJ, Brettle RP, Hughes GRV. Polyarteritis nodosa: a clinical and angiographic analysis of 17 cases. Semin Arthritis Rheum 1979;8:184.
53. Futrell N, Millikan C. Frequency, etiology, and prevention of stroke in patients with systemic lupus erythematosus. Stroke 1989;20:583.
54. Devinsky O, Petito CK, Alonso DR. Clinical and neuropathological findings in systemic lupus erythematosus: the role of vasculitis, heart emboli, and thrombolic thrombocytopenic purpura. Ann Neurol 1988;23:380.
55. Fauci AS, Haynes BF, Katz P, Wolff SM. Wegener's granulomatosis: prospective clinical and therapeutic experience with 85 patients for 21 years. Ann Intern Med 1983;98:76.
56. Asherson RA, Khamashta MA, Ordi-Ros J. The "primary" antiphospholipid syndrome: major clinical and serological features. Medicine (Baltimore) 1989;68:366.
57. Ostergaard JR, Hog E. Incidence of multiple intracranial aneurysms: influence of arterial hypertension and gender. J Neurosurg 1985;63:49.
58. Prestigiacomo CJ, Connolly ESJ, Quest DO. Use of carotid ultrasound as a preoperative assessment of extracranial carotid artery blood flow and vascular anatomy. Neurosurg Clin N Am 1996;7(4):577.
59. Hacke W, Kaste M, Fiesche C, et al. Intravenous thrombolysis with a recombinant tissue plasminogen activator for acute hemispheric stroke: The European Cooperative Acute Stroke Study (ECASS). JAMA 1997;274:1017.
60. The National Institute of Neurological Disorders and Stroke r-tPA Stroke Study Group. Tissue plasminogen activator for acute ischemic stroke. N Engl J Med 1995;333:1581.
61. North American Symptomatic Carotid Endarterectomy Trial Collaborators. Beneficial effect of carotid endarterectomy in symptomatic patients with high-grade carotid stenosis. N Engl J Med 1990;323:1505.
62. European Carotid Surgery Trialists' Collaborative Group. MRC European carotid surgery trial: interim results from symptomatic patients with severe (70–90%) or mild (0–29%) carotid stenosis. Lancet 1991;337:1235.
63. Executive Committee for the Asymptomatic Carotid Atherosclerosis Study. Endarterectomy for asymptomatic carotid artery stenosis. JAMA 1995;273:1421.
64. Stroke Prevention in Atrial Fibrillation Investigators. Stroke Prevention in Atrial Fibrillation Study: final results. Circulation 1991;84:527.
65. The Boston Area Anticoagulation Trial Fibrillation Investigators. The effect of low-dose warfarin on the risk of stroke in patients with nonrheumatic atrial fibrillation. N Engl J Med 1990;323:1505.
66. Petersen P, Boysen G, Godtfredsen J, et al. Placebo-controlled, randomised trial of warfarin and aspirin for prevention of thromboembolic complications in chronic atrial fibrillation: The Copenhagen AFASAK Study. Lancet 1989;1:175.
67. Matchar DB, McCrory DC, Barnett H, Feussner JR. Medical treatment for stroke prevention. Ann Intern Med 1994;121:41.

68. Hart RG, Foster JW, Luther MF, Kanter MC. Stroke in infective endocarditis. Stroke 1990;21:586.
69. Antiplatelet Trialist's Collaboration. Collaborative overview of randomised trials of antiplatelet therapy—I: Prevention of death, myocardial infarction, and stroke by prolonged antiplatelet therapy in various categories of patients. BMJ 1994;308:81.
70. Farrell B, Godwin J, Richards S, Warlow C. The United Kingdom Transient Ischemic Attack (UK-TIA) Aspirin Trial: final results. J Neurol Neurosurg Psychiatry 1991;54:1044.
71. Sorensen PS, Pedersen H, Marquardsen J, et al. Acetylsalicylic acid in the prevention of stroke in patients with reversible cerebral ischemic attacks. Stroke 1983;14:15.
72. The American-Canadian Co-operative Study Group. Persantine aspirin trial in cerebral ischemia, part II: endpoint results. Stroke 1985;16:406.
73. The Canadian Cooperative Study Group. A randomized trial of aspirin and sulfinpyrazone in threatened stroke. N Engl J Med 1978;299:53.
74. The Dutch TIA Trial Study Group. A comparison of two doses of aspirin (30 mg vs. 283 mg a day) in patients after a transient ischemic stroke. N Engl J Med 1991;325:1261.
75. The SALT Cooperative Group. Swedish Aspirin Low-dose Trials (SALT) of 75-mg aspirin as secondary prophylaxis after cerebrovascular ischemic events. Lancet 1991;338:1345.
76. Candelise L, Landi G, Perrone P, et al. A randomized trial of aspirin and sulfinpyrazone in patients with TIA. Stroke 1982;13:175.
77. Gent M, Blakely JA, Hachinski V, et al. A secondary prevention, randomized trial of suloctidil in patients with a recent history of thromboembolic stroke. Stroke 1985;16:416.
78. Gent M, Blakely JA, Easton JD, et al. The Canadian American Ticlopidine Study (CATS) in thromboembolic stroke. Lancet 1989;1:1215.
79. Grotta JC, Norris JW, Kamm B. Prevention of stroke with ticlopidine: who benefits most? TAAS Baseline and Angiographic Data Subgroup. Neurology 1992;42:111.
80. Harbison JW. Ticlopidine versus aspirin for the prevention of recurrent stroke: analysis of patients with minor stroke from the Ticlopidine Aspirin Stroke Study. Stroke 1992;23:1723.
81. Hass WK, Easton JD, Adams HPJ, et al. A randomized trial comparing ticlopidine hydrochloride with aspirin for the prevention of stroke in high risk patients. N Engl J Med 1989;321:501.
82. Hirsh J, Poller L, Deykin D. Optimal therapeutic range for oral anticoagulants. Chest 1989;95(suppl 5):S-11.
83. Poller L. The effect of low-dose warfarin on the risk of stroke in patients with nonrheumatic atrial fibrillation. N Engl J Med 1991;325:129.
84. Ille O, Woimant F, Pruna A, et al. Hypertensive encephalopathy after bilateral carotid endarterectomy. Stroke 1995;26:488.
85. Schwartz RB, Jones KM, Kalina P, et al. Hypertensive encephalopathy: findings on CT, MR imaging and SPECT imaging in 14 cases. Am J Roentgenol 1992;159:379.
86. Calhoun DA, Oparil S. Treatment of hypertensive crisis. N Engl J Med 1990;323:1177.
87. Durand ML, Calderwood SB, Weber DJ, et al. Acute bacterial meningitis in adults. a review of 493 episodes. N Engl J Med 1993;328:21.
88. Dyck PJ, Kratz KM, Kaines JL, et al. The prevalence by staged severity of various types of diabetic neuropathy, retinopathy and nephropathy in a population-based cohort: The Rochester Diabetic Neuropathy Study. Neurology 1993;43:817.

# 17
# Neurologic Consultation in the Medical Intensive Care Unit

Mustapha Ezzeddine and Walter J. Koroshetz

The primary goal of medical intensive care is to preserve neurologic function while treating patients with life-threatening conditions or multiorgan failure. The brain and peripheral nervous system are commonly affected in the critically ill patient. A large proportion of patients admitted to critical care units have neurologic dysfunction as a complication of a primary systemic disease, but many are critically ill because of injury or disease of the brain, nerves, or muscle. Several studies have examined the prevalence of neurologic disease in the intensive care unit (ICU), including a study by Isensee and colleagues [1] in which 18 of 100 patients were admitted to an ICU with a primary neurologic problem. Twenty-seven had neurologic complications, the most common of which was metabolic encephalopathy. Interestingly, mortality was much higher in the group with nervous system involvement. Bleck and colleagues reported their prospective experience with 1,850 patients admitted to the medical ICU in a large academic medical center. The prevalence of neurologic complications in this series was 12.3%, excluding 92 patients (4.9%) who were admitted with a primary neurologic disorder. Common complications were metabolic encephalopathy, hypoxic-ischemic encephalopathy, seizures, and stroke. Again, neurologic dysfunction lengthened the stay in the ICU and was associated with increased mortality.

## GENERAL APPROACH TO THE INTENSIVE CARE UNIT PATIENT

### History

The complete neurologic evaluation of critically ill patients is often a daunting task in view of the usually complex patterns of illness. A review of the chart is necessary to establish the range of medical abnormalities. A review of the patient's history of previous neurologic illnesses, previous medical illnesses, and current medical problems sets the stage for attacking the neurologic issue. Especially for questions relating to mental status, the nurses' notes are often most informative. Physical therapists' notes may give excellent information on motor function. Direct discussion of patient behavior with the primary nurse can establish an accurate mental picture of the patient's prior state, fluctuations in the mental status, pattern of response to medications, paroxysmal events, and so on. In the haste to stabilize the critically ill patient, ICU staff frequently abbreviate or even omit the neurologic history. There may be little or no information about the baseline neurologic functioning. A phone call to the patient's family can sometimes dramatically redirect the neurologic diagnosis. An accurate neurologic assessment may require information from eyewitness accounts of the patient's medical decline; baseline functional status; and history of previous neurologic disease such as encephalopathy, dementia, cerebrovascular disease, peripheral nervous system disease, epilepsy, depression, substance abuse, or trauma.

An essential part of the evaluation is to review the patient's medications and to consider primary adverse drug effects, side effects resulting from common drug interactions, as well as drug toxicity resulting from impairment of hepatic or renal drug metabolism. Also of importance are drugs used by the patient before admission, including sedatives, alcohol, antidepressants, anticonvulsants, and recreational drugs; the possibility of withdrawal symptoms should be entertained. History of unusual drug reactions such as neuroleptic malignant syndrome or porphyria is often evident only after discussion with the family.

Baseline and current nutritional status may provide clues to the presence of a nutritional deficiency as the cause of the neurologic complication. Wernicke's encephalopathy may be precipitated in the hospital after administration of glucose-containing solutions to a patient with thiamine deficiency. Laboratory data should be reviewed for indications of metabolic abnormalities. It is often useful to review not only the discrete numbers but also the trends in the laboratory values; acute changes are often more significant. Invasive procedures, including surgery, central line placement, balloon pump placement, angiography, use of ventricular-assist devices, extracorporeal membrane oxygenation, and epidural catheter placement may be causally linked to the neurologic conditions. Correlating abnormalities in the vital signs chart with the onset of neurologic abnormalities is important; for example, episodes of hypotension or hypoxia might contribute to brain injury; patterns of fever suggest the presence of a systemic infection versus a central nervous system (CNS)-induced pyrexia.

## Examination

General Examination

Neurologic examination should include a general physical examination, including evaluation of the skin for evidence of hemorrhage, icterus, needle tracks, vesicular herpetic rash, palpable purpura, petechial rash, trauma (Battle's sign), livedo reticularis, peripheral emboli, stigmata of chronic liver disease, and markers of phakomatoses. Spider angiomata and the odor of fetor hepaticus may suggest liver disease. A sallow, doughy skin with loss of lateral aspect of the eyebrows suggests hypothyroidism. Hyperpigmentation of the palmar creases or axilla suggests Addison's adrenal insufficiency. Petechiae in the patient with low platelets and renal dysfunction might suggest thrombotic thrombocytopenic purpura. Vascular examination, including palpation of internal and external carotid, peripheral pulses, and carotid bruit, may reveal the presence of atherosclerotic carotid disease. Funduscopic evaluation might reveal papilledema, subhyaloid hemorrhage, diabetic or hypertensive changes, or evidence of emboli such as Hollenhorst plaques. Otologic examination is useful to rule out hemotympanum or otitis media. The head and neck should be examined for evidence of trauma. If there is a possibility of significant trauma, then the neck should be immobilized until cervical spine instability can be ruled out.

## Mental Status Evaluation

The main purpose of the neurologic examination of the patient with altered sensorium is to establish the level of consciousness, test the integrity of brain stem function, and look for lateralizing signs. If the patient is breathing spontaneously, breathing patterns can help in localizing the problem (Table 17.1). A proportion of patients in medical ICUs are treated with continuous infusions of fast-acting anesthetic agents or morphine. In many cases a brief cessation of these very sedating medications can be tolerated for the purpose of performing a neurologic examination.

The patient should be observed for spontaneous movement; the examiner should look for blinking, asymmetry, abnormal movements, reflex posturing, and movements linked to phases of ventilation. The level of consciousness is established by attempting to arouse the patient, first with verbal stimulation, then, if unsuccessful, with shaking of the trunk, and, if still unsuccessful, with progressively more noxious stimuli; the patient is observed for voluntary responses versus reflexive responses versus no response at all. A patient with abulia resulting

*Table 17.1*  Breathing patterns in comatose or encephalopathic patients

| Pattern | Description | Localization |
|---------|-------------|--------------|
| Posthyperventilation apnea | >12 secs apnea following voluntary five deep breaths | Bihemispheric dysfunction |
| Cheyne-Stokes respiration | Crescendo-decrescendo alternating apnea/hyperpnea | Bilateral dysfunction above the pons, commonly in diencephalon |
| Central neurogenic hyperventilation | Sustained rapid deep breathing with low $pCO_2$ (rare) | Central nervous system lymphoma is most common cause; possible lesion in paramedian reticular formation between lower midbrain and middle one-third of the pons |
| Apneustic breathing | Prolonged inspiratory pause at full inspiration | Dorsolateral pons |
| Ataxic breathing | Irregular pattern, usually slow rate | Medullary lesion or compression, central caudal medulla |

Source: Modified with permission from F Plum, JB Posner. Diagnosis of Stupor and Coma (3rd ed). Philadelphia: Davis, 1982;32–39.

from frontal lobe dysfunction or hydrocephalus may exhibit long delays before responding. A patient who responds should then be challenged by simple tests of memory function and orientation to place and time. Aphasia can be evaluated by assessing the ability to converse normally, name objects or people, repeat words after the examiner, and read. Attentional disorders are often best demonstrated by testing the patient's ability to count sequentially. Comprehension can be quickly tested by use of a standard command, such as, "Point to the source of illumination in the room." Delirium is often characterized by inappropriate speech, hyperactivity, disorientation as to time and place, inability to form new memories, and easy distractibility, and sometimes by delusions and hallucinations.

## Cranial Nerve Evaluation

The evaluation of brain stem reflexes starts with the testing of pupillary reactions; asymmetry in pupil size as well as the magnitude and rapidity of change in response to light should be recorded. Lesions in the brain stem or third nerve involving the parasympathetic innervation of the iris (constrictors) lead to sluggish pupillary dilation or lack of response to light. Dysfunction of sympathetic innervation of the pupil (as in Horner's syndrome with miosis and ptosis) is best detected in the dark. Midposition unreactive pupils are seen in midbrain lesions, pinpoint pupils in pontine lesions, and small and sluggishly reactive pupils in many drug intoxications, commonly opioid intoxication. Vision should be checked by confrontational testing in which the examiner looks for blinking as the extended finger is brought close to the eye sequentially from each visual hemifield. Care must be taken not to push air onto the cornea, which will stimulate blinking via the corneal reflex. The oculocephalic reflex (or doll's eye reflex) tests the integrity of the vestibulo-ocular connections. It cannot be overemphasized that this test should not be performed unless the integrity of the cervical spine is confirmed. Cold caloric testing, which consists of infusing ice water into the ear canal and observing for forced deviation of the eyes toward the cooled ear, uses a stronger stimulus to engage vestibular-ocular reflexes that cause eye movement. Corneal reflexes should also be tested. Absence of the corneal reflex signifies brain stem pathology; asymmetry can sometimes be seen with hemispheric lesions.

## Motor Examination

Observation of spontaneous and reflexive eye movements is often quite useful. Conjugate eye deviation has great localization value. Intermittent driving of the eyes to one side with nystagmoid jerks may be the only clue to subclinical seizures; sometimes there are small-amplitude twitches of the eyelids or frontalis muscle. Roving, fish-tail–like eye movements are frequently encountered in comatose patients as a result of bihemispheric dysfunction. Eyes often deviate toward the side of cerebral lesions and are unable to look to the side of brain stem lesions. Refractory nystagmus, convergence nystagmus, vertical nystagmus, and ocular bobbing are highly suggestive of intrinsic brain stem lesions. Opsoclonus suggests an inflammatory brain stem process—paraneoplastic or viral encephalitis. Macro-square-wave jerks, ocular dysmetria, and hypometric or hypermetric saccades suggest cerebellar dysfunction; downbeat nystagmus in primary gaze suggests a low medullary lesion. Asymmetry of grimace, eyelid opening or eyelid tone, or flattening of the nasolabial fold is seen with facial weakness. In an intubated patient, the gag reflex can be checked by moving the endotracheal tube.

In the obtunded or comatose patient motor examination is performed by testing for tone and response to progressively more noxious stimuli, such as nail-bed pressure or sternal rub, applied to each limb. Extensor or flexor posturing should be noted. Increased limb resistance to increasing passive force exerted by the examiner, so-called paratonia, is common in metabolic encephalopathy. A pitfall is considering a triple flexion response or other spinal cord reflex to be a sign of higher brain function. Testing of deep tendon reflexes, as well as Babinski's sign, might further aid in localization [2,3]. Grasp, suck, or snout reflexes suggest frontal lobe dysfunction. Deep tendon reflexes are lost in many patients with peripheral neuropathy. Patients with spinal cord injury commonly have a spinal level below which sensation is diminished, poor rectal tone, and absent sacral reflexes.

## THREE COMMON CONSULTS IN THE MEDICAL INTENSIVE CARE UNIT

### Altered Mental Status

The term *altered mental status* usually encompasses the whole spectrum from mild confusion to coma. The differential diagnoses are very wide, but three major groups are identified: (1) those associated with *brain injury,* such as may occur in brain ischemia, intracranial hemorrhage, intracranial tumor, meningitis, encephalitis, raised intracranial pressure (ICP), hypoglycemia, and carbon monoxide poisoning; (2) those caused by *metabolic encephalopathy* secondary to sepsis, electrolyte disorders, endocrine disorders, respiratory failure [4], drug toxicity, hepatic failure, renal failure, and hyperglycemia; and (3) those caused by *epileptiform activity.*

A few core issues should be addressed by the consultant. One of the most helpful historical features is a history of a previous similar event, for instance, one caused by drug withdrawal or overdose, or a hypoglycemic episode. An eyewitness account of seizure activity, complaint of headache, hemiparesis, and unusual body or eye movements can sometimes lead to the correct diagnosis. Next, it should be determined whether the change in mental status correlated in time with the initiation of a new medicine, a medical or surgical procedure, a change in vital signs, or some other condition. Finally, key laboratory values should be checked, including levels of blood glucose, sodium, calcium, and magnesium; drug levels (especially of digoxin, lithium, tricyclic antidepressants, hypnotics, and sedatives); results of liver function and renal function tests; vitamin $B_{12}$ level; results of thyroid function tests; morning cortisol level; results of screen for toxins; and red and white blood cell counts, platelet count, prothrombin time, and partial prothrombin time. Cyanide levels should be checked in patients who have been on nitroprusside for prolonged periods. Carbon monoxide levels should be checked in patients with the appropriate exposure history.

The examination is as described above. Focal findings suggesting localized neurologic dysfunction usually are indications for brain imaging. A basic goal is to be sure that brain hemorrhage or intracranial mass effect of some other origin is not the underlying cause of the patient's altered mental status. Suspicion of intracranial hemorrhage must be high in patients who are on anticoagulant therapy, have a primary coagulopathy, complain of headache or have a history of head trauma. Suspicion of massive cerebral edema must be low in patients who become obtunded with hyponatremia, severe hypertension, severe hepatic failure, meningitis or encephalitis, or stroke. Fever or other signs of infection, especially with nuchal rigidity, are indications for examination of the spinal fluid. The consultant must be very suspicious of meningitis in the immune-suppressed patient with altered mental status. Cerebrospinal fluid (CSF) should be cultured for bacterial, fungal, and tuberculous organisms. Cryptococcal antigen titer can be helpful.

The diagnosis of encephalitis can be difficult. Seizure and acute onset of behavioral or memory disorder, accompanied by fever and red and white cells in the CSF, can occur in acute herpes encephalitis, which should be treated with acyclovir. Petechial rash followed by headache and brain swelling occurs in patients with a tick bite who contract Rocky Mountain spotted fever. Petechial rash may also denote meningococcemia. Magnetic resonance imaging (MRI) demonstrating a distribution of lesions, usually affecting hippocampus and synaptically connected structures, is helpful in the diagnosis of herpes encephalitis. MRI is also useful in diagnosing the newly described but probably common condition termed *posterior leukoencephalopathy*. Patients with this condition become subacutely blind and encephalopathic; patients often have hypertension or hyponatremia or have used cyclosporine or FK 506. The electroencephalogram (EEG) shows epileptiform activity in the occipital lobe, and the MRI shows diffuse edema, most extensively in the posterior cerebral white matter.

## Weakness

The first step in evaluation of a patient with "weakness" is to attempt to localize the process in the neurologic axis. This step may be difficult if a concomitant decreased level of consciousness is present.

## Lesions of the Central Nervous System

The most common cause of a CNS lesion in the critically ill patient is a cerebrovascular accident, either ischemic or hemorrhagic. Multiple factors place critically ill patients at high risk of suffering a stroke; these factors include new-onset atrial fibrillation, subacute bacterial endocarditis, marantic endocarditis, acute myocardial infarction, and systemic hypotension that results in a low-flow stroke (which can produce unilateral or bilateral symptoms in the distribution of a stenosed cerebral vessel). Critically ill patients also commonly undergo diagnostic procedures that carry risk of stroke, including cardiac catheterization and direct angiography, which may be complicated by cholesterol or tip-of-catheter emboli. Deep venous thrombosis in immobile patients can lead to a paradoxical brain embolus via a cardiac right-to-left shunt (most commonly a patent foramen ovale). Hypercoagulable states can be produced or exacerbated by systemic disease and can result in a stroke [5]. Such an occurrence has been described in patients with malignancy (especially involving the pancreas, colon, lung, ovaries, and gallbladder) [6,7], nephrotic syndrome (caused by depletion of anticoagulant proteins involved in the fibrinolytic pathways), acute liver dysfunction, myeloproliferative disorders (including polycythemia vera, essential thrombocythemia, chronic myelogenous leukemia, and myelofibrosis), systemic vasculitis (including systemic lupus erythematosus, polyarteritis nodosa, Behçet's disease, rheumatoid arthritis, and scleroderma), and heparin-induced thrombocytopenia, as well as in patients undergoing certain chemotherapeutic regimens.

Determining the cause of the acute stroke is of extreme importance for establishing the optimal plan for treatment. Thus, evaluation of the brain and cerebrovascular system becomes crucial. In critically ill patients, worsening of previous compensated deficits or occurrence of nonischemic strokelike events can occur. An MRI technique for brain imaging called *diffusion-weighted imaging* can be particularly useful [8] in this setting. Diffusion-weighted imaging permits the identification of acute stroke, even if only an hour old, and distinguishes it from more chronic lesions. One algorithm for diagnostic evaluation is proposed in Figure 17.1 [9].

Other CNS lesions to be considered in the appropriate setting include cerebral hemorrhage, venous sinus thrombosis (frequently with seizure as well as focal deficit), spinal cord infarction, and spinal cord compression by epidural abscess or hematoma. Epidural abscesses can complicate systemic infection, and hemorrhage can complicate anticoagulant therapy or coagulopathy. The latter may be extremely difficult to diagnose in a patient who cannot report back pain [10]. Spinal cord infarction can be seen in the ICU in patients suffering from aortic dissection, aortic thrombosis, coagulopathies, systemic lupus erythematosus, and global ischemia secondary to cardiac arrest [11].

## Lesions of the Peripheral Nervous System

Involvement of the peripheral nervous system in ICU patients in the form of critical-illness polyneuropathy and critical-illness myopathy is increasingly being recognized (Table 17.2) [12]. Other entities to be considered include acute and chronic infectious demyelinating polyneuropathy, compression mononeuropathies, traumatic neuropathies and plexopathies secondary to invasive procedures in the ICU, porphyric neuropathy, heavy metal or organophosphate poisoning, steroid-induced myopathy, complications of long-term use of neuromuscular agents, myasthenic syndromes, neuroleptic malignant syndrome [13], aminoglycoside-induced neuromuscular blockade, hypermagnesemia [14], botulism, and underlying rare neuromuscular diseases (acid maltase deficiency [15], muscular dystrophies, amyotrophic lateral sclerosis) that were previously undiagnosed or are exacerbated by the critical illness. Systemic diseases associated with a mononeuritis multiplex include many of the vasculitides, such as Wegener's granulomatosis, Churg-Strauss syndrome, and polyarteritis nodosa. Severe peripheral neuropathy occurs in human immunodeficiency virus (HIV) or can be caused by HIV medications. Electromyography and nerve conduction studies are essential for the diagnosis of either neuropathy, neuromuscular junc-

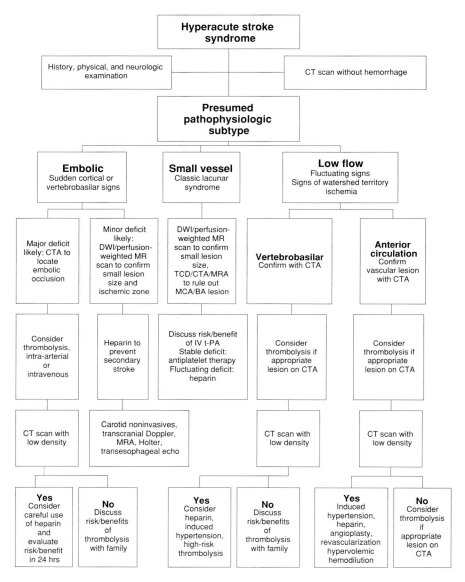

*Figure 17.1*   An algorithmic approach to the evaluation and treatment of the hyperacute stroke patient. (CT = computed tomography; CTA = computed tomoangiography; DWI/perfusion weighted MR = diffusion/perfusion-weighted magnetic resonance; TCD = transcranial Doppler; MRA = magnetic resonance angiography; MCA = middle cerebral artery; BA = basiliar artery; t-PA = tissue plasminogen activator.) (Reprinted with permission from WJ Koroshetz, H Ay. Diagnosis and Evaluation of Stroke. In R Sacco [ed], The American Journal of Medicine Continuing Education Series: New Approaches to the Treatment of Ischemic Stroke. Part I. Ischemic Stroke: A Disease Update. Bell Mead, NJ: Exerpta Medica, 1996;18–23.)

*Table 17.2*   Neuromuscular weakness in critically ill medical patients

| Entity | Clinical characteristics | Treatment |
|---|---|---|
| **Nerve disorders** | | |
| Critical-illness neuropathy | Use of steroids or neuromuscular blockers, sepsis, or multiorgan failure for more than 1 wk; predominantly axonal neuropathy | Supportive therapy? Nutrition? |
| Acute inflammatory demyelinating polyneuropathy | Areflexia, demyelinating neuropathy, increased cerebrospinal fluid protein | Plasmapheresis, IV immune globulin (IVIg) |
| Organophosphate poisoning | Altered mental status, vomiting | Atropine sulfate |
| Diphtheria | Diphtheric membrane, recent upper-respiratory-tract infection, positive throat culture | Antibiotics |
| Botulism | Dilated pupils, bulbar signs, constipation and abdominal pain, food poisoning or wound infection | Supportive care, antibiotics |
| Heavy metal poisoning | Positive urine test | Chelation therapy |
| Acute intermittent porphyria | Abdominal pain, increased urine porphobilinogen | Avoidance of drugs that precipitate crisis, glucose |
| Traumatic neuropathies and plexopathies | Spontaneous retroperitoneal hematoma, internal jugular vein cannulation, radial arterial line insertion, femoral vein/artery cannulation; post–coronary artery bypass graft | Decompression if worsening |
| **Neuromuscular junction diseases** | | |
| Myasthenia gravis | Fatigable weakness, positive edrophonium test, acetylcholine receptor antibodies | Plasmapheresis, IVIg, pyridostigmine bromide (Mestinon), steroids |
| Aminoglycoside or polymixin B sulfate induced | — | Cessation of drug |
| Tick paralysis | Tick exposure | Tick removal |
| Hypermagnesemia | Serum level, cathartics | IV calcium |
| Prolonged neuromuscular blockade | Persistent metabolites of vecuronium bromide | Support |
| **Muscle disorders** | | |
| Acute steroid-induced myopathy | Steroid exposure | Weaning off steroids |
| Critical-illness myopathy | Absent myosin filaments | Support, weaning off steroids and paralytics |
| Hypokalemia | Low serum level | Supplementation |
| Hypophosphatemia | Low serum level | Supplementation |
| Acidmaltase deficiency | Muscle enzyme essay | |
| Hypothyroidism or hyperthyroidism | Abnormal thyroid function tests | Correction of thyroid function tests |

Source: Modified with permission from RAC Hughes, D Behari. Acute neuromuscular respiratory paralysis. J Neurol Neurosurg Psych 1993;58:339–363.

tion dysfunction, or myopathy. In some cases, nerve or muscle biopsy may also be necessary to correctly diagnose the peripheral cause of diffuse muscular weakness.

Occasionally, the peripheral nervous system dysfunction manifests in difficulty weaning the patient off mechanical ventilation. It is important to realize that diaphragmatic dysfunction can be the sole clinical manifestation of these entities. Also, patients with previous chronic neuromuscular disease may develop severe hypercapnia and loss of respiratory drive following administration of supplemental oxygen therapy [16]. This phenomenon is similar to that in patients with chronic hypercapnia secondary to chronic obstructive lung disease.

## Abnormal Movements

A number of movement disorders are seen in critically ill patients. Asterixis occurs commonly in metabolic encephalopathy, especially hepatic failure and hypercarbia. Tremor with delirium, tachycardia, and diaphoresis is the hallmark of delirium tremens. Paratonia with some cogwheeling rigidity is common in metabolic encephalopathy. Stimulus-sensitive (sometimes linked to ventilator phase), diffuse, multifocal myoclonus is common in patients with anoxic and renal encephalopathy. Chorea occurs in patients with hypocalcemia, lupus cerebritis, and lesions of the basal ganglia. Severe stimulus-sensitive muscular spasms and trismus occur in patients with tetanus. Dystonia occurs most commonly as a drug side effect in ICU patients treated with neuroleptic agents for agitation. Metoclopramide is also a known cause of dystonia.

## COMMON NEUROLOGIC DISORDERS ENCOUNTERED IN MEDICAL INTENSIVE CARE UNITS

### Metabolic Encephalopathy

Metabolic encephalopathy is extremely common in medical patients with critical illness. In patients with positive blood cultures and fever, severe encephalopathy occurs in almost one-half and is associated with a 50% mortality rate [17]. The cause of encephalopathy in sepsis is not clear. Drug-induced encephalopathy is also very common (Table 17.3). For diagnostic purposes, narcotic encephalopathy can be reversed with naloxone hydrochloride, and benzodiazepine encephalopathy can be reversed with flumazenil. Hepatic and renal failure, hypertension, hyperosmolar states, and hypoglycemia are the next most common causes of encephalopathy in the medical ICU [18]. Hyponatremia and hypercalcemia should also be considered.

The EEG can be helpful in certain instances in evaluating the patient with encephalopathy. In mild metabolic encephalopathy, generalized continuous slowing of the EEG is expected, and a change in the EEG toward faster lower amplitude is expected with patient arousal. Frontal intermittent rhythmic delta activity that is blocked by stimulation is common in initial stages of metabolic coma. Triphasic waves are characteristic of hepatic coma. Rarely, periodic lateralizing

*Table 17.3*   Central nervous system drug effects in critically ill medical patients

| Drug | Effect | Comments |
|---|---|---|
| Aminoglycoside | Hearing loss | |
| Penicillin and its derivatives, especially imipenem | Seizure | May be dose related or idiosyncratic |
| Narcotic | Encephalopathy seizure, withdrawal state on discontinuation | Can reverse with naloxone hydrochloride if patient will tolerate |
| Aminophylline | Tremor, encephalopathy, seizure | Check levels |
| Lithium | Tremor, encephalopathy, seizure | Check levels; often profound effect on electroencephalogram |
| Lidocaine, flecainide acetate | Delirium, seizure | |
| Cimetidine | Encephalopathy | |
| Nitroprusside | Encephalopathy | Check cyanide levels |
| Beta blockers | Hallucinations | |
| Metoclopramide | Dystonia | |
| Prochlorperazine edisylate (Compazine) | Dystonia | |
| Haloperidol and other neuroleptics | Parkinsonism, seizure | Can cause torsades de pointe in high doses |
| Tricyclic antidepressants | Seizure, anticholinergic encephalopathy | Anticholinergics poorly tolerated in patients with Alzheimer's disease, Parkinson's disease |
| Cyclosporine | Seizure, reversible posterior leukoencephalopathy (RPLE) | RPLE associated with cortical blindness, status epilepticus, coma, pyramidal tract signs |
| Benzodiazepine | Encephalopathy | Abrupt withdrawal can cause seizure |
| Corticosteroids | Delirium, mania | Mania may be helped by treating with lithium |

epileptiform discharges are found on EEG that relate to focal brain injury. Deeply comatose patients can exhibit bursts of high-voltage slow waves interspersed with periods of almost no EEG activity, a so-called burst-suppression pattern. A diffuse, steady, monotonous EEG rhythm that does not change with stimulation is seen in some anoxic encephalopathies. On occasion—especially in patients with a previous seizure disorder, encephalitis, or known CNS lesion—an EEG is necessary to diagnose nonconvulsive status epilepticus as a primary cause of stupor or coma.

It is not uncommon to encounter patients in the medical ICU with a clinical state most consistent with a metabolic encephalopathy but without a clearly measurable metabolic abnormality and with normal CSF, EEG, and brain imaging. Sepsis is considered by some to be the major cause of encephalopathy in ICU patients. In unexplained cases of encephalopathy, the consultant may consider treating the patient empirically with thiamine and then following the patient clinically. The consultant should consider stopping medications occasionally associated with encephalopathy and replacing needed ones with drugs that have alternative mechanisms of action or side effect profiles.

## Seizure

Seizure is common in ICU medical patients, affecting as many as 28% of patients [18]. Many of the causes of metabolic encephalopathy can also lead to seizure activity (see Table 17.3). Anoxic encephalopathy and azotemia are not uncommonly accompanied by seizure activity. Penicillin applied to the brain is commonly used to create seizures in animal models. Seizure may also occur as a sign of brain injury resulting from stroke, tumor, or CNS infection (meningitis or encephalitis). A CT scan and a CSF examination are required in most patients to search for the more destructive causes. Intravenous loading with phenytoin or fosphenytoin sodium is the most commonly used first-line anticonvulsant therapy.

Correctable metabolic abnormalities should be attended to quickly to avoid worsening seizure disorder or status epilepticus. Hyponatremia, hyperosmolar states, hypocalcemia, hypoglycemia, and hypomagnesemia may cause seizure in the ICU.

## Cerebrovascular Disease

Cerebral ischemia causes stupor or coma if it affects both hemispheres (as in systemic hypotension or bilateral carotid disease) or if it affects the reticular activating system in the dorsum of the midbrain and in the thalamus. Ischemic stroke is not uncommon in medical ICUs. In one study series, 22% of critically ill patients suffered stroke [18]. Atherosclerotic heart disease is a common condition leading to ICU admission. Infection, hypotension, hypercoagulable conditions, and invasive procedures probably increase the risk of ischemic stroke during the period of critical care illness. Administration of anticoagulants and thrombolytic drugs, as well as hematologic disorders probably increase the risk of intracranial hemorrhage.

Transient symptoms of neurologic dysfunction are common in critically ill patients and are often difficult to ascribe to a specific cause. Waxing and waning encephalopathy, drug effects, seizure, and transient cerebral ischemia are the common considerations. Noninvasive carotid studies, CT scan or MRI to detect previous stroke, transcranial Doppler ultrasonography, or even magnetic resonance angiography may be necessary to establish whether or not the event represents a warning of a serious underlying risk for upcoming neurologic injury. Carotid endarterectomy and carotid or vertebrobasilar angioplasty may be hazardous to perform in the critically ill patient but must be considered if the alternative is massive stroke. Thrombolysis with intravenous administration of tissue-type plasminogen activator has been approved for use in acute stroke patients as long as fairly strict criteria are followed to ensure safety. Intra-arterial thrombolysis for large-artery (internal carotid artery, major coronary artery stem, vertebrobasilar) occlusion has the advantage that the systemic dose of thrombolytic agent is lower than with intravenous thrombolysis, it can be combined with angioplasty if necessary, and the probability of successful large-clot lysis is higher.

## Critical Care Neuropathy and Myopathy

Critically ill patients are at risk for the development of profound quadriparesis resulting from neuromuscular weakness. Not uncommonly, patients with severe asthma treated with steroids and neuromuscular blocks, as well as patients with sepsis or respiratory failure managed with (or sometimes without) paralytic drugs, may first be noted to be weak when they fail to wean from the respirator. A variety of causes should be considered, including: (1) prolonged neuromuscular blockade, which can occur after paralytic agents are stopped in patients with metabolic acidosis, elevated magnesium levels, and renal failure [19]; a contribution to a myasthenic syndrome from aminoglycoside or polymixin B sulfate antibiotics as well as the appearance of a primary neuromuscular disease (myasthenia gravis, Lambert-Eaton syndrome) should also be considered; (2) acute myopathy, characterized by variable elevation in creatine kinase levels and selective loss of myosin fibers on muscle biopsy [20,21]; (3) acute, primarily axonal, motor neuropathy [22]; and (4) Landry-Guillain-Barré syndrome with slowed conduction velocities and albuminologic and cytologic differentiation in the CSF [23]. Except in cases of the latter, which often responds to plasmapheresis or intravenous gamma globulin, management of patients with critical care motor neuropathy or myopathy is primarily supportive. The consultant should attempt to eliminate the use of paralytic agents and steroids and to treat infection. Weakness may last for weeks in patients with critical-illness myopathy or neuropathy.

## Intracranial Mass Lesions and Raised Intracranial Pressure

A variety of conditions may be associated with an acute introduction of mass into the cranial cavity. As mass is introduced, the ICP may be kept constant by redistribution of CSF or blood volume. Further increases in intracranial mass, however, cause increased ICP. In fact, once mass effect causes increased ICP, brain compliance may be so reduced that small additional increases in intracranial mass cause dramatic rises in ICP. Such additional intracranial mass may occur as a result of decreased venous outflow because of tracheal suction, fever, increase in transmitted chest pressure to the spinal space, and so on. In such instances, there is often a reflexive increase in blood pressure. Global cerebral perfusion pressure (CPP) is the difference between mean arterial blood pressure (MAP) and ICP. Normally CPP exceeds 70 mm Hg. Below a CPP of 60 mm Hg, brain ischemia may occur, the saturation of oxygen in jugular venous blood may fall, and the patient deteriorates rapidly. In addition to this effect on CPP, mass lesions also cause destructive compression or distortion of midline structures, so-called herniation syndromes. Patients with mass effect in the posterior fossa are in the most precarious condition, because compression of the brain stem is followed rapidly by cardiorespiratory collapse and brain stem injury. Secondary stroke may occur as a result of compression of the posterior cerebral artery against the lateral wall of the midbrain or as a result of anterior cerebral artery compression by subfalcial herniation of brain tissue.

Patients with dangerously elevated ICP almost always show an obvious mass effect on CT scan. One exception to this rule is patients with brain edema whose ventricles are not compressed because of concomitant communicating hydrocephalus (e.g., patients with cryptococcal meningitis). Because of bone artifact, significant mass effect in the posterior fossa can be missed on CT scan. Decompressive cerebellar surgery can be lifesaving, and patients can have substantial recovery.

In addition to being caused by tumor, ischemic brain swelling, and hemorrhage, increased ICP in medical patients can be due to hepatic failure, hyponatremia, encephalitis, meningitis, and the postanoxic state. Rational management is difficult without an ICP monitor. Elevation of the head without kinking of jugular veins, control of fever, avoidance of hyponatremia, use of hyperosmolar therapy or furosemide (Lasix), use of barbiturates to induce burst suppression or flat EEG pattern, and decompressive surgery are the means used to preserve brain viability in the face of dangerous mass effect. In some instances vasopressor substances may be used to increase MAP to maintain CPP (ICP minus MAP) at greater than 70 mm Hg. Hyperventilation is the quickest maneuver for lowering intracranial pressure, but chronic lowering of $pCO_2$ below 30 mm Hg may actually exacerbate the ischemic insult.

## Postanoxic Encephalopathy

Patients who survive a cardiac arrest have variable patterns of recovery. In general the most severe insults cause loss of brain stem reflexes—absent pupillary, corneal, and cold caloric reflexes. The patient is initially flaccid. If the patient is to attain a good neurologic outcome, the brain stem reflexes must begin to return within hours. Decerebrate posturing may be replaced by decorticate posturing and finally by purposeful withdrawal reaction to pain. In a study of 210 patients with hypoxic-ischemic coma, Levy and colleagues reported that the lack of return of the pupillary light response on day 1, the lack of purposeful motor response, and spontaneous or roving eye movements after 24 hours all predicted either death or persistent vegetative state [24]. Only 3 of 33 patients who were vegetative at 1 week attained any independent level of function. Generalized myoclonus or generalized seizures may also occur in the postarrest patient. In some patients cortical injury can occur that leads to selective memory loss (hippocampal injury) or ataxia with or without intention myoclonus (cerebellar injury).

Treatment of the postarrest patient is supportive. It is controversial whether control of raised ICP in the postarrest patient leads to improved functional outcome.

## Brain Death

Death of the brain is a legally accepted definition of death. This criterion must be met to obtain organs for donation from persons who have irreversible, complete brain injury. In cases in which the cause is known and is consistent with irreversible, total brain death, and in which there are no complicating factors, clinical criteria for brain death suffice [23,25,26]. Complicating factors that preclude a clinical diagnosis of brain death include the presence of barbiturate or other drug intoxication, hypothermia, and shock. The clinical criteria for a brain death diagnosis include: (1) absent brain stem reflexes (i.e., no pupillary response to light, no corneal response, no extraocular movements with head turning or ice water calorics, no gag reflex, no blink to threat); (2) absent motor response to painful stimulation; (3) failed apnea test. In the apnea test, the patient is ventilated with 100% oxygen for at least 10 minutes to increase $pO_2$ and the respiratory rate is altered to obtain a $pCO_2$ of approximately 40 mm Hg. The patient is then disconnected from the ventilator and a catheter is placed into the trachea that sufflates the lung with 100% oxygen at a rate of about 6 liters per minute. The blood pressure and oxygen saturation must be maintained as the chest wall is observed for any sign of respiratory movement. If the $pCO_2$ rises by more than 20 mm Hg or the pH drops by more than 0.2 pH units without any observable respiratory effort, then the apnea test is considered failed. Another sign of brain stem dysfunction is required for the diagnosis of brain death.

Special attention must be paid to the conditions that may make the brain death criteria inappropriate. The patient who has brain stem injury and is in a "locked-in" state is not brain dead. Hypothermia, hypotension, hypoglycemia, paralytic drug treatment, and sedative drug overdose are possibly reversible conditions that may produce a neurologic examination simulating brain death. Head injury with ocular trauma, vestibular trauma, and concussion may also simulate brain death. Electrocerebral silence on an EEG, cerebral angiography showing lack of dye passage into the arteries and veins, radionuclide brain scan without tracer entry into brain, and transcranial Doppler ultrasound study of the middle cerebral arteries showing spikes of to-fro flow with no flow, or reversed flow, in diastole are all confirmatory tests in the diagnosis of brain death.

## SUMMARY

The neurologic consultant can play an extremely important role in the management of the critically ill medical patient. The illnesses that lead to intensive care admission, along with the unstable course of these patients, are major threats to the nervous system. Neurologic injury, especially to the brain, is a common cause of permanent loss of function, and brain injury is a common event that leads to the termination of critical care. Appropriate diagnosis and management of the neurologic issues results in improved functional outcome. The cases encountered in the medical ICU are often neurologically complex and tragic, and require a high level of clinical expertise and clinical effort.

## REFERENCES

1. Isensee LM, Weiner LJ, Hart RG. Neurologic disorders in a medical intensive care unit: a prospective survey. J Crit Care 1989;4:208–210.
2. Bates D. The management of medical coma. J Neurol Neurosurg Psychiatry 1993;56:589–598.
3. Samuels MA. The evaluation of comatose patients. Hosp Pract 1993;28:165–182.
4. Chikatara RJ, Kahn FA. Systemic manifestation of pulmonary disease: neurologic manifestation of lung disease. Semin Respir Med 1988;9:395–402.
5. Schafer AI. The hypercoagulable states. Ann Intern Med 1985;102:814–828.
6. Bick RL. Alterations of homeostasis associated with malignancy. Semin Thromb Hemost 1978;5: 1–26.

7. Hart RG, Kanter MC. Hematologic disorders and ischemic stroke: a selective review. Stroke 1990; 21:1111–1121.
8. Koroshetz WJ, Gonzales G. Diffusion-weighted MRI: an ECG for "brain attack"? Ann Neurol 1997;41:565–566.
9. Koroshetz WJ, Ay H. Diagnosis and Evaluation of Stroke. In R Sacco (ed), The American Journal of Medicine Continuing Education Series: New Approaches to the Treatment of Ischemic Stroke. Part I. Ischemic Stroke: A Disease Update. Bell Mead, NJ: Exerpta Medica, 1996;18–23.
10. Danner RL, Hartman BJ. Update on spinal epidural abscess: 35 cases and review of the literature. Rev Infect Dis 1987;9:265–274.
11. Cheshire WP, Santos CC, Massey EW, et al. Spinal cord infarction: etiology and outcome. Neurology 1996;47:321–330.
12. Chad DA, Lacomis D. Critically ill patients with newly acquired weakness: the clinicopathological spectrum. Ann Neurol 1994;35:257–259.
13. Caroff SN, Mann SC. Neuroleptic malignant syndrome. Med Clin North Am 1993;77:185–202.
14. Swift TR. Weakness from magnesium-containing cathartics: electrophysiologic studies. Muscle Nerve 1979;2:295–298.
15. Felice JK, Alessi AG, Grunnet ML. Clinical variability in adult-onset acid maltase deficiency: report of affected sibs and review of the literature. Medicine 1995;74:131–135.
16. Gay PC, Edmonds LC. Severe hypercapnia after low-flow oxygen therapy in patients with neuromuscular disease and diaphragmatic dysfunction. Mayo Clin Proc 1995;70:327–330.
17. Young GB, Bolton C, Austin TW, et al. The encephalopathy associated with septic illness. Clin Invest Med 1990;13:287–304.
18. Bleck TP, Smith MC, Pierre-Louis S, et al. Neurologic complications of critical medical illnesses. Crit Care Med 1993;21:98–103.
19. Segredo V, Caldwell J, Matthay M, et al. Persistent paralysis in critically ill patients after long-term administration of vecuronium. N Engl J Med 1992;327:524–528.
20. MacFarlane IA, Rosenthal FD. Severe myopathy after status asthmaticus. Lancet 1977;2:615.
21. Hirano M, Ott BR, Raps EC, et al. Acute quadriplegic myopathy: a complication of treatment with steroids, nondepolarizing blocking agents or both. Neurology 1992;42:2082–2087.
22. Zochodone DW, Bolton C, Wells GA, et al. Critical illness polyneuropathy: a compilation of sepsis and multiple organ failure. Brain 1987;110:819–842.
23. Preston DC, Logigian EL. Guillain-Barré syndrome during high dose methylprednisolone therapy. Muscle Nerve 1991;14:378–379.
24. Levy DE, Caronna JJ, Singer BH, et al. Predicting outcome from hypoxic ischemic coma. JAMA 1995;253:1420–1426.
25. Wijdicks EFM. Determining brain death in adults. Neurology 1995;45:1003–1011.
26. Report of the Quality Standards Subcommittee of the American Academy of Neurology: practice parameters for determining brain death in adults. Neurology 1995;45:1012–1014.

## SUGGESTED READING

Anonymous. Guidelines for the Determination of Death. Report of the Medical Consultants on the Diagnosis of Death of the President's Commission for the Study of Ethical Problems in Medicine and Biomedical and Behavioral Research. JAMA 1981;246:2184–2186.
Bass E. Cardiopulmonary arrest: pathophysiology and neurologic complications. Ann Intern Med 1985;103:920–927.
Bolton CF, Young GB, Zochodne DW. The neurological complication of sepsis. Ann Neurol 1993;33:94–100.
Chen R, Bolton C, Young BG. Prediction of outcome in patients with anoxic coma: a clinical and electrophysiologic study. Crit Care Med 1996;24:672–678.
Crippen D. Pharmacologic treatment of brain failure and delirium. Crit Care Clin 1994;10:733–766.
Hamel MB, Goldman L, Teno J, et al. Identification of comatose patients at high risk for death or severe disability. JAMA 1995;273:1842–1848.
Heiman-Patterson TD. Neuroleptic malignant syndrome and malignant hyperthermia: important issues for the medical consultant. Med Clin North Am 1993;77:477–492.
Hughes RAC, Behari D. Acute neuromuscular respiratory paralysis. J Neurol Neurosurg Psych 1993;56:339–363.

Kelly BJ, Matthay MA. Prevalence and severity of neurologic dysfunction in critically ill patients: influence on need for continued mechanical ventilation. Chest 1993;104:1818–1824.

Krumholz A, Stern BJ, Weiss HD. Outcome from coma after cardiopulmonary resuscitation: relations to seizures and myoclonus. Neurology 1988;38:401–405.

Leijten FS, Harinck-de Weerd JE, Poortvliet D, et al. The role of polyneuropathy in motor convalescence after prolonged mechanical ventilation. JAMA 1995;274:1221–1225.

Lowenstein DH, Aminoff MJ. Clinical and EEG features of status epilepticus in comatose patients. Neurology 1992;42:100–104.

Mayo-Smith MF. Pharmacological management of alcohol withdrawal: a meta-analysis and evidence-based practice guideline. JAMA 1997;278:144–151.

Messing RO, Closson RG, Simon RP. Drug-induced seizures: a 10-year experience. Neurology 1984;34:1582–1586.

Plum F, Posner JB. Diagnosis of Stupor and Coma (3rd ed). Philadelphia: Davis, 1982;32–39.

Saitz R, Mayo-Smith MF, Roberts MS, et al. Individualized treatment for alcohol withdrawal: a randomized double-blind controlled trial. JAMA 1994;272:519–523.

Saper CB, Breder CD. The neurologic basis of fever. N Engl J Med 1994;330:1880–1885.

Spitzer AR, Giancarlo T, Maher L, et al. Neuromuscular causes of prolonged ventilator dependency. Muscle Nerve 1992;15:682–686.

Steiner T, Mendoza G, De Georgia M, et al. Prognosis of stroke patients requiring mechanical ventilation in a neurological critical care unit. Stroke 1997;28:711–715.

Watling SM, Dasta JF. Prolonged paralysis in intensive care unit patients after the use of neuromuscular blocking agents: a review of the literature. Crit Care Med 1994;22:884–893.

Young BG, Gilbert JJ, Zochodne DW. The significance of myoclonic status epilepticus in postanoxic coma. Neurology 1990;40:1843–1848.

# 18
# Geriatrics

Jerome E. Kurent

Gerontology is the study of aging from broad scientific, biological, and social perspectives. Geriatric medicine represents the comprehensive and humane approach to providing medical care to the elderly patient. It also defines the natural history of diseases occurring during later life and provides for their management and prevention. The existence of clinical geriatrics as a viable entity was scarcely recognized in the United States until relatively recently. Geriatrics has become increasingly influential in American medicine and is now a major priority of our national health care initiatives.

Two-thirds of all the people in the entire history of the world who have reached age 65 are alive today. One-half of the women in the United States alive at 65 today will survive to 85 years. From 1980 to 1990, the U.S. population older than 85 years increased by 40%. The number of centenarians has doubled.

The aging of America has profound implications for the allocation of health care resources and the manner in which health care services will be provided. The fastest growing segment of the U.S. population is represented by individuals aged 85 years and older, who are referred to the as the *very old*. Approximately 20% of these elderly people have dementia. Many other illnesses that disproportionately affect the elderly are often associated with neurologic and cognitive disability.

An estimated 30% of U.S. health care costs are devoted to the medical needs of patients 65 years of age and older. Forty percent of the national Medicaid budget is used to provide nursing home care, most of it for elderly disabled patients. A large neurologic disease burden falls on the geriatric population. Neurologists are consulted to provide recommendations for diagnostic evaluation and management of disabled elderly patients.

Ageism persists in our society, as evidenced by widespread negative attitudes toward the elderly that may have contributed to a resistance toward the development of geriatrics in this country. Many neurologic conditions affect the members of the geriatric population with much greater frequency than middle-aged adults including dementia, delirium, stroke, and Parkinson's disease. Historically, the neurologist has played a vital role in diagnosing and managing patients affected with these disorders. The role of the neurologist is expected to become increasingly important as the number of aging patients with associated neurologic diseases increases.

## NEUROLOGIC DISABILITY IN THE ELDERLY

Neurologic disability of the elderly is a public health problem of immense proportions. Diseases of the nervous system have been estimated to account for almost 50% of disability experienced by patients 65 years and older. The neurologist involved in the care of the elderly patient has unprecedented opportunity to combine advances of modern neuroscience with the art of patient care in a manner unique to the practice of geriatric neurology. Elderly patients experience many of the same neurologic diseases as do young adults. In addition, progressive cognitive decline, compromised balance and coordination, and impairment of central and peripheral motor and sensory functions are common in the geriatric population. Major causes of morbidity in the elderly include immobility, gait instability, incontinence, and intellectual impairment, all of which often have a neurologic basis.

## PRINCIPLES OF GERIATRIC MEDICINE AND THEIR RELATIONSHIP TO GERIATRIC NEUROLOGY

### Illness Behavior in the Elderly

Several features of illness behavior in the elderly represent significant challenges to the clinician. Underreporting of illness by the elderly patient reflects the widely held impression that advancing age is inevitably associated with illness and progressive functional decline. Elderly patients may therefore choose not to obtain medical evaluation, even in a setting of progressive disability. Underreporting of illness may also be a result of impaired cognitive function, fear of discovery of serious underlying disease, or financial concerns related to obtaining medical evaluation.

### Multiple Medical Illness Burden

Surveys have indicated that the hospitalized elderly patient averages six underlying medical and neurologic conditions, all of which may not be clinically evident. Complex interactions exist between medical and neurologic illnesses in the elderly patient and may complicate the evaluation process.

## Atypical Presentation

Atypical presentation of disease occurs frequently in the elderly patient. Non-localizing signs and symptoms, as seen in delirium, may be the first indication of illness related to underlying medical nonneurologic disease. Thus, delirium may be caused by myocardial infarction, metabolic abnormalities, underlying malignancy, or infection, in addition to many other unrelated conditions. Atypical presentation of disease in the elderly usually affects the organ system made most vulnerable by previously sustained organ pathology. The most vulnerable organ system is often different from that suggested by the clinical presentation. For example, in the cognitively impaired patient, delirium may be the primary manifestation of underlying urinary tract infection, myocardial infarction, or fecal impaction. In many elderly individuals, the brain, lower urinary tract, and musculoskeletal system may be compromised at baseline, so that confusion, depression, incontinence, or falls become the presenting symptom of pathology involving other organ systems.

## Homeostenosis

*Homeostenosis* refers to the progressive constriction of organ system homeostatic reserves as it occurs in the normal aging individual. Gradual loss of organ function probably begins during the third decade, is slowly progressive and linear over time, and varies among individuals. Specific organ system decline is independent of changes occurring in other organs of the same individual and is probably influenced by genetics, diet, personal habits such as tobacco and alcohol use, and environmental factors.

In the normal aging individual, subtle and gradual compromise of homeostatic reserves does not usually cause acute symptoms. The abrupt onset of impaired organ function is usually attributable to acute superimposed pathology and not to normal aging.

## ROLE OF THE NEUROLOGIC CONSULTANT IN GERIATRIC MEDICINE

The neurologist is frequently requested to evaluate elderly patients in the acute inpatient setting. Common neurologic problems include stroke, delirium, and worsening dementia. Effective neurologic consultation requires prompt and thorough evaluation of the elderly patient. The evaluation often occurs in a setting of family anxiety; this must be considered during interactions between family members and the consultant.

The initial written neurologic consult should be supplemented by follow-up discussion with the requesting physician that is initiated by the neurologist. Timely, appropriate follow-up is highly valued by the requesting physician. In the current practice environment, which emphasizes cost-effective care, the neurologic consultant should consider recommending diagnostic tests that have relatively high yield and measurable effects on patient management.

## NEUROLOGIC EXAMINATION DURING NORMAL AGING

The neurologic examination often changes as a function of normal aging. Approximately one-half to one-third of abnormalities found in the neurologic examination of elderly individuals are not attributable to identifiable clinical disease and usually do not have therapeutic implications. Published estimates vary regarding the prevalence of specific abnormal neurologic findings in the elderly.

Absent deep tendon reflexes of the ankle among persons 85 years and older have been noted in 0–78% of individuals, depending on the study population. Although neurologists frequently observe the absence of ankle myotatic reflexes in elderly individuals who have no evidence of neurologic disease, no consistent figure is present in the neurologic literature that would reflect the true prevalence of this phenomenon.

The challenge facing the consultant neurologist is to interpret unexpected abnormal neurologic findings in the elderly patient. Should the apparent abnormalities be attributed to underlying neuropathology or simply recorded to be of uncertain significance? Decreased arm swing and increased tone of the lower extremities may be present in clinically normal individuals 85 years of age and older. This finding usually has no specific implications for underlying neurologic disease. The underlying basis of most age-related changes in neurologic function observed in normal elderly individuals is unclear at this time.

Grasp reflexes may be present in up to 28% of individuals 85 years of age and older. Snout reflexes may be noted in up to 32% of the very old in the absence of clinically evident neurologic disease. Vibratory sense perception of the great toe has been reported as decreased in approximately 21% of normal individuals 85 years and older.

Neurologic findings considered suspicious or abnormal in many clinical settings should be interpreted with caution when evaluating the geriatric patient. The clinician should determine their potential significance in the context of symptoms and associated general physical findings, while bearing in mind the high incidence of deviation from the normal neurologic examination in the geriatric population.

## DEMENTIA

Dementia affects an estimated 3–4% of the population aged 65 years and older. Dementia is sometimes mistakenly considered to be a normal consequence of aging by many families of affected patients. Cognitive impairment is usually a consequence of neuronal or vascular pathology. Alzheimer's disease is the most common cause of dementia, and ischemic brain damage occurring alone or in combination with Alzheimer's pathology is the next most frequent cause of cognitive impairment. Lewy body disease has received much attention as another cause of dementia in the elderly. Other causes of dementia occur less commonly in the geriatric population and are considered elsewhere.

Alzheimer's disease increases in frequency with increasing age and affects at least 20% of the population over age 85 years. Approximately 50–70% of demented patients have Alzheimer's disease pathology. Duration of life varies following onset of Alzheimer's disease; most patients survive between 6 and 10 years. Most patients die severely demented, often in a neurovegetative state, and usually in a nursing home.

A diagnosis of pathologically confirmed Alzheimer's disease as verified by autopsy study can be achieved in up to 85–90% of patients diagnosed clinically with probable Alzheimer's disease. This relatively high degree of diagnostic accuracy has been demonstrated in tertiary health care centers and research facilities where evaluation by clinical neurologists and use of neuropsychologic testing have been essential components of the diagnostic effort. It is uncertain whether an equivalent degree of diagnostic accuracy can be achieved in the primary health care setting in the absence of clinicians possessing a high degree of neurologic expertise and personnel capability of performing high-quality neuropsychologic testing.

Variable estimates suggest that 5–15% of demented patients may have potentially reversible features to their illness. The lower estimates are likely more reflective of the true incidence of reversible dementing illness in elderly patients. Potentially treatable causes of dementia include vitamin $B_{12}$ deficiency, hypothyroidism, neurosyphilis, and other chronic central nervous system infections, as well as pseudodementia observed in depressed patients. However, evidence suggests that a high proportion of patients diagnosed with pseudodementia eventually develop frank dementia. Pseudodementia may therefore actually be a predictor of subsequent dementia for some patients.

Published estimates of potentially treatable intracranial structural lesions diagnosable in demented patients usually suggest an incidence of less than 1%. Possible abnormalities include normal pressure hydrocephalus (NPH), brain tumor, and chronic subdural hematoma. Even when structural brain lesions are identified with brain-imaging procedures such as computed tomography (CT) or magnetic resonance imaging (MRI), subsequent treatment of these potentially reversible causes of dementia is only rarely associated with significant sustained clinical improvement.

Published reports also suggest that NPH has been overestimated in its significance as a potentially treatable cause of dementia. Uncertainties associated with arriving at a precise clinical and radiologic diagnosis of NPH along with risk-benefit considerations associated with unpredictable results following ventriculoperitoneal shunting should be considered. These should be discussed in detail with the patient and family as an informed consent issue before aggressively pursuing this diagnosis in the demented geriatric patient.

Vascular dementia as a result of multiple small strokes, or multi-infarct dementia (MID), is responsible for an estimated 8–12% of all cases of dementia. MID has been reported to occur in greater than 30% of patients in some series, however. Neuropathologic evidence of coexisting Alzheimer's disease and MID occurs in at least 15% of elderly demented patients diagnosed with Alzheimer's disease.

Patients with MID usually develop dementia of insidious onset, but may also experience abrupt changes in neurologic or cognitive function in association with acute ischemic events. The pathophysiology of dementia in patients with ischemic brain damage may be caused by loss of brain volume complicated by damage to critical brain structures or neural pathways. A loss of 50–100 cc of brain volume has been strongly correlated with dementing illness.

The primary neuropathology of MID consists of multiple small lacunes. The number and size of lacunes, however, do not correlate with the degree of clinical dementia. Brain imaging with CT or MRI may provide evidence of ischemic injury that suggests underlying MID, but it does not rule out the possibility of coexisting Alzheimer's disease. Attempts to distinguish demented patients with Alzheimer's disease from those having MID during life or to identify those with coexisting disease have not been successful. An imperfect correlation also exists between ischemic damage demonstrated by brain-imaging techniques and clinical dementia. Many normal elderly individuals have evidence of small-vessel disease on CT scans or brain MRI but have no evidence of significant cognitive impairment.

Prevention of further decline of patients with MID should be a primary goal. Treatment of risk factors for MID, such as hypertension and diabetes mellitus, represents an important management strategy. Although no evidence demonstrates that specific interventions actually affect the natural history dementia in patients with MID, it seems prudent to employ measures with potential benefit that pose no harm to the patient. These include control of hypertension and hypercholesterolemia. The importance of maintaining serum cholesterol in the normal range as a means of managing this risk factor for cerebrovascular disease in the geriatric patient is controversial.

Taking a detailed history is critical when evaluating the elderly patient with dementia. The history should include information on the present and past use of medications, particularly drugs with anticholinergic properties as well as benzodiazepines, barbiturates, and neuroleptics. History of head trauma, alcohol abuse, or illicit drug use should be obtained. Human immunodeficiency virus (HIV) infection and neurosyphilis can also cause dementia in the elderly. A family history of dementia may occur in geriatric patients with Alzheimer's disease, but is more typical of patients having earlier age of onset.

Neurologic evaluation of patients with Alzheimer's disease may demonstrate varying degrees of impaired cognitive function. Short-term memory impairment, confusion, and visuospatial problems are common early features. These often advance to a neurovegetative state over subsequent years. Focal neurologic signs are usually absent, and Babinski's sign is not present. Cortical release signs are often present, including suck, palmomental, and grasp reflexes. Formal neuropsychologic evaluation will confirm the clinical impression of dementia.

Laboratory investigation of the elderly demented patient should include complete blood cell count, erythrocyte sedimentation rate (ESR), and electrolytes, including sodium and calcium determinations, liver function tests, and serum $B_{12}$ and folate levels. Urinary heavy metal and drug screens may be requested for selected patients. The clinical utility of serum apolipoprotein E determinations in the evaluation of patients with suspected Alzheimer's disease is controversial. Medical-ethical issues have also been raised in the use of this test in individuals who are clinically normal but who have a family history of Alzheimer's disease. No therapeutic implications exist for measuring serum apolipoprotein E in demented geriatric patients.

The value of brain imaging in evaluating dementia in the elderly patient is controversial. Survey questionnaire data indicate that neurologists usually request CT or MRI brain scans to evaluate patients with dementia, including those who already have a diagnosis of probable Alzheimer's disease. This practice may be modified as studies of cost effectiveness encourage the more selective use of brain imaging in the evaluation of geriatric patients with dementia.


## DELIRIUM

*Delirium* is the accepted term for acute, transient, global organic disorders of higher nervous system function. It implies impairment of consciousness and attention and is synonymous with acute confusional state of the *International Classification of Diseases, Ninth Revision*. Neurologists often use the term *encephalopathy* to describe delirium. The four key features associated with delirium are acute change in mental status with a fluctuating course, inattention, disorganized thinking, and change in level of consciousness. Delirium in the geriatric patient may sometimes be distinguished by an akinetic and apathetic state and is in contrast to the hyperkinetic state younger patients usually manifest.

Delirium in the elderly is a common syndrome with high associated morbidity and mortality. The frequency of delirium increases with age and has an incidence of at least 17% in hospitalized elderly patients. Patients often fail to return to their premorbid baseline and experience high risk of death over the ensuing weeks to months following onset of delirium.

Multiple etiologies have been associated with delirium, but the underlying pathophysiology is poorly understood. The final common pathway in delirium leading to neuronal dysfunction is thought to relate to impairment of central cholinergic function. The nature of specific cellular and molecular mechanisms responsible for the syndrome of delirium are obscure. Oxidative stress may be a factor.

Acute infections, hip fracture, postoperative states, electrolyte and other metabolic disturbances, and hypoxia and hypercapnia have all been associated with the development of delirium. Stool impaction as well as sensory deprivation and overstimulation have also been associated with delirium. The confused elderly patient in the intensive care unit is a common example of a patient with sensory overload. Delirium may also be a nonspecific and nonlocalizing indicator of acute life-threatening conditions such as myocardial infarction, particularly when pain is not a prominent feature. Hyperthyroidism, hypothyroidism, and occult malignancy may also present as delirium.

Cognitive impairment is a risk factor for the development of delirium. Delirium is also a risk factor for the development of dementia. On first encounter with the confused elderly patient, the neurologist may not be able to determine the relative contributions of dementing illness and superimposed delirium to the confusional state manifested by the patient. A history of cognitive impairment provided by a family member or documented in the medical record will be invaluable.

Evaluation of the elderly patient with delirium should focus on identifying potentially treatable causes of delirium. Many elderly patients who develop delirium have no specific identifiable risk factor. This situation is problematic in terms of management and recommendation of specific therapeutic interventions. Identification of a specific precipitant of delirium, such as urinary tract infection, can lead to a prompt therapeutic intervention that increases the likelihood of recovery.

Predicting whether, how soon, and to what extent recovery from delirium will occur is difficult. Up to 30% of patients will not have returned to their premorbid baseline mental status months after initial presentation. Reasons for failure to fully recover are poorly understood.

## GAIT DISORDERS

The neurologist may be requested to evaluate the elderly patient with gait instability, imbalance, or a history of falls. Gait disorders occur with high prevalence in the elderly and affect approximately 15% of individuals older than 60 years of age. The presence of gait disorders increases with age, and gait disorders affect 25% or more of the very old aged 85 years or more. Gait instability predisposes individuals to falls, with associated risk of hip fracture and high morbidity and mortality.

### Normal Gait

Normal gait results from a synthesis of locomotor and dynamic balance. Locomotion associated with normal gait refers to the phasic advance resulting from loading and unloading of the limbs. *Dynamic balance* refers to the maintenance of the center of gravity in relationship to the base of support during the gait cycle. Sensory input from the visual and vestibular systems as well as proprioception contribute to the maintenance and stability of balance.

Normal elderly individuals often experience modest changes in gait as they age. Reduction in velocity of approximately 15–20% occurs, along with reduction in stride length. Changes in gait morphology also occur. Elderly individuals have a shorter and more broad-based stride than young and middle-aged adults. Reduced pelvic rotation and joint excursions with increased dependence on double limb support are more prominent in the elderly. Non-neurologic factors, such as those resulting from increased muscle and joint stiffness, are partially responsible for these changes. No consensus has been reached regarding the impact of underlying subtle progressive neuropathology on age-related changes in gait.

### Age-Related Changes in Gait

A defensive posture of gait may occur even in the normal elderly individual because of reduced confidence and anxiety related to a sense of biomechanical instability. A cautious gait is manifested as a forward posture with a broad base of support, shortened stride, and reduced cadence. Mildly compromised gait present in the elderly may be aggravated by superimposed cervical spondylosis, stroke, or peripheral neuropathy leading to clinically significant gait disorder. Determining one specific cause of gait disturbance in the geriatric patient may be impossible because of coexisting multiple contributing factors. Certain types of gait impairment are characteristic of underlying pathology, however, and are usually obvious to the neurologist. A spastic hemiparetic gait is a common consequence of stroke. A slow, shuffling gait is a hallmark of the patient with parkinsonism. Ataxia may be a result of ischemic injury to the cerebellum or hydrocephalus. Sensory ataxia may be a result of severe sensory peripheral neuropathy, spinal cord disease or, rarely, primary sensory ganglionopathy.

## Senile Gait

The term *senile gait* is controversial but has been used to refer to the unsteady gait present in the elderly patient where no specific cause can be established. It is characterized by a stooped posture, reduced arm swing, and increase in double stance. Impaired coordination of cyclical limb movements with reduced hip and knee rotations may also be present. Although hydrocephalus has been implicated as the cause in some patients with senile gait, there is no consensus regarding the presence of specific underlying neuropathology.

Senile gait has been suggested to result from the cumulative loss of Betz's cells, cerebellar Purkinje's cells, dopaminergic neurons, and spinal cord motor neurons. Age-related impairment of strength, sensation, and vestibular balance mechanisms, as well as difficulties with control of body sway, may also contribute to the development of senile gait.

## FALLS

Falls are a major cause of morbidity in the elderly. Approximately 35–40% of elderly individuals residing in the community experience at least one fall annually. Some 10–15% of falls in the elderly result in serious injury. At least 50% of falls do not have a clear etiology. Hip fractures represent the major cause of morbidity and mortality. Falls in the elderly are frequently a consequence of gait disorder and contribute to most of the estimated 200,000 hip fractures that occur annually in the United States.

Falls in the elderly patient can be a manifestation of many different underlying pathologies. Falls may be a result of mechanical locomotor problems or to a variety of unrelated pathophysiologic mechanisms such as those associated with syncope or seizures. Fear of falling may characterize the elderly patient who has experienced one or more falls. Consequently, this fear can severely limit the elderly patient's ability to ambulate.

Most falls in the elderly probably result from a combination of different factors, such as postural instability, prolonged reflex reaction time, postural hypotension, and reduced peripheral sensory input resulting from impaired proprioception, vision, or hearing. Inattention to obstacles in the home environment, such as electrical cords and thresholds, and difficulty descending stairways also contribute to fall risk. Defects in central processing as well as underlying neuropathology caused by Parkinson's disease, dementia, or delirium may predispose the elderly patient to falls. Patients with gait disorders are also particularly at high risk for falling.

Other underlying conditions predisposing the elderly patient to falls include neuromuscular diseases such as peripheral neuropathy, myasthenia gravis, and amyotrophic lateral sclerosis. Cervical spondylosis and foot problems related to bunions, toe deformities, and poorly fitting footwear are also significant risk factors. Acute infections of the urinary tract and lungs can be associated with dehydration, generalized malaise, and weakness, which may predispose to falls. Weakness associated with advancing age caused by physical deconditioning predisposes to falls.

Medications are a major risk factor for falls in the elderly. The use of benzodiazepines, neuroleptics, and barbiturates is clearly associated with increased fall risk. It is possible that antidepressant medications may also predispose to falls in the elderly. Limiting the initial use of pharmacologic agents that have the potential to cause falls and periodically reviewing medications and eliminating those no longer necessary is prudent.

A detailed history should be obtained when evaluating elderly patients with a history of falls. This should include inquiry about specific symptoms that may have preceded the fall, such as dizziness, near-syncope, or sense of impaired balance. A complete medication history should be requested, including the use of over-the-counter drugs. Specific attention should be directed to detecting underlying medical and neurologic conditions that predispose to falls. The geriatric patient's home environment should be reviewed and possibly inspected to identify possible obstructions in the household, including telephone cords, throw rugs, elevated thresholds, and slippery floors.

Evaluation of the elderly patient who has fallen should include determination of postural pulse and blood pressure in the supine, sitting, and standing positions. A drop in systolic blood pressure of 20 mm Hg or more should be noted, as it may represent clinically significant hypotension predisposing to falls.

The focused physical examination should include assessing for signs of dehydration and malnutrition. Decreased skin turgor is of questionable clinical significance in the elderly patient because of age-related decrease in skin elasticity. The integument should nevertheless be evaluated in the context of other factors such as serum electrolyte levels and blood urea nitrogen level. The musculoskeletal system of the elderly patient who has fallen should be carefully evaluated. Special attention should be directed to detecting possible limitations about the joints as well as foot deformities and use of unsafe footwear.

Mobility of the elderly patient can be assessed with the "up and go" test. The patient is asked to rise from a chair, walk 3 m across the room, turn around, walk back to the chair, and sit down. The test is scored as follows: 1 = normal; 2 = very slightly abnormal; 3 = mildly abnormal; 4 = moderately abnormal; 5 = severely abnormal. Although the "up and go" test is not highly quantitative, it can be of value in longitudinal follow-up of the elderly patient with gait problems or a history of falling.

Performing a detailed neurologic examination is critical when evaluating the elderly patient with a history of falls. Focal or generalized weakness should be identified. Evaluation should be performed for increased tone or frank rigidity of the extremities and trunk. A detailed sensory examination should be performed to detect impairment of tactile sensation, proprioception, visual acuity, and hearing. Recommendations for fall prevention should be based on the identification of risk factors. Minimizing environmental hazards and treating diagnosed neurologic and medical illness help reduce the risk of falling. Gait and balance training, as well as exercise and physical therapy with assistive devices, are valuable fall-prevention measures.

## PARKINSON'S DISEASE

Parkinson's disease is a common neurodegenerative disorder that increases in incidence with age. Parkinson's disease affects 1% of the population over the age of 50 and 2% over the age of 70. Resting tremor, rigidity, bradykinesia, and eventually postural instability are the hallmarks of this disorder. Onset typically consists of asymmetric tremor and is followed by relentless progression. Treatment of patients with early-onset Parkinson's disease with L-dopa in combination with a peripheral dopa decarboxylase inhibitor is associated with gratifying clinical improvement. Most patients eventually develop side effects, including on-off phenomenon, dyskinesias, and other motor fluctuations. Confusion and hallucinations often occur with higher dosage schedules. The elderly are probably more susceptible to these side effects than younger adults.

The stereotypical case of Parkinson's disease would appear to represent a straightforward clinical diagnosis. Autopsy studies suggest, however, that there is less than a 70% correlation between the clinical diagnosis of Parkinson's disease and neuropathologic findings determined at time of autopsy. Idiopathic parkinsonism syndromes encompass Parkinson's disease and Parkinson's-plus syndromes, including progressive supranuclear palsy, Shy-Drager syndrome, striatonigral degeneration, and related conditions. Secondary parkinsonism may be drug induced or related to ischemic brain injury, infections, head trauma, and structural brain lesions.

Management of the geriatric patient with idiopathic Parkinson's disease usually parallels that of younger adults with the disease, but with special considerations. Anticholinergic medications should be avoided in Parkinson's disease patients 65 years and older and should be used only with caution in younger patients who have a history of confusion or impaired cognitive function. The elderly are particularly susceptible to the toxic side effects of most antiparkinsonism medications and should be closely monitored.

Antiparkinsonism medications are of limited, if any, benefit for patients with Parkinson's-plus syndromes. The ability of a patient with parkinsonism to demonstrate a favorable response to L-dopa is thought to offer strong indirect support for the diagnosis of idiopathic Parkinson's disease.

Parkinson's disease in the elderly is a significant cause of morbidity and mortality. Patients are particularly susceptible to falls caused by a combination of factors including gait instability and postural hypotension associated with the pathophysiology of Parkinson's disease; postural hypotension secondary to antiparkinsonism medications; reduced vasomotor tone related to prolonged motor inactivity; weakness as a result of deconditioning; confusion; and the frequent presence of multiple medical diseases in the elderly patient. Fall-prevention strategies should be employed in patients with Parkinson's disease.

Drugs are the most common cause of secondary parkinsonism. A careful history should be obtained from the geriatric patient and family to determine if the patient has been taking a drug associated with parkinsonism. Neuroleptic medications such as phenothiazines and butyrophenones are leading causes of drug-induced parkinsonism. Metoclopramide is a commonly used drug and has been associated with the development of parkinsonism. Treatment of drug-induced parkinsonism consists of removing the offending drug.

Co-administration of an anticholinergic or a neuroleptic medication is a common practice when treating patients with psychosis. This practice should be avoided as a management strategy when treating the geriatric patient. Clozapine has been used successfully for the management of psychosis in patients with Parkinson's disease because of its $D_2$-receptor–sparing effect.

Dementia occurring in the elderly patient with advanced Parkinson's disease may be difficult to distinguish from that associated with Alzheimer's disease. Neuropathologic evidence of both Alzheimer's disease and Parkinson's disease occurs in 25% or more of patients with dementia. Determining the specific cause of dementia in many elderly patients that have clinical features of both these conditions may be impossible.

## MOVEMENT DISORDERS

Movement disorders affecting the elderly are challenging management problems. Movement disorders may reflect damage to the basal ganglia and extrapyramidal system. Essential tremor and parkinsonian tremor are particularly common among the elderly, and drug-induced dyskinesias occur frequently. Diagnosis of movement disorders is relatively straightforward. Management strategies are essentially those used for younger adults.

## STROKE

Stroke is a major cause of death and disability, affecting 500,000 patients annually in the United States. Each year 300,000 deaths result from stroke. Many other patients are left severely disabled. The greatest negative impact of cerebrovascular disease is experienced by the elderly. The incidence of stroke and associated mortality increase exponentially with age, and the risk of stroke doubles each decade after age 55. Stroke is the third leading cause of death in the United States in individuals aged 65–84 years, and the second leading cause of death in persons 85 years and older. The annual incidence of stroke is 2.1 per 1,000 persons aged 55–64 years; 4.5 per 1,000 aged 65–74 years; and 9.3 per 1,000 aged 75–84 years. Stroke is usually a result of embolism or thrombosis and may be associated with hemorrhage. Specific stroke syndromes and management strategies are discussed in Chapter 7.

Although overall death rates from stroke have decreased significantly, the geriatric population continues to be at much greater risk than younger adults. The reduction in stroke incidence has been attributed to effective and aggressive treatment of hypertension. Diabetes mellitus, atrial fibrillation, history of transient ischemic attack, and prior stroke are additional stroke risk factors.

Smoking and hypercholesterolemia probably represent additional risk factors for stroke, but evidence for causality is less definitive. The value of managing hypercholesterolemia in the geriatric population is unproven; it is a subject of considerable debate and in need of resolution. Definitive evidence is not yet available to indicate that aggressive reduction of serum cholesterol in the elderly has measurable impact on lowering cerebrovascular risk.

Implementation of prevention and health maintenance programs are clearly the preferred approach to lowering cerebrovascular morbidity and mortality from a population-based public health perspective. Diagnostic and management strategies for the symptomatic geriatric patient parallel those for the adult patient population. A detailed present and past medical history with assessment of risk factors for stroke must be obtained, and complete general physical and neurologic examinations must be performed. Laboratory evaluations should consist of complete blood cell count with differential, ESR, blood glucose level, serum electrolytes, blood urea nitrogen, creatinine, serologic test for syphilis, and serum cholesterol. The value of obtaining serum antiphospholipid antibody determinations in the geriatric patient population is uncertain.

Carotid ultrasound testing is indicated for patients with symptoms of anterior circulation ischemia. Echocardiography is indicated for patients with atrial fibrillation and where there is suspicion of mural thrombus. The value and cost-effectiveness of performing echocardiography as routine evaluation of patients with stroke or symptoms of transient cerebral ischemia in the absence of more specific indications is debated. CT scan of the brain is adequate for the study of most geriatric patients who have experienced stroke. In the acute clinical setting, CT is the procedure of choice in view of its ability to detect recent blood, as in hemorrhagic stroke, subarachnoid hemorrhage, or small hematomas. MRI is clearly more sensitive in detecting subtle evidence of ischemic injury. Increasing pressures related to cost-benefit considerations may limit the use of MRI brain imaging for the routine study of elderly patients with cerebral ischemia. It is not clear that there is value added from MRI use versus CT brain imaging in the study of most elderly patients with cerebrovascular disease. Clear exceptions include use of MRI for the identification of small lacunar infarctions that may escape detection by CT brain imaging. The decision to use CT brain imaging as opposed to MRI should be made by the neurologist on a case-by-case basis.

Guidelines that apply to the use of cerebral angiography in younger adults generally serve the needs of the geriatric patient population. Risk-benefit considerations are pre-eminent when making the decision to perform cerebral angiography in the elderly patient. Patients who have high multiple medical disease burdens or who have isolated but severe cardiac or pulmonary disease usually do not represent acceptable surgical candidates and should not be subjected to angiography. Preoperative evaluation of the geriatric patient by the internal medicine consultant should be requested in advance of any contemplated surgical intervention such as carotid endarterectomy.

The neurologist's choice of a specific surgeon to perform carotid endarterectomy when this intervention is indicated is clearly a most critical decision to be made on the patient's behalf. The neurologist must have a clear knowledge of the surgeon's skills and success rate measured by morbidity and mortality statistics. This matter should not be left to chance. Medical management options available to the elderly patient are similar to those of younger patients with cerebrovascular disease. These include antiplatelet therapy with aspirin or ticlopidine hydrochloride. The latter agent is appropriate for patients who are allergic to aspirin or who have not responded to aspirin therapy. Thrombolytic therapy will revolutionize the treatment of patients with acute nonhemorrhagic strokes. Geriatric patients are expected to benefit from this therapy if they present within the 3-hour time window necessary to be considered candidates for treatment.

## SEIZURES

The incidence and prevalence of epilepsy increase with advancing age. The incidence of new-onset seizure disorders after age 60 is 3.5 per 1,000. Seizures must be distinguished from other conditions associated with transient neurologic symptoms, loss of consciousness, and falls.

Partial seizures account for up to 80% of new-onset seizure disorders in patients older than 60 years. Lesions causing partial seizures in the geriatric population are usually secondary to focal ischemic injury. Patients with simple partial seizures maintain an intact level of consciousness. Complex partial seizures are characterized by impaired consciousness during the ictal episode. Complex partial seizures usually last 1–2 minutes and are often characterized by automatisms such as lip smacking, picking at one's clothing, and other semipurposeful movements.

Most complex partial seizures originate from a temporal lobe focus. Simple partial seizures may also originate from other regions of the brain, such as the frontal and occipital lobes. Partial seizures may generalize to tonic-clonic seizures. Absence seizures, atonic seizures, and tonic seizures are rare in elderly adults.

The history is invaluable in establishing a clinical diagnosis of seizure disorder. Differential diagnoses of seizures in the elderly include syncope, falls, transient ischemic attacks, and pseudoseizures. The absence of aura, automatisms, tonic-clonic activity, or postictal confusion favors a diagnosis of syncope rather than partial seizure but does not rule out the latter. A cardiogenic cause such as arrhythmia is usually responsible for syncope in the elderly patient when a cause can be established. Syncope may be difficult to distinguish initially from seizures causing loss of consciousness. Evaluation of seizures and their management are discussed in Chapter 5.

## NEUROMUSCULAR DISEASES

Neuromuscular diseases commonly affect the geriatric population. Some disorders are clearly age-related and increase in frequency with advancing age. Neuromuscular diseases are conditions that affect the motor unit. The motor unit consists of the spinal cord anterior horn cell, axon, motor nerve root, peripheral nerve, neuromuscular junction, and myofibril.

Amyotrophic lateral sclerosis (ALS) is the prototype anterior horn disorder but also includes upper motor neuron pathology as evidenced by involvement of the corticobulbar and corticospinal tracts. Median age of onset is the mid-50s, with most cases occurring between the ages of 40 and 70 years. The incidence increases with age, however, so that increasing numbers of older patients are expected to be seen as the elderly population increases in number.

Patients with ALS typically present with asymmetric lower motor neuron weakness and atrophy of the distal upper or lower extremity. Evidence of upper motor neuron pathology is often present during early stages of the disease or evolves soon thereafter. This pathology is manifested as hyperreflexia, Babinski's sign, and spasticity. Electromyography (EMG) eventually demonstrates evidence of diffuse denervation. Typical EMG findings include fibrillations, positive sharp waves, fasciculations, giant motor unit potentials, and reduced recruitment with maximal voluntary effort. Peripheral nerve studies are within normal limits except for reduced amplitude of evoked motor action potentials reflecting severe axonal dropout.

The diagnosis of ALS is essentially a clinical diagnosis. EMG is simply an extension of the clinical examination and must be interpreted with caution. Evidence of focal denervation, although sometimes consistent with clinical ALS, does not define it as a clinicopathologic entity. The neurologist must consider alternative diagnoses to explain abnormal neurologic findings observed in patients with suspected ALS. An extensive list of conditions can mimic ALS, although it is not within the scope of this chapter to discuss them.

In the geriatric population, cervical spinal cord lesions occur commonly and may mimic ALS by showing the clinical manifestations of combined lower and upper motor neuron abnormalities. These may be caused by spinal cord and cervical root compression caused by cervical spondylosis, cervical stenosis, or meningioma, all potentially treatable conditions. Lumbar stenosis can also present with clinical manifestations similar to ALS. Parasagittal meningioma can cause spastic monoparesis of the lower extremity that resembles the occasional case in which the suspected ALS patient presents with primarily upper motor weakness and signs and symptoms involving the lower extremity. MRI imaging studies are extremely important to rule out structural lesions of the spinal cord and brain. A second neurologic opinion is often requested by the initial consultant for diagnostic confirmation of this fatal condition. More extensive discussion of the variable clinical manifestations of ALS and differential diagnosis and management can be found elsewhere.

Peripheral neuropathy is a common neuromuscular disorder affecting elderly patients. Numerous possible etiologies exist. The most common identifiable causes of peripheral neuropathy in the developed world are diabetes mellitus and chronic alcohol abuse. Many other causes of neuropathy are broadly categorized as metabolic; for example, there is neuropathy caused by vitamin $B_{12}$ deficiency; toxic neuropathy, such as that caused by occupational and recreational exposure to toxic hydrocarbons; disimmune neuropathy caused by monoclonal gammopathies and vasculitis; paraneoplastic syndromes caused by occult carcinoma, most commonly of the lung and breast; and hereditary neuropathies. Because it is highly unusual for inherited neuropathies to present in the later years of life, these disorders are an unlikely possibility for most geriatric patients. Systemic or localized amyloidosis is a rare cause of painful small-fiber peripheral neuropathy that is often associated with autonomic symptoms.

Evaluation of elderly patients with peripheral neuropathy should include taking a detailed present and past medical history. A history of glucose intolerance and alcohol abuse should be noted, and possible toxic exposure should be considered. The neurologic examination may reveal distal sensory impairment to pain, light touch, temperature, vibration, and position sense. Distal motor weakness may be present in patients with pathologic involvement of motor fibers. Myotatic reflexes are usually hypoactive or absent but may occasionally remain intact. Preserved deep tendon reflexes can occur in a setting of predominantly small-fiber axonal neuropathy.

There appears to be a subset of geriatric patients who experience painful small-fiber axonal peripheral neuropathy for which no specific cause can be determined once diabetes and alcohol have been excluded as potential causes. Neurophysiologic studies usually reveal evidence of axonal neuropathy. Sural nerve biopsies generally do not disclose specific pathology except for evidence of axonal damage. Rarely, a biopsy may reveal evidence of vasculitis. The etiology of the painful small-fiber neuropathy observed in geriatric patients is unknown. A possible role for ischemia has been suggested but a definitive cause-and-effect relationship is unproven.

The pain associated with neuropathy caused by diabetes can often be successfully managed. Carbamazepine, phenytoin, valproate sodium, gabapentin, and topical capsaicin may be of benefit. Amitriptyline hydrochloride if used in the elderly, should be administered with great caution and at low doses because of potential anticholinergic toxicity. Acupuncture is of unproven value. Use of minor analgesics such as acetaminophen in combination with carbamazepine may be of modest value in some patients.

Myasthenia gravis is an uncommon neuromuscular disorder but does not spare the elderly population. Elderly men may have some predisposition to developing ocular myasthenia with mild to moderate manifestations of systemic involvement. General principles employed to manage younger patients with myasthenia gravis usually apply to geriatric patients. Elderly patients should be closely monitored for side effects of medication, particularly corticosteroids and cytotoxic agents. Homeostatic reserves are compromised, and the elderly are probably more prone to toxicity, including osteoporosis associated with corticosteroid administration.

Polymyositis is a rare cause of weakness in the geriatric patient. Proximal muscle weakness of the lower and upper extremities, and elevated serum creatine phosphokinase are the hallmarks of this disorder. EMG may be helpful in supporting the clinical impression. Muscle biopsy should be obtained for confirmation of this disorder; characteristic inflammatory pathology will be noted. The possibility of underlying malignancy should be entertained in newly diagnosed patients with polymyositis, and a search for occult malignancy should be considered.

Geriatric patients with immune-mediated neuromuscular diseases such as disimmune peripheral neuropathies, myasthenia gravis, and polymyositis are often frail and present complex medical management issues. These patients may benefit from additional consultation provided by a neurologic subspecialist with special expertise in the management of neuromuscular disorders.

## SPINAL CORD DISEASES

Spinal cord diseases that affect younger adults may likewise affect the elderly, but the rates of susceptibility differ. The incidence of ALS increases with advancing age, whereas the incidence of multiple sclerosis greatly decreases. Myelopathies resulting from degenerative changes affecting the vertebral column increase greatly with age. Radiographic evidence of cervical spondylosis is found in an estimated 50% of individuals over age 45 and 75% of individuals over age 65. The incidence of clinically significant cervical spondylosis likewise increases. The coexistence of cervical spondylosis in a patient with suspected ALS is a common occurrence and presents challenges to the neurologist in attempting to make a definitive diagnosis. The patient may ultimately prove to have one condition or both conditions concurrently.

The range of clinical manifestations of spinal cord disease is relatively limited and may consist of upper and lower motor neuron weakness and spasticity with or without sensory abnormalities. The neurologist must consider extensive differential diagnoses that reflect an array of underlying neuropathologic processes capable of affecting the spinal cord. A detailed history and neurologic examination assists greatly in limiting the differential diagnoses and localizing the anatomic site of neuropathology.

The differential diagnoses of spinal cord disease include degenerative conditions such as ALS and syringomyelia; mechanical compression caused by cervical spondylosis; spinal cord extradural tumor such as meningioma, schwannoma, and metastatic tumor; rarely, intramedullary glioma; infections such as extradural abscess, necrotizing myelopathy caused by varicella-zoster virus, HIV, and human T-lymphotropic virus type 1 myelopathy; ischemic injury resulting from embolic occlusion of the anterior spinal artery and watershed infarction; and subacute combined degeneration of the spinal cord caused by vitamin $B_{12}$ deficiency. Lumbar stenosis may be associated with weakness and atrophy of the lower extremities. Relatively minor trauma to the spinal cord secondary to a fall in a patient with unsuspected cervical stenosis may result in severe neurologic deficit.

Diagnostic evaluation is dictated by the history and clinical examination. The potential for successful outcome is a direct reflection of the specific underlying neuropathology. Some spinal cord entities are eminently treatable. For example, subacute combined degeneration of the spinal cord can be treated with vitamin $B_{12}$, and surgical intervention is successful in selected patients with cervical spondylosis. Other conditions, such as ALS, have more limited treatment options. The diagnostic acumen and determination of the geriatric neurologist are critical in arriving at a specific diagnosis.

## URINARY INCONTINENCE

Urinary incontinence is a common problem in the elderly population. Urinary incontinence occurs in approximately 5–15% of community-residing elderly; in 35% of acutely hospitalized elderly; and in 40–66% of long-term-care patients. Risk factors associated with urinary incontinence include neurologic disease and impaired mobility; women are also at greater risk. Although it is important to rule out acute neurologic disease as the cause of urinary incontinence, most elderly patients have a non-neurologic basis for their problem.

Other risk factors associated with transient urinary incontinence in the elderly include delirium, infection of the urinary tract or other organ systems, atrophic vaginitis and urethritis, restricted mobility such as being bedfast, and stool impaction. Medications may also contribute to transient urinary incontinence. These include potent diuretics, adrenergic agents, and sedative hypnotics.

A neurologic basis for urinary incontinence should always be considered. Spinal cord lesions should be ruled out. These include primary and metastatic tumors, abscess, and spinal cord trauma. Pain, weakness, increased deep tendon reflexes, Babinski's sign, or a spinal cord sensory level could represent evidence for the presence of a spinal cord lesion.

A targeted neurologic examination of the incontinent elderly patient should include mental status testing, motor examination, evaluation of muscle tone and deep tendon reflexes, and sensory examination, including a determination of whether a spinal cord sensory level is present. External rectal sphincter tone, anal wink, bulbocavernosus reflex, and perineal sensation should also be tested.

Although normal aging affects the lower urinary tract, incontinence should not be considered part of the aging process. Incontinence is highly treatable in the elderly patient. More aggressive approaches to this common problem have been developed. Age-related changes in elderly men and women include reduced bladder capacity, decreased ability to postpone voiding, and reduced urinary flow rate. Aging women experience a decline in maximal urethral closure pressure as well as reduction of urethral length. Uninhibited bladder contraction also occurs with increased prevalence as a function of aging. Postvoid residual volume also increases, up to 50–100 ml.

Transient incontinence commonly occurs in the elderly and affects up to one-half of hospitalized elderly patients. The causes of transient incontinence include delirium, infection, atrophic urethritis or vaginitis, pharmaceuticals, depression (psychological), excess urinary output, restricted mobility, and stool impaction, and can be remembered using the mnemonic *DIAPPERS*. Medications associated with urinary incontinence include sedative hypnotics, diuretics, and those with anticholinergic properties, as well as adrenergic agents.

## HEADACHE

Evaluation of headache in the geriatric patient population should include consideration of disease states that occur more commonly in this patient subgroup than in younger adults. Systemic illness may be related to headache in older patients more often than in the general population. Certain headache variants such as migraine and muscle-contraction headache are unlikely causes of new-onset headache syndromes in the elderly patient. Temporal arteritis and headache related to cervical spine disease occur much more frequently in elderly patients than in younger individuals. Structural compressive lesions of the brain and spine should be considered as possible serious underlying causes of headache. Hypertensive headaches usually do not occur in the absence of significant prolonged elevations of blood pressure. These headaches are usually most symptomatic early in the morning and improve as the day goes on. Prolonged headache in an acutely hypertensive patient should alert the clinician to the possibility of hypertensive hemorrhage or subarachnoid hemorrhage.

Diagnosis of temporal arteritis is usually straightforward. Elevated ESR in an elderly patient with headache who also demonstrates tenderness to palpation over the temporal arteries represents presumptive evidence for the diagnosis of this condition. The patient may also experience jaw claudication with anemia and show elevated values on liver function tests. Polymyalgia rheumatica may precede or accompany temporal arteritis. Temporal artery biopsy usually provides confirmatory evidence for the diagnosis.

Corticosteroid therapy should be initiated once a preliminary diagnosis of temporal arteritis is made and should not be delayed while temporal artery biopsy results are pending. The risk of blindness for patients with temporal arteritis makes initiation of corticosteroid therapy urgent.

Treatment regimens for temporal arteritis vary but usually consist of high doses of prednisone. The drug may be provided as 60 mg daily for the first week while clinical status and follow-up ESR are monitored. Prednisone can be tapered while monitoring the patient and the ESR but may be required for several months or longer. Temporal arteritis appears to be a self-limiting condition, and the patient will eventually no longer require corticosteroid therapy.

The decision to use brain imaging in the evaluation of headache in the elderly patient is made case by case and is based on several factors. These include the presence or absence of focal neurologic signs and symptoms, the presence of papilledema, the severity of the headache, and evidence of systemic illness. The decision to perform lumbar puncture with cerebrospinal fluid examination and culture is based on essentially the same factors considered in making this decision with younger patients.

## DIZZINESS

An estimated two-thirds of all patients over the age of 65 have complained of dizziness or have experienced a sense of imbalance. The diagnostic yield for establishing the cause of dizziness or true vertigo is relatively low, probably no greater than 25%. Presbyataxis, or dysequilibrium of aging, is a clinical diagnosis of exclusion. This diagnosis implies that all benign and serious causes of the patient's complaints have been ruled out.

Other causes of dizziness in the geriatric patient include postural hypotension related to underlying medical or neurologic conditions and to drug side effects. Benign postural vertigo increases in incidence with age and is a self-limiting condition. Vestibular neuronitis occurs secondarily to acute inflammation of the vestibular nerve. It is considered to be of viral origin, though definitive evidence is lacking. The acute vertigo usually improves over several weeks and resolves completely within 3 months. Ischemia of the posterior cerebral circulation can cause symptoms resembling vestibular neuronitis and should be considered in the differential diagnosis.

Menière's disease is manifested by tinnitus, vertigo, and hearing loss. It has a peak incidence during the sixth and seventh decades of life. The mainstay of medical therapy is diuretics, usually acetazolamide. This controls vertigo in 80% of patients, but does not prevent progressive hearing loss. It is vitally important to rule out structural lesions such as acoustic neuroma and glomus jugulare tumor, which could mimic Menière's disease.

Other causes of dizziness and vertigo in the elderly include labyrinthitis caused by viral or bacterial infection, tertiary syphilis, trauma, and vestibulotoxic drugs. A detailed history and neurologic examination are critical in determining the cause of the patient's complaints. Postural pulse and blood pressure determinations should be obtained in the dizzy patient. Formal vestibular testing can be accomplished when a specific diagnosis cannot be established. Available procedures include electronystagmography, vestibulo-ocular reflex testing, and posturography.

Management should be directed toward the specific cause of the dizziness or vertigo. Antivertigo medications such as meclizine hydrochloride are effective for nonspecific control of symptoms. These should be administered with caution in elderly patients, as side effects can occur at relatively low dosages. The "start low and go slow" principle should be applied when prescribing most medications for geriatric patients.

## SYNCOPE

*Syncope* is defined as the sudden and transient loss of consciousness, loss of tone, and unresponsiveness. Syncope usually results from transient reduction of blood supply in association with impaired delivery of oxygen and glucose to the brain. Spontaneous recovery occurs and resuscitation is not required. Many causes of syncope exist.

A yearly incidence of syncope of 6% in the elderly has been reported, and recurrent syncope has been found to occur in up to 30% in some studies. Cardiovascular causes were identified in most patients with recurrent syncope. Morbidity rates associated with syncope vary. Among the very old, injury rates are less than 5%, but syncope itself is correlated with functional decline. A 10% rate of major complications was reported with syncope affecting the elderly that was associated with automobile accidents. A study of patients 65 years and older experiencing recurrent syncope indicated an injury rate of 56%. Determining a cause for syncope in the elderly patient is not possible in 30–50% of instances.

Cardiovascular causes of syncope include cardiac arrhythmia, Stokes-Adams attack, and carotid sinus hypersensitivity. Seizures are a rare cause of syncope. Syncope has been associated with vasovagal, micturitional, postprandial, and defecational mechanisms. Cases of patients experiencing syncope while eating have been reported. The nature of the association of eating with syncope is unclear. Syncope in the elderly may also occur in association with myocardial infarction, angina, pulmonary embolism and, rarely, glossopharyngeal neuralgia.

Evaluation of syncope in the elderly should include taking a detailed history and conducting a physical examination. History and physical examination alone allow determination of the presumptive cause of syncope in elderly patients in up to 25% of the cases in which a cause is eventually determined. Dizziness after standing up abruptly or after eating a meal offers clues to the cause of subsequent syncopal episode. Chest pain or shortness of breath suggests cardiac or pulmonary etiologies. Nausea in association with a flushed sensation may suggest vasovagal syncope. Clonic jerking may occur after syncope and cerebral hypoperfusion and does not necessarily imply the presence of seizure as the cause of syncope. A prolonged postictal period in association with urinary incontinence may provide some indirect evidence for seizure as the cause of syncope.

Determination of pulse and blood pressure in the supine, sitting, and standing positions should be made. A thorough general physical and neurologic examination should be performed. Laboratory evaluation of the elderly patient with syncope is essentially the same as that for the younger adult.

## SLEEP DISORDERS

Complaints concerning sleep are common among the elderly. There may be difficulty falling asleep and then staying asleep. Patients may experience transient or chronic insomnia, which may be associated with depression. Rebound insomnia may occur with withdrawal of sedative hypnotic medications. Clinical suspicion of obstructive sleep apnea can be confirmed by sleep laboratory evaluation, which usually provides confirmatory evidence to support the diagnosis. Interventions appropriate for younger adults are applicable to the elderly. Other sleep disorders affecting the elderly include restless legs syndrome and periodic limb movement disorder.

Sleep may be disrupted in patients with dementia, in those who have disabling medical conditions causing pain, or in those who have cardiac or respiratory compromise. A detailed history usually provides the information required to diagnose the cause of the sleep disturbance and may be supplemented with a formal sleep study.

Further diagnostic evaluation and specific interventions appropriate to the needs of the individual patient can be provided.

## VISUAL AND HEARING DISORDERS

Visual impairment is a common disabling condition affecting the elderly. The same conditions affecting younger patients often affect the elderly but some occur with increased frequency. Some causes of visual impairment, such as macular degeneration and cataracts, preferentially affect the elderly. Others, such as glaucoma, occur with increased frequency. Anterior ischemic optic neuropathy is caused by infarction of the optic nerve head. The arteritic form is typical of temporal arteritis.

Age-related macular degeneration is a leading cause of vision loss in the elderly. It occurs in over 28% of persons over age 75. Some studies have found an association with lifetime sun exposure. There is presently no effective therapy for macular degeneration. Suggestions that oxidative stress may be related to the pathophysiology of this condition may offer hope for the development of preventive and therapeutic approaches.

Hearing impairment is one of the most common disorders affecting the elderly. Almost one-third of people over age 65 experience significant hearing loss. Up to 50% of those over 75 are candidates for hearing rehabilitation. The significance of hearing impairment and its negative impact on functional status in the elderly are underestimated. Conductive hearing loss as a result of cerumen impaction is common and is easily treated. Sensorineural hearing loss implies cochlear or retrocochlear pathology. Injury to the cochlear hair cells by long-term noise exposure is a common cause of hearing impairment in the elderly. Other causes of hearing loss in the geriatric patient population include serous otitis media, tympanic membrane perforation, and otosclerosis. Perilymphatic fistula, cochlear otosclerosis, acoustic neuroma, infection, and cerebrovascular disease also cause hearing deficit in the geriatric patient.

Presbycusis is the most common cause of hearing impairment in the elderly. Sensorineural hearing loss as a result of presbycusis is an age-related problem often occurring in association with a history of significant noise exposure. Several different audiometric patterns of presbycusis have been described. Hearing amplification is the primary treatment for this condition. Many elderly patients are reluctant to use hearing aids because of their cumbersome nature and negative cosmetic appearance. Refinements in electronics have resulted in improved fidelity with smaller hearing aid units. Elderly patients should be strongly encouraged to use these devices when appropriate for their hearing problem. Formal consultation with an ear, nose, and throat specialist should be obtained to evaluate hearing impairment in the elderly. Quality of life can be greatly improved in many instances.

## PRINCIPLES OF MEDICATION USE

There are important age-related features of drug metabolism that may predispose the elderly individual to adverse drug reactions. Simultaneous use of multiple medications or polypharmacy in the elderly may further complicate use of drugs. Gastrointestinal absorption of most drugs in the elderly does not differ significantly from that in the nongeriatric population. Hepatic phase I or oxidative reactions become impaired, however, even as a result of normal aging, whereas phase II or conjugation reactions are relatively spared. Renal drug clearance is reduced by approximately 30% in the elderly; this reduced clearance is obviously an important consideration when treating geriatric patients with medications excreted by the kidney.

Drug half-life is proportional to volume of distribution over clearance. The fact that fat increases as a proportion of body weight in the elderly as lean body mass decreases has implications for the administration and dosage of fat-soluble drugs. Although serum albumin does not decrease significantly in the healthy aging individual, low albumin frequently occurs in the malnourished or chronically ill patient and may affect circulating drug levels when protein binding occurs. The normal elderly are also more sensitive to many different drugs, including benzodiazepines and anticholinergic agents, opiates, and warfarin sodium. As mentioned earlier, "start low and go slow" is an important guiding principle when prescribing medications for the elderly.

Prescriber knowledge of metabolic pathways, pharmacokinetics, and pharmacodynamics is important when treating the elderly patient. Use of medications in a long-term-care setting such as a nursing home presents special challenges. Low staff-to-resident ratios and the absence of an on-site physician to monitor adverse drug reactions have the potential to delay identification of a medication problem.

## PAIN MANAGEMENT

The consultant neurologist is frequently asked to evaluate an elderly patient who is experiencing pain. Nonmalignant pain in the elderly patient is common but is underreported and undertreated. Pain has been erroneously considered an inevitable consequence of aging. Malignant pain caused by cancer is common but is also often undertreated because of unfounded concerns regarding possible narcotic addiction. Clinical practice guidelines for pain management are available through the Agency for Health Care Policy and Research.

## COMMON PAIN SYNDROMES

Many neurologic and non-neurologic causes of pain affect the elderly patient, including disorders of the spinal column such as cervical osteoarthritis, lumbosacral spine disease, and compression fractures associated with osteoporosis.

Headache secondary to temporal arthritis, trigeminal neuralgia, shingles and postherpetic neuralgia, and pain secondary to underlying malignancy are also common causes of pain in the geriatric patient. More common causes of pain include muscle strain and degenerative joint disease, which are both benign.

Providing effective pain management is best accomplished by identifying the specific cause of the elderly patient's symptoms. Minor analgesics such as acetaminophen or aspirin taken at the rate of 650 mg every 4 hours on a regular basis provide effective pain relief for many patients. More specific interventions such as carbamazepine administration may be required to treat neuropathic pain complicating conditions such as postherpetic neuralgia. Although amitriptyline hydrochloride is effective for the treatment of this condition compared with a placebo in double-blind trials, it has significant anticholinergic side effects and should be used with great caution, if at all, in the geriatric patient. The elderly patient may become confused or may experience side effects such as dry mouth, blurred vision, and urinary retention, even when relatively low doses are administered. Elderly men with benign prostatic hypertrophy are at particular risk for developing the latter complication. Alternative medications should be considered, such as desipramine hydrochloride, which has less tendency to cause anticholinergic drug toxicity.

Other potentially useful drugs include nonsteroidal anti-inflammatory agents, topical capsaicin, and lidocaine. Nonsteroidal anti-inflammatory drugs have significant potential for causing gastrointestinal bleeding and renal toxicity in the elderly, particularly when used on a long-term basis. Use of these helpful but potentially toxic medications in the elderly should be closely monitored, and long-term use should be avoided if possible.

Acupuncture may be of benefit for pain control, but its efficacy has not been demonstrated in controlled clinical trials. Most patients with postherpetic neuralgia eventually experience spontaneous improvement of pain. Pharmacologic management of pain should be attempted until this occurs, however. A cautious approach is advisable when initiating drug therapy in the elderly patient. Start with the lowest potentially effective dose and slowly increase over days to weeks until the desired clinical benefit is achieved.

Cutaneous varicella-zoster infection may be associated with severe burning, itching, and lancinating pain. Central nervous system invasion may occur in the elderly or immunosuppressed patient. Postherpetic neuralgia occurs with increased frequency in the elderly population, because cutaneous zoster increases with increasing age. Postherpetic neuralgia may occur in up to 50% of patients over age 60 years who have experienced cutaneous infections, compared with 15% of younger patients affected by acute cutaneous varicella-zoster infection.

Oral acyclovir is frequently used in the treatment of cutaneous zoster. Parenteral use should be avoided unless overwhelming or life-threatening infection occurs. Oral corticosteroids may reduce the duration of pain during active cutaneous varicella-zoster infection and may also reduce the risk of postherpetic neuralgia. Published reports suggest that the risks associated with corticosteroid therapy in this setting are not significant.

Acupuncture has been associated with pain relief in some patients with postherpetic neuralgia. A transcutaneous nerve stimulation unit can benefit some patients. Capsaicin cream has been associated with symptomatic improvement in patients with postherpetic neuralgia. However, localized burning and the requirement for frequent application may limit patient compliance. It is usually necessary to apply capsaicin four times daily for at least 4 weeks for maximal clinical efficacy.

Surgical procedures—including rhizotomy, neurectomy, dorsal root entry zone lesions, cordotomy, and thalamotomy—have been used in the treatment of chronic postherpetic neuralgia. Surgical interventions should be considered only for patients who have refractory and severe manifestations of postherpetic neuralgia. Surgery may be associated with significant morbidity and has unpredictable results.

## END-OF-LIFE DECISIONS

The challenging issues of withholding and withdrawing life-sustaining treatment for terminally ill patients are commonplace in clinical practice. The neurologist often plays a prominent role in helping to determine the competency of the elderly patient when critical end-of-life decisions must be made. Advance directives should address issues of withholding and withdrawing medical interventions and are designed to eliminate the confusion often associated with unexpected life-threatening events in the elderly patient. Prolonging the dying process by providing futile care should be avoided.

The neurologist may be asked to determine the integrity of central nervous system function following an acute catastrophic event, such as cardiac arrest or hypertensive intracerebral hemorrhage. Determining the level of existing brain function as it relates to the patient's short- and long-term prognosis is often key in making the decision to withhold or withdraw supportive medical therapies.

Patient autonomy should be respected when the patient's wishes are known to medical caregivers. Surrogate decision making may be necessary in the absence of explicit directives provided by the patient. Family members, as legal next of kin, usually serve as surrogates.

Intrafamily conflict can make this process more difficult. Institutional ethics committees serve a vital role in helping resolve medical-ethical dilemmas when clear indications of patient preference are not available or when family consensus is not possible.

## SUGGESTED READING

Alexander NB. Comprehensive review of gait disorders and treatment in older adults. J Am Geriatr Soc 1996;44:434–451.

Barclay L. Clinical Geriatric Neurology. Philadelphia: Lea & Febiger, 1993.

Folstein MF, Folstein SE. Neuropsychiatric Assessment of Syndromes of Altered Mental State. In WR Hazzard, et al. (eds), Principles of Geriatric Medicine and Gerontology (3rd ed). New York: McGraw-Hill, 1994.

Folstein MF, Folstein SE. Syndromes of Altered Mental State. In WR Hazzard, et al. (eds), Principles of Geriatric Medicine and Gerontology (3rd ed). New York: McGraw-Hill, 1994.

Francis J, Kapoor WN. Delirium in hospitalized elderly. J Gen Intern Med 1990;5:65–79.

Gillick M. Choosing Medical Care in Old Age: What Kind, How Much, When to Stop. Boston: Harvard University Press, 1996.

Kaye JA, Oken BS, Howieson DB, et al. Neurologic evaluation of the optimally healthy oldest old. Arch Neurol 1994;51:1205–1211.

King MB, Tinetti ME. Review of falls in community-dwelling older adults. J Am Geriatr Soc 1995;43:1146–1154.

Koller WC, et al. A description of senile gait disorders. Ann Neurol 1983;13:343–344.

Levkoff SE, Evans DA, Lipzin B, et al. Delirium: the occurrence and persistence of symptoms among elderly hospitalized patients. Arch Intern Med 1992;152:334–340.

Lipsitz L. Syncope in the elderly. Ann Intern Med 1983;99:92–105.

Lipsitz L, Pluchino FC, Wei JY, et al. Syncope in institutionalized elderly: the impact of multiple pathological conditions and situational stress. J Chronic Dis 1986;39:619–630.

Lipsitz LA, Nyquist P, Wei J, Rowe J. Postprandial reduction of blood pressure in the elderly. N Engl J Med 1983;309:81–83.

Marcantonio ER, Goldman L, Mangione CM, et al. A clinical prediction rule for delirium after elective noncardiac surgery. JAMA 1994;271:134–139.

Odenheimer G, Funkenstein HH, Beckett L, et al. Comparison of neurologic changes in successfully aging persons vs. the total aging population. Arch Neurol 1994;51:573–580.

Pompei P, Foreman M, Rudberg MA, et al. Delirium in hospitalized older persons: outcomes and predictors. J Am Geriatr Soc 1994;42:809–815.

Posiado D, Richardson S. Timed "up and go": a test of basic functional mobility for frail elderly persons. J Am Geriatr Soc 1991;39:142–148.

Resnick NM. Urinary incontinence in older adults. Hosp Pract 1992;27(10):139–150.

Resnick NM. Geriatric Medicine. In K Isselbacher, et al. (eds), Harrison's Principles of Internal Medicine (13th ed). New York: McGraw Hill, 1994.

Rubenstein LZ, Robbins AS, Josephson KR, et al. The value of assessing falls in an elderly population. Ann Intern Med 1990;113:308–316.

Sudarsky L. Etiologic Classification of Gait Disorders. In J Marsden, L Sudarsky, L Wolfson (eds), Gait Disorders of Aging. Boston: Little, Brown, 1995.

Sudarsky L. Geriatrics: gait disorders in the elderly. N Engl J Med 1990;322:1441–1446.

Tag M, Maestre G, Tsai W, et al. Relative risks of Alzheimer disease and age-at-onset distributions, based on APOE genotypes among elderly African Americans, Caucasians and Hispanics in New York City. Am J Hum Genet 1996;58:574–584.

Tinnetti ME. Factors associated with serious injury during falls by ambulatory nursing home residents. J Am Geriatr Soc 1987;35:644–648.

Tinetti ME, Speechley M, Ginter SF. Risk factors for falls among elderly persons living in the community. N Engl J Med 1988;319:1701–1707.

Tinetti ME, Williams TF, Mayewski R. Fall risk index for elderly patients based on number of chronic disabilities. Am J Med 1986;80:429–434.

# II
## Surgery

# 19
# Cardiothoracic Surgery

Jon Brillman

For neurologists at tertiary care institutions, a major source of consultation requests is the cardiothoracic service, because increasing numbers of elderly patients require invasive procedures for cardiovascular disorders. Regrettably, most of these consultations are for postoperative complications. Coronary revascularization procedures (coronary artery bypass graft [CABG]) and valve replacement surgery, commonly performed on older patients, give rise to the largest number of neurologic consultations. An estimated 500,000 cardiopulmonary bypass procedures are performed in the United States and Canada annually. Approximately 10% require the advice of a neurologist for problems that range from severe encephalopathy and stroke to traumatic neuropathies. The consulting neurologist must therefore become familiar with the risks of cardiopulmonary bypass (CPB) surgery, the particular problems associated with the bypass apparatus, the surgical maneuvers in the operating room, and problems that patients develop postoperatively. Accurate and timely consultative services for these patients assist the cardiothoracic surgeon, inform and reassure anxious families, and direct nursing care postoperatively. This chapter reflects more than 20 years of experience in examining postoperative cardiothoracic patients and highlights the major neurologic syndromes seen in this setting. In addition, circumstances in which a neurologist may be asked to render an opinion preoperatively, such as whether prophylactic endarterectomy should be performed in patients scheduled for open heart surgery, are reviewed.

## CORONARY REVASCULARIZATION PROCEDURES

The nervous system of a patient undergoing CPB procedures is exposed to unique hazards not common to other surgeries. The length of the surgery associated with bypass, aortic cross-clamping, artificial circulation and oxygenation, hypothermic cardiac arrest, hemodilution, and manipulation of the heart and aorta pose

433

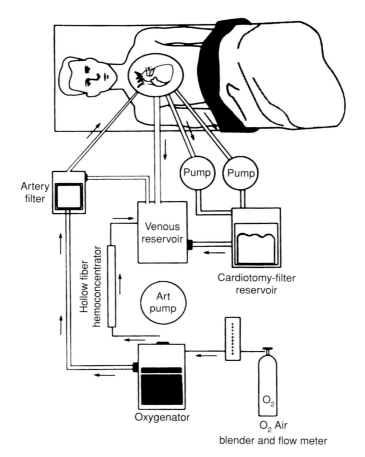

*Figure 19.1*   The basic cardiopulmonary bypass apparatus. (Reprinted with permission from PA Casthely. The Anatomy of Cardiopulmonary Bypass. In PA Casthely, D Bregman [eds], Cardiopulmonary Bypass: Physiology Related Complications and Pharmacology. Mount Kisco, NY: Futura, 1991;24.)

particular threats. Additional risks are caused by the administration of general anesthesia (fentanyl and isoflurane), which lowers cerebral blood flow already reduced with intraoperative hypothermia. Hemodilution with crystalloid prime reduces the hematocrit by 50% and may contribute to intraoperative hypotension. The transfer onto cardiopulmonary bypass alters the circulation from pulsatile to laminar flow and substitutes an altered arterial waveform that also may put the brain at risk. The consulting neurologist, therefore, should be acquainted with the series of events that transpires in the operating room so that he or she may be able to identify a possible source of the neurologic disturbance.

The basic CPB apparatus is illustrated in Figure 19.1. Deoxygenated blood is drained by gravity from the right atrium into a large reservoir, where it is diluted

*Table 19.1*  Common intraoperative events and possible adverse consequences

| Intraoperative event | Consequence |
| --- | --- |
| Induction of anesthesia (fentanyl and isoflurane) | Decreased cerebral blood flow |
| Hemodilution | Hypotension |
| On bypass | Altered arterial waveform characteristic (laminar flow) |
| Hypothermia | Decreased cerebral blood flow |
| Aortotomy and cross-clamp application | Microemboli, macroemboli |
| Cardioplegia | Microemboli (air) |
| Partial cross-clamp on or off | Microemboli |
| Elevation of heart to inspect integrity of grafts | Microemboli (air) |
| Cross-clamp off | Microemboli |
| Rewarming of patient | Hypotension |
| Bubble oxygenator[a] (if used) | Microemboli |
| pH stat[b] (if used) | Disordered autoregulation, microemboli |

[a]A type of oxygenator in which gaseous exchange takes place without a membrane.
[b]The addition of carbon dioxide during the procedure to increase cerebral blood flow.

to approximately 50% of its hematocrit value by crystalloid prime. A centrifugal or roller pump—producing laminar, nonpulsatile flow in most cases—directs the blood through the oxygenator. The blood is returned to the patient through a 25- or 40-μm arterial line filter. Oxygenated blood is then circulated through the aortotomy to the various organs. Pumps continually drain the left ventricle so the surgeon can operate in a bloodless field with a decompressed heart. Nearly all medical centers in the United States and Canada use membrane oxygenators to minimize the generation of bubbles.

Table 19.1 lists the sequence of events in CPB surgery and the altered physiology that results and may lead to neurologic complications.

When asked to see a patient postoperatively, the neurologist is likely to encounter either a stroke or what is called post-CABG encephalopathy. The incidence of the latter condition is estimated to be 5–15%; the condition carries a mortality of approximately 30%. Delayed extubation and emergence from anesthesia; small, reactive pupils; restlessness; and agitation are the clinical features of this condition. Normally, the condition tends to improve over a week's time. The neurologist should first inspect the operating room flow sheet to identify untoward events, such as intraoperative hypotension. The latter is rarely identified, however. Hypotension may occur perioperatively as a result of left ventricular failure, arrhythmia, or blood loss, but during the operation the blood pressure is controlled by the perfusionist. The pressure is normally maintained at 60–80 mm Hg (mean), but lower pressures, although rare, are well tolerated and are not normally associated with neurologic complications. Nevertheless, occasional mishaps occur that may be attributed to hemodilution with crystalloid prime, anesthesia, and warming of the hypothermic patient. Hypotension is poorly correlated with neurologic outcome. Although a decline in cerebral blood flow of about 1% per minute is expected during the procedure (Figure 19.2), cerebral autoregulation remains intact unless $CO_2$ is added (pH stat). Under this circumstance, cerebral blood flow increases but the cerebral metabolic rate

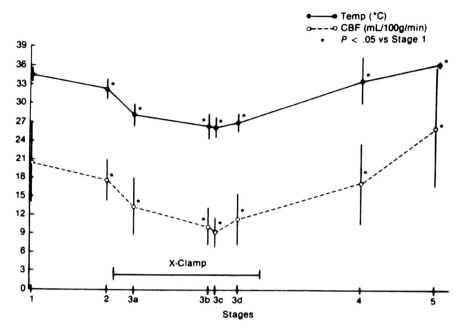

*Figure 19.2*   The changes in temperature and cerebral blood flow (CBF) during cardiopulmonary bypass surgery. Note the relationship between hypothermia and CBF. (Reprinted with permission from G Rodewald. Introduction to the Subject. In AE Willner, G Rodewald [eds], Impact of Cardiac Surgery on the Quality of Life. New York: Plenum, 1990;175.)

of oxygen remains unchanged; patient outcome has been shown to be unaffected by this maneuver.

Most feel that microemboli are a significant factor in the pathogenesis of post-CABG encephalopathy. Small-capillary arterial dilatations (Figure 19.3) have been identified in postmortem brain specimens and presumably reflect vestiges of microemboli. Numerous cerebral and retinal microemboli have been detected by transcranial Doppler ultrasonography (Figure 19.4) and fluorescein angiography during CPB surgery. A strong positive correlation exists between the number of microemboli and neurologic and neuropsychiatric complications. In addition, microemboli that result from surgical maneuvers, especially cross-clamp removal and aortotomy, are probably particulate emboli associated with neurologic and neuropsychiatric decline, whereas those that come from the CPB apparatus, which are primarily air emboli, are better tolerated by the patient. Air emboli may be related to bubble oxygenators or lack of filtration; however, membrane oxygenators and arterial line filtration are in common use in the United States.

Minor cognitive decline is also a well-recognized postoperative problem that possibly affects 60% of patients. It can be measured by neuropsychiatric testing, but it is also reported by many individuals and their families as difficulty in concentrating and remembering. Although this complication would not involve the

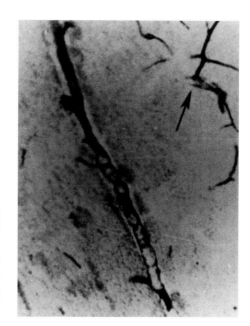

*Figure 19.3* Small-capillary arterial dilatations present in a medium-sized arteriole in a patient who underwent cardiopulmonary bypass surgery. (Note the clear swollen area and the intact vascular walls.) (Reprinted with permission from DM Moody, MA Bell, VR Challa, et al. Brain microemboli during cardiac surgery or aortography. Ann Neurol 1990;28:480.)

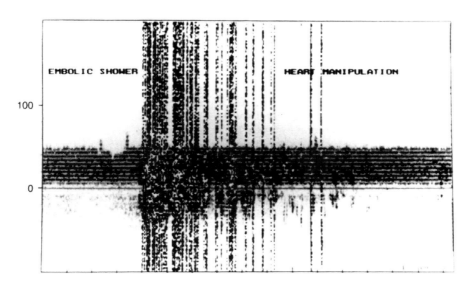

*Figure 19.4* A shower of microemboli as assessed by transcranial Doppler analysis toward the end of a coronary artery bypass graft procedure when the heart is manipulated during graft inspection.

consultant immediately, evidence exists that those patients that have neurologic complications will have cognitive disturbances many years later.

The patient with post-CABG encephalopathy must be observed carefully. Agitation should be treated with short-acting benzodiazepines; resistance to the respirator can be treated with morphine. The dose and timing of these agents must be monitored, because they contribute to encephalopathy and confound the neurologic picture. If improvement in cognitive status is not observed in 4–5 days, a more ominous prognosis is indicated.

A rare phenomenon described as hyperperfusion may occur in the initial stage of the bypass procedure. When this happens, transcranial Doppler monitoring has detected a greater than 50% increase in mean flow velocities lasting 1–2 minutes. Though the cause for this sudden occurrence of apparent dysautoregulation is unknown, it has been associated with post-CABG encephalopathy and death.

## VALVE REPAIR

Valve repair, usually aortic and mitral, may be performed as an isolated procedure or in conjunction with CABG. Because these are open-ventricle operations, additional hazards are possible, including the introduction of air into the circulation if adequate de-airing procedures and venting are not carried out. In addition, biomechanical valves, especially those placed in the aortic region, are often associated with the formation of platelet emboli. In patients with biomechanical valves, the incidence of cerebral emboli is approximately 3% per year, even when patients are given full anticoagulation with warfarin sodium (international normalized ratio of 3.5–4.5). The addition of 81 mg of aspirin per day further reduces the risk of embolic events. Bioprosthetic valves such as porcine valves are associated with a low incidence of emboli. The risk of cerebral emboli in patients with these valves is approximately 3% per year, and anticoagulant therapy is used for a short period, perhaps 3–6 months, after which the patient may take aspirin or dipyridamole (Persantine). Dipyridamole, widely recognized to be ineffective in prevention of arteriosclerotic stroke, is of value in reducing the incidence of cerebral emboli in patients with biomechanical valves.

Intraoperative transcranial Doppler ultrasound evaluation of patients undergoing valve replacement surgery shows numerous microembolic events; by far, the majority of these occur toward the end of the procedure when the heart fills with blood and begins to beat again, and the cross-clamp is removed. This finding suggests that air is trapped within the heart during open-ventricle surgery.

## STROKE

Stroke remains a devastating complication of CPB procedures and occurs in 5–10% of cases. The majority of these are territorial infarcts; however, occasionally multiple infarcts are seen in regions of the brain where borderline perfusion occurs, possibly as a result of perioperative hypotension. Approximately 20%

of strokes occur intraoperatively or in the first perioperative day; 50% occur in the second to the tenth postoperative day; and 30% occur thereafter. Late-onset strokes are most commonly associated with postoperative atrial fibrillation. The cause for post-CPB strokes is not always clear and is rarely anticipated. Carotid stenosis is a risk factor, but the incidence of postoperative stroke is only slightly greater (by 2.9%) in patients with asymptomatic carotid stenosis than in patients without carotid narrowing. In light of the Asymptomatic Carotid Artery Study data, it would seem prudent to consider carotid endarterectomy in CABG candidates if 60% or greater carotid stenosis can be identified. The proper timing of carotid endarterectomy is unknown, however. Anecdotal evidence suggests that simultaneous carotid endarterectomy and CABG surgery are dangerous, but vascular surgeons have long insisted that both operations can be done during the same period with safety. A clinical trial in progress may serve to settle this issue. At this time, waiting 4 weeks between surgeries unless the CABG procedure is an emergency is recommended. Although perioperative stroke may be caused by macroemboli from valves, hypotension, prothrombic states, and carotid disease, atheroma from the ascending aorta has emerged as a principal cause. Numerous studies have shown a correlation between atheroma in the ascending aorta and cerebral atheromatous emboli in patients undergoing open-heart surgery. Intraoperative epiaortic echocardiography or transesophageal echocardiography has been used to identify patients at risk for microemboli, and sites of aortotomy and cross-clamp placement have been changed on this basis. Several investigations have shown that aortotomy and cross-clamp application and removal are a prominent source of microemboli signals as detected by transcranial Doppler ultrasonography monitoring during surgery. With respect to prothrombic factors, thromboxane $B_2$, the stable metabolite of thromboxane $A_2$, has been shown to be transiently elevated during CPB procedures but falls to normal by the end of the operation. Other prothrombic factors have not been demonstrated to be altered during the procedures.

The cardiothoracic surgeon commonly asks the neurologist if anticoagulants should be used in patients with postoperative stroke. If a computed tomographic scan excludes hemorrhage and if the infarct promises not to be too large, anticoagulant therapy is generally recommended, because the stroke is most likely to be cardioembolic or aortogenic. If postoperative atrial fibrillation is present with or without stroke, anticoagulation with heparin sodium or warfarin sodium should be started and should be continued indefinitely until reversion to normal sinus rhythm.

Regrettably, stroke can ruin an otherwise uneventful operation. Because of generalized atherosclerosis, all patients undergoing CPB surgery are stroke prone, and those with significant carotid stenosis, aortic atheroma, atrial fibrillation, and left ventricle failure are at particular risk.

## CEREBRAL ISCHEMIC OR ANOXIC ENCEPHALOPATHY

In some circumstances the neurologist is asked to see a patient who does not awaken after surgery and in whom an episode of hypotension could be identified during the operation or the immediate postoperative period. As previously noted, intraoperative hypotension is uncommon, but in certain individuals cerebral blood

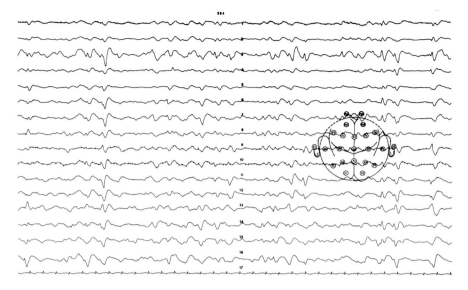

*Figure 19.5*   Burst-suppression pattern seen in a patient with severe anoxic encephalopathy.

flow could fall to critically low levels (10–15 ml/100 g/minute) if an adverse reaction to anesthesia or hemodilution occurs. Under these conditions, there is a rapid decline in peripheral vascular resistance, and the anesthesiologist may attempt to correct the problem by administering phenylephrine hydrochloride (Neo-synephrine). The hypotensive episode should be identified on the operative record. Perioperatively, hypotension may result from blood loss in the intrathoracic cavity (often undetected), hemopericardium, left ventricular failure, and atrial or ventricular arrhythmias. Occasionally, a cardiac arrest may occur requiring resuscitation and even left-ventricle-assist devices. Patients with severe anoxic or ischemic encephalopathy are ordinarily in deep coma and, unlike patients with post-CABG encephalopathy, are much more difficult to arouse. Under these circumstances, the patient often requires ventilatory assistance and may have dilated, light-fixed pupils, increased extremity tone, and bilateral Babinski's signs. Seizures may occur and are usually myoclonic, either with rhythmic jerking of the extremities or twitching of the mouth and facial muscles. These types of seizures are notoriously difficult to control and may require high dosages of phenytoin, phenobarbital, or benzodiazepines. The electroencephalogram (EEG) may show burst-suppression patterns (Figure 19.5), an ominous prognostic sign. Whether these seizures should be vigorously treated is under some debate. Ordinarily, phenytoin, 1,000 mg, is given (18 mg/kg); however, if the seizures continue, as is often the case, phenobarbital, diazepam, or lorazepam is frequently added. Unfortunately, although the seizures may frequently be controlled by the administration of these agents, they may make it difficult to accurately assess improvement in the patient's level of consciousness.

Briefer and less severe episodes of hypotension result in lighter states of coma. Here patients may seem agitated, restless, or confused. The condition commonly improves after 2 or 3 days. The EEG may be normal (alpha-theta coma) or show generalized slowing. At times, the patient may demonstrate no significant alterations in level of consciousness or cognitive function, but may show varying degrees of extremity weakness. Curiously, in many cases, the arms may be disproportionately weaker than the legs ("man-in-barrel syndrome"), most likely because of ischemia in the cortical arterial boundary zones where terminal flow is meager and where the arms are represented on the cortical surface. Patients who have disproportionate arm weakness ordinarily progress slowly and may need prolonged periods of rehabilitation, including physical and occupational therapy. The prognosis is generally favorable.

## MECHANICAL (LEFT-VENTRICULAR-ASSIST) DEVICES

Mechanical circulatory devices are occasionally used to support a failed heart until a suitable donor for cardiac transplantation may be found. These devices include centrifugal pumps, the Jarvik artificial heart, and a variety of other ventricular-assist devices. The most frequent neurologic complication of these devices relates to thromboembolism caused by promotion of prothrombic factors and platelet activation in regions of low flow, thrombogenesis in areas of recirculation, and stagnation. Poor convection occurs near device valve rings; high shear-induced platelet aggregation is also a problem. Unquestionably, altered blood flow patterns generated by these devices is the key factor in the genesis of thromboembolic complications. Rheologic factors may also be important. It has been demonstrated, for example, that the Jarvik artificial heart increases blood viscosity, as well as increasing fibrinogen concentration. Other artificial devices have also been shown to increase blood viscosity. Infection is also another possible source of thromboembolism and may form as vegetation on the valves of the artificial heart. The surfaces of the prosthetic devices and their conduits initiate and enhance coagulation through a variety of processes, including increased thrombin generation, platelet activation, reduction in protein C levels, and absorption of factor XII. One study demonstrated that nearly 50% of patients with an artificial device suffered strokes. Although anticoagulant therapy may control some of these events, its exact benefit is uncertain in this setting. Despite this fact, left-ventricular-assist devices are an important development and serve as a therapeutic bridge until donor hearts may be found.

## DISORDERS OF THE AORTA

At times, the consulting neurologist is asked to see a patient with the consequences of aortic dissection or a surgically corrected abdominal aortic aneurysm. Because patients with dissections of the ascending or thoracic aorta most commonly present with chest pain or hemorrhagic shock, the neurologist may become involved only when the dissection occurs between the intima and the media, disrupting the ostia of the innominate, carotid, or vertebral arteries, and the patient presents with a stroke. Neurologic complications resulting from dissection of this portion of the aorta occur at a rate of approximately 20–30%. In the hospital setting, it is much more common to see a patient who is paraplegic or paraparetic following surgery for an unruptured abdominal aortic aneurysm. The cervical spinal cord is amply supplied with collateral arterial feeders and is relatively resistant to ischemia, but the thoracic and lumbar segments are less well endowed. The anterior spinal artery and the paired posterior spinal arteries supply the substance of the cord and have an anastomotic ring that is supplemented by radiculomedullary branches of the segmental arteries from the aorta. The great anastomotic artery of Adamkiewicz is a key collateral in the blood supply of the lower thoracolumbar spinal cord. It most commonly arises from T9 through T12 on the left side and also contributes to the anastomotic ring encircling the conus medullaris, which is supported by the lumbar and iliolumbar arteries from the external iliac artery. Most vascular insults to the spinal cord are anterior spinal artery syndromes. These conditions present with an initially flaccid paraplegia or paraparesis, Babinski's sign, and a loss of pain and temperature sensation below the lesion with preservation of joint-position sense. Vascular lesions confined to the posterior one-third of the cord do not exist. Many patients have complete loss of all motor and sensory function below the ischemic lesion, which results from intraoperative hypotension or ischemic interruption of the radiculomedullary arteries in the suprarenal aorta by crossclamping and surgical sacrifice or interruption of the anastomotic artery of Adamkiewicz in the infrarenal aorta. Regrettably, the incidence of paraplegia or paraparesis following aneurysmectomy has been reported at 15%. It is particularly disheartening to have successful surgery for potentially life-threatening aneurysm result in what is generally an irreversible paraparesis or paraplegia. It has been suggested that postoperative paraplegia can be minimized if spinal fluid drainage is carried out or if the great radicular artery of Adamkiewicz is identified and revascularized at the time of surgery. Little evidence exists to confirm this view, and most centers do not conduct the neuroradiographic procedures required to identify the presence of this artery. Intraoperative somatosensory evoked potentials are measured in some centers to ascertain when the surgeon may be rendering the spinal cord ischemic, but this monitoring technique has not improved outcome overall. Occasionally, when paraparesis occurs it is unclear whether the ischemic insult is to the spinal cord, lumbar roots, or peripheral nerves. In the latter case, which is actually more common than myelopathy, the patient has a cold extremity with weakness and loss of deep tendon reflexes. An ischemic monomelic neuropathy may occur if occlusion of the proximal arteries occurs near the aorta. Asymmetry of findings may help distinguish ischemic radiculopathy from myelopathy. Hematoma formation in the retroperitoneal space may compress the femoral, sciatic, and obturator nerves, and the clinical syndromes therefore are confined to the distribution of these nerves.

The prognosis for patients with ischemic myelopathy is poor, and, if paraplegia occurs, improvement is not likely. High dosages of corticosteroids as well as hyperbaric oxygenation may be used, but these therapeutic measures have done little to improve the outcome. The prognosis for patients with ischemic neuropathy is more favorable, with a gradual improvement expected in some cases over time.

## CARDIAC TRANSPLANTATION

When the cardiothoracic service performs cardiac transplantation, a neurology consultation is likely requested because neurologic complications occur in 50–60% of transplant patients. Apart from the intraoperative complications of thromboembolism and encephalopathy similar to those seen in valve surgery or CABG procedures, long-term complications from immunosuppression and the use of immunosuppressive drugs, as discussed in Chapter 20, may occur.

## PERIPHERAL NERVOUS SYSTEM COMPLICATIONS OF CARDIOPULMONARY BYPASS PROCEDURES

Generally, several days pass after CPB procedures before a consultation is requested for peripheral nerve damage. Fortunately, most of the neuropathies and plexopathies that result from such surgical procedures are transient and reversible. The most common peripheral neurologic injury reported in cardiopulmonary bypass procedures is brachial plexus damage. In most cases, the lower trunk or medial cord fibers are involved, as confirmed by clinical and electrodiagnostic evaluation. The injury has been reported to be attributable either to traumatic cannulation of the internal jugular vein on the side of the injury or to excessive traction on the brachial plexus following sternotomy with fracture of the first cervical rib. Ulnar neuropathies, usually reversible after 4–6 weeks, are fairly common and result from compression of the nerve at the elbow, particularly during prolonged procedures. Peroneal neuropathies as well as saphenous neuropathies have also been reported and are a result either of direct compression of the peroneal nerve around the fibular head or of stretching of the saphenous nerve. The extent to which hypothermia renders the peripheral nervous system susceptible to damage during these procedures is conjectural, but both axonal degeneration and myelin breakdown may occur during exposure to extreme cold.

An additional problem involving the peripheral nervous system that has more serious consequences is hemidiaphragmatic paralysis resulting from phrenic nerve injury. Such injury results from exposure of the phrenic nerve to the topical ice-saline slush that is commonly used to maintain cardiac hypothermia during cardioplegic arrest. In one study series, 54% of patients undergoing CABG surgery exhibited abnormal diaphragmatic motion. Postoperatively, phrenic nerve conduction studies demonstrated a high percentage of abnormalities ipsilaterally. Although some degree of diaphragmatic paresis may persist in up to one-fourth of the patients in such cases, it appears to have little morbidity, although prolonged hospital stays have been noted in individuals with phrenic nerve injuries. Care to insulate the nerve during these procedures may limit damage to the phrenic nerve.

Unilateral Horner's syndrome has been described following CABG surgery and occurs in approximately 8% of cases. The condition disappears in 6 months in most patients, although it may persist indefinitely in some.

## CAROTID ENDARTERECTOMY

In many institutions, cardiothoracic surgeons perform carotid endarterectomies. Occasionally, neurologists may be asked to give advice concerning the appropriateness of performing carotid endarterectomy before CABG procedures or in patients with isolated carotid stenosis. Most vascular surgeons are familiar with the well-established criteria regarding the use of carotid endarterectomy for high-grade symptomatic carotid stenosis as issued by the North American Symptomatic Carotid Endarterectomy Trial (NASCET); however, the criteria for surgical intervention for asymptomatic carotid stenosis are less clear. The Veterans Administration trial and Asymptomatic Carotid Artery Study have demonstrated that surgical intervention may be appropriate in certain patients with asymptomatic carotid disease. The data in these studies that favor surgical intervention do not, however, carry the statistical certitude demonstrated in the NASCET study. Accordingly, some patients with asymptomatic carotid stenosis have surgery and others do not. Evidence exists, however, that the appearance of progressive stenosis on successive Doppler ultrasonography examinations indicates an increased risk factor for stroke and may tip the balance toward surgical intervention.

Because a small (2–3%) but definite risk of stroke exists in patients with asymptomatic carotid stenosis who undergo cardiopulmonary bypass procedures, prophylactic carotid endarterectomy should be performed before open-heart operations if the arterial narrowing is greater than 60%. The best timing for this procedure is yet to be determined. The consulting neurologist may also be asked about the best method to determine cerebral function intraoperatively. Many surgeons still perform carotid endarterectomy under local anesthesia, in which case the patient's clinical condition may be directly monitored. Surgeons who use general anesthesia may wish to monitor their patients with either EEG or transcranial Doppler sonography. In the former case, cerebroprotective barbiturates may be used that produce burst-suppression patterns. A focal isoelectric EEG implies ischemic brain injury. When transcranial Doppler sonography is used, a 2-MHz probe is fixed over the appropriate temporal window throughout the procedure. Both mean flow velocities and microembolic events are monitored, and adverse outcomes have been well correlated with increased numbers of microembolic counts as revealed by transcranial Doppler sonography. Surgical maneuvers (such as shunt placement) may be altered if the ultrasonographer detects increased numbers of microembolic events.

Postoperatively, the major risks of carotid endarterectomy are stroke, myocardial infarction, and death. Appropriately selected patients who are operated on by qualified surgeons should have a combined morbidity and mortality of less than 3% in most circumstances. Minor complications of the procedure should also be recognized by the neurologist. Among these are local bleeding with compressive hematoma, wound infection, and cranial nerve palsies, including temporary tongue weakness with deviations on the side of the surgery resulting from trauma to the ansa hypoglossus and temporary numbness of the face and neck. Cerebral hemorrhage may also occur postoperatively as a result of hyperperfusion or hypertension. Careful follow-up of blood pressure is important, because postoperative severe hypertension may occur as a result of damage to the baroreceptor reflex in the carotid sinus. Occasionally focal brain edema may also occur as a result of hyperperfusion and must be treated aggressively with antiedemic agents and occasionally internal decompressive surgery. Immediate postoperative stroke occurs occasionally as a result of local thrombus formation. Under these circumstances, the vascular surgeon frequently inspects the site of surgery for thrombus formation.

## SUGGESTED READING

Barbut D, Giold JP, Heinemann MH, et al. Horner's syndrome after coronary artery bypass surgery. Neurology 1996;19:181.

Berger MP, Tegeler CH. Transcranial Doppler Detection of Emboli. In V Babikian, L Weschler (eds), Transcranial Doppler Ultrasonography: Clinical and Research Application. St. Louis: Mosby–Year Book, 1993;232.

Blauth CI, Arnold JV, Schulenberg WE, et al. Cerebral microembolism during cardiopulmonary bypass: retinal microvascular studies in vivo with fluorescein angiography. J Thorac Cardiovasc Surg 1988;95:558.

Brillman J. CNS complications of coronary artery bypass surgery. Neurocardiology 1993;11:474.

Clark RE, Brillman J, Davis DA. Microemboli during CABG: genesis and effect on outcome. J Thorac Cardiovasc Surg 1995;109:249.

Coffey CE, Massey EW, Roberts KB, et al. Natural history of cerebral complications of coronary artery bypass graft surgery. Neurology 1983;33:1416.

DeVita MA, Robinson LR, Rehder J, et al. Incidence and natural history of phrenic neuropathy occurring during open heart surgery. Chest 1993;103:850.

Eidelman BH, Obrist WD, Wagner WR, et al. Cerebrovascular complications associated with the use of artificial circulatory support services. Neurol Clin 1993;11:463.

Gilman S. Neurological complications of open heart surgery. Ann Neurol 1990;28:475.

Hanson MR, Bever AC, Furian AJ, et al. Mechanism and frequency of brachial plexus injury in open-heart surgery: a prospective analysis. Ann Thorac Surg 1983;36:675.

Harris DNF, Bailey SM, Smith PLC, et al. Brain swelling in first hour after coronary artery bypass surgery. Lancet 1993;342:586.

Hise JH, Nipper ML, Schmitker JC. Stroke associated with coronary artery bypass surgery. Am J Neuroradiol 1991;12:811.

Lederman RJ, Brever AC, Hanson MR, et al. Peripheral nervous system complications of coronary artery bypass graft surgery. Ann Neurol 1982;12:297.

Lynch DR, Dawson TM, Raps EC, Galetta SL. Risk factors for the neurologic complications associated with aortic aneurysms. Arch Neurol 1992;49:284.

Moody DM, Bell MA, Challa VR, et al. Brain microemboli during cardiac surgery or aortography. Ann Neurol 1990;28:477.

Pedrini L, Paragona O, Pisano E, et al. Morbidity and mortality following carotid surgery. J Cardiovasc Surg 1991;32:720.

Reed GL, Singer DE, Picard EH, DeSanctis RW. Stroke following coronary artery bypass surgery. N Engl J Med 1988;319:1246.

Wareing TH, Davila-Roman VG, Brazilai B, et al. Management of the severely atherosclerotic ascending aorta during cardiac operations: a strategy for detection and treatment. J Thorac Cardiovasc Surg 1992;103:453.

Willner AE, Rodewald G. Impact of Cardiac Surgery on the Quality of Life: Neurologic and Psychological Aspects. New York: Plenum, 1990.

# 20
# Neurologic Complications of Organ Transplantation

Martin A. Samuels and Roy A. Patchell

Organ transplantation, begun in the mid–twentieth century with renal transplantation, is one of the greatest advances in medicine. Considerable advances in immunology have allowed longer survival for transplant recipients, but because of this longer survival time, a number of neurologic problems have emerged in these patients.

Three types of transplants exist: syngenic transplants (between identical twins), allogenic transplants (between persons of different genetic origins), and autologous transplants (with the patient's own tissue). When a new organ is implanted in place of an old one (e.g., in liver transplantation), the transplant is said to be *orthotopic*. In most cases, the transplants are allogenic, and therefore the recipients require some form of lifelong immunosuppressive therapy to prevent rejection. The neurologic complications of organ transplantation may be divided into two major categories: (1) those common to all allogenic transplants, resulting primarily from the effect of long-term immunosuppression, and (2) those specific to particular transplant procedures, resulting either from the underlying disease that leads to the need for the transplant or from some phenomenon that is peculiar to the specific transplantation technique.

## NEUROLOGIC COMPLICATION RESULTING FROM LONG-TERM EFFECTS OF IMMUNOSUPPRESSIVE DRUGS

*Cyclosporine*, the drug most commonly used to prevent rejection, works by inhibiting lymphokine release. Its major toxicity is renal. The hypertension that almost always complicates cyclosporine use is the result in part of renal toxicity, but results to a larger extent from the tendency of cyclosporine to stimulate the sympathetic nervous system by an unknown mechanism. Most, if not all, of its neurologic toxicity results from its tendency to produce hypertension. The encephalopathy of cyclosporine toxicity is roughly correlated with blood levels (the therapeutic level is 250–500 ng/ml of whole blood or 50–300 ng/ml

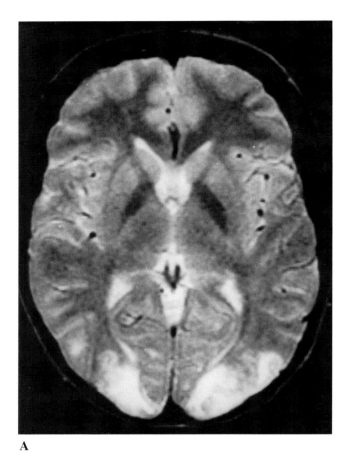

**A**

*Figure 20.1*   (**A**) Magnetic resonance image (MRI) of a patient with cyclosporine toxicity shows T2-bright areas in the parieto-occipital junction representing water leakage through poorly autoregulated cerebral vessels. (**B**) MRI taken after patient was treated with magnesium sulfate and cyclosporine shows resolution of the abnormality in just 3 hours.

of plasma), but it is more strongly correlated with the rate of change in blood pressure from the patient's baseline level. Cyclosporine neurotoxicity may be thought of as a *forme fruste* of hypertensive encephalopathy. It is characterized by tremor, abnormalities in mental state ranging from mild inattention to coma, seizures, and various visual syndromes characteristic of dysautoregulation in the posterior circulation distal arterial territories. These include visual hallucinations, visual field deficits, visual agnosias, Balint's syndrome (i.e., the triad of simultanagnosia, abnormalities in visually directed reaching, and difficulties with voluntary eye movements), and cortical blindness with denial of deficit (i.e., Anton's syndrome). Magnetic resonance imaging (MRI) shows increased signal on T2-weighted images in the occipital white matter, a finding that may be quite evanescent and does not represent stroke (Figure 20.1). Flow studies such as single photon emis-

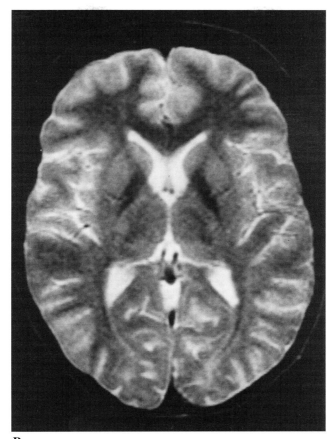

**B**

sion computed tomography demonstrate that this finding is a result of increased flow with extravasation of water. These findings are identical to those seen in patients with hypertensive encephalopathy, including the syndrome of toxemia of pregnancy. It should be emphasized that the patient's blood pressure need not be very high (i.e., in the range of malignant hypertension) for this syndrome to occur. The pathogenesis appears to be related to the rate of change of blood pressure combined with loss of cerebral autoregulation rather than to the absolute level of blood pressure. Lowering the blood pressure by any means, such as (but not limited to) decreasing the blood level of cyclosporine, will result in resolution of the clinical syndrome and the imaging abnormalities.

*FK 506* is a newer antirejection drug that works by a mechanism similar to cyclosporine. Although experience with this drug is limited, the range of side effects seems identical to that for cyclosporine and is probably due to the same effects on blood pressure.

*OKT3* is a monoclonal antibody directed against T cells. Its major neurologic side effect is aseptic meningitis, which occurs in about 1 in 20 patients during the first 3 days of exposure to the drug. Cerebrospinal fluid analysis shows a lymphocytic pleocytosis with normal glucose and normal or slightly elevated protein. The syndrome is self-limiting and benign; however, the clinician should be certain to perform a lumbar puncture and culture the spinal fluid to exclude a bacterial or fungal meningitis before settling on the more benign diagnosis of OKT3-induced aseptic meningitis. The mechanism of the meningeal inflammation is probably an allergic response similar to that seen in some patients placed on nonsteroidal anti-inflammatory drugs such as ibuprofen or treated with intravenous immunoglobulin. The ibuprofen syndrome appears to be more common in patients with rheumatic diseases such as systemic lupus erythematosus. Whether the same is also true for meningitis induced by intravenous immunoglobulin and OKT3 is still unknown. A more severe syndrome characterized by variable degrees of mental status derangement, including seizures, may occur very rarely. It is associated with evidence of cerebral edema on neuroimages, but it is also self-limiting and benign, even if the OKT3 is continued. The long-term serious side effect of OKT3 use is the development of lymphoma, which appears to be dosage related.

*Antithymocyte globuli* and *antilymphoblast globulin* are antisera directed against thymocytes or lymphocytes. Rarely, patients on these drugs develop an aseptic meningitis similar to that seen with OKT3. It is also self-limiting and benign in nature.

*Corticosteroids*, the immunosuppressive drugs longest in use, are less specific in their actions than the agents listed above. Neurologic complications include psychosis and mania, a proximal myopathy, and, rarely, spinal cord compression resulting from epidural lipomatosis. Long-term use of steroids also predisposes to glucose intolerance, gastrointestinal bleeding, and osteoporosis, all of which have their own secondary neurologic effects.

*Neurologic infections* occur in about 10% of all transplant recipients but are more important clinically than this number suggests, because about one-half of the central nervous system infections that occur in immunocompromised patients result in death. Nearly every conceivable organism has been reported to infect transplant recipients, but about 80% of the cases are a result of infection with *Listeria monocytogenes*, *Cryptococcus neoformans*, or *Aspergillus fumigatus*. Central nervous system infections in immunocompromised hosts may be difficult to recognize, because the usual signs of infection, such as fever and meningismus, depend in part on a vigorous immune response to the infection and may be minimally present or absent in such patients. Because the usual signs of central nervous system infection may be absent, and because nearly any organism (bacterium, fungus, parasite, or virus) may be responsible, the clinician should have a high index of suspicion for infectious causes of neurologic deterioration in any transplant recipient. A few clues may be of help in determining the likely predominant organism.

An infection outside the nervous system should alert the clinician to a possible neurologic infection. Skin lesions may be found to harbor *Cryptococcus* and lung infection suggests *Aspergillus*, *Nocardia*, or *Cryptococcus*.

Acute meningitis is often caused by *Listeria monocytogenes,* whereas chronic meningitis, often with cranial nerve palsies, suggests *Mycobacterium tuberculosis* or fungal organisms. A progressive multifocal syndrome with hemiparesis, visual symptoms, ataxia, dysarthria, and dementia should raise the specter of progressive multifocal leukoencephalopathy caused by the JC polyomavirus. A localized mass lesion (e.g., a brain abscess) is often caused by multiple organisms, including anaerobes, but the predominant organism in the immunocompromised patient is usually *Aspergillus, Nocardia,* or *Toxoplasma.*

Another clue to the causative organism comes from the time after transplantation at which the infection occurs. In the early period (i.e., up to 1 month) infections are caused by organisms common in the nonimmunocompromised patient. In the intermediate period (i.e., between 1 and 6 months post-transplantation), the risk of neurologic infection peaks, and infection is usually caused by either a virus (e.g., cytomegalovirus, Epstein-Barr virus) or opportunistic bacteria and fungi (e.g., *Listeria, Aspergillus,* and *Nocardia*). Late infections (i.e., more than 6 months post-transplantation) are related to the chronic use of potent antirejection medications such as steroids, monoclonal antibodies, and cyclosporine. The most common organisms are *Cryptococcus, Listeria,* and *Nocardia.*

Lymphoproliferative syndromes occur after prolonged immunosuppression and range from apparently benign polyclonal lymphoid hyperplasia to monoclonal lymphoma. The nervous system is involved in about 20% of patients with such conditions. When the central nervous system is involved, it is the only apparent site of involvement 85% of the time. Post-transplant lymphoproliferative syndromes are strongly associated with Epstein-Barr virus infection, whereas primary central nervous system lymphomas in immunocompetent people are not associated with Epstein-Barr virus infection. These B cell lymphomas arise deep in the brain and have a propensity for the perivascular spaces. Central nervous system lymphoma is distinguished from progressive multifocal leukoencephalopathy by the fact that the former produces mass effect and shows enhancement with gadolinium in MRI scans.

## NEUROLOGIC COMPLICATIONS ASSOCIATED WITH SPECIFIC TRANSPLANT TYPES

*Renal transplantation* is most often performed in patients with glomerulonephritis (membranous or membranoproliferative), diabetes mellitus, and hypertensive renal disease. Other underlying diseases include polycystic kidney disease, systemic lupus erythematosus, amyloidosis, analgesic nephropathy, and obstructive nephropathy.

Most of the neurologic complications of renal transplantation are a result of the underlying disease for which the transplant was performed. For example, polycystic kidney disease may be associated with multiple cerebral berry aneurysms; hypertension, with ischemic and hemorrhagic stroke; systemic lupus erythematosus, with antineuronal antibodies and mental state changes; and uremic encephalopathy, with hepatorenal syndrome. Rapid correction of hyponatremia may lead to central pontine myelinolysis, a syndrome that can range in severity from mild tetraparesis to deep coma or even death and can now be easily demonstrated in the pons or extrapontine sites by MRI.

The renal transplantation procedure itself is the oldest of all the organ transplant procedures and now rarely causes any neurologic problems. Occasionally, peripheral nerve injuries (e.g., to the lateral femoral cutaneous nerve of the thigh) may be caused by retractors or patient positioning during the surgical procedure, but these are usually reversible without specific treatment.

The most common post–renal transplantation neurologic complication is stroke caused by underlying cerebrovascular or cardiac disease. Such stroke is related to the risk factors of hypertension and diabetes that are so often present in renal transplant recipients.

*Bone marrow transplants* are performed for two major indications: (1) The bone marrow is abnormal or absent (as in aplastic anemia; genetic diseases such as lysosomal storage diseases or thalassemia major; acute leukemia, such as acute myelocytic, acute lymphoblastic, or chronic lymphocytic leukemia; or combined immunodeficiency disease), and (2) hazard to the marrow is the limiting factor in aggressive treatment of a disease (as in lymphoma, solid-tumor autologous marrow programs for breast cancer, glioblastoma multiforme, and neuroblastoma).

Neurologic complications occur in about 70% of bone marrow transplant recipients and are the cause of death in 6%. The most common problem is metabolic encephalopathy caused by respiratory failure, hepatic failure, electrolyte disorders, or renal failure. The drugs used to prepare patients for the transplantation—including intrathecal methotrexate sodium, busulfan, cyclophosphamide, and adriamycin—may also contribute to the metabolic encephalopathy. Total-body irradiation is often used (2,000 cGy or less), which can lead to long-term cognitive dysfunction, particularly in children.

Graft-versus-host disease (GVHD) occurs in about one-third of HLA-matched and two-thirds of HLA-mismatched transplants. Acute GVHD, which occurs within 3 months of transplantation, consists of rash, diarrhea, and hepatic dysfunction, but no neurologic complications have been reported. Chronic GVHD occurs in about one-third of patients who survive more than 3 months after transplantation. It may have an autoimmune pathogenesis and has been associated with polymyositis, myasthenia gravis, and chronic inflammatory demyelinating neuropathy.

A leukoencephalopathy occurs in bone marrow transplant recipients who have been treated with methotrexate sodium and total-body irradiation. It appears that high-dose intravenous or intrathecal methotrexate sodium must be combined with radiation therapy to produce the leukoencephalopathy. Hemorrhages are usually related to severe thrombocytopenia (i.e., platelet count of fewer than 20,000/mm$^3$). Cerebral infarcts are largely caused by emboli from endocarditis, either infective endocarditis or nonbacterial thrombotic endocarditis, which can occur as part of a generalized hypercoagulable state in bone marrow transplant recipients.

*Cardiac transplantation* is used to treat patients with medically intractable dilated, hypertrophic, restrictive, and ischemic cardiomyopathies as well as some patients with rheumatic heart disease. Neurologic complications are very common, occurring in 50–60% of patients. The cardiac transplantation procedure is associated with variable periods of extracorporeal circulation, which may result in diffuse hypoxic-ischemic injury or focal cerebral infarction related to thromboembolism or air embolism. Damage to the brachial plexus is also commonly seen as a result of retraction of the chest wall, and the phrenic nerve may be damaged when the heart is packed in ice during the procedure.

*Liver transplantation* is used to treat chronic advanced liver disease (e.g., cholestatic diseases such as primary biliary cirrhosis and sclerosing cholangitis; hepatocellular diseases such as alcohol-induced disease or viral hepatitis; and vascular diseases such as Budd-Chiari syndrome), hepatic malignancies (e.g., hepatoma, cholangiocarcinoma, and isolated hepatic metastasis such as may be seen in carcinoid), fulminant hepatic failure (e.g., caused by viral hepatitis or liver damage induced by halothane or gold), and metabolic liver diseases (e.g., alpha$_1$-antitrypsin deficiency, Wilson's disease, glycogen storage disease type I and type II, and protoporphyria).

Many neurologic complications are related to the underlying liver disease. Most patients have some degree of portosystemic encephalopathy. In patients with Wilson's disease or acquired hepatocerebral degeneration, the neurologic syndrome is usually dramatic and consists of dysarthria, movement disorder, dementia, and spasticity.

The transplantation procedure is particularly traumatic and is often associated with a great deal of blood loss that requires aggressive replacement of blood product and fluid. Hypotension is common and often results in some degree of hypoxic-ischemic cerebral damage. Coagulation is frequently defective, a state that can lead to cerebral hemorrhages, and intraoperative cerebral infarctions may occur as a result of air or arterial embolism. Central pontine myelinolysis is particularly common in liver transplant patients and probably occurs in approximately 10% of cases. This occurrence is probably related to the fact that fluid and blood replacement often results in a rapid rise in serum sodium concentration, the presumed cause of central pontine myelinolysis.

*Pancreas transplantation* is used to treat patients with type I diabetes who have severe end-organ damage. Often, it is done in conjunction with renal transplantation, with the aim of making the patient insulin independent and reversing some of the end-organ damage. Neurologic complications are very common and occur in perhaps as many as two-thirds of patients. Much of the neurologic difficulty is related to the fact that all pancreas transplant recipients have retinopathy and neuropathy at the time of the transplantation. In addition, nearly all patients have cerebrovascular disease related to the premature atherosclerosis associated with type I diabetes. The procedure involves either transplanting the whole pancreas into the abdomen or transplanting free islet cells. The former procedure is thus by far the most successful in correcting the diabetes and reversing or retarding damage to end organs. No unique neurologic complications are caused by the procedure itself.

Because *lung transplantation* is a relatively new procedure, experience with neurologic complications is limited. Single- and double-lung transplantation as well as combined heart-lung transplantation are now being performed in specialized centers. No specific neurologic complications have been identified, although the usual neurologic effects of metabolic encephalopathy are particularly common in patients undergoing these very complex procedures.

## SUGGESTED READING

Adams HP, Dawson G, Coffman TJ, Corry MD. Stroke in renal transplant recipients. Arch Neurol 1986;43:113–115.
Estol CJ, Pessin MS, Martinez AJ. Cerebrovascular complications after orthotopic liver transplantation. Neurology 1991;41:815–819.
Hotson JR, Pedley T. The neurological complications of cardiac transplantation. Brain 1976;99:673–694.

Lacomis D, Samuels MA. Adverse neurologic effects of glucocorticosteroids. J Gen Intern Med 1991;6:367–377.

Openshaw H, Slatkin NE. Differential diagnosis of neurological complications in bone marrow transplantation. Neurologist 1995;1:191–206.

Patchell RA. Neurological complications of organ transplantation. Ann Neurol 1994;36:688–703.

Patchell RA, White CL, Clark AW, et al. Neurologic complications of bone marrow transplantation. Neurology 1985;35:300–306.

Samuels MA, Patchell RA. The Neurologic Complications of Organ Transplantation. In MA Samuels, S Feske (eds), Office Practice of Neurology. New York: Churchill Livingstone, 1996.

Textor SC, Canzanello VJ, Taler SJ, et al. Cyclosporine-induced hypertension after transplantation. Mayo Clin Proc 1994;69:1182–1193.

Vogt DP, Lederman RJ, Carey WD, Broughan TA. Neurologic complication of liver transplantation. Transplantation 1988;45:1057–1061.

# 21
## Consultations in the Operating Room and for Pain Management
Lawrence Rodichok and Garfield B. Russell

### INTRAOPERATIVE NEUROPHYSIOLOGIC MONITORING

#### General Principles

Monitoring one or more neurophysiologic parameters during a surgical procedure can serve one or more purposes, as follows:

1. Protection of the nervous system from injury
2. Identification of systemic changes such as hypoxia or hypotension that might have a global effect on the nervous system
3. Identification of the location of a lesion along the course of a tract or nerve
4. Identification of neural tissue
5. Anatomic localization

The success of intraoperative neurophysiologic monitoring (IONPM) is dependent on the selection of the appropriate pathway(s) to be monitored. Many false-negatives in monitoring are in reality not failures of monitoring but rather failures to monitor. It is the responsibility of the consulting neurophysiologist to advise the surgeon as to the most reliable technique to accomplish the desired goal. Sometimes the technical aspects of the surgery do not permit the use of the ideal neurophysiologic technique, and a compromise is necessary. This interaction with the surgeon should be included in the monitoring record. Some institutions may also play a role in the imposition of neurophysiologic monitoring, because they share in the medical and legal risks. The neurophysiologic consultant should be familiar with institutional and regional standards of care as they apply to the surgical procedure being monitored. Several textbooks can serve as useful guides to IONPM [1–3].

IONPM presupposes that a change in the physiologic parameter being monitored can be recognized soon enough to permit a reversal of the injury. Several time delays are inherent in this process, which must be kept to a minimum when possible. For example, one must use the minimum time possible to acquire evoked potentials so that frequent updates can be viewed. When changes in the neuro-physiologic signal are seen, one must be prepared to eliminate any possible technical factors quickly. In some instances, the anesthesiologist plays a critical role in maintaining a stable physiologic state, especially during critical stages of the procedure. IONPM cannot be successful without a good working relationship with the anesthesiologist, who should be familiar with the techniques being employed.

In general, the mechanisms of injury in the operating room (OR) are as follows:

1. Mechanical compression or stretching by instruments such as retractors
2. Interruption of the blood supply by compression or ligation
3. Excessive application of heat, such as from a laser or Bovie coagulator

## Personnel and Equipment

Requests for neurologic consultation in the OR are likely to be for the purpose of providing neurophysiologic monitoring during a surgical procedure. Many neurologists are not familiar with this relatively new field. At various centers this expertise may be provided by anesthesiologists or doctoral neurophysiologists. Proper intraoperative monitoring demands the supervision of a trained neurophysiologist (MD, PhD, or DO) with special expertise in the neurophysiologic techniques employed and their unique application to the OR setting. This expertise should include experience with the surgical procedures to be monitored, so that the appropriate physiologic parameters can be chosen for that particular case. The monitoring physician must also be aware of the critical parts of the surgery when the nervous system is most vulnerable. In general, proper IONPM requires that the physician be physically present in the OR during the surgery. In some instances, monitoring from a remote location by means of computer or video link may be acceptable. Such monitoring is not a substitute for prior experience in the OR itself. If remote monitoring is attempted, the physician must be available to come to the OR at a moment's notice. A neurologist who agrees to provide intraoperative neurophysiologic monitoring must be aware of the exceptional level of medical and legal exposure involved. Although the incidence of serious postoperative deficit is not high, the gravity of any deficit—for example, paraplegia after spine surgery or stroke after endarterectomy—is such that a lawsuit is very possible and any potential judgment will be very damaging financially. Almost equally critical is that the surgeon be familiar with the techniques being used. False expectations on the part of the surgeon can render monitoring useless, if not dangerous, to the patient and physicians involved.

The monitoring team generally includes a technologist. Like the physician/neurophysiologist, this individual must have extensive experience in electroencephalography (EEG) and measurement of evoked potentials. Such a technologist must also have special expertise and experience in the OR. The American Board of Registration in Electroneurodiagnostic Technology offers an examination in this field.

The equipment used for IONPM must also be appropriate for the OR. It should incorporate special safety standards as well as a number of modifications required for the continuous display of data. For example, some instruments are capable of multimodal acquisition, such as collecting free-running electromyographic

(EMG) data in some channels at the same time that evoked responses are acquired in others. Such multimodal acquisition can be very advantageous in the OR. It cannot be assumed that equipment used in the diagnostic laboratory can be used for intraoperative monitoring as well.

## Anesthesia-Related Considerations

Normal neurophysiologic responses form the basis of much of neuroanesthesia. Normal cerebral function is dependent on adequate cerebral blood flow (CBF) and energy substrate delivery. Maintenance of normal cerebral perfusion pressure—the difference between mean arterial pressure (MAP) and intracranial pressure (ICP)—is vital here. ICP depends on a balance between intracranial tissue mass, blood volume, and cerebral spinal fluid volume. CBF is maintained in the normal range of 50–60 ml/100 g per minute by autoregulatory mechanisms. That is, CBF is normally unchanged at MAP values of 50–150 mm Hg and at arterial oxygen partial pressures of 50–300 mm Hg, but it correlates positively with carbon dioxide partial pressure ($pCO_2$). This relationship allows ICP to increase or decrease as a patient's $pCO_2$ increases or decreases, respectively, in direct relation to changes in CBF. This relationship is obviously also manipulated therapeutically.

CBF and cerebral metabolism (represented by consumption of oxygen and glucose) are normally coupled; CBF increases or decreases in response to metabolic demands. This relationship can be pharmacologically uncoupled by anesthetic agents, however, or pathologically uncoupled by disorders such as tumors or intracerebral or subarachnoid hemorrhages.

### Cerebral Function and Anesthetic Agents

Whether a specific anesthetic agent is chosen for a particular patient because of its effect on CBF, its associated hemodynamic stability, or its speed of onset, cerebral metabolism is altered. Anesthetic agents depress metabolism through inhibition of the synthesis of transmitter substances (acetylcholine, catecholamines), inhibition of glycolysis, and changes in citric-acid-cycle intermediates and amino acids [4]. There is not always coupling between the anesthetic state and cerebral metabolism, however, let alone between metabolism and CBF.

### Volatile Anesthetics

The halogenated anesthetic gases produce a dose-related depression of cerebral metabolism [5]. At the same time, CBF increases, uncoupling flow and metabolism. Cerebral metabolism is reduced more by isoflurane and enflurane than by halothane at the minimum alveolar concentration (MAC) preventing movement to skin incision, which is approximately 45%, 50%, and 30%, respectively, for the three gases. The maximum metabolic suppression by isoflurane occurs with EEG isoelectricity at about 2 MAC. Enflurane increases metabolism about 50% or more when seizures are induced at high concentrations during hypocapnia. Three percent enflurane reduces metabolism 50%, but the onset of seizure activity returns it to baseline. Halothane decreases metabolism globally. Isoflurane produces a more regional effect, with less reduction within the cerebral subcortex than within the neocortex.

The halogenated ethers sevoflurane and desflurane have cerebral metabolic rate (CMR) depressant effects similar to those of isoflurane [6]. At 0.5–2.0 MAC, desflurane can decrease metabolism approximately 20%. This decrease is similar to the changes seen with isoflurane. Regional distribution of changes has not been evaluated. EEG depression occurs at equipotent dosages of desflurane and isoflurane. Development of EEG tolerance to neuroelectric depression may be seen.

Nitrous oxide is commonly used in combination with intravenous and volatile anesthetics. When nitrous oxide is given along with baseline sedation or other anesthetic agents, no changes or slight decreases (about 15%) in cerebral metabolic rate have been noted. Regional increases may occur in the thalamus, hippocampus, and caudate and putamen nuclei.

## Intravenous Anesthetics

Most intravenous anesthetic agents cause a dose-related decrease in cerebral metabolism as well as neuroelectric depression. No direct flow-metabolism coupling occurs across agents. Indeed, ketamine hydrochloride can increase metabolism. Barbiturates may decrease evoked potential amplitude, while etomidate may amplify it. Intravenous anesthetics vary widely in pharmacologic type and relative potency, so that some variations in dose-response relationships are expected.

## Induction Agents

The barbiturates (thiopental sodium, methohexital sodium, thiamylal sodium) all produce a maximum 50–55% decrease in brain metabolism; the effect reaches a maximum at the dosage that results in isoelectricity and is not reduced after electrical silence is induced [7]. The onset of general anesthesia is associated with a 30% reduction in cerebral oxygen consumption. This strong metabolic depressant effect has led to barbiturate use for cerebral protection.

EEG changes induced by barbiturates are similar to those induced by other anesthetic agents. After low barbiturate doses, low-voltage, fast EEG activity is seen, followed by increasing waveform amplitude. A generalized slowing with delta and theta activity follows. Burst suppression or isoelectricity occurs at higher doses.

Etomidate is an imidazole derivative used for anesthetic induction [8]. It is associated with greater hemodynamic stability than barbiturates. With stimulation of central gamma-aminobutyric acid inhibition, it reduces metabolic rate up to 50%; the maximum reduction is also coincident with isoelectricity. Etomidate can activate the EEG and has been shown to increase epileptiform activity detected with depth electrodes in epileptic patients. It results in some prolongation of somatosensory evoked potential latency, but doses of 0.1 and 0.2 mg/kg augment the evoked waveform amplitude.

Ketamine hydrochloride produces both cerebral excitation and depression. The effects are regional. Activation of thalamic and limbic structures has been demonstrated, as have ketamine-induced electrical seizure activity. There may be no change in metabolism, however, despite a 60% increase in CBF.

Propofol is also a metabolic depressant. Injection as a bolus (2 mg/kg) and administration as an infusion (0.2 mg/kg/minute) decrease cerebral metabolism by 36%. EEG depression and isoelectricity are easily attained.

The benzodiazepines are most frequently used to sedate, but at times they (particularly midazolam hydrochloride) are used for induction of general anesthesia. Diazepam, lorazepam, and midazolam hydrochloride all decrease metabolism by 20–35% when given to sedating effect. This reduction in metabolism is less than that produced by barbiturates. The EEG is activated with sedation; the somatosensory evoked responses (SERs) show decreased amplitudes, but there is minimal effect on latency.

## Opioids

Narcotics are used as a part of most anesthetic regimens administered to patients for surgical procedures. The type of narcotic and the dosage received can vary widely. Although the narcotics as a group seem either not to effect CMR or to slightly reduce it, most studies have been done when multiple agents have been interacting in subjects.

## Adjunctive Anesthetic Agents

Many medications used as part of anesthetic regimens may affect cerebral metabolism. Droperidol is commonly used as an antinauseant or in combination with a narcotic in neuroleptanesthesia. The vasodilating properties linked primarily to its mild alpha-blocking activity may decrease systemic blood pressure. Even when this occurs, administration of 0.25 mg/kg of droperidol with 5 μg/kg of fentanyl does not change cerebral metabolism.

The benzodiazepine receptor antagonist flumazenil is used to antagonize residual sedation. When it is given without benzodiazepines and with background anesthesia from isoflurane and nitrous oxide, brain metabolism does not change. When midazolam hydrochloride has been given with a resulting decrease in brain metabolism, flumazenil returns the metabolic rate to baseline levels; however, it can also increase CBF and ICP.

Muscle relaxants themselves have no direct effect on cerebral metabolism. Associated histamine release can result in dilation of cerebral vasculature and increased ICP, with a concomitant decrease in blood pressure and cerebral perfusion pressure. The relaxant with the greatest histamine release, dimethyl tubocurarine iodide, has the largest effect. The epileptogenic metabolite of atracurium, laudanosine, does not reach significant blood levels in patients given therapeutic doses. The use of the depolarizing muscle relaxant succinylcholine chloride in neurosurgical patients with increased ICP is controversial. It does not increase cerebral metabolism, but ICP may increase about 5 mm Hg for about 10 minutes. This effect is probably secondary to afferent activity from the muscle spindle apparatus and is prevented or blunted by defasciculation, deep anesthesia, and hyperventilation.

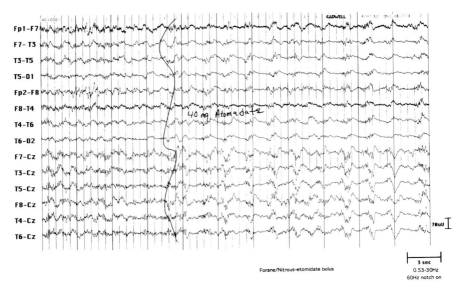

*Figure 21.1*    Burst-suppression electroencephalogram pattern during induction with etomidate.

## Electroencephalography

The EEG is still generally recorded on conventional multichannel free-running instruments with either analog paper or digital outputs. "Processed" EEGs are also available using a variety of outputs that have the potential to provide a simple visual indication of a significant change. The authors prefer the use of traditional free-running raw EEG. The use of mathematically processed EEG signals is not a substitute for an adequate understanding of basic EEG interpretation. Raw EEG signals must be available in such systems so that the role of various types of artifact in the signal analysis can be evaluated. We have generally used silver–silver chloride or gold cup electrodes applied with collodion, although subdermal needles may be appropriate in some situations. The full set of 19 electrodes (omitting A1 and A2) is preferable. A minimum of eight channels should be available, and in most instances the more standard 16-channel output is desirable.

EEG activity undergoes a gradual change with induction and maintenance of anesthesia. For the most part, the patterns seen are the same for all anesthetic agents at equivalent concentrations. It is not unusual to see a brief period of burst-suppression with induction (Figure 21.1). This pattern may last for several minutes and then gradually evolve to a more stable and continuous pattern with maintenance anesthesia (Figure 21.2). During the early phases a prominent anterior rhythmic slow frequency is usually present that at first may be in the alpha range but that gradually slows to the theta and even delta ranges, depending on the depth of anesthesia desired. These rhythmic slow frequencies become more generalized as the procedure progresses.

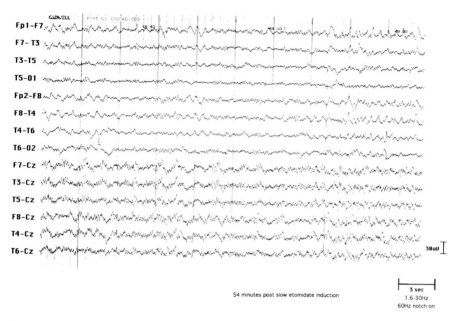

Fp1-F7

F7-T3

T3-T5

T5-O1

Fp2-F8

F8-T4

T4-T6

T6-O2

F7-Cz

T3-Cz

T5-Cz

F8-Cz

T4-Cz

T6-Cz

30uU

54 minutes post slow etomidate induction

3 sec
1.6-30Hz
60Hz notch on

*Figure 21.2*    Typical electroencephalogram pattern during early maintenance anesthesia.

Carotid endarterectomy is the most common indication for the use of EEG in the OR. It is important that an adequate array of electrodes be used with carotid endarterectomy, because changes may be confined to a restricted vascular territory not covered by a limited two- or four-channel placement. EEG activity may be expected to change when blood flow is below 20 ml/100 g per minute and certainly will change below 10 ml/100 g per minute [9–12]. It is important that the anesthesiologist maintain a stable and normal carbon dioxide level [13]. Alterations in EEG activity may be seen in 10–30% of cases. The EEG change may take the form of either voltage attenuation or high-amplitude slowing. The changes may be focal, hemispheric, or generalized (Figure 21.3). The most common time to see acute changes is during cross-clamping of the common carotid artery. The delay is usually about 20 seconds, although longer delays may be seen. In general, the longer the delay to the EEG change, the less the clinical significance of the change. EEG changes are usually reversed when a shunt is placed. When such a reversal does not occur, the patient is at higher than normal risk for postoperative neurologic deficit [14,15]. Changes at other times during the procedure are less common and may be a result of changes in perfusion pressure, unexpected occlusion of the shunt, or thrombosis of the artery after it is closed.

EEG may be requested during hypothermic circulatory arrest. A characteristic evolution of cortical activity occurs during this process [16]. It is the same for patients of all ages. A brief burst of high-amplitude slowing may be seen as the patient is placed on the bypass pump. This slowing is probably caused by the sudden change in temperature of the perfusion fluid. Thereafter, amplitudes

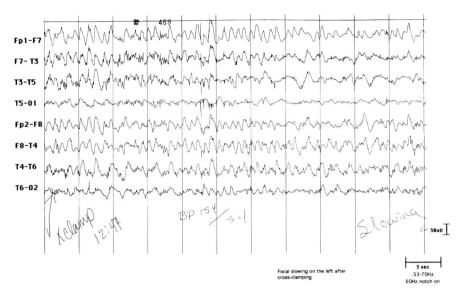

*Figure 21.3* Focal voltage attenuation and slowing on the left 6 seconds after placement of the common carotid clamp.

gradually decline and frequencies slow until a temperature of approximately 20°C is reached, at which time a pattern of periodic complexes may be seen (Figure 21.4). The period between these complexes lengthens until activity is minimal. Activity is often present, however, even at the desired minimum temperature of about 15°C. If it is desirable to have all EEG activity suppressed at this point in the procedure, administration of thiopental sodium may be necessary. The need for EEG monitoring during hypothermic circulatory arrest is by no means generally accepted.

## Electrocorticography

Direct recording of cortical activity is most commonly used during surgery for epilepsy, although it may be useful during other neurosurgical procedures as well. Recordings are usually made using metal ball electrodes attached to a ring so that they may be directed to various locations on the cortex. Subdural strips or grids of electrodes are used for this purpose as well, although contact with the cortex may be less satisfactory. During cortical mapping, the corticogram is important in order to identify "afterdischarges," which are trains of high-frequency spikes that occur after stimulation of the cortex, usually with a hand-held stimulator. Afterdischarges usually suggest that the stimulation intensity should not be increased further or a clinical seizure may be induced. Seizure induction is undesirable when the patient is awake for the functional mapping and therefore not intubated. Afterdischarges may also indicate the presence of an area

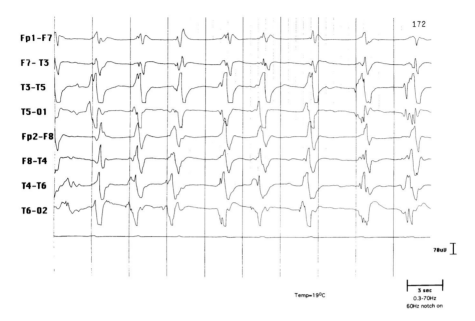

Fp1-F7
F7-T3
T3-T5
T5-O1
Fp2-F8
F8-T4
T4-T6
T6-O2

172

70uV

Temp=19°C

3 sec
0.3-70Hz
60Hz notch on

*Figure 21.4* Patterned periodic activity during hypothermia.

with an abnormally low seizure threshold, although their occurrence is not by itself a reliable means of finding a seizure focus for resection. It is important that the neurosurgeon allow enough time between individual periods of stimulation for the neurophysiologist to make a determination regarding the presence or absence of an afterdischarge. Making such a determination requires at least 3–5 seconds until the artifact from the stimulus itself subsides. We have found it useful to record free-running EMGs from appropriate muscle groups during cortical mapping as a supplement to the observations of the anesthesiologist and patient.

## Evoked Responses

### Somatosensory Evoked Responses

When the spinal cord is in jeopardy, as during surgery on the spine, SERs may provide a means to prevent irreversible injury. SER monitoring does appear to significantly reduce the morbidity of major spine surgery and is the standard of care in these cases [3]. Responses are elicited from both upper and lower extremities, bilaterally if at all possible. The success of SER monitoring is influenced by the choice of anesthetic agent. This choice must be made primarily by the anesthesiologist, although it is usually possible to use agents friendly to the acquisition of SERs. Balanced nitrous oxide with narcotics and low concentra-

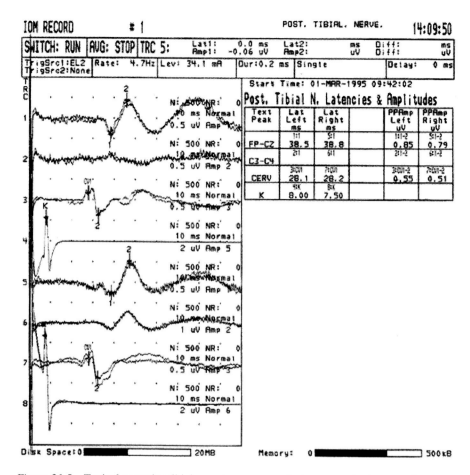

*Figure 21.5*   Typical posterior tibial somatosensory evoked response in the operating room with cortical (1, 2), subcortical (CV1) and peripheral nerve (K) responses.

tions of isoflurane (preferably below 0.2%) is usually satisfactory. Nevertheless, it is imperative that potentials of subcortical origin be recorded to minimize dependence on cortical responses that are very sensitive to anesthetic technique (Figure 21.5). Acquisition of an SER after induction of anesthesia but before incision provides a baseline for the procedure. It may be necessary to ask the surgeon to delay incision until this can be accomplished, because Bovie coagulator artifact will prohibit acquisition for some time thereafter. Although there is some debate as to what constitutes a significant change in the SER, a 50% or greater reduction in amplitude or a 10% or greater increase in latency should be reported to the surgeon. The neurophysiologist must always interpret results within the context of the procedure. Lesser changes may be important to communicate if they occur at critical parts of the procedure, especially when the spine is being distracted during scoliosis surgery. It is also important to document all interactions with the surgeon and others on the record.

Success in SER monitoring assumes that the posterior columns are anatomically appropriate to monitor, because the SER is largely an indication of conduction along that pathway. When the spinal cord is mechanically disrupted, such as by compression by bone or an instrument, the SER is likely to be sufficiently sensitive. The change in SER is likely to be prompt as well. When the blood supply to the spinal cord is compromised, however, which is probably the more common mechanism of injury, then the SER may fail, because the ischemia will occur in the distribution of the anterior spinal artery and will spare the posterior columns [17,18]. Furthermore, when the mechanism is vascular, it may take as long as 20 minutes for a change in the neurophysiologic signal to occur [19,20]. Measurement of motor evoked potentials may therefore be necessary in most cases to adequately monitor the integrity of the spinal cord. Such measurement may be accomplished by electrical stimulation of the spinal cord or the motor cortex or by magnetic stimulation. We measure responses elicited by electrical stimulation of the cord by means of electrodes placed intraoperatively by the surgeon in adjacent rostral spinous processes. Occasionally, stimulation can be accomplished by percutaneous placement of electrodes in the base of the lamina. Particular difficulty is encountered when the upper cervical cord is the surgical site. A nasopharyngeal electrode may be used as an anode in such instances. With these types of stimulation, responses may be recorded from the sciatic nerve in the popliteal fossa (Figure 21.6). In general, motor evoked responses are more reliable and more sensitive when the spinal cord is at risk [21,22].

SER monitoring may be useful during other types of procedures. It is commonly used to locate the primary sensory strip during functional cortical mapping. For this purpose, the median nerve is stimulated at the wrist and responses are recorded from a four- or six-contact subdural strip placed lengthwise over the region of the central sulcus. The contact at which the phase reversal of the polarity of the response occurs is closest to the sensory strip (Figure 21.7).

Other applications of SER monitoring include monitoring during vascular procedures such as carotid endarterectomy, for which it is probably not superior to EEG monitoring. During aneurysm surgery, alteration in the SER with placement of the clip may indicate compromise of the parent vessel and suggests that the clip should be repositioned [23]. SERs have also been used to monitor the integrity of peripheral nerves when they are in danger of stretch injury, as in distraction of the pelvis for fractures [24].

## Brain Stem Auditory Evoked Potentials

Brain stem auditory evoked potentials (BAEPs) are employed to monitor conduction via the auditory nerve through the pontomedullary junction rostrally to the lower midbrain. BAEP monitoring is most commonly used during surgery

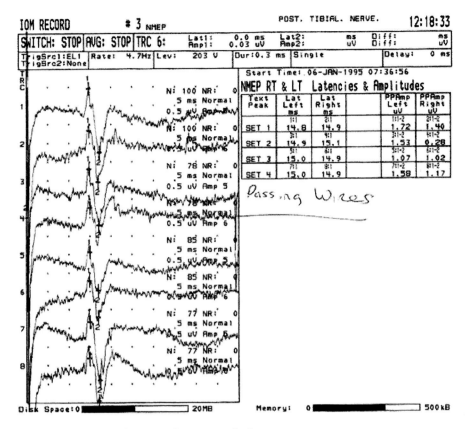

*Figure 21.6*    Series of neurogenic motor evoked responses.

for vestibular neurilemomas. It is also very useful during other types of posterior fossa surgery in which auditory function is at risk. The 10% incidence of hearing impairment with microvascular decompression for hemifacial spasm or tic douloureux can be reduced to nearly zero by monitoring the BAEP. As with the application of other evoked potentials in the OR, technical modifications are essential to the successful use of this technique [25]. Although there is some debate as to what constitutes a significant change in the BAEP, most consider a greater than 1-ms prolongation in the latency of wave V, especially if it occurs over a short period or at a critical point in the procedure, or a 50% or greater reduction in the amplitude of wave V worthy of a warning to the surgeon. The use of BAEP monitoring appears to result in an improvement in the preservation of hearing during procedures involving the acoustic nerve [26,27]. It is usually combined with EMG monitoring of cranial nerves to preserve their integrity as well.

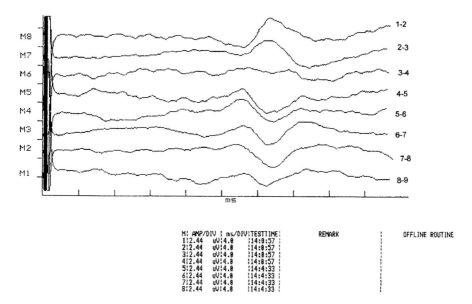

```
M! AMP/DIV ! ms/DIV!TESTTIME!        REMARK        !    OFFLINE ROUTINE
1!2.44   uV!4.0   !14:0:57 !                       !
2!2.44   uV!4.0   !14:0:57 !                       !
3!2.44   uV!4.0   !14:0:57 !                       !
4!2.44   uV!4.0   !14:0:57 !                       !
5!2.44   uV!4.0   !14:4:33 !                       !
6!2.44   uV!4.0   !14:4:33 !                       !
7!2.44   uV!4.0   !14:4:33 !                       !
8!2.44   uV!4.0   !14:4:33 !                       !
```

*Figure 21.7* Localization of the primary sensory strip by median nerve somatosensory evoked response monitoring. Recorded with multicontact subdural strip using a linked chain montage. Note electroneural response in third trace suggesting that the sensory strip is midway between two contacts in that channel.

## Nerve Conduction and Electromyography

Direct stimulation of a nerve may be used either to identify an area of injury or to simply identify the presence of nervous tissue. It is usually accomplished by using a bipolar stimulator (oriented along the length of the nerve, with the cathode closest to the recording site) and recording either from a distal segment of nerve or from the muscle innervated. If recording is from the muscle, neuromuscular blockade must be minimized or eliminated altogether. Compound nerve action potentials are much smaller in amplitude and thus are not as easily detected. A minimum of 4 cm between stimulating and recording sites is required to recognize the compound nerve action potential after the stimulus artifact.

Free-running EMG is employed in a wide variety of circumstances, often in combination with other modalities such as evoked responses. It is usually accomplished through the use of subdermal needle electrodes placed in the appropriate muscles. For example, during posterior fossa surgery, it is appropriate to monitor several divisions of the facial nerve as well as the trigeminal nerve, and often portions of cranial nerves IX, X, XI, and XII (Figure 21.8). During surgery for tethered spinal cord, multiple lower-extremity muscles may be monitored, along with the anal sphincter, to aid in the identification of

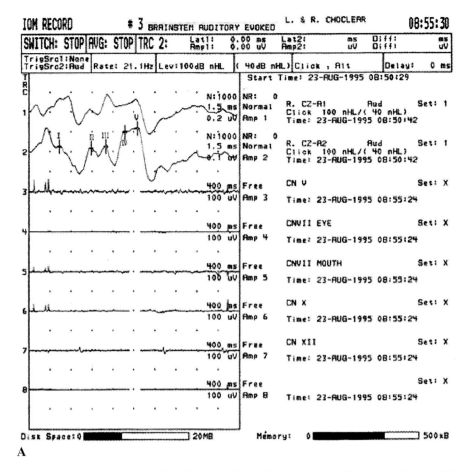

*Figure 21.8* (**A**) Typical multimodal recording with brain stem auditory evoked potentials in channels 1 and 2 and electromyographic signals from multiple cranial nerves in the remaining channels. (**B**) Response from the facial nerve (traces 2 and 3).

neural tissue. Evoked EMG may be used to evaluate the placement of pedicle screws [28] (Figure 21.9).

## PAIN: ETIOLOGY AND MANAGEMENT

The normal patient's pain-free state is a balance between noxious input received and the physiologic modulatory mechanisms generated by the noxious input, which suppress it. Increased input or reduced modulation results in pain. Pain control strives to maintain or control this balance. The noxious stimuli may be

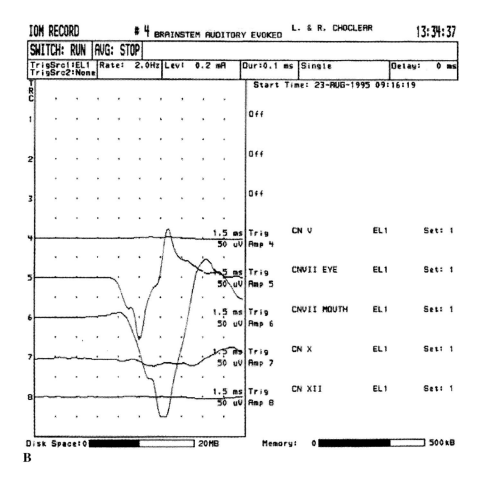

**B**

(1) peripheral, with activation of nociceptors by direct tissue injury (such as postoperative surgical pain), or (2) central, which are usually either psychogenic or result from sensory deafferentation. Deafferentation pain is triggered by a specific lesion that interferes with input into the somatosensory system [29]. A lack of consistency exists, however, in some pain-lesion relationships, treatment responses, and onset. Postherpetic neuralgia, amputation and stump pain, and pain associated with strokes are grouped in this category. This discussion focuses on the treatment of chronic pain; treatment of acute pain is not considered. Specific pain syndromes and treatments are used as examples and should not be considered to be all-inclusive.

Pain treatments can interrupt pain input. For example, tic douloureux can be treated by a variety of measures. Medical treatment may consist of mild analgesics and carbamazepine gabapentin administered orally. When the pain persists, however, the treatment becomes invasive. The trigeminal nerve may receive percutaneous radio-frequency coagulation, which is a selective and focused tech-

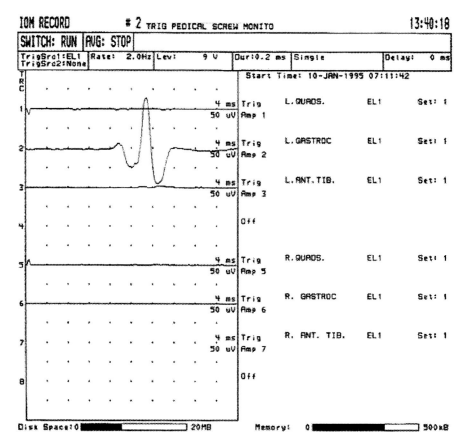

*Figure 21.9*   Response from the left gastrocnemius muscle with stimulation of old pedicle screw at left S1 using 9 V. The response suggests that the wall of the pedicle is breached. The screw was replaced.

nique [30]. A radiologically guided needle is inserted into the foramen ovale with the patient under sedation or short-duration anesthesia. Stimulation at 50–100 Hz is then carried out with the patient awake so that paraesthesias are induced in the area of pain. When the pain is duplicated, the patient is again briefly anesthetized, and a radio-frequency lesion is made by increasing needle current flow (150–250 mA) and temperature (70–90°C). When medically appropriate, intermittent anesthesia can be induced with small doses of barbiturates (thiopental sodium or methohexital sodium) or, more commonly, propofol. Percutaneous injection of glycerol and percutaneous balloon ablation are used. Last-resort patients may have a posterior fossa craniotomy for trigeminal nerve resection. Microvascular decompression for trigeminal neuralgia and possibly for other similar disorders appears to be promising as well [31].

Other pain syndromes can also require aggressive therapy to improve quality of life. A percutaneous intercostal neurectomy can be performed to treat cancer pain of the sternum, ribs, or parietal pleura. Radio-frequency lesion-creating equipment is used to identify the nerve through stimulation of the muscle so that responses can be monitored and is then used to perform the ablation. Visceral pain secondary to cancer (cancer of the pancreas is an example) can be treated by per-cutaneous sympathectomy. Alcohol or phenol can be injected into the celiac plexus with radiologically guided needle placement. Success rates can be greater than 90%, although complications such as a hypotension and somatic nerve damage can occur. Dorsal rhizotomies, cordotomies, commissurotomies, and other percutaneous and open surgical procedures may at times be indicated.

Techniques that interrupt pain input are not always possible or may not always succeed. Directing efforts at pain modulation may then be necessary. This approach must often be taken for both nociceptive and deafferentation pain mechanisms.

Opiates affect nociception at both the spinal cord and brain level. Chronic pain syndromes may be treated with long-term placement of either intrathecal or epidural catheter systems [32]. These catheters are inserted under strictly sterile conditions and are connected to refillable reservoirs or pumps. The catheters can be tunneled and externalized. Few reports exist of fistula formation or epidural abscess development. Totally implanted systems offer the advantages of greater sterility and comfort and less external interference with daily activities. Reser-voirs can be refilled percutaneously.

Morphine is usually the drug of choice for patients with cancer who require long-term administration of pain-killing medication. For patients who have been on oral morphine, the initial epidural bolus is usually one-tenth of the oral dose. This dose provides analgesia for about 12 hours. With time, doses generally have to be increased substantially. Infusions may also be given to avoid changing dosage levels. External pumps for externalized catheters are more acceptable for bed-ridden patients. Implanted pumps are better for mobile patients. A reservoir of 20 ml minimum with a wide range of administrable doses is required. Examples of functional pump types include continuous-flow pumps, peristaltic pumps, and pulsatile pumps. Some are programmable. These pumps are much more expen-sive than simple portal drug-delivery systems.

Complications include meningitis, epidural abscess, fistula development, and dural puncture headache [33]. Epidural catheters may migrate into the subdural or subarachnoid space; this migration increases central drug delivery and raises the risk of inadvertent overdose. Some side effects can be drug specific. For example, urinary retention and emesis may be caused by any opioid.

Epidural and intrathecal delivery of opioids exert a powerful analgesic effect secondary to spinal action. Their effectiveness has not been demonstrated for all types of pain, however. Effectiveness may also decrease with time as nociception increases, tolerance develops, and the catheter produces an inflammatory response that alters drug delivery.

Deafferentation pain may also require modulation, because the creation of destructive lesions in pain pathways is seldom effective. Chronic nervous system stimulation was developed for pain treatment. This stimulation has been shown to be more effective for deafferentation pain than for nociceptive pain. Various techniques are employed. Peripheral nerve stimulation can be used for the trigeminal nerve. Dorsal spinal cord stimulation is used in other cases. If a percutaneous trial of stimulation works, then long-term treatment can be undertaken with long-term implantable stimulators. Dorsal cord stimulators are inserted under monitored anesthesia and sedation or during short periods of general anesthesia with the patient in the prone position and with periods of arousal for paraesthesia induction and site identification. A Tuohy needle is inserted into the epidural space, and a suitable stimulating electrode is inserted in the midline with fluoroscopic confirmation to the area where appropriate paraesthesias are produced. One-half to three-quarters of patients whose initial tests suggest improvement have pain relief.

The treatment of pain is multifactorial. The psychogenic, nociceptive, and deafferentation aspects must be delineated. Assessment and treatment are complex and often require skilled diagnostic evaluations by psychologists, neurologists, neurosurgeons, orthopedists, and anesthesiologists with pain management expertise. Patient assessment and treatment must be individualized.

# REFERENCES

1. Moller A. Intraoperative Neurophysiologic Monitoring. Philadelphia: Harwood Academic, 1995;343.
2. Russell G, Rodichok L. Primer of Intraoperative Neurophysiologic Monitoring. Boston: Butterworth–Heinemann, 1995.
3. Nuwer M, et al. Somatosensory evoked potential spinal cord monitoring reduces neurologic deficits after scoliosis surgery: results of a large multicenter survey. Electroencephalogr Clin Neurophysiol 1995;96:6.
4. Siesjo J. Brain metabolism and anesthesia. Acta Anaesthesiol Scand 1978;60:883.
5. Todd M, Drummond J. A comparison of the cerebrovascular and metabolic effects of halothane and isoflurane in the cat. Anesthesiology 1984;60:276.
6. Scheller M, et al. The effects of sevoflurane on cerebral blood flow, cerebral metabolic rate for oxygen, intracranial pressure, and the electroencephalogram are similar to those of isoflurane in the rabbit. Anesthesiology 1988;68:548.
7. Michenfelder J. The interdependency of cerebral function and metabolic effects following massive doses of thiopental in the dog. Anesthesiology 1974;41:231.
8. McPherson R, Sell B, Traystman R. Effects of thiopental, fentanyl and etomidate in upper extremity somatosensory evoked potentials in humans. Anesthesiology 1986;65:584.
9. Sharbrough F, Messick JJ, Sundt TJ. Correlation of continuous electroencephalograms with cerebral blood flow measurements during carotid endarterectomy. Stroke 1973;4:674.
10. Sundt T, et al. Cerebral blood flow measurements and electroencephalograms during carotid endarterectomy. J Neurosurg 1974;41:310.
11. Zampella E, et al. The importance of cerebral ischemia during carotid endarterectomy. Neurosurgery 1991;29:727.
12. Trojaborg W, Boysen G. Relation between EEG, regional cerebral blood flow and internal carotid artery pressure during carotid endarterectomy. Electroencephalogr Clin Neurophysiol 1973;34:61.
13. Kalkman C, et al. Influence of changes in arterial carbon dioxide tension on the electroencephalogram and posterior tibial nerve somatosensory cortical evoked potentials during alfentanil/nitrous oxide anesthesia. Anesthesiology 1991;75:68.
14. Blume W, Ferguson G, McNeill D. Significance of EEG changes at carotid endarterectomy. Stroke 1986;17:891.
15. Redekop G, Ferguson G. Correlation of contralateral stenosis and intraoperative electroencephalogram change with risk of stroke during carotid endarterectomy. Neurosurgery 1992;30:191.
16. Rodichok L, et al. The evolution of EEG changes during extracorporeal circulation and progressive hypothermia with or without circulatory arrest. Am J EEG Technol 1994;34:66.
17. Zornow M, et al. Preservation of evoked potentials in a case of anterior spinal artery syndrome. Electroencephalogr Clin Neurophysiol 1990;77:137.

18. Lesser R, et al. Postoperative neurological deficits may occur despite unchanged intraoperative somatosensory evoked potentials. Ann Neurol 1986;19:22.
19. Owen J, et al. Relationship between duration of spinal cord ischemia and postoperative neurologic deficits in animals. Spine 1990;15:618.
20. Ueta T, Owen J, Sugioka Y. Effects of compression on physiologic integrity of the spinal cord, on circulation, and clinical status in four different directions of compression: posterior, anterior, circumferential, and lateral. Spine 1992;17(8S):S217.
21. Owen J, et al. Sensitivity and specificity of somatosensory and neurogenic-motor evoked potentials in animals and humans. Spine 1988;13:1111.
22. Kai Y, et al. Use of sciatic neurogenic motor evoked potentials versus spinal potentials to predict early-onset deficits when intervention is still possible during overdistraction. Spine 1993;18:1134.
23. Friedman W, et al. Monitoring of somatosensory evoked potentials during surgery for middle cerebral artery aneurysms. Neurosurgery 1991;29:83.
24. Vrahas M, et al. Intraoperative somatosensory evoked potential monitoring of pelvic and acetabular fractures. J Orthop Trauma 1992;6:50.
25. Erwin C, Erwin A. The Use of Brain Stem Auditory Evoked Potentials in Intraoperative Monitoring. In G Russell, L Rodichok (eds), Primer of Intraoperative Neurophysiologic Monitoring. Boston: Butterworth–Heinemann, 1995;135.
26. Harper C, et al. Effect of BAEP monitoring on hearing preservation during acoustic neuroma resection. Neurology 1992;42:1551.
27. Radtke R, Erwin C, Wilkins R. Intraoperative brainstem auditory evoked potentials: significant decrease in postoperative morbidity. Neurology 1989;39:187.
28. Calancie B, Madsen P, Lebwohl N. Stimulus-evoked EMG monitoring during transpedicular lumbosacral spine instrumentation. Spine 1994;19:2780.
29. Tasker R. Deafferentation. In P Wall, R Melzack (eds), Textbook of Pain. Edinburgh: Churchill Livingstone, 1984.
30. Sweet W, Wepsic S. Controlled thermocoagulation of trigeminal ganglion and results for differential destruction of pain fibers. J Neurosurg 1974;29:143.
31. Barker F, et al. The long-term outcome of microvascular decompression for trigeminal neuralgia. N Engl J Med 1996;334:1077.
32. Poletti C, et al. Cancer pain relieved by long-term epidural morphine with permanent indwelling systems for self-administration. J Neurosurg 1981;55:581.
33. Zenz M, et al. Long-term peridural morphine analgesia in cancer pain [Letter]. Lancet 1981;1(91): 8211.

# 22
# Ophthalmology
## Misha Pless and Nasrollah Samiy

A neurologist who is asked to render an opinion on a patient with an ophthalmic or neuro-ophthalmic complaint will ordinarily have to address questions related to diplopia, vision loss, ocular pain, ocular oscillations, and pupil size. The following is a practical neuroanatomic approach based on differential diagnosis that can be used to address the most common questions encountered in the hospital consultation environment.

## DIPLOPIA

Caution must be exercised in distinguishing monocular from binocular diplopia at the outset of an evaluation. Diplopia occurs when the subject sees an object in two different places at the same time. Diplopia is said to occur, with a few exceptions, when one image falls on the fovea of a fixating eye while it falls on the nonfoveal portion of the fellow eye; this noncorrespondence causes an unpleasant sensation. This phenomenon takes place when both eyes are open, and it disappears when either eye is closed. It is known as *binocular diplopia*, and it must be distinguished from the monocular variety: Binocular diplopia implies ocular misalignment, whereas *monocular diplopia* usually occurs without foveal misalignment. Monocular diplopia is thought to involve multiple images or ghost images of a single object falling on the retina. Monocular diplopia almost always occurs as a result of irregularities in the media of one eye, and the overwhelming majority of causes are optical. Occasionally, subtle diplopia may be misconstrued as blurred vision or difficulty in focusing by the unsuspecting patient.

The following questions may help in distinguishing monocular from binocular diplopia: Is the symptom present with one or both eyes open? Covering which eye abolishes or enhances the symptom? On occasion, a patient who has media abnormalities in both eyes may experience binocular or bilateral monocular diplopia. In addition, oscillatory eye movement disorders such as nystagmus may occasionally be sensed by the individual as diplopia.

## Diplopia with Ocular Misalignment

A series of steps should be taken to delineate the type of misalignment leading to binocular diplopia. Often the diagnosis can be suggested by history alone. A perception of images that fall side by side suggests horizontal diplopia, whereas object duplication in the vertical plane suggests vertical diplopia. Straight edges or lines that appear oblique suggest a torsional mechanism such as one encounters in a fourth-nerve palsy or a supranuclear vertical skew deviation. Pain and an acute change in the external appearance of the eyes should be investigated thoroughly, because the cause may range from external ocular disease to cavernous sinus pathology. A history of strabismus or eye muscle surgery may offer an explanation for a decompensated problem that appears new and acute. The distance between duplicated objects in near vision versus the distance between them in far vision offers important information about the mechanism of diplopia. Diplopia with a diurnal variation suggests neuromuscular disease.

Saccadic eye movements and range of motion should be tested with both eyes open and should also be tested in each individual eye with alternating monocular occlusion. Even when full ocular range of motion is present, unilateral saccadic slowing may be seen, for instance, in adduction slowing that is a sign of an incipient or subtle internuclear ophthalmoplegia.

Binocular diplopia can be divided into concomitant (or comitant) and noncomitant (or incomitant) diplopia. In either case, ocular misalignment is present. Each type will be discussed in detail below. Binocular diplopia can rarely occur without loss of alignment. Aniseikonia is an example, and it occurs when the size of the object being viewed is perceived as different in the two eyes. Large differences in refraction between the eyes may lead to aniseikonia, a phenomenon known as anisometropia. A substantial difference in axial length between the eyes can also lead to anisometropia as, for instance, when one eye is myopic and the other hyperopic.

## Concomitant Ocular Misalignment

*Concomitance* (or *comitance*) is defined as the persistence of the same degree of ocular misalignment in all fields of gaze. Ophthalmoplegia is usually absent.

### Skew Deviation

Skew deviation can be incomitant at the onset, but if it persists it usually becomes concomitant. Patients with vascular disease and stroke are at risk to develop a vertical skew deviation, but such a deviation may also be a manifestation of demyelinating disease and, occasionally, of neoplasm. Skew deviation results from lesions at any level of the vestibulo-ocular pathways in the brain stem. It is occasionally associated with downbeat nystagmus. Skew deviation can occur acutely and can be easily mistaken for a fourth-nerve palsy because of the torsional deficit that accompanies a skew deviation. Lesions in locations as rostral as the midbrain and as caudal as the cervicomedullary junction have been identified by magnetic resonance imaging (MRI) as associated with vertical skew deviation. The clinical neuroanatomic localization, however, is nonspecific unless an internuclear ophthalmoplegia is present as well, in which case the ventromedial pons is implicated.

## Convergence Paresis

Diplopia at near vision with normal distance vision is known as convergence paresis and is considered also to be a supranuclear bilateral medial rectus paresis. Absence of miosis is said to support the diagnosis but should not be relied on heavily. Demyelination, vascular malformations, hypertensive bleeds, brain stem stroke, and head trauma have been described as causes of acute convergence paresis. Volitional and hysterical loss of convergence should be considered in patients with diplopia who have otherwise normal versions and ductions but who have diplopia at near distances. Some authors differentiate convergence paresis from convergence insufficiency. Pupillary miosis in a patient attempting near fixation and convergence supports the diagnosis of hysterical convergence insufficiency, a diagnosis of exclusion.

## Divergence Paresis

Divergence paresis, which can be considered a form of bilateral supranuclear lateral rectus insufficiency, is characterized by unimpaired horizontal versions and ductions at near vision but esotropia at distance vision. The result is horizontal binocular diplopia at distance fixation. Divergence paresis must be differentiated from sixth-nerve palsy, not only on the basis of examination, but by history as well. Unless an abducens palsy is minimal, normal vision at near fixation would be unusual and not expected. As in convergence paresis (and both entities can coexist), in divergence paresis, cerebrovascular and neoplastic etiologies are the leading causes, but head trauma has also been implicated in this disorder. Divergence paresis can herald bilateral sixth-nerve palsies in demyelinating disease. Other rare causes of divergence paralysis include postinfectious demyelination and neurosyphilis. Spasm of the near reflex, an associated entity, is seen mainly in the outpatient setting but should be suspected in patients with headaches, blurred vision, and diplopia at distance vision. Occasionally a diagnosis of overreaction of the near reflex can be made. Preservation of miosis when attempting to view distant objects is a helpful aid in this diagnosis.

## Decompensated Phoria

Decompensated phorias are relatively common and quite easy to diagnose using the cover-uncover test. Normal ductions and versions should be present. Intermittent symptoms of diplopia can be experienced for a lifetime without any neuro-ophthalmic pathology. Imaging usually proves fruitless.

## Incomitant Ocular Misalignment

*Incomitance* (or *noncomitance*) is defined as a lack of ocular alignment as gaze changes direction and is generally associated with ophthalmoplegia. The differential diagnosis of diplopia due to congenital or acquired ophthalmoplegia is daunting. A hierarchic approach is necessary for neuroanatomic localization. Incomitant eye movement disorders can be divided in descending neuroanatomic order into supranuclear or internuclear, nuclear, and infranuclear or fascicular. Subsequently, one must consider peripheral etiologies such as neuromuscular junction diseases, myopathies, and orbital pathology.

### Oculomotor Nerve Disorders

The oculomotor nucleus lies in the dorsomedial aspect of the midbrain, anterior to the periaqueductal grey. The somatic oculomotor nucleus contains subnuclei with fibers innervating four muscles involved in eye movement (medial, superior, and inferior recti and inferior oblique). It also contains subnuclei of fibers innervating the superior levator palpebrae. In primates, and probably in humans, the superior rectus subnucleus innervates the contralateral superior rectus muscle. The subnucleus involved in levator function has fibers that end bilaterally. Hence, a pure unilateral nuclear lesion could lead to bilateral ptosis. This condition needs to be distinguished from apraxia of eyelid opening, a supranuclear phenomenon. The visceral component of the nucleus subserves parasympathetic pupillary function (constrictor muscles) as well as accommodation (ciliary body muscles). This function appears to be purely ipsilateral in the human. Several varieties of third-nerve palsy exist. Involvement of all components results in ptosis, mydriasis, and an eye that is depressed and abducted. Intorsion may be observed by asking the patient to adduct the eye while it is infraducted. Selective involvement of the superior rectus and the superior levator palpebrae muscles indicates a lesion in the superior division of the peripheral oculomotor nerve as it enters the orbit. A third-nerve palsy does not always begin with diplopia. If levator function is impaired early, a patient may lose vision in one eye by virtue of total lid dysfunction and not experience double vision.

Aneurysms are among the leading causes of third-nerve palsies in adults, and it is important to recognize them early because of the potential morbidity and mortality. Painful ophthalmoplegia is characteristic. The pupil is almost universally involved. The causes of adult third-nerve palsies are, in descending order of frequency, diabetic or hypertensive small-vessel disease, aneurysm, trauma, neoplasm, and infection. Cranial neuropathies related to human immunosuppressive virus that are not associated with other opportunistic infections have been described. Paget's disease and collagen vascular disease can potentially cause oculomotor ophthalmoplegia. Atherosclerotic vascular disease and end-arterial lipohyalinosis are involved in the pathophysiology of pupil-sparing third-nerve palsies. In this setting, the lack of pupillary involvement is apparently only clinical, because microscopic techniques almost invariably show relative pupillary involvement in all cases.

## Trochlear Nerve Disorders

Diplopia caused by a fourth-nerve palsy can manifest with symptoms of loss of balance and dizziness, because an unpleasant oblique perception of the environment is introduced. The diagnosis of a fourth-nerve palsy is facilitated by the Bielschowsky three-step test. Trauma is the most common cause of isolated, unilateral or bilateral, acquired palsies of the trochlear nerve when a cause can be determined. The localization of lesions of the trochlear nerve to the nucleus or fascicles (or both), subarachnoid space, cavernous sinus and superior orbital fissure, or orbit depends on the associated damage to neighboring neurologic structures. Contrary to third-nerve palsies, fourth-nerve palsies are rarely caused by aneurysms. Some individuals harbor a small congenital fourth-nerve palsy, which may become clinically apparent intermittently throughout their lifetime.

## Abducens Nerve Disorders

The cardinal feature of sixth-nerve palsies is horizontal diplopia that is present at near fixation but gets worse at distance fixation and that is worse in one direction of gaze. The cause of sixth-nerve palsies is undetermined in approximately 30% of cases (depending on the study series), although aneurysms, vascular disease, and neoplasm can lead to dysfunction of the abducens nerve. By virtue of its long course, the sixth nerve is very vulnerable to compression and injury by adjacent inflammation along its path over the clivus and through the cavernous sinus.

Duane's syndrome is a sixth-nerve palsy look-alike that should be recognized, because it carries a benign prognosis and needs no investigations. Patients with this congenital disorder do not usually complain of diplopia. The patient may be brought to medical attention by a family member who has just noticed a "crossed eye," which may wrongly suggest an acute process. In Duane's syndrome, there is failure of abduction of one eye; with attempted abduction, the affected eye may elevate or retract by virtue of co-contraction of the medial rectus. Agenesis of the ipsilateral sixth-nerve nucleus was encountered in a case of Duane's syndrome brought to postmortem examination.

## Ocular Myasthenia

Ocular myasthenia should always be suspected in any patient with diplopia. Myasthenia is a relatively rare disorder, and its ocular variety is rarer yet. Intravenous edrophonium chloride testing should be considered in patients who have an ophthalmoplegia that does not fit a specific neurogenic pattern, a history of relapsing and remitting diplopia, symptoms that have a diurnal variation, and lid fatigue. One must keep in mind that ocular myasthenia can mimic any pupil-sparing ophthalmoplegia.

## Miller Fisher Variant

Progressive diplopia and associated loss of eye movements may be a peculiar manifestation of acute polyradiculoneuropathy or Guillain-Barré syndrome. In honor of the original description by Dr. C. Miller Fisher, the concomitant appearance of ophthalmoplegia and ataxia have been labeled the *Miller Fisher syndrome*. The ophthalmoplegia can take any guise. It can be unilateral or bilateral; it usually appears incomitant, but cases of concomitant ocular misalignment have been described. The eye movement disorder may begin insidiously with the loss of function in individual muscles and precede loss of deep tendon reflexes by days.

## Monocular Diplopia

Most causes of monocular diplopia are optical and should be abolished by viewing through a pinhole. The differential diagnosis for monocular diplopia is quite large and includes a host of corneal and lenticular abnormalities. These can potentially cause changes in the refractive index of the media that lead to irregularities in the light rays falling on the retina. Astigmatism is one of the most common causes of monocular diplopia. Patients may sense a "ghost" image around the objects and letters. Some forms of cataract can also lead to irregular light refraction. The neurologist and other nonophthalmic specialists should be alert to the possibility of lenticular subluxation, such as may occur in Marfan syndrome and metabolic disorders such as homocystinuria.

Polyopia and palinopsia are symptoms rarely encountered in practice. Polyopia is characterized by the presence of double or multiple binocular or monocular images. A homonymous or lateralizing distribution is possible in binocular cases. Polyopia and palinopsia usually result from structural lesions at the level of the parieto-occipital junction and inferior occipital regions. Palinopsia and polyopia have been described in brain tumors, arteriovenous malformations, stroke, and toxic-metabolic disorders. In selected cases the perceptual aberration may also be associated with metamorphopsia. If so, one must search diligently for retinal disease, which can also lead to monocular diplopia and metamorphopsia. The phenomenon of metamorphopsia is revealed when the straight lines of an Amsler grid appear wavy or distorted. Metamorphopsia should raise the suspicion of retinal disease. Retinal detachment is a typical entity in which the peripheral nature of the disorder may not be apparent to the unsuspecting neurologist unless full-dilated funduscopy is performed to exclude it.

Persistence of monocular diplopia in a patient with no evidence of structural abnormalities on neuro-ophthalmic examination suggests a psychogenic or hysteric etiology. All efforts should be taken to make somatization and malingering diagnoses of exclusion. One should remember that, although it may occasionally appear easy to uncover a case of psychogenic visual symptoms, "real" disease is usually hidden within.

## VISION LOSS

Patients may occasionally describe a homonymous versus a heteronymous visual field defect, specific marching spectral lines, or monocular versus binocular positive visual phenomena. The luxury of such detailed descriptions is not usually forthcoming, and the physician is usually left with a series of symptoms to be investigated with directed questioning. When a patient presents with vision loss, one of the most important decision forks is to determine whether the problem is retinal or neurogenic, whether the symptoms are optical or neurogenic, and finally whether the problem is prechiasmal, chiasmal, or postchiasmal.

### Prechiasmal Vision Loss

Monocular symptoms are suggestive but not pathognomonic of prechiasmal localization. Bilateral symptoms represent a greater challenge. Bedside aids may be used to differentiate retinal from optic nerve diseases. Retinal disorders tend not to cause a relative afferent pupillary defect unless there is widespread retinal destruction. Conversely, even small optic nerve lesions may cause a swinging flashlight sign. Optic nerve damage tends to cause dyschromatopsia, whereas retinal disorders cause nyctalopia, photopsias, and metamorphopsia. In general, optic nerve lesions tend to cause central or paracentral visual field defects. Mid-peripheral and peripheral defects are more likely to be caused by retinal disorders. Persistence of positive symptoms such as photopsias with eye closure are suggestive of retinal pathology.

Retinovascular disorders such as central retinal artery occlusion (CRAO) or branch retinal artery occlusion (BRAO) have to be distinguished from vascular diseases of the optic nerve, such as anterior ischemic optic neuropathy (AION). CRAO typically presents as paroxysmal, painless, monocular visual loss. It tends neither to improve nor to worsen with time. If the area of retina compromised is large, there may be an afferent pupillary defect. One is generally not present, however, and it is not necessary for the diagnosis of CRAO or BRAO. The amount of retinal compromise is directly proportional to the vascular distribution of retinal infarction; most of it is apparent on dilated funduscopy, which is of paramount importance to make the diagnosis. A focal area of infarction may be identified on funduscopy; otherwise a cherry-red spot may be seen if the area of the retina that is infarcted is in the macula. Anterior chamber paracentesis, carbon dioxide inhalation, vasodilating agents, and nitrates have been used in the treatment of CRAO and BRAO, with modest success. CRAO and BRAO can also occasionally be the initial presentation of giant cell arteritis. Thus, the following discussion of the diagnosis and management of suspected giant cell arteritis is relevant for these retinovascular disorders as well.

AION is one of the leading causes of neurogenic vision loss in the elderly. Arteritic AION, a consequence of giant cell arteritis, needs to be differentiated from its nonarteritic variety, and both should be promptly recognized in the elderly. Both types of optic nerve pathology can present in exactly the same manner. The proper diagnosis of arteritic AION depends on systemic findings. Vision loss is usually central or paracentral in AION. Dyschromatopsia and an afferent pupillary defect represent the hallmark findings in this entity. Inferior altitudinal defects are commonly seen that can often be correlated with focal superior optic disk edema. The latter is an indispensable feature of AION, without which the diagnosis should not be made. Peripapillary hemorrhages are also frequently seen. Approximately one-third of affected individuals experience worsening of vision loss, and another one-third experience modest improvement. Unchanged long-term vision function characterizes the relative majority of patients. Patients with AION in one eye have a 30% chance of experiencing AION in the fellow eye over 5 years. The risk of recurrence in the affected eye is unknown, but it is estimated to be lower than for the fellow eye. The risk factors for nonarteritic AION are vascular disease, lipohyalinosis, hypertension, and diabetes. As of yet, no cardiac valvular or cardioembolic risk factors have been proved to be significantly linked to AION, although they have long been suspected and sought. Treatment with aspirin is commonly recommended, but it has no proven long-term benefit.

The diagnosis of arteritic AION is based on systemic findings that define giant cell arteritis. Any patient over the age of 65 years who has AION (or any other form of unexplained vision loss) must be suspected of having giant cell arteritis. The associated findings include weight loss, fatigue, myalgias and arthralgias, polymyalgia rheumatica, headache, scalp tenderness, and jaw claudication. Anemia and high erythrocyte sedimentation rates may be seen, although giant cell arteritis is a clinical diagnosis, and laboratory testing is employed to support the diagnosis. Temporal artery biopsy constitutes the gold standard for diagnosis. Bilateral temporal artery biopsies may sometimes be appropriate in selected high-risk patients with negative initial biopsies.

Giant cell arteritis must be suspected in any patient over 65 years of age who experiences transient or permanent vision loss. If not recognized and treated, this disorder has significant morbidity and can be fatal. In addition to arteritic AION, other manifestations of giant cell arteritis include CRAO, BRAO, transient monocular blindness, disk edema without vision loss, and ophthalmoplegia resulting from cranial mononeuropathies or polyneuropathies. If giant cell arteritis is suspected, high-dose corticosteroids should be given to the patient pending a temporal artery biopsy. Unless absolutely contraindicated, treatment should be given immediately and should not be delayed pending biopsy results.

Insidious onset of painless vision loss associated with dyschromatopsia, afferent pupillary defect, and central or paracentral visual field defects should raise the possibility of compressive or infiltrating optic neuropathy. Metastatic disease causes relatively rapid progression of vision loss if the lesions are in the anterior visual pathways. Regardless of findings on slit-lamp biomicroscopy, and regardless of lack of systemic evidence of a lymphoproliferative disorder or primary neoplasm, an infiltrating lymphomatous or carcinomatous optic neuropathy should be excluded. Primary optic nerve tumors such as optic nerve glioma and optic nerve sheath meningioma are relatively more common in young and middle-aged patients. Optic neuropathies resulting from vasculitis or collagen vascular diseases are known and have been described, although they seldom present in the absence of systemic disease. It is customary to seek systemic evidence of collagen vascular disease in patients who present with unexplained optic neuropathy. A history of pulmonary symptoms raises the possibility of sarcoidosis. Gadolinium-enhanced MRI may aid in the diagnosis.

Patients who experience painless vision loss in one eye followed in weeks to months by vision loss in the fellow eye should be suspected of having Leber's hereditary optic neuropathy. Characteristically present is disk edema with rubeosis, a feature of the optic disk resulting from intrapapillary and peripapillary telangiectasis. Unlike in most forms of disk edema, fluorescein angiography fails to show leakage of fluorescein in optic disk edema associated with Leber's optic neuropathy. Thus patients with unexplained monocular or binocular vision loss should have a test to detect one of the several mitochondrial DNA mutations that may lead to the phenotype of this disorder.

Occasionally the diagnosis of nutritional and toxic-metabolic optic neuropathy may be made in patients with bilateral, symmetric vision loss. Current and past drug regimens need to be reviewed. Chronic concomitant use of alcohol and tobacco may be more toxic than either alone. Bilateral centrocecal scotomata must be present for the diagnosis of tobacco-alcohol amblyopia. Vitamin $B_{12}$ level should be measured in individuals with bilateral, cecocentral vision loss and in patients without satisfactory explanation for prechiasmal vision loss. Vitamin $B_{12}$–associated optic neuropathy is a very rare disorder, and it may occasionally be present without subacute combined degeneration or dementia.

Fungal and viral infections are among the leading causes of vision loss in the hospitalized and immunosuppressed population, particularly in patients with acquired immunodeficiency syndrome. A complete discussion of infections of the anterior visual pathways is beyond the scope of this chapter. Cytomegalovirus, varicella-zoster virus, and human immunosuppressive virus have been linked to progressive optic neuropathy. The most common fungi that may affect the optic nerve include *Aspergillus*, *Cryptococcus*, and *Candida*. Diagnosis is often difficult and requires multiple attempts at spinal fluid serologic examination and culturing. Syphilis can cause an optic neuropathy that can closely resemble optic neuritis.

Traumatic optic neuropathies are evident from the history. In the elderly and very young, mild closed-head trauma may occasionally cause damage to the optic nerve. Physical abuse, falling, and alcoholism increase the incidence of traumatic optic neuropathy. Intravenous corticosteroids should be considered, along with optic canal decompression, which may be of benefit.

Acute demyelinating optic neuritis is a diagnosis usually made in the outpatient setting, though occasionally a patient with multiple sclerosis hospitalized for a different reason may develop it. Central or paracentral vision loss and dyschromatopsia may be heralded by painful eye movements in this disorder.

## Chiasmal Vision Loss

Chiasmal compression typically causes a bitemporal visual field cut, although the exact nature of the bitemporal field defect is determined by the degree of chronicity of chiasmal compression. Whereas chiasmal lesions in young patients suggest the presence of a pituitary tumor, in the older age groups metastases are relatively more prevalent. Possibly because of its rich vascular supply, the pituitary gland is particularly prone to seeding by those tumors that spread through a hematogenous route. Pituitary gland tumors tend to have a highly insidious course. The type and extent of field defect do not correlate with the size of the tumor. Rapidly progressive vision loss associated with bitemporal field loss suggests a neoplastic process unless diagnosed otherwise by MRI, the radiologic study of choice to visualize the chiasm. Pregnancy may promote growth of an otherwise asymptomatic pituitary adenoma or parasellar meningioma. Craniopharyngioma has a bimodal age distribution and is more common in young adults and older patients. In the elderly, it may present insidiously with vision loss, optic disk atrophy, and dementia. Typically this tumor is calcified on computed tomographic (CT) scanning, and it can be cystic. Complete resections are sometimes achieved. Large cavernous sinus carotid artery aneurysms can grow superiorly and cause chiasmal compression.

The rapid onset of vision loss associated with bitemporal defects or junctional defects (the latter are defects characterized by a central defect in one eye and a supratemporal depression or defect in the fellow eye) in association with a severe headache suggests the diagnosis of pituitary apoplexy. Evidence of long-standing endocrinopathy is occasionally evident. A hemorrhage within a sellar tumor can cause sudden enlargement of the sellar contents and chiasmal compression. If not treated promptly with surgical decompression, the hemorrhage can be fatal. Pituitary abscess, an entity often suspected and seldom diagnosed, presents as a perisellar ring-enhancing lesion. It may be necessary to perform a trans-sphenoidal biopsy for diagnosis, because the spinal fluid does not always yield evidence of inflammation.

## Postchiasmal Vision Loss

Optic tract lesions, characterized by incongruous homonymous hemianopia, are uncommon. Neoplasm, metastasis, and infarction are the most common causes of optic tract lesions.

Hallucinations are common reasons for consultation in the hospital setting. Toxic-metabolic causes should be excluded first. Although well-formed hallucinations are usually nonorganic, they can occasionally result from lesions in the parietal and occipital lobes. Presence of hallucinations in a hemianopic field is suggestive of migraine in young patients, although generally a structural lesion needs to be sought. Parieto-occipital arteriovenous malformations may occasionally bleed and result in homonymous quadrantanopsic or hemianopic field cuts. Asymmetries in ocular response to a rotating optokinetic drum aid in the diagnosis and confirm localization. A headache may herald the bleed, but the visual symptoms are the hallmark. The same is true for embolic or hemorrhagic strokes, common reasons for admission to the hospital. Patients do not usually complain of hemianopic vision loss but rather perceive the problem as monocular.

Other lesions that can lead to postchiasmal vision loss include tumors and metastases in the optic radiations or occipital cortex. The further posterior the lesion is along the optic radiations, the more congruous the hemianopia becomes. Formal visual field testing is of paramount importance in the evaluation of such patients. Giant cell arteritis can occasionally involve the posterior circulation and present with a stroke involving the optic radiations.

## TRANSIENT VISION LOSS

*Transient monocular blindness* (TMB), as its name implies, is defined as loss of vision in one eye lasting for minutes to hours. This condition is different from the phenomenon of *transient visual obscuration* (TVO), which may also have monocular features but generally lasts seconds. TVOs are reported by patients with optic disk edema and are believed to have a different pathophysiology. TMB is thought to represent a thromboembolic event in distal carotid branches, namely, in the distribution of the ophthalmic or central retinal artery. Classically it presents as a dark "shadow" that descends "like a curtain," but it can also present as sudden loss of vision in the entire visual area of one eye. Results of funduscopic examination usually prove normal during an attack. An embolic cause for TBM must be sought in most patients over the age of 40 and in selected younger patients. If embolic particles are found in retinal arterioles, an embolic cause must be assumed.

Extensive investigations for an embolic source in young individuals who experience TMB usually prove fruitless. Conversely, in the geriatric population one is likely to find ipsilateral carotid disease. The combination of magnetic resonance angiography (MRA) and carotid flow ultrasonography to find internal carotid stenosis is extremely helpful and has high sensitivity. Symptomatic internal carotid stenosis greater than 70% is now considered an indication for internal carotid endarterectomy. If carotid disease is not evident, a search for embolic sources elsewhere is undertaken. Studies currently recommended to search for embolic sources include cardiac echocardiography with intravenous agitated saline injection, 24- to 48-hour Holter monitoring, and transesophageal-echocardiography if the patient is an appropriate candidate. The last technique yields clearer visualization of the left atrium, the aorta, and the takeoff portion of the carotids.

Chronic, recurrent TMB with negative investigations for embolic source has been described. The cause is thought to be vasospasm, and in some cases arterial attenuation has been observed during the attack. Treatment with calcium channel blockers and nitrates can be of benefit.

## OCULAR PAIN

Ocular and periocular pain can be a portent of devastating vision loss for the hospitalized patient and can aid the neurologist in making a diagnosis. On the one hand, ocular pain may be the result of a trivial corneal abrasion. On the other hand, such pain can be a manifestation of a systemic disease with broader implications.

Following is a review of some of the ocular diseases that may emerge in the consultation setting and that can produce ocular pain. Entities such as migraine, intracranial aneurysm, trigeminal neuralgia, and central nervous system tumors are covered elsewhere and thus are not included in this discussion. Narrow-angle (or angle-closure) glaucoma requires the immediate attention of an ophthalmologist, although it must always be suspected by the consulting neurologist who sees a patient with a severely painful, red eye.

## Ocular Surface Disease

The cornea has rich neural innervation, and thus it is exquisitely sensitive to the slightest disturbance. Any perturbation of the central cornea, ranging from slight punctate keratopathy to full-thickness edema, can result in blurred vision. In addition, the patient may complain of a foreign-body sensation, in spite of the fact that a foreign body is clearly absent. Severe pain secondary to a corneal abrasion or inflammation is accompanied by conjunctival injection, reflex tearing, and even lid edema.

An abnormality of the facial nerve can result in lagophthalmos (poor lid closure) and subsequent desiccation of the ocular surface secondary to exposure. Corneal exposure is most blatant while the patient is asleep, especially if the patient has a poor Bell's phenomenon. With facial nerve dysfunction, the lid usually covers the upper part of the cornea and leaves the inferior cornea exposed. The conjunctiva may be diffusely or sectorially injected with associated tearing. Without aggressive lubrication and lid taping, an ulcer can form in the exposed area and can become secondarily infected.

Ocular pain can be the major presenting symptom in herpes zoster neuropathy (herpes zoster ophthalmicus), which involves the ophthalmic division of the trigeminal nerve. The pain is akin to that of postherpetic neuralgia and can occur in advance of or in the absence of an obvious dermatomal vesiculopustular rash. During full-blown herpes zoster ophthalmicus, considerable eye pain can result from corneal surface or intraocular inflammation or glaucoma. The pain can persist once all skin and ocular inflammation has resolved. The risk of developing postherpetic neuralgia appears to be reduced by starting the patient on oral acyclovir within the first 3–5 days of onset of the rash.

Like varicella-zoster virus, herpes simplex virus can produce painful corneal or intraocular inflammation. Once again, ocular pain may precede any overt sign of ocular involvement. The ulcer characteristically exhibits a dendritic pattern, but herpetic keratitis can also take the form of punctate keratitis, a geographic ulcer, or interstitial or disciform keratitis. Herpetic ocular disease may be associated with intraocular inflammation or glaucoma, both of which can produce eye pain.

## Ocular and Orbital Inflammation

Any ocular inflammation can produce significant ocular pain in addition to subnormal vision. The inflammation may cause intense spasm of the ciliary muscle, and the pain can thus be diminished with instillation of a topical cycloplegic agent. The inflammation, as in the form of sclerosis, may involve the long ciliary nerves that carry sensory fibers. In addition to pain, ocular inflammation produces other symptoms, such as photophobia and the appearance of floaters. Ocular inflammation is of special importance to the neurologist because many of the diseases that produce ocular inflammation can produce inflammation within the central nervous system as well.

Occasionally, giant cell arteritis can present with ocular pain alone, but signs of intraocular inflammation are seldom if ever present. Conversely, intraocular inflammation is quite prominent in Behçet's disease, an idiopathic systemic vasculitis. The ocular manifestations of Behçet's disease are protean and span from the anterior chamber (hypopyon) to the posterior pole (retinitis). A strong correlation exists between ocular and central nervous system involvement. Other diagnostic criteria of Behçet's disease include erythema nodosum, genital and oromucosal ulcers, and arthralgias.

Although usually not prominent, ocular pain can also accompany the inflammation associated with intraocular lymphoma. The patient may also complain of decreased vision and floaters. The ocular process is bilateral in 80% of cases and portends concurrent or subsequent central nervous system involvement in 80–90% of patients.

The ocular pain associated with scleritis is characterized as "boring" and "dull." The eye exhibits a violaceous hue secondary to dilation of the scleral and episcleral vessels. Severe ocular pain can also develop in posterior scleritis, in which there are often no discernible changes on the anterior ocular surface. The diagnosis of posterior scleritis is based on careful dilated fundus and posterior pole ultrasound examinations.

The list of conditions associated with scleritis (and intraocular inflammation) is daunting, but many of the diseases have neurologic implications. Among them are rheumatoid arthritis, Behçet's disease, Wegener's granulomatosis, infection with herpes simplex and varicella-zoster viruses, syphilis, and tuberculosis.

Ocular pain is one of the cardinal features of idiopathic or inflammatory orbital pseudotumor. This condition is characterized by inflammation of the orbit, including the extraocular muscles, adipose tissue, fibrous connective tissue, and the lacrimal gland. The typical presentation is characterized by the acute onset of ocular pain, proptosis, lid edema, and injected conjunctiva. Because of extraocular muscle involvement, the patient often experiences painful diplopia. When orbital inflammation is present, one should exclude the possibility of an infectious orbital cellulitis, which is an ophthalmic emergency that requires immediate administration of systemic antibiotics. The treatment for orbital pseudotumor consists of oral or intravenous corticosteroids. A rapid response is usually seen within the first 24 hours of therapy.

Pain with eye movement is not limited to orbital pseudotumor but can be an important feature of trichinosis that involves an extraocular muscle. The nematode *Trichinella spiralis* reaches the orbit by the hematogenous route. The patient may have mild to severe orbital signs, including conjunctival edema, subconjunctival hemorrhage, and pain on eye movement. Diagnosis is based on peripheral leukocytosis and eosinophilia and, conclusively, on the presence of larvae in a biopsy of involved tissue.

Over one-half of patients experiencing acute demyelinating, or idiopathic, optic neuritis experience ocular pain, which is typically described as a "dull ache." In 16% of patients, the pain precedes visual problems. Not unlike in trichinosis, the pain occurs predominantly with eye movement. The proximity of the rectus muscles to the inflamed optic nerve at the orbital apex constitutes the anatomic basis for this phenomenon. Ophthalmoplegic cranial neuropathies associated with hypertensive or diabetic microvascular disease may also present with eye pain on eye movement.

## Vascular Diseases

Severe pain of usually subacute or chronic nature can develop in the setting of a condition known as *ocular ischemic syndrome*. This condition is almost always unilateral and results from chronic low perfusion that results, in turn, from stenosis of the ipsilateral common carotid artery. Parallel internal and external carotid critical stenoses can lead to the same scenario. As a result, the eye appears red, and intraocular inflammation and low intraocular pressure are present. Neovascularization can develop, but is less likely than in a condition such as a central retinal vein occlusion. Visual prognosis is poor if the disease is not recognized early enough. In most cases a vascular surgeon should be consulted concomitantly.

Carotid cavernous sinus fistula may also present with pain. Antecedent trauma usually occurs, and much of the pain can be attributed to secondary elevation of intraocular pressure. The eye itself is proptotic and exhibits dilated and tortuous surface vessels. The fundus reveals an edematous optic disk and dilated retinal veins, occasionally in association with intraretinal hemorrhage. A carotid cavernous fistula can be diagnosed by either MRA or conventional angiography. A similar entity in which there is usually no history of trauma is a fistulization between meningeal branches of the internal or external carotid and the cavernous sinus (cavernous dural fistula). The clinical presentation of this condition may be less dramatic than that of a carotid cavernous fistula, and in a significant percentage of patients the cavernous dural fistula resolves spontaneously.

Oculosympathetic dysfunction heralded or followed by pain can result from dissection of the internal carotid artery. This dissection may occur spontaneously or may follow trauma. In addition to ptosis, miosis, and variable anhydrosis, pain is a prominent feature and is usually not localized to the eye but radiates from the neck to the face. The pain may be described as "gnawing" or "toothache-like." Diagnosis is confirmed by MRA or conventional angiography. Anticoagulant therapy for stroke prevention is controversial, though accepted in most practices.

## Tumors

Two tumors involving the periorbital and orbital structures are particularly capable of producing ocular orbitofacial pain. Both nasopharyngeal carcinoma and lacrimal gland adenoid cystic carcinoma can produce pain out of proportion to clinical findings because of their propensity for perineural invasion. In fact, both of these tumors travel posteriorly by way of nerves into the sinuses, orbits, and cranium. Pain in both conditions tends to be chronic. Diagnosis is made by facial and orbital CT scanning and biopsy.

## OCULAR OSCILLATIONS

The term *nystagmus* is specific and is used widely to describe a form of rhythmic ocular phenomena; however, its use is generous, and it has often been used to describe other ocular disorders such as flutter, myoclonus, and opsoclonus that have nystagmoid features. In addition to examining ductions and versions, one should also examine smoothness of slow and fast pursuit, saccadic jerks, the response to optokinetic stimulus, and suppression of the vestibulo-ocular reflex.

Pendular and phasic nystagmus are discussed below. By convention, the direction in phasic nystagmus is defined by the direction of the fast phase. Nystagmus in which the fast component remains in the same direction regardless of direction of gaze is known as *unidirectional*. *Bidirectional nystagmus*, also known as *direction-changing nystagmus*, is characterized by a change in the direction of the fast component on gaze change. For unilateral nystagmus, an additional sub-classification by degree may sometimes be found. It refers to and usually correlates with the severity of unilateral nystagmus.

## Nystagmus with Symmetric and Conjugate Features

The consulting neurologist is frequently preoccupied by the potential of nystagmus to be a manifestation of central nervous system disease. This preoccupation is a result of the difficulty in distinguishing central from peripheral causes of spontaneous nystagmus. The fear of not recognizing posterior fossa tumor or hemorrhage prompts imaging studies of most patients who present with symptoms of dizziness or vertigo and exhibit nystagmus. This course may no longer be possible in our cost-conscious environment. A few aids can guide in diagnosis.

The medulla, which contains the vestibular nuclei, receives information from both vestibular otolith end organs and the semicircular canals. The information is in turn relayed rostrally to the cranial nuclei controlling eye movements via complex pathways. Maintenance of primary gaze is achieved by the cancellation of equal-intensity, bilateral stimulation in the steady state. Dysfunction in one vestibular system (end organ, sensory nerve, or nucleus) leads to overreaction by the contralateral system. The net effect is a slow conjugate eye movement toward the side of pathology. An uncomfortable sensation of movement in the direction opposite to eye movement is sensed. A cortical reflex involving the inferior parieto-occipital junction is thought to lead to the fast, corrective jerks that characterize nystagmus. Intact cortex is essential for this compensatory reflex; it is absent in comatose patients. In unidirectional nystagmus, the direction of the slow component is usually to the side of pathology. Nystagmus caused by peripheral pathology often has a rotatory component, can fatigue, and has the same direction in all positions of gaze. Nystagmus caused by central lesions tends to be direction changing, and it does not fatigue. In general, peripheral lesions are more symptomatic.

### Physiologic Nystagmus

Phasic nystagmus can be seen in individuals without any pathology. It characteristically has low amplitude, lasts for a few beats, and extinguishes spontaneously with change in gaze. To be called *physiologic*, the nystagmus must be present on eccentric gaze only. Fatigue and extinction are its cardinal features. To distinguish physiologic nystagmus from other forms of nystagmus, the clinician asks the patient to look to the extreme end gaze and then to look medially by a few degrees but not as far as primary gaze. This maneuver should abolish the oscillations.

## Drug-Induced Nystagmus

Medications arguably constitute the most common cause of nystagmus in the hospitalized population. Ethanol, benzodiazepines, lithium, and anticonvulsants are the most common culprits. Psychoactive medications are a common cause of horizontal nystagmus, and they constitute by far the most common cause of vertical nystagmus. Drug-induced nystagmus is upbeating more frequently than downbeating. It is gaze evoked, although it may persist in primary gaze, regardless of drug level. Phenytoin can cause cerebellar atrophy with long-term use. If such atrophy has occurred, nystagmus may be permanent despite discontinuation of the drug.

## Positional Nystagmus

Positional nystagmus can be peripheral or central. It is defined as the presence of jerk nystagmus on alteration of head position. It is not always associated with vertigo, but, if positional vertigo is present, the cause is usually peripheral. Habituation with repetition is a cardinal feature of peripheral positional nystagmus. Symptoms, unfortunately, may not always habituate. Habituation is observed after testing repeatedly with change in head position. The nystagmus may diminish in intensity and frequency. Peripheral positional nystagmus is usually benign and is associated with disease in the vestibular end organ. Habituation is rarely seen in the central variety. Central positional nystagmus can be caused by a variety of lesions, such as demyelination, stroke, and neoplasm. Patients with multiple sclerosis frequently exhibit positional nystagmus. Localization is nonspecific. For patients with positional vertigo and no nystagmus on gross examination, electronystagmography may be required for further diagnosis.

## Gaze-Paretic Nystagmus

Gaze-paretic nystagmus is characterized by an inability to maintain eccentric gaze, which may occur, for example, during recovery from a gaze palsy. An attempt is made to maintain eccentric gaze, but it is interrupted by slow return to the original position, closer to primary gaze. Saccadic jerks toward the intended direction of gaze may be seen. Gaze-paretic nystagmus can sometimes be observed in some normal subjects in darkness. Unlike in other forms of nystagmus, the fast component beats toward primary gaze.

## Rebound Nystagmus

*Rebound nystagmus* is defined as the appearance of nystagmus on return of the eyes to primary position from eccentric gaze, where nystagmus may or may not be apparent. It is frequently encountered in patients with alcohol-related brain disease or with unilateral cerebellar hemispheric lesions of any type. In patients with cerebellar lesions who have rebound nystagmus, the fast phase may occur in a direction opposite to that from which the eyes are moved.

Vertical Nystagmus

Vertical nystagmus may be upbeating or downbeating. The direction is defined by the direction of the fast vector. Downbeating nystagmus may be present in the primary position, but one must always look for it in downgaze. A lesion at the level of the craniocervical junction should be sought. A variety of lesions can cause downbeating nystagmus, including tumors around the foramen magnum and bony disorders like platybasia. New-onset downbeating nystagmus in a young patient should suggest the diagnosis of Chiari malformation or posterior fossa tumor. Degenerative cerebellar disorders and multisystem atrophies should be considered in the differential diagnosis as well. Other causes of downbeating nystagmus include stroke and drugs. Patients with new-onset vertical nystagmus should have screening for toxic substances in the serum, even if reassurances are given by the patient that extraneous substances play no role.

Upbeating nystagmus is less localizing neuroanatomically. Many types of nystagmus are rotational but have an upward vector. Any type of lesion involving the cerebellar vermis or the pons can cause it. Upbeating nystagmus has been described in lesions from the most rostral to the most caudal regions of the posterior fossa. If upbeating nystagmus is acute, special care must be given to excluding the involvement of cranial nerves. If cranial nerve abnormalities are found, imaging is mandatory. Tobacco, alcohol, and psychoactive drugs routinely cause upbeating nystagmus; however, efforts should be made to seek alternative explanations, and these should be diagnoses of exclusion.

Mention must be made of the dorsolateral medullary syndrome. Commonly caused by a stroke in the distribution of the posterior-inferior cerebellar artery as a result of ipsilateral vertebral artery embolism or atheroma, this syndrome is characterized by horizontal, unidirectional rotatory nystagmus with eyes open. When the eyes are closed, a reversal of direction may be observed. Other signs include ipsilateral Horner's syndrome, dysphagia, dysarthria, ipsilateral loss of pain and temperature in the face, and contralateral loss of sensation in the body. Lateropulsion, a tendency of the eyes to move tonically toward the side of the lesion on vertical or horizontal saccades, may also be seen with such a lesion.

Pendular Nystagmus

Most often seen in the pediatric population, to-and-fro oscillations of the eyes, mostly in the horizontal plane, are known as *pendular nystagmus*. An adult with acquired pendular nystagmus should undergo diagnostic imaging, because the differential diagnosis includes neoplasia and demyelination in the brain stem. Neonatal pendular nystagmus may be an early manifestation of bilateral vision loss or compressive lesions of the afferent visual pathways. In patients with normal vision, the most common type of pendular nystagmus is ocular myoclonus.

Ocular myoclonus has been observed in association with palatal and facial myoclonus persistent in sleep. Its features include conjugate, low-frequency, rhythmic movements of the eyes, usually vertically. Oculopalatal myoclonus is a manifestation of a rare disorder caused by lesions in the region of the olivary and red nuclei and the central tegmental tract.

Patients with abnormal afferent visual pathways may also have ocular myoclonus. It must be kept in mind, however, that loss of vision from any cause can lead to conjugate, pendular nystagmus. Nystagmus from visual deprivation can occur with vision loss at any age, but the overwhelming majority of such cases are found in the pediatric population.

Latent Nystagmus

The phenomenon of latent nystagmus is induced by monocular occlusion. It is congenital in most cases. When both eyes are open, no nystagmus is seen. Occlusion of one eye causes nystagmus in which the fast phase beats toward the covered eye. It may occur in either eye. Because visual acuity is routinely measured monocularly, decreased monocular visual acuity may occasionally be incorrectly diagnosed. Incomplete or intermittent foveation in the oscillating uncovered eye results in diminished visual acuity.

## Nystagmus with Symmetric but Disconjugate Eye Movements

Convergence-Retraction Nystagmus

Frequently associated with limited upgaze and light-near dissociation, convergence and retractory nystagmus can be seen with lesions of the dorsal midbrain. Both eyes develop simultaneous, medially beating fast phases. Any lesion that causes compression, ischemia, or mass effect acting upon the dorsal mesencephalon can lead to this triad or to parts of it. Retraction and convergence can sometimes be precipitated by attempts at upgaze or by viewing a moving optokinetic drum. A rare disorder known as *oculomasticatory myorrhythmia* may be a cryptic manifestation of Whipple's disease. Converging eye movements are synchronized with rotatory mandibular motions in patients who have a dementia. This disorder is treatable with antibiotic therapy.

Seesaw Nystagmus

Seesaw nystagmus is characterized by simultaneous downbeating and extortion in one eye and upbeating and intorsion in the fellow eye. Any patient with acquired seesaw eye movements should undergo diagnostic imaging. Seesaw nystagmus has been described in chiasmal optic nerve or brain stem intrinsic glial tumors, and in extra-axial chiasmal compression. This disorder has also been reported as a result of pontine and midbrain strokes and in septo-optic dysplasia.

## Asymmetric or Monocular Nystagmus

Spasmus Nutans

Spasmus nutans usually presents in the first months of life and is characterized by head nodding, torticollis, and nystagmus. The nystagmus is characteristically unilateral and horizontal, but slit-lamp magnification may show finer conjugate nystagmus in the fellow eye. A similar type of monocular pendular nystagmus, with or without the head nodding, has been seen in infants with chiasmal glioma. Spasmus nutans may occur in fetal alcohol syndrome and other developmental disorders. Any form of monocular pendular nystagmus requires MRI with special attention to the inferior third ventricle and chiasm.

Monocular vision loss can lead to monocular vertical pendular nystagmus much more commonly in children than in adults.

## Superior Oblique Myokymia

A relapsing-remitting monocular oscillation or monocular tremor, sensed as an intermittent tilting of the environment, is suggestive of superior oblique myokymia. The symptoms are intermittent, and it is not unusual for the patient to experience clusters of episodes and then to experience no symptoms for months or years. Occasionally an eye twitch can be observed; it can be elicited by having the involved eye look repeatedly in the direction of action of the superior oblique muscle. Electromyography can sometimes be of use, but the diagnosis is generally made on the basis of history alone. The disorder has no specific etiology, although there have been reports of midbrain astrocytomas that purportedly caused superior oblique myokymia. The large majority of patients with superior oblique myokymia have normal investigations. Carbamazepine can be of benefit in treating the symptoms.

## Nystagmoid or Nystagmus-Like Oscillations

### Flutter

Horizontal oscillations precipitated by fixation or by a change in eye position constitute the cardinal feature of flutter. The oscillations are fast and saccadic. Flutter can be confused with pendular nystagmus. In the latter, the oscillations may be horizontal or vertical. Ocular flutter occurs in the horizontal plane. The frequency of oscillation is higher in flutter, as is the velocity of the saccadic movements involved. Flutter can be observed in a variety of degenerative cerebellar disorders. It is not as frequently seen with neoplasms, but flutter has been described in association with focal lesions of the posterior fossa or lesions involving the cerebellar peduncular connections. Ocular flutter should be viewed as part of a continuum with ocular dysmetria at one end and opsoclonus at the other. No successful treatment has been identified for flutter, although reversible features have been described in forms of self-limiting cerebellar disease, such as postencephalitic demyelination of the cerebellum.

### Opsoclonus

Continuous, dart-like conjugate eye movements characterize the eye-movement disorder known as *opsoclonus*, which is sometimes labeled *saccadomania*. The movements tend to persist during sleep. In children, opsoclonus is frequently a manifestation of neuroblastoma, and a thorough search for this tumor should be undertaken. In adults, opsoclonus associated with polymyoclonus suggests a paraneoplastic disorder and is sometimes linked to breast-ovarian carcinoma or oat cell lung cancer. Adult opsoclonus has also been seen in association with demyelinating disease and postinfectious encephalitis. Medications that have been tried, with varying degrees of success, for both flutter and opsoclonus include clonazepam, diazepam, carbamazepine, baclofen, reserpine, and thiamine. Intravenous immunoglobulin has also been used with success to treat opsoclonus.

Ocular Bobbing

Bobbing has been described in association with catastrophic brain stem lesions such as pontine glioma and large intraparenchymal brain stem bleeds. Its features include tonic and fast, phasic downward movements of both eyes, which may occur symmetrically or asymmetrically. In ocular bobbing, loss of horizontal eye movements usually occurs. This disorder has also been seen in association with toxic-metabolic encephalopathies, Wernicke's encephalopathy, and rhombencephalitis.

## PUPILLARY SIZE ABNORMALITIES

In this section we discuss some of the common abnormalities of pupillary size that occur in the hospital setting: the acutely mydriatic pupil and oculosympathetic dysfunction or Horner's syndrome. The pupil must be examined directly and consensually in both light and dark conditions. It is preferable to use a collimated source of light, such as a thin-beam, variable-brightness source, rather than a source of diffuse light, which may produce an irregular beam and fail to provide adequate stimulation of the retina. Near synkinesis should always be tested.

Consultation is frequently requested regarding anisocoria. Physiologic anisocoria is present in up to 15% of the population. If the degree of discrepancy in pupillary size is the same in light and dark conditions and both pupils have normal direct and consensual reaction, if no lid abnormality is present, and if near synkinesis is normal, the condition is benign physiologic anisocoria.

The presence of ptosis ipsilateral to the miotic pupil in the anisocoric patient is suggestive of oculosympathetic dysfunction. The deficit in the function of the upper eyelid may sometimes be subtle and may also be accompanied by dysfunction of the lower eyelid, the position of which may be slightly higher than in the fellow eye. In Horner's syndrome, both pupils react normally to direct and consensual light. In darkness, the amount of anisocoria must increase, thus demonstrating insufficient sympathetic innervation of the pupillary dilator muscles of the iris. Dilute cocaine testing is used to cause an increase in the relative magnitude of the anisocoria. A discrepancy in size of greater than 0.5 mm between pupils after negative cocaine testing is diagnostic of oculosympathetic dysfunction. If the cause of such pathology is not already apparent from ancillary studies and the rest of the neurologic examination is not revealing, then hydroxyamphetamine testing can be performed to further localize the site of the lesion.

Light-near dissociation is rarely found, much talked about, and not always accurately diagnosed. Paralysis of the miotic response of the direct light reflex needs to be verified with magnification and slit-lamp examination for accurate diagnosis. Acute light-near dissociation in the absence of convergence-retractory nystagmus or upgaze paresis is exceedingly uncommon.

In a hospital setting, a unilateral mydriatic pupil that responds poorly to direct light or does not respond at all should be deemed a result of accidental instillation of a parasympatholytic agent until proven otherwise. The use of parasympatholytic bronchodilators is exceedingly common in intensive care and pulmonary settings. Not uncommonly, the face mask is placed on the face in a way that allows gases to escape asymmetrically. Even minute amounts of uninhaled bronchodilator could cause prolonged dilation of a single pupil. In some cases, both eyes become accidentally contaminated by these agents and bilateral poorly reactive pupils may be encountered. Parasympatholytic agents such as atropine sulfate may occasionally be instilled in one eye by an unsuspecting health care worker or volitionally by an individual with ulterior gains in mind. In such cases, the 1% (nondilute) pilocarpine hydrochloride test can be used. Constriction of the affected pupil rules out acute accidental or otherwise spurious parasympatholytic pharmacologic causes and suggests possible use of sympathomimetic agents or existence of a preganglionic parasympathetic lesion, a rare condition. Adie's syndrome or postganglionic parasympathetic denervation is diagnosed by history, slit-lamp examination, and the 0.1% (dilute) pilocarpine hydrochloride test. The majority of patients are young or middle-aged women, who frequently experience periorbital pain days before the pupil dilates. Slit-lamp examination may show sectorial paralysis of the constrictor mechanism of the iris. Cholinergic supersensitivity is diagnostic of Adie's syndrome; it is demonstrated by the dilute pilocarpine hydrochloride test, in which the affected pupil becomes more myotic.

## SUGGESTED READING

Albert DM, Jakobiec FA. Principles and Practice of Ophthalmology: Clinical Practice. Philadelphia: Saunders, 1994.

Berlit P. Isolated and combined pareses of cranial nerves III, W and VI: a retrospective study of 412 patients. J Neurol Sci 1994;103:10–15.

Brazis PW. Palsies of the trochlear nerve: diagnosis and localization—recent concepts. Mayo Clin Proc 1993;68:501–509.

Burde RM, Savino PJ, et al. Clinical Decisions in Neuro-Ophthalmology. St. Louis: Mosby–Year Book, 1992.

Carlow TJ. Paresis of cranial nerves III, W, and VI: clinical manifestation and differential diagnosis. Bull Soc Belg Ophthalmol 1989;237:285–301.

Hayreh HH. Anterior ischemic optic neuropathy: differentiation of arteritic from non-arteritic type and its management. Eye 1990;4:25–35.

Hoyt CS, Nickel BL, et al. Ophthalmological examination of the infant: developmental aspects. Surv Ophthalmol 1982;26(4):177–189.

Jakobiec FA. Non-Infectious Orbital Inflammations. In WH Spencer (ed), Ophthalmic Pathology: An Atlas and Textbook (3rd ed). Philadelphia: Saunders, 1986;2777–2795.

Keane JR. Fourth nerve palsy: historical review and study of 215 inpatients. Neurology 1993;43: 2439–2443.

Keane RK. Ocular skew deviation: analysis of 100 cases. Arch Neurol 1975;32:185–190.

Kennerdell JS, Dresner SC. The nonspecific orbital inflammatory syndromes. Surv Ophthalmol 1984; 29:93–105.

Kodsi SR, Younge BR. Acquired oculomotor, trochlear, and abducent cranial nerve palsies in pediatric patients. Am J Ophthalmol 1992;114:568–574.

Miller NR. Walsh and Hoyt's Clinical Neuro-Ophthalmology. Baltimore: Williams & Wilkins, 1991.

Newman NM. The prechiasmal afferent visual pathways. Int Ophthalmol Clin 1977;17(1):1–38.

Nussenblatt R, Palestine AG. Uveitis: Fundamentals in Clinical Practice. Chicago: Year Book, 1989.

Pavan-Langston D. Viral Diseases: Herpetic Infections. In G Smolin, R Thoft (eds), The Cornea. Boston: Little, Brown, 1992.

Rush JA, Younge BR. Paralysis of cranial nerves III, IV, and VI: cause and prognosis in 1,000 cases. Arch Ophthalmol 1981;99(1):76–79.

Spalton DJ, Hitchings RA, et al. Atlas of Clinical Ophthalmology. London: Mosby–Year Book, 1994.

# 23
# Neurologic Issues in Obstetrics and Gynecology

Steven K. Feske

Pregnancy in women with neurologic disease raises many important issues regarding diagnosis and safe therapy. Pregnant women can develop any of the many neurologic disorders to which any young woman is subject. In addition, pregnancy predisposes patients to certain disorders and modifies the course of other chronic or recurrent disorders. Exposure of the developing fetus or nursing infant to illness in the mother and to medications restricts the range of available pharmacotherapies. This chapter addresses many of the problems that a neurologist confronts in an obstetric hospital. It also discusses some of the neurologic issues arising in regard to patients with gynecologic tumors and tumors affected by hormonal therapies. Aspects of the neurologic disorders that are not distinctly related to pregnancy or other gynecologic conditions are largely omitted in the interest of saving space, and the reader is referred to the other chapters of this book to supplement the discussion here.

## HEADACHE AND PREGNANCY

### Spectrum of Headaches in Pregnancy

As in the general population, most pregnant patients who present with headache will have benign headache syndromes, especially migraine. Pregnancy and the puerperium, however, predispose patients to several more severe disorders that should always be considered when headache occurs in this context. Table 23.1 lists the major diagnoses to consider. Other less common causes include rapid growth of brain tumors and central nervous system infections. When features of the headache raise concerns about a significant underlying lesion or when the neurologic examination is abnormal, brain imaging by computed tomographic (CT) scan or magnetic resonance imaging (MRI),

*Table 23.1*   Most common causes of headache during pregnancy and the puerperium

---

Migraine and other benign headache syndromes
Intracranial hemorrhage
   Aneurysmal hemorrhage
     Subarachnoid
     Intraventricular
     Parenchymal
   Arteriovenous malformation
   Other vascular malformations
   Venous sinus thrombosis with hemorrhagic infarction
Ischemic stroke
   Venous sinus thrombosis
   Arterial infarction
Hypertensive encephalopathy, with or without pre-eclampsia–eclampsia
Pseudotumor cerebri

---

and in some cases lumbar puncture, should be performed to seek important underlying causes.

## Migraine in Pregnancy

Effect of Pregnancy on Migraine Frequency and Severity

Susceptibility to migrainous attacks is greatly influenced by estrogen. It is after menarche that the relative frequency in females compared to males increases from unity to two to three. Approximately 60% of women with migraine complain of headaches precipitated by the premenstrual state. Although the relationship of estrogen to migraine is complex and probably involves interactions with endorphins, catecholamines, serotonin, other centrally active amines, and prostaglandins, it is clear that the late luteal-phase physiologic decline of estrogen is an important trigger of premenstrual migraine [1]. For this withdrawal headache to occur, it is necessary to have the priming provided by the high luteal-phase estrogen levels. Menstrual migraine may be successfully treated with estrogen supplementation at the time of the premenstrual drop [2,3]. Inhibition of the luteal-phase estrogen rise with danazol or of estrogen effects with tamoxifen citrate can also prevent menstrual migraine [4,5]. Although these therapies are not routine, their reported success supports the hypothesis that estrogen withdrawal precipitates migraine. Many patients with migraine will experience an increase in the frequency and severity of their headaches during early pregnancy [6]. Estimates of the risk vary and depend greatly on the definition of migraine; many series with low estimates exclude milder vascular headaches [7]. For most patients, this tendency wanes in the second and third trimesters, and most, especially those with a history of primarily menstrual migraine, experience improvement compared to their nonpregnancy pattern [6,8]. A large minority experience no change, and fewer still experience worsening of the condition [9,10]. Typical headache patterns usually return shortly after delivery; lactation provides no protection [9].

Migraine Therapies during Pregnancy

It is desirable to limit the exposure of pregnant patients to multiple medications, even though there is little established danger to the fetus from many of the medications that are commonly used. Certain drugs are clearly contraindicated during pregnancy. Ergot alkaloids are potent vasoconstrictors that can compromise placental perfusion and stimulate uterine contraction. These should be strictly avoided. Sumatriptan succinate is also a vasoconstrictor. Although it does not have the prolonged elimination half-life of ergotamine tartrate and there is no systematic experience with it during human pregnancy, animal studies and theoretical considerations suggest potential harmful effects, and it too is best avoided. Agents that inhibit prostaglandin synthesis and platelet function, such as aspirin and nonsteroidal anti-inflammatory agents, may increase the risk of hemorrhage. They may also affect fetal development, for example by inducing early closure of the ductus arteriosus when given in late pregnancy. Although these agents may be used during pregnancy to treat certain diseases, they are best avoided for treatment of migraine. Methysergide should be avoided because of its potential to cause vascular complications and fibrosis. Anticonvulsants, especially valproic acid, should be avoided for this indication, because they increase the risk of congenital malformations. Combination preparations containing isometheptene (e.g., Midrin) should be avoided, because they cause vasoconstriction and may compromise placental circulation.

These restrictions leave a limited number of available drugs for acute analgesic therapy of attacks of headache. Acetaminophen has a well-established history of safe use and can be given as a rectal suppository when nausea accompanies the headache. Medications combining acetaminophen, caffeine, and butalbital are safe and effective for intermittent use in cases in which acetaminophen alone is inadequate. If used sparingly, the barbiturate doses should not be large enough to cause teratogenicity or fetal sedation. If stronger medications are needed for headache, oral narcotics are safe for intermittent use. Although, under most circumstances, narcotics are a poor choice for treatment of this chronic or recurrent pain syndrome, in pregnancy where the terminus is clear they are safe and effective when strong analgesics are sought. Oral meperidine, 25–100 mg every 4–6 hours or oxycodone can be used for severe and refractory recurrent headaches. Although it is unproven, some retrospective data raise questions of an association between codeine use and congenital malformations, and this drug is best avoided [11]. When a prolonged headache is resistant to treatment, a brief course of oral corticosteroids is safe and often effective. These should be given with the patient free of narcotics. We have used a 3-day tapering course of 15 mg three times a day, 10 mg three times a day, and 5 mg three times a day; each dosage is given for 1 day, and then therapy is discontinued. Even when nausea is not prominent, patients often have gastroparesis during migraine attacks, and they may benefit from antiemetic medication. Trimethobenzamide may be given as a rectal suppository for this purpose.

The prophylactic agents most commonly used for migraine can be tried, if necessary. These include beta blockers, calcium channel blockers, and tricyclic agents. Beta blockers are vasoconstrictors and have been associated with intrauterine growth retardation, so the severity and frequency of the headaches should clearly justify their use [12]. If given near delivery, they may also cause newborn hypoglycemia, bradycardia, respiratory depression, and hyperbilirubinemia. Calcium channel blockers are probably safe; however, there are no systematic studies to confirm this impression, and they, too, should be used only when the severity and frequency of the headaches are debilitating enough to justify their use. Tricyclic agents are also usually safe. Although various congenital anomalies have been reported with amitriptyline, there is no clear evidence of a causal relationship. A neonatal withdrawal syndrome characterized by colic, rapid respirations, and irritability has been reported in association with nortriptyline and could occur with other tricyclic agents. Newborn urinary retention may also occur when tricyclics are used near term [11]. Therefore, tricyclics should be used only when indicated by the degree of suffering and when the patient understands these risks. As noted above, valproic acid should not be used because of the established risk of teratogenicity, including neural tube defects, associated with its use for epilepsy. Table 23.2 lists drugs that may be used for migraine attacks and prophylaxis.

## Oral Contraceptive Agents and Migraine

As occurs during a normal menstrual cycle, the withdrawal of estrogen during the administration of cyclic oral contraceptive agents can precipitate a migraine attack. Many women with migraine experience more frequent headaches when taking oral contraceptives, though some benefit [13]. Continuous use may eliminate the problem caused by cyclic withdrawal, but this approach increases the risk of dysfunctional uterine bleeding and raises issues concerning cancer risk. The risk of stroke is slightly greater in patients with migraine and in those on estrogen-containing contraceptives. In most young women, the absolute risk is low enough that this increase does not constitute a contraindication (Table 23.3). In patients with complex migraine, a history of prior stroke, or risk factors for early stroke, however, oral contraceptives are best avoided. The issue of stroke and migraine is discussed below.

## Pseudotumor Cerebri

Headache, papilledema, and an MRI or CT scan of the brain that is either normal or shows only small ventricles or an empty sella suggest pseudotumor cerebri. The cerebrospinal fluid (CSF) pressure is measured to demonstrate the presence of intracranial hypertension. CSF analysis is typically normal, except for a low total protein. The major underlying diagnosis that should be considered in this setting is venous sinus thrombosis, which may present with isolated intracranial hypertension and the symptoms and signs that follow from it. With venous thrombosis, the CSF will often be abnormal, with an elevated protein, red blood cells, and a mild pleocytosis; however, it can also be normal. For this reason, evaluation of

*Table 23.2*  Medications used for headache during pregnancy

| Drug | Dose | Caveat |
| --- | --- | --- |
| **Acute attacks** | | |
| Acetaminophen | 325–500 mg q4h prn | |
| Acetaminophen + caffeine + butalbital | For example, 325 mg, 40 mg, and 50 mg, respectively, in combination preparations | In high doses, barbiturates may increase the risk of congenital malformations; they may also cause newborn sedation and withdrawal. High dosages of caffeine have been associated with low birth weight and spontaneous abortion. |
| Narcotics | — | Overuse may lead to addiction and to newborn sedation. |
| Meperidine hydrochloride | 25–100 mg q4h prn | |
| Oxycodone hydrochloride | 5 mg (usually in combination with acetaminophen) | |
| Prednisone | 15 mg tid for 1 day, 10 mg tid for 1 day, 5 mg tid for 1 day | Corticosteroids may exacerbate hypertension and glucose intolerance. |
| Trimethobenzamide hydrochloride | 250 mg PO/IM tid–qid prn 200 mg PR tid–qid prn | |
| **Prophylaxis** | | |
| Beta blockers | — | Vasoconstriction may lead to fetal growth retardation. Near term, they may cause fetal hypoglycemia, bradycardia, respiratory depression, and hyperbilirubinemia. |
| Propranolol hydrochloride | 60–160 mg qd | |
| Verapamil hydrochloride | 120–480 mg daily (slow release) in one or two doses | May cause uterine relaxation, prolonging labor, if used near term. |
| Amitriptyline hydrochloride May use other tricyclics (nortriptyline hydrochloride, desipramine hydrochloride) with fewer side effects. | 25–100 mg qd at hs | Some reported anomalies, but not clearly caused by amitriptyline hydrochloride. Potential for neonatal withdrawal syndrome and urinary retention if used near term. |

suspected pseudotumor cerebri should also include MRI, preferably with a magnetic resonance venogram, to rule out possible venous sinus thrombosis. These studies are safe during pregnancy and reliably demonstrate venous thrombosis, unless it is confined to the cavernous sinus or to a cortical vein.

As in all patients with pseudotumor, vision loss is the primary concern, and careful monitoring of visual acuity and visual fields is critical to determine the

*Table 23.3*   Oral contraceptives: estrogen dose, age, and stroke risk

| Estrogen dose | Absolute attributable risk: strokes per 100,000 |
|---|---|
| 20-yr-old women | |
| 50 µg | 6 |
| 30–40 µg | 4 |
| 40-yr-old women | |
| 50 µg | 40 |
| 30–40 µg | 60 |

Source: Data used with permission from Ø Lidegaard. Oral contraception and risk of a cerebral thromboembolic attack: results of a case-control study. BMJ 1993;306:956–963.

need for intervention. Treatment generally includes weight loss, lumbar puncture, administration of acetazolamide, and in some cases operative intervention with either optic nerve sheath fenestration or lumboperitoneal shunt to preserve vision. Pregnant patients should not try to lose weight; however, careful control of weight gain to 20 lb or less is recommended. Acetazolamide is not an established teratogen and appears to be safe during pregnancy; however, its use is best delayed until after the first trimester. When vision is stable, lumbar punctures may be performed to temporize until delivery. In severe cases, where osmotic diuretics such as mannitol and glycerol are needed for more aggressive medical therapy, careful monitoring of electrolytes and fetal growth is necessary. In cases with progressive vision loss or other severe effects of intracranial hypertension, surgical decompression should be performed during pregnancy. When there is vision loss, this surgery may be optic sheath fenestration or lumboperitoneal shunt. With more severe effects of intracranial hypertension, such as altered consciousness with no other reversible cause, CSF shunting should be done. Also, when relief of headache is a major goal of surgical intervention, the patient will more likely benefit from shunting than from optic sheath fenestration.

Sometimes the elevation of intracranial pressure will resolve shortly after delivery. In cases where there has been a good response to lumbar puncture and acetazolamide or both during pregnancy, it may be possible to stop the acetazolamide at the time of delivery. Acetazolamide is excreted in small amounts in breast milk, and newborn exposure is low. The manufacturer recommends that it not be given to nursing mothers, however, because of the potential problems with fluid, electrolyte, and acid-base balance in the infant. Therefore, if it is needed for treatment of the mother, formula feeding is necessary.

It has been reported that pregnancy may promote pseudotumor cerebri both in patients with and without a prior history of it. Digre and colleagues found, however, that 8.3% of 109 women were pregnant at the onset of pseudotumor and argued that this rate does not exceed the chance rate in women between 15 and 44 years of age [14]. In their patients, pseudotumor did not affect the outcome of pregnancy, and pregnancy did not increase the risk of vision loss. It is also not clear that subsequent pregnancies promote the recurrence of symptomatic pseudotumor cerebri. Therefore, in general, patients need not be counseled to avoid future pregnancies.

In his series, Digre did not find a relationship between oral contraceptive use and pseudotumor [14]. Claims of such a relationship have been made in the past; however, there are no systematic studies of this issue, and interpretation of such claims is complicated by the widespread use of these drugs.

## SEIZURES AND PREGNANCY

The coexistence of epilepsy and pregnancy and the desire of patients with epilepsy for effective contraception raise many important questions concerning both mother and child. There are a multitude of studies addressing these issues. Two publications offering concise guidelines for clinicians are included in the chapter references [15,16].

### Risks of Seizures during Pregnancy

The risks to the mother of seizures during pregnancy are the same as the risks at any time. The main risks are trauma related to sudden loss of consciousness and falls or tongue biting, the debated potential for seizures to promote more seizures, and the risks of the potentially severe medical and neurologic effects of status epilepticus in patients prone to this condition.

The risks to the fetus of seizures per se are mainly the risks of direct trauma, as from a blow to the gravid uterus during a fall and tonic-clonic activity, and the risks of fetal hypoxia and other metabolic effects resulting from prolonged seizures. In addition, in patients with idiopathic epilepsy, the risks of developmental malformations, cognitive deficits, and seizures in the offspring are statistically increased. This increase may be a result of hereditary factors transmitted by either the affected or the unaffected parent or of psychosocial factors that cluster with epilepsy.

### Risks of Antiepileptic Drugs

Teratogenesis

The fetus exposed to antiepileptic drugs (AEDs) during development is at a slightly increased risk for many major malformations that cause significant dysfunction or death, including neural tube defects, congenital heart lesions, orofacial clefts, intestinal atresia, and urogenital malformations. Although there is a voluminous literature on the risks of various agents, the available information is conflicting, and, with a few exceptions, it is difficult to differentiate the relative risks of the various AEDs in this regard. Despite the well-known reports of teratogenicity of phenytoin, termed *fetal hydantoin syndrome* [17], phenytoin does not clearly convey a higher teratogenic risk than other agents. Valproic acid is associated with a 1–2% risk of neural tube defects, most commonly spina bifida aperta [18,19]. Carbamazepine is associated with a risk of neural tube defects of approximately 0.5–1.0% [20,21]. Phenytoin and phenobarbital prob-

*Table 23.4*   Relative timing and developmental pathology of certain malformations

| Tissues | Malformations | Approximate interval after first day of last menstrual period |
|---|---|---|
| Central nervous system | Meningomyelocele | 28 days |
| Face | Cleft lip | 36 days |
|  | Cleft maxillary palate | 10 wks |
| Heart | Ventricular septal defect | 6 wks |

Source: Reprinted with permission from AV Delgado-Escueta, D Janz. Consensus guidelines: preconception counseling, management, and care of the the pregnant woman with epilepsy. Neurology 1992;42(suppl 5):152.

ably most commonly cause ventricular septal defects and cleft lip and palate. The common use of multiple drugs in combination complicates the analysis of the effects of single agents. It is clear, however, that combinations of drugs entail greater risks than single agents, especially for congenital heart defects and facial clefts, and single agents should be used wherever possible. In particular, valproic acid and carbamazepine increase the risk of neural tube defects, and combinations of these two agents with phenobarbital caused a very high rate of malformations (58%) in one small series [22]. Trimethadione has been associated with a particularly high rate of malformations, and this drug should be avoided altogether during pregnancy [23]. Many studies have tried to quantify the risk of a major malformation. This risk is roughly 6–8% with monotherapy and higher with polypharmacy [18,24,25]. The timing of exposure also greatly influences risk (Table 23.4).

Minor defects that cause less severe degrees of dysfunction and minor dysmorphisms that have no significant medical consequences may also occur at an increased rate in the infants of mothers on AEDs. This association has been questioned, however, and it will take further large-scale studies to establish a definite connection. The fetal hydantoin syndrome was first described and is best known. Later authors, however, have reported similar syndromes in patients taking other AEDs. Moreover, infants of mothers with epilepsy who are unexposed to AEDs in utero have a higher rate of minor malformations than the general population [26], and many of the features reported in the original description of the syndrome may be associated with inheritance from epileptic mothers or the infants' fathers. Most of these defects become increasingly less apparent with maturity [27].

Hanson and Smith described the fetal hydantoin syndrome in 1975 [17]. Their description included craniofacial anomalies (epicanthal folds, hypertelorism, and others), limb defects (digital hypoplasia and others), growth deficiency, and mental deficiency. As noted, similar findings have since been reported to accompany in utero exposure to other AEDs; these findings suggest that the syndrome as originally reported was not specific to phenytoin. Hypertelorism and digital hypoplasia have retained the greatest claim to a true and specific association [26].

Neural tube closure is completed with closure of the posterior neuropore at approximately 29 days of gestation [28]. Both valproic acid and carbamazepine have been associated with an increased risk of spina bifida aperta [18–21]. Risk of neural tube defects is increased when there is a family history of defects. Therefore, such a history should be sought in the families of both parents. When a family history is uncovered, it is best to avoid the use of valproic acid and carbamazepine.

Sedation of the infant resulting from administration of barbiturates and benzodiazepines to the mother can lead to early medical complications and to poor feeding and slow weight gain. Infants may also develop irritability and seizures as a result of withdrawal from these agents after in utero exposure [29].

Ethosuximide is most commonly used in children with absence epilepsy and has only limited use in adults. Therefore, the issue of its effect on pregnancy arises only occasionally. Malformations have been reported in a few of the in utero exposures to ethosuximide; however, because of limited information and multiple drug exposures, a causal relationship cannot be confirmed.

Several new AEDs have become available, including lamotrigine, gabapentin, vigabatrin, and felbamate. The use of felbamate has been greatly restricted because of cases of severe marrow failure. None of the agents has been clinically tested in pregnant patients. Lamotrigine has caused toxicity in fetal rats at doses near the maximum antiepileptic dose. Although it has not shown evidence of teratogenicity in animal studies, it does lower fetal folate levels in rats. Gabapentin has been associated with an increased risk of malformations in animals at doses higher than those used in humans. Felbamate has not been shown to increase the risk of malformations in animals. No specific recommendation can be made for these drugs, except that they should be used in pregnancy only when the clinical need is clear and the patient understands that the risk is undefined.

Although reliable information concerning the effects of single-agent exposure in utero has been somewhat elusive, it is clear from the available studies that polypharmacy significantly increases the risk of major malformations [18,24,30]. Particularly implicated as increasing risk is the combination of valproic acid, carbamazepine, and phenobarbital. The infants of patients on monotherapy are more likely to have spinal defects and glandular hypospadias than to have the heart, facial, cognitive, and dysmorphic abnormalities seen with polypharmacy [18,27].

Studies of mice have found reduced levels of metabolites of tetrahydrofolate in animals treated with valproic acid at doses adequate to produce exencephaly. Treatment with folate reduces the risk of the malformation [31]. Low serum folate levels before pregnancy and in early pregnancy in women with epilepsy have been correlated with fetal malformations and spontaneous abortions [30]. A dose-response relation has been shown between decreased folate levels in pregnant women and AED levels and malformations at birth. In a study of women having a child with a neural tube defect, the use of folate supplements (4 mg/day) before the diagnosis of a subsequent pregnancy provided a 72% protective effect when compared to the use of no therapy and other vitamins in control subjects [32]. Given this information, it is best to recommend folate supplementation in all women with child-bearing potential who are taking AEDs and to supplement folate in all pregnant women taking AEDs. The optimal dose for supplementation has not been established, and recommendations vary from 1 to 5 mg per day. When particular concern arises, red blood cell and serum levels can be measured to ensure adequate supplementation.

## Hemorrhagic Risks

AEDs can cause depletion of the vitamin K–dependent clotting factors II, VII, IX, and X in newborns [33,34]. Hemorrhagic complications can occur in mothers and especially in the newborns of mothers treated with AEDs. Such complications are most common with phenobarbital, primidone, and phenytoin but can occur with other agents, including carbamazepine, benzodiazepines, and ethosuximide.

Risk to the mother is relatively low and usually limited to increased bleeding during delivery. The greater risk is to the newborn. Intracranial, intrathoracic, and intra-abdominal bleeding can occur, and the mortality may be very high [16,34]. Unlike other types of neonatal hemorrhage, which usually occur on the second or third day of life, hemorrhage caused by AED exposure in utero often occurs in the first 24 hours.

It is generally agreed that newborns exposed to these drugs in utero should receive 1 mg of intramuscular vitamin K immediately after birth to prevent hemorrhage. When the prothrombin time and partial thromboplastin time of cord blood are severely prolonged or when bleeding occurs, intravenous vitamin K and fresh frozen plasma should be given [33,34]. There is less consensus regarding the prophylactic treatment of the mother. Many authors recommend treatment with oral vitamin $K_1$ at 20 mg per day during the last month of pregnancy [16,33,35].

## Breast-Feeding Risks

The excretion of anticonvulsant medications into breast milk depends primarily on their molecular size, charge, and degree of protein binding. Drugs that are highly protein bound show much lower levels in breast milk than in plasma. The levels achieved in the serum of the feeding infant also depend on the half-life of the drug. All of the main drugs are excreted to some degree in breast milk. In most cases the excretion is low enough to avoid significant levels in the infant, and therefore these drugs can be used in the breast-feeding mother (Table 23.5). As an example, carbamazepine is excreted into milk with a milk to plasma ratio of roughly 0.40. Assuming a therapeutic serum level of 10 mg/liter, one would expect a concentration of 4 mg/liter in breast milk. If an infant then drinks 1 liter of milk per day, he

*Table 23.5*　Excretion of anticonvulsant drugs in breast milk

| Drug | Percentage unbound in serum | Percentage of plasma level in breast milk | Breast milk concentration range (mg/liter) |
|---|---|---|---|
| Phenytoin | 10 | 18 | 1.8–3.6 |
| Carbamazepine | 25 | 41 | 1.6–4.1 |
| Phenobarbital | 40 | 36 | 5.4–10.8 |
| Valproic acid | 5–10 | 2.5 | 1.25–2.25 |
| Primidone | 80 | 70 | 2.5–8.4 |
| Ethosuximide | 97 | 86 | 4.3–8.6 |

or she will receive a daily dose of 4 mg of carbamazepine. Assuming a weight of 5 kg, the dose is 0.8 mg/kg per day, roughly one-tenth of the recommended therapeutic dose. In most cases, doses in this range have no significant effect on the infant. The main problem that arises is central nervous system depression of infants with the sedating agents. Both phenobarbital and the commonly used benzodiazepines have long enough half-lives for infants to accumulate significant levels over time. In such cases, sedation and drug withdrawal can occur. In particular, phenobarbital has a longer half-life in infants than in adults (40–300 hours), as well as a lesser bound fraction; these characteristics make it a relatively common problem for breast-feeding mothers. With the caveat that the infants of mothers on phenobarbital, primidone, and benzodiazepines should be observed for sedation, all of the commonly used AEDs are compatible with breast-feeding. Little is known about the newer agents lamotrigine, gabapentin, felbamate, and vigabatrin.

## Managing Antiepileptic Drug Therapy in Anticipation of and during Pregnancy

When patients with epilepsy who are planning a pregnancy have been seizure-free for 2 years, it is reasonable to try a slowly tapering withdrawal of their AEDs. For patients with controlled or rare but more recent seizures, an individualized decision weighing risks and benefits of the discontinuation of AEDs must be made. When AEDs are indicated during pregnancy, it is best to attempt to move to therapy with a single agent before conception. This transfer can be accomplished by first achieving the desired level of the chosen drug and then tapering the other AEDs over a period of 1 to 3 months. Although it is certainly best in principle to maintain the lowest effective dose and level, this dose may be difficult to determine in practice.

### *Alterations in Pharmacokinetics*

Several physiologic changes during the course of pregnancy affect the pharmacokinetics and levels of AEDs. These changes may affect drug absorption, distribution, elimination by metabolic conversion and renal clearance, and protein binding. The effects become increasingly important as the pregnancy progresses. Pregnancy reduces gastric motility and thus compromises AED absorption. Also, antacid medications are commonly prescribed during pregnancy, and these may decrease absorption of drugs that are weak acids by causing ion trapping within the gut lumen. Intravascular and extracellular volumes increase. The increased cardiac output is distributed to many organs, including the placenta and kidneys, so that increased metabolic conversion and renal clearance are promoted. The increased volume of distribution creates a need for higher loading doses of AEDs. The placenta contains enzyme systems for oxidation, reduction, hydrolysis, and conjugation, including cytochrome P-450 enzymes responsible for the bulk of phenytoin metabolism. These systems greatly increase the metabolic mass and promote more rapid conversion of many AEDs. Fetal metabolism adds only a small amount to the increased metabolic rate. Renal blood flow and clearance increase, and this increase causes a more rapid elimination of AEDs that exit unchanged in the urine. The serum albumin level falls, and there is a corresponding decrease in protein binding of drugs. Because many AEDs are highly protein bound, this change may significantly affect total levels and the unbound fraction of drug. As a result, a given total level, as commonly measured, corresponds to a higher free and effective level during pregnancy. What one typically witnesses clinically is a demonstrable fall in the total level with maintenance of the free level.

Phenytoin has been most extensively studied and appears to undergo the most dramatic increase in dose-to-level ratio during pregnancy. During the first 32 weeks of pregnancy, there is a gradual rise until, during the last 8 weeks of pregnancy, it is common to see a twofold increase in the dose needed to maintain an adequate level. Increased metabolic conversion accounts for the bulk of this increased clearance. Phenytoin is a weak acid, and it may also be absorbed inefficiently, especially when antacids are given. It is also highly protein bound, approximately 90%. Binding decreases through the first 16 weeks of pregnancy and then returns to normal over the 5–7 weeks postpartum [36]. There may be an immediate rise in phenytoin levels after delivery that compensates for a large part of the altered metabolism. This increase may occur because placental metabolism accounts for most of the change during pregnancy.

Valproic acid may also undergo a much-increased metabolic clearance as a result of conversion and enhanced renal elimination. By the third trimester, a dose doubling may be necessary as with phenytoin [36]. Also, like phenytoin, valproic acid is highly protein bound (85–90%) and the free ratio increases with increasing levels [36].

Other AEDs are affected to a lesser extent. Carbamazepine is metabolized through the active carbamazepine-10,11-epoxide metabolite. Because this metabolite may have toxic and teratogenic as well as anticonvulsant effects, its concentration should be considered when adjusting doses. Increased metabolic conversion probably accounts for the increased dose-to-level ratio. The effect is smaller for carbamazepine than for phenytoin. Carbamazepine is about 75% protein bound, so the effect of altered binding is also less. The effect of pregnancy on phenobarbital is also slight compared to its effect on phenytoin and valproic acid. Protein binding is not significantly changed. Primidone is metabolized through the active compounds phenobarbital and phenylethylmalonamide, and these substances should be measured when adjusting doses.

### Monitoring Recommendations

When AEDs are used during pregnancy, levels should be checked periodically and maintained at the lowest effective dose. When levels are low, noncompliance should be considered, as with any patient. It should be remembered that late in pregnancy, lower protein binding dictates that a lower total level will reflect a given active level, so that doses should not be excessively increased to maintain a stable total level. Measurement of free levels can help determine the proper dose. As the pregnancy progresses, it is most common for the effective level to fall so that there is a need to increase the dose—with phenytoin, by 50–100%. In late pregnancy, it is prudent to check levels approximately every other week, or more often if there is any instability in the epileptic condition. During the 4–8 weeks after delivery, the required dose will gradually decline to the dose required before the pregnancy. Levels must be checked and appropriate dose reductions made during this period. Phenytoin may represent an exception to this postpartum course.

Its level may abruptly rise after delivery, perhaps caused by loss of placental metabolism or by increased absorption. Therefore, it is reasonable to immediately lower the phenytoin dose by half of the supplemental increment that was given during the pregnancy and then gradually taper the other half.

### Use and Timing of Ultrasonography and Amniocentesis for Alpha-Fetoprotein

Three major tests are used to monitor pregnancy for the possible early diagnosis of fetal abnormalities: ultrasonography, measurement of maternal serum alpha-fetoprotein (AFP) levels, and amniocentesis with measurement of amniotic fluid AFP levels. In experienced hands, high-resolution ultrasonography and measurement of serum AFP levels can detect more than 94% of neural tube defects [37]. This expertise is not available in most centers, however, and measurement of amniotic fluid AFP levels remains the standard for early diagnosis of such defects. Referral centers offer amniocentesis with amniotic fluid AFP testing at approximately 15–17 weeks, based on the poor sensitivity of serum AFP testing [38]. Ultrasonography can identify other malformations, such as those of the heart and face. When performed at about 20 weeks, it optimally allows identification of defects with time to repeat a questionable result and safely terminate pregnancy. The decision to perform such tests will depend on the patient's attitude concerning the termination of a pregnancy. The patient and obstetrician should discuss these issues and determine the need for and timing of tests.

## PRE-ECLAMPSIA AND ECLAMPSIA

Pre-eclampsia is a multisystem disorder of mid- to late pregnancy (generally after 20 weeks of gestation) characterized by hypertension, edema, and proteinuria. The criteria for diagnosis as published by the American Congress of Obstetrics and Gynecology are shown in Table 23.6.

In addition to these abnormalities, many patients will develop an accompanying thrombocytopenia, microangiopathic hemolytic anemia, and abnormalities of liver and, sometimes, renal function. The acronym HELLP has been

*Table 23.6*   Criteria for the diagnosis of pre-eclampsia and eclampsia

*Pre-eclampsia*

   Hypertension: diastolic blood pressure ≥90 mm Hg or systolic blood pressure ≥140 mm Hg or rise of diastolic blood pressure by 15 mm Hg or systolic blood pressure by 30 mm Hg on at least two readings 6 hrs apart *and*

   Proteinuria: ≥300 mg protein/24 hrs or ≥1 g/liter protein in at least two random specimens ≥6 hrs apart *or*

   Edema: >1+ pitting edema after 12 hrs bed rest or weight gain of ≥5 lb in 1 wk

*Eclampsia*

   Seizures: convulsions not caused by any coincidental neurologic disease, such as epilepsy, in a woman who meets the criteria for pre-eclampsia

Source: Reprinted with permission from PW Kaplan, JT Repke. Eclampsia. Neurol Clin 1994;12:566.

coined to refer to the hemolytic anemia, elevated liver function tests, and low platelet counts seen in some women with severe pre-eclampsia. This pattern of findings suggests a pathogenic role for endothelial cells in this disorder on analogy with disorders that it resembles, such as thrombotic thrombocytopenic purpura (TTP) and hemolytic uremic syndrome [39]. Various abnormalities of endothelial cell function have been found to accompany pre-eclampsia, although none has been established as the primary underlying disorder. It is likely that a placental factor initiates a cascade of dysfunction that compromises control of vascular tone and permeability [39]. The abnormalities in vascular tone and permeability underlie the neurologic complications that are common in pre-eclampsia–eclampsia.

Eclampsia is defined as pre-eclampsia complicated by seizures or coma and may occur when there are few other signs of pre-eclampsia [40]. Risk factors include nulliparity, poor nourishment, multiparity and age greater than 35 years, extrauterine pregnancy, and molar pregnancy.

## Eclamptic Seizures

The cause of eclamptic seizures has not been fully elucidated, but they emerge in the context of eclamptic encephalopathy. The pathologic state of brain underlying them appears to be the cerebral edema and possibly ischemia that result from the hypertension and vasculopathy of eclampsia. The seizures can be focal or generalized, although in the latter case there is probably secondary generalization after an inapparent focal onset.

Traditional therapy of pre-eclampsia–eclampsia has included the infusion of magnesium sulfate. The effectiveness of magnesium for anticonvulsant therapy is controversial [41,42,43], and it is best to treat seizures with an effective traditional antiepileptic drug, such as phenytoin, phenobarbital, or lorazepam. Two studies, however, validate the traditional wisdom and argue strongly for the effectiveness of magnesium sulfate in preventing eclamptic seizures. In one study, magnesium sulfate was compared to phenytoin and diazepam and appeared to have a greater effect than either of these in preventing seizure recurrence [44]. In another study, women with pregnancy-induced hypertension were given either magnesium sulfate or phenytoin and followed for the occurrence of seizures. Magnesium sulfate strongly outperformed phenytoin for seizure prevention [45]. The possible role of excitotoxicity mediated by $N$-methyl-D-aspartate (NMDA) receptors in the pathogenesis of seizures and the function of magnesium as a physiologic NMDA blocker provide a potential mechanism of action to be further investigated [46]. With the available information, it can be recommended that magnesium sulfate be given for pre-eclampsia to prevent seizures. Once seizures occur, there is no reason to withhold traditional antiepileptic drugs. The best choice is phenytoin, because it can be given intravenously and does not cause neonatal sedation, as do phenobarbital and the benzodiazepines. These latter two drugs, however, may also be chosen when phenytoin allergy contraindicates its use. Magnesium sulfate may be continued while phenytoin is given, although care must be taken to avoid side effects such as cardiac arrhythmia, sedation, and respiratory depression that can occur with high magnesium levels [40].

## Hypertensive Encephalopathy

Although probably more common than seizures, toxemic encephalopathy as a result of hypertensive encephalopathy and resultant cerebral edema is less widely recognized. The cerebral blood flow is normally maintained within relatively narrow bounds despite large fluctuations in the mean arterial pressure. This maintenance of cerebral blood flow is accomplished by the autoregulatory capacity of the cerebral blood vessels. When the upper threshold of autoregulation is exceeded, cerebral blood flow increases. The underlying endothelial dysfunction that is thought to contribute to pre-eclampsia–eclampsia may result in both impaired vascular relaxation (and hence systemic hypertension and local vasospasm with resultant cerebral ischemia) and early breakthrough of autoregulation at mean arterial pressures significantly below the 150–160 mm Hg tolerated by normal vessels (and hence excessive cerebral blood flow with resultant cerebral edema and sometimes hemorrhage). These lesions are most commonly seen in the territory of the posterior circulation, although other regions may be affected [47].

Affected patients commonly develop headaches and visual symptoms, including scintillations, scotomas, and cortical blindness. More severe degrees of encephalopathy may affect other structures, primarily those in the posterior fossa, producing corresponding deficits: cranial nerve deficits and motor and sensory deficits involving the extremities (pons and midbrain), ataxia (cerebellum), and depressed level of consciousness (midbrain, thalamus, or hemispheres). Where the ultimate pathology is vasogenic edema and microhemorrhage, the lesions will be reversible. Some patients, however, develop persistent deficits caused by larger hemorrhage or infarction.

Evaluation of patients with headache, cranial nerve deficits, focal signs, confusion, or depression of the level of consciousness in the context of late pregnancy should include an examination and laboratory studies to look for features of eclampsia. Brain imaging may show evidence of cerebral edema as areas of high signal on T2-weighted MRI scans or areas of low density on CT scans (Figure 23.1) Sometimes lesions enhance slightly with contrast agents. They are most commonly seen in the white matter of the occipital and parietal lobes. Lesions involving grey matter and extending throughout the territory of the posterior circulation and into areas of the anterior circulation also occur, however. Areas of infarction and hemorrhage may be present. Magnetic resonance angiography and venography clarify the diagnosis when arterial occlusion or venous infarction is a possible competing diagnosis. Single photon emission computed tomography can help to differentiate between the hyperperfusion usually seen with hypertensive encephalopathy and the hypoperfusion seen with arterial occlusion; however, this study is not usually needed in clinical situations. Patients with the HELLP syndrome and hypertensive encephalopathy may fulfill all of the traditional criteria for the diagnosis of TTP. The latter is more likely to affect the kidneys and to have accompanying fever. In some cases the ultimate diagnosis may depend on the clinical context and course.

The most important therapy in cases of severe pre-eclampsia–eclampsia is aggressive control of blood pressure and administration of magnesium sulfate. Many patients will have a low intravascular volume, and renal function should be monitored and fluid therapy carefully managed as hypertension is brought quickly under control. Significant thrombocytopenia increases the risk of

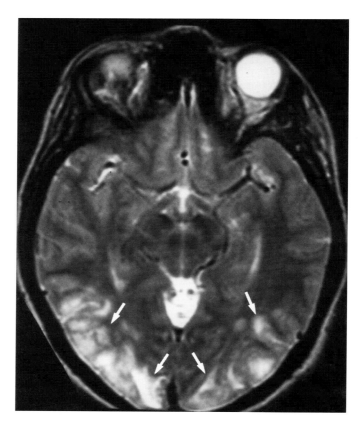

*Figure 23.1*    Magnetic resonance image (MRI) of a 35-year-old woman who developed a severe headache followed by a generalized tonic-clonic seizure 3 days after a normal-term delivery. Her blood pressure on admission was 160/84 mm Hg. The axial T2-weighted MRI shows increased signal intensity involving the grey and white matter of both occipital lobes and extending forward into the posterior temporal lobes consistent with hypertensive encephalopathy (*arrows*) (1.5 Tesla, TR/TE/NEX = 3000/80 eff/1).

intracranial hemorrhage and complicates management. Platelet transfusions will restore safe counts. In the majority of cases, deficits result from brain edema, and even extensive ones are reversible with supportive care.

## CEREBROVASCULAR DISEASE AND PREGNANCY

Pregnancy increases the risk of stroke by several mechanisms. Ischemic stroke may accompany toxemic encephalopathy, as noted above, although most such deficits are reversible. Pregnancy and delivery cause a state of hypercoagulability that can promote arterial occlusion or venous thrombosis. Patients with toxemic encephalopathy may have intracranial hemorrhage with or without thrombocytopenia. Also, some vascular anomalies may bleed at an increased rate during pregnancy.

## Hypercoagulability

Normal pregnancy causes several changes that promote hypercoagulability. Platelet reactivity is increased. Levels of coagulation factors VII, VIII, and X rise. Levels of protein S fall, while levels of protein C remain unchanged [48,49]. Fibrin generation is increased, and fibrinolysis is inhibited by high levels of endothelially derived plasminogen activator inhibitor type 1 (PAI-1) and placentally derived PAI-2, especially in the third trimester [48,49]. Risk of venous thrombosis is increased by any underlying predisposition to thrombosis, such as resistance to activated protein C resulting from a point mutation in the gene coding for factor V (Leiden mutation) or antiphospholipid antibody syndrome.

Arterial Cerebral Infarction

Arterial infarction is an uncommon complication of pregnancy. There is some controversy concerning the absolute risk. Wiebers found the risk of ischemic stroke to be 33 per 100,000 pregnancies, an estimated thirteenfold increase above the expected rate among women of childbearing age; the large majority of strokes were caused by arterial occlusion [50]. Several other studies have found a lower risk of ischemic stroke during pregnancy and the puerperium of about 4–5 per 100,000, although these figures still represent an increased risk of severalfold [51–53]. A large-scale population-based study differentiated the risk during pregnancy, when no increased risk was found, and the risk during the puerperium, when an almost ninefold increased risk was found [54]. The risk conferred by the hypercoagulable state of pregnancy may be augmented during the puerperium by the rapid decrease in blood volume. There is evidence for a vasculopathy in preeclampsia as noted above, and changes intrinsic to the vessel wall may also contribute to risk in a way that has not been clearly defined. When investigating the cause of arterial occlusion during pregnancy, the clinician should seek evidence of cardioembolism, paradoxical embolism through a patent foramen ovale, and in situ thrombosis at a site of vascular abnormality, including vascular dissection; the clinician should also look for early atherosclerosis as well as drug abuse and other causes of stroke in young patients.

Pregnant women who have the antiphospholipid antibody syndrome with or without lupus erythematosus are at risk for spontaneous abortion, stillbirth, and pre-eclampsia and for thrombotic events, including stroke. Because of the risk of fetal loss, low dosages of aspirin (≤150 mg/day), with or without prednisone, are often given to such patients during the second and third trimesters. Studies of low-dose aspirin use for pregnancy-induced hypertension suggest that such therapy is safe for the newborn and mother [55]. When there is a history of prior stroke or another thrombotic event, anticoagulant therapy is recommended. If a prolonged course of anticoagulants is needed before delivery, a regimen of adjusted-dose, subcutaneous heparin should be given to maintain an activated partial thromboplastin time of 1.5–2.5 times the control value [56,57]. Low-molecular-weight regimens provide the safety of heparin for the fetus with the added benefit that they allow once-daily dosing and do not cause thrombocytopenia. These regimens will probably be substituted as clinical experience with them increases. Warfarin crosses the placenta and is contraindicated during pregnancy because of its teratogenicity, though heparin, which does not cross the placenta, is relatively safe. Heparin does increase the risk of maternal bleeding complications. In most cases in which heparin is used to reduce stroke risk, it is reasonable to discontinue it 24 hours before electively induced labor. Protamine sulfate can be used when needed because of persistent anticoagulant effect during labor.

## Venous Sinus Thrombosis

Venous sinus thrombosis causes 20–40% of ischemic strokes related to pregnancy. The great majority of these occur during the first few postpartum weeks [50,51]. Venous sinus thrombosis should be considered whenever a pregnant or postpartum woman presents with a depressed level of consciousness, persistent headache, seizure, or focal neurologic symptoms. The presentation is the same as that for nonpregnant patients with evidence of increased intracranial pressure or with focal symptoms and signs. Onset may be insidious and findings minimal. Some patients may present with findings identical to those in pseudotumor cerebri. Especially suggestive are bilateral focal deficits with recurrent seizures. Cerebral venous thrombosis can also present with findings of cavernous sinus thrombosis; however, this presentation usually results from regional spread of a local bacterial infection and not from systemic hypercoagulability. Because the presentations are varied and the symptoms and signs nonspecific, it is important to maintain a high index of suspicion for cerebral venous thrombosis.

When this diagnosis is suspected, noncontrast CT may show a hyperdense superior sagittal or lateral sinus or a subtle dense cortical vein. There may be indirect evidence of thrombosis, such as infarction, edema, or hemorrhage. A contrast CT may show an empty delta sign—enhancement of the dura forming the superior sagittal sinus seen in cross-section around the low signal of a luminal clot—or tentorial or gyral enhancement. MRI will typically show subacute clot as hyperintense signal within the sinus on T1- and T2-weighted images. A magnetic resonance venous flow study demonstrates the lack of flow in the involved sinus (Figure 23.2).

Heparin has been shown to improve outcome of cerebral venous sinus thrombosis [58]. This appears to be true even when hemorrhagic venous infarction is present, although special care is necessary, because there is a risk of promoting frank hemorrhage. General issues of heparin use in pregnancy apply as discussed above for arterial cerebral infarction. Heparin does not cross the placenta, and it should be given as for nonpregnant patients. The heparin can be held at the onset of uterine contractions and restarted after delivery to minimize hemorrhagic risks. Warfarin should not be used during pregnancy because it crosses the placenta and can produce teratogenic effects when given early in pregnancy and, more to the point here, fetal and neonatal hemorrhage and placental abruption later [59].

## Cerebral Hemorrhage

Intracranial hemorrhage is an important cause of maternal death during pregnancy, accounting for 5–12% of the total [60]. Many possible causes may underlie cere-

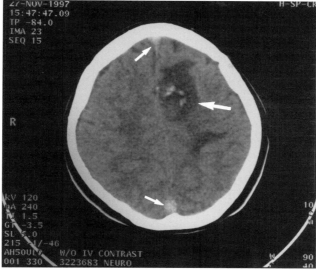

A

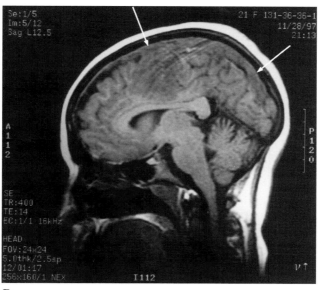

B

*Figure 23.2*   Scans of a 21-year-old woman who developed a headache, right hemiparesis, and focal seizure 1 week after a term delivery complicated by pre-eclampsia. Computed tomography (CT) and magnetic resonance imaging (MRI) reveal typical findings of superior sagittal sinus (SSS) thrombosis. **(A)** Noncontrast axial CT scan at presentation shows a parasagittal left frontal hemorrhagic infarct and extensive surrounding edema (*large arrow*) and hyperdensity of the SSS anteriorly and posteriorly (*small arrows*). **(B)** Sagittal T1-weighted MRI 48 hours after onset shows isointense signal along the length of the SSS (*arrows*) consistent with acute thrombosis (1.5 Tesla, TR/TE=400/14).

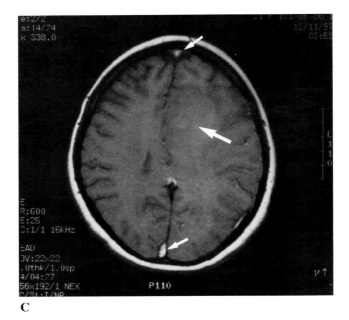

**C**

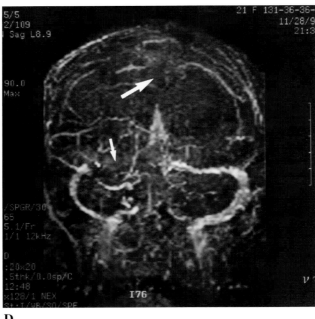

**D**

*Figure 23.2* (continued) **(C)** Axial T1-weighted MRI 2 weeks after onset shows hyperintensity in the SSS anteriorly and posteriorly (*small arrows*) consistent with subacute thrombosis and mass effect from the left frontal hemorrhagic infarct (*large arrow*) (1.5 Tesla, TR/TE=600/25). **(D)** Frontal projection of a magnetic resonance venous flow study reveals the absence of flow signal in the SSS (*large arrow*) and the right transverse sinus (*small arrow*).

bral hemorrhage during pregnancy. These include pre-eclampsia–eclampsia, aneurysm, vascular malformations, and the various other causes of hemorrhage in young adults. Special issues arise when considering the risk of hemorrhage of established lesions, such as aneurysms or arteriovenous malformations (AVMs), and the timing of surgical therapy.

Aneurysm

Subarachnoid hemorrhage resulting from rupture of an arterial aneurysm is the most common cause of intracranial hemorrhage during pregnancy; it is slightly more common than rupture of an AVM [60,61]. As with any aneurysm, the risk of rupture during pregnancy depends on its size. Risk also appears to rise with maternal age and increasing gestational age. Several physiologic changes accompanying pregnancy might underlie this progressive risk. Blood volume increases by about 45%, reaching a maximum around 32 weeks and then leveling off until delivery. Blood pressure begins falling by 7 weeks, reaches a nadir at about 24–28 weeks, and then slowly rises toward normal by term. Stroke volume and cardiac output increase, peaking at 20–24 weeks. Heart rate increases, reaching its maximum at 32 weeks, after which it is maintained until delivery [62]. Hormonal changes mediate an increased laxity of blood vessels during pregnancy. Because the risk continues to rise after the peak of blood volume, blood pressure, and stroke volume, intrinsic changes in vessel walls probably contribute significantly to this increased bleeding risk. The risk of recurrent bleeding from an untreated aneurysm after subarachnoid hemorrhage is probably high. Estimates quoted are 33–50% (this number includes AVMs, which bleed at a lower rate; see below [60]). Although many authors have reported that labor and delivery do not pose an increased risk of rupture [63], when analysis is made of the risk of rupture per day, this daily risk is found to increase severalfold on the day of delivery [61].

When subarachnoid hemorrhage is considered because the patient has experienced headache, syncope, or presyncope, the patient should have a CT scan to look for blood. If no blood is seen, lumbar puncture, including analysis for xanthochromia, should be performed to take a more sensitive look. When aneurysm is expected on clinical grounds, including after subarachnoid hemorrhage, the woman should undergo cerebral angiography with proper shielding of the fetus. Iodinated contrast may be given without significant risk to the fetus if maternal hydration is maintained. When an aneurysm is identified, it should be treated based on neurosurgical principles. When there is a large and accessible aneurysm and no neurologic devastation from a prior subarachnoid hemorrhage, surgical clipping during the pregnancy is indicated in most cases to avoid the high mortality associated with nonsurgical care. Nimodipine is given to reduce the risk of vasospasm. After successful clipping and recovery to a stable neurologic condition, vaginal delivery is preferable. In patients who do not undergo operative therapy before delivery, it is advisable to deliver the patient by cesarean section even though cesarean delivery has not been shown to improve outcome. Cesarean delivery is also advised if labor begins during the acute recovery phase after surgical clipping. However, this recommendation also remains unsupported by systematic data.

## Arteriovenous Malformation

AVMs may present with seizures or intracranial hemorrhage. There has been some controversy concerning the risk of hemorrhage of AVMs during pregnancy. In a much-quoted paper, Robinson and colleagues reported an incidence of hemorrhage of 33% between the thirtieth week of gestation and the sixth postpartum week in patients with AVMs discovered after subarachnoid hemorrhage. Based on this interpretation of the data, they recommended elective cesarean delivery at 38 weeks [64]. The method of discovery in their series, however, does not allow a calculation of the risk of hemorrhage of AVMs. Later series suggest that the rate of hemorrhage is much lower and may not be significantly increased by pregnancy and delivery. Horton and colleagues reported a retrospective analysis of 540 pregnancies in 451 women with known AVM [63]. They found a rate of hemorrhage of 0.035 per person-year or 3.5% per year, a rate no greater than that among nonpregnant women without a prior hemorrhage. They found the rate of hemorrhage to be uniform throughout pregnancy and the puerperium. Among other differences from Robinson's series, Horton and colleagues reported on all AVMs, while Robinson and colleagues reported on AVMs identified after hemorrhage, when the bleeding risk is probably greater. Weir and Macdonald noted the ratio of aneurysm to AVM causing intracranial hemorrhage during pregnancy to be 1.3 to 1 compared to 6.4 to 1 for these lesions in all patients (pregnant and nonpregnant) or 8.4 to 1 for all patients with intracranial hemorrhage. They argued that pregnancy has a greater effect on the bleeding rate of AVM; however, this argument does not take into account the age differences in the two groups—that is, that a younger population would be expected to have a higher proportion of AVMs [61].

Search for an AVM usually begins after a seizure or intracranial hemorrhage. In most cases an AVM will be seen on contrast CT scan; however, MRI is a more sensitive test. After identification by CT or MRI, a contrast angiogram is done to define the AVM and to look for evidence of simultaneous aneurysms. As in the workup of aneurysmal hemorrhage, the determination of the need for these tests should be made based on neurosurgical principles, as in nonpregnant patients.

Two major operative goals must be considered: the operative evacuation of an intracranial hemorrhage and the excision of the AVM. In most cases, surgery is deferred until after delivery. When there is major mass effect, however, especially with a cerebellar hematoma unresponsive to ventricular drainage and medical therapy, surgical evacuation of the clot is indicated during pregnancy. Given the data suggesting a relatively low rate of hemorrhage during pregnancy, in most cases surgical excision of the AVM may be deferred until after delivery, although neurosurgeons will differ in their interpretation of the data and approach. It is prudent to begin anticonvulsant therapy when the AVM presents with a seizure or involves the cortex, although there are no data to support the need for anticonvulsants in the latter case. Surgical excision is undertaken during pregnancy when multiple hemorrhagic events occur or when a small AVM is present and surgery is being done to treat a hematoma with mass effect. Both Horton and Dias found no added risk from vaginal delivery in patients with AVMs. Based on these data, vaginal delivery with epidural anesthesia is preferred unless obstetric considerations dictate a need for cesarean section. In the weeks following delivery, after maternal circulatory physiology has normalized, definitive therapy of the AVM should be undertaken.

## Pre-Eclampsia–Eclampsia and Thrombotic Thrombocytopenic Purpura

As noted above, hemorrhage may complicate pre-eclampsia–eclampsia and TTP, two disorders promoted by pregnancy. Hemorrhages of pre-eclampsia–eclampsia are most often lobar and posterior in the occipital and parietal lobes. They usually result from hypertensive encephalopathy and the vascular disease of pre-eclampsia–eclampsia. TTP may cause small petechial hemorrhages throughout the cerebral grey and hemispheric white matter or larger lobar or deep hemorrhages. In all cases, decisions concerning surgical or medical therapy should be based on a consideration of the medical issues (e.g., coagulopathy) and surgical issues (site, size, and risk of herniation). Although differentiation of these two disorders may present a clinical challenge because of their many overlapping features, it is important to do so as promptly as possible so that appropriate medical therapy can be initiated.

## Cerebrovascular Disease and Oral Contraceptive Agents

Oral contraceptive agents have been shown to increase the risk of ischemic stroke in young women. The risk varies with the estrogen content. The older tablets containing 50 μg or more of estrogen caused a significantly increased risk of thrombotic events, including stroke. This risk has been greatly diminished by lowering the estrogen content of the pills. The absolute risk remains quite low in this large population of young women; however, in those with other risk factors for thrombosis, it may be significant. The risk rises with age; it increases tenfold over the two decades from age 20 to age 40 [65] (see Table 23.3).

## MULTIPLE SCLEROSIS AND PREGNANCY

Young women of childbearing age are at highest risk to develop multiple sclerosis (MS). Most women with multiple sclerosis will remain stable or even improve during pregnancy. It has been hypothesized that this remission of multiple sclerosis, and of other autoimmune diseases, results from the physiologic immune suppression that fosters maintenance of normal pregnancy [66,67]. The risk of attacks appears to be increased during the postpartum period. Several retrospective studies argue that approximately 20–40% of women with MS have postpartum relapses, usually during the first 3 months after delivery. This incidence is roughly two to three times the expected rate [68]. However, this increased postpartum risk was not confirmed in a prospective study, which found risks to be unchanged during the first and second trimesters and during the 6 months postpartum and to be decreased during the third trimester [69]. Most studies agree that pregnancy conveys no long-term adverse effect, although the populations studied may reflect a selection bias for those with milder disease who choose to get pregnant. Multiple sclerosis does not appear to affect fertility, outcome of pregnancy, or ability to nurse. Patients with major disabilities, however, especially gait disorder and weakness, may find it difficult to care for their infants independently [70].

There is no consensus concerning the proper treatment of acute attacks of multiple sclerosis, although there is now evidence of improved early outcome in patients with acute optic neuritis treated with intravenous methylprednisolone followed by a tapering course of prednisone over 2 weeks. Although short-term use of moderate to low dosages of corticosteroids appears to be safe in mid- and late pregnancy, early use, high dose, or prolonged use may increase risks of fetal malformation, virilization, and adrenal suppression. If the physician chooses to treat attacks with corticosteroids, it is prudent to choose the lowest doses and briefest courses compatible with the clinical therapeutic goal. Other immunosuppressive drugs, such as cyclophosphamide and azathioprine, should be avoided until after delivery. Patients should also be advised of their potential effect on fertility.

Two new therapies have emerged for the treatment of relapsing-remitting multiple sclerosis: interferon-β-1b (Betaseron) and interferon-β-1a (Avonex). It is likely to become more common for women to become pregnant or to desire pregnancy while taking these medications. Pregnant and nursing patients have been excluded from the major studies of these drugs. Information concerning their safety in these contexts is limited. Animal data indicate that these drugs may have abortifacient effects at doses much higher than those recommended for therapy. The manufacturers recommend that patients discontinue therapy with them if they become pregnant or are planning pregnancy.

Other drugs are commonly used for symptomatic treatment of multiple sclerosis. Baclofen is an agonist of the inhibitory central neurotransmitter gamma-aminobutyric acid used for the skeletal muscle spasticity of MS. At doses many times greater than those used for therapy, it has been associated with developmental abnormalities in animals, but there is no evidence of human teratogenicity. Oxybutynin chloride is an antimuscarinic agent that promotes smooth muscle relaxation and is commonly used to treat the spastic neurogenic bladder of MS. Little is known about its influence on pregnancy or breast-feeding. Its mechanism of action suggests that it might impair uterine contractions. Amantadine hydrochloride has been used to counteract the debilitating fatigue of MS. Its mechanism of action is unclear, and little is known about its effect in pregnancy or during breast-feeding. The central nervous system stimulants methylphenidate hydrochloride and pemoline have also been used for fatigue. Little is known about their use in pregnancy or during breast-feeding, and they are best avoided.

MS demands little modification of obstetric care. Neurogenic bladder is common, and the obstetrician should follow closely for evidence of urinary tract infection. Infections should be treated promptly; when they are recurrent, prophylactic antibiotic administration should be considered. It is prudent to encourage adequate rest during and after delivery. Delivery is also largely unaffected by MS. Magnesium sulfate and intravenous anesthetics can be given. Although it has been suggested that spinal anesthesia may be associated with relapses, the available data do not allow a clear recommendation concerning the choice of anesthetic methods. "Stress dose" steroids (e.g., hydrocortisone at 100 mg intravenously every 8 hours) are recommended if the patient has taken more than 10–20 mg of prednisone for more than 2 weeks in the preceding year [66].

There is no contraindication to breast-feeding, unless high-dose corticosteroids or other immunosuppressive therapies are being used. All mothers should be encouraged to get sufficient rest, although there is no evidence that this will lower the postpartum relapse rate. When disability is significant, the mother should be encouraged to find adequate assistance with childcare.

## PERIPHERAL NEUROPATHIES AND PREGNANCY

### Isolated Neuropathies

Facial Palsy

The incidence of idiopathic facial palsy is increased during pregnancy. Most cases occur during the third trimester and first two postpartum weeks. Adour quoted a threefold increase in incidence in pregnant versus nonpregnant women, with six times as many cases occurring in the third trimester as in the first and second trimesters [71]. The course and prognosis are not known to differ from those of nonpregnant patients and depend largely on the initial severity. The best available evidence suggests that an early course of prednisone lessens denervation and ultimate disability [72]. This short-term use of corticosteroids is safe in late pregnancy. If there are no contraindications, we recommend a 10-day course of therapy in which 30 mg is given twice a day for 5 days with the dose tapered over the subsequent 5 days. Adour has recommended an additional 10 days of therapy for patients who show no improvement after 5 days [73]. Polymerase chain reaction evidence suggests that reactivation of herpes simplex type 1 infection is responsible for many cases of facial palsy [74]. No clinical studies of antiviral therapy have yet established its early use. In cases that occur within a week before delivery or postpartum, however, acyclovir 200 mg five times daily (or one of its analogues) can be given over 7–10 days after delivery, unless the mother is breast-feeding.

Meralgia Paresthetica

Meralgia paresthetica is a compressive neuropathy of the lateral femoral cutaneous nerve. This nerve arises from the L2 root in the lumbar plexus and travels along the pelvic wall to emerge beneath the lateral end of the inguinal ligament just medial to the anterior superior iliac spine. The pressure of the gravid uterus can cause compression of the nerve at this site. The nerve is purely sensory, supplying a wide area of the anterolateral thigh. The typical complaint is of unpleasant paresthesias or pain and numbness in the skin of the anterolateral thigh. There is a patch of hypesthesia and usually a larger area of altered sensation in this same location. Typically, the area of altered appreciation of light touch is larger than that of altered pinprick and pain sensation. There may be tenderness at the site of the nerve's emergence medial to the anterior superior iliac spine, and tapping at this site may elicit paresthesias. The motor and reflex examinations should be normal. Clinical diagnosis is adequate in most cases. For electrophysiologic confirmation, one can usually demonstrate the absence of sensory potential on the affected side. Because the normal lateral femoral cutaneous nerve cannot be reliably isolated on nerve conduction studies, however, the diagnostic value of its absence is questionable. Electrophysiologic testing is usually unnecessary unless another diagnosis is suspected. The major alternative diagnoses to consider are radiculopathies at the L2–L4 levels, femoral neuropathy, and lumbar plexopathy. Such lesions are usually accompanied by motor and reflex changes and abnormalities of motor conduction and electromyography. Intraspinal lesions may rarely cause diagnostic confusion. Treatment is directed at minimizing pressure on the nerve and alleviating pain. Pressure at the vulnerable site is lessened by avoiding constricting clothing and resting lying on the opposite side during the pregnancy. Delivery most successfully removes the offending pressure. Pain can be relieved most directly by a local nerve block applied just medial and inferior to the anterior superior iliac spine. Analgesia with tricyclic agents, carbamazepine, or gabapentin may be used to treat the neuropathic pain after delivery. Before delivery, safe analgesics, such as short-term narcotics, may be used when pain demands treatment. Recovery depends on the degree of injury. Demyelinating injury heals over 6–8 weeks. More severe compressive lesions with axonal loss may require many months to recover by axonal regeneration.

## Carpal Tunnel Syndrome

Carpal tunnel syndrome is common during late pregnancy. Up to one-third of pregnant women report hand symptoms in some series [75]. It is caused by compression of the median nerve beneath the flexor retinaculum at the wrist. The reason for the high incidence in pregnancy is not clear but is probably related to fluid retention and increased tissue pressure. The typical symptom is waking with an aching, tingling numbness in the hand. Symptoms usually affect the thumb and first three fingers respecting the median distribution, but patients commonly describe paresthesias involving all of the fingers. The aching pain may extend up the volar forearm. Elevating the hand may afford relief, and, when mild, the pain often resolves after rising. There is often little to find on examination. Tinel's sign (paresthesias and pain in the median distribution on tapping the site of the median nerve on the volar aspect of the wrist) and Phalen's sign (provocation of symptoms by flexion of the wrist for 30–60 seconds) may be positive. Median compression at the wrist may compromise the bulk and power of the abductor pollicis brevis, opponens pollicis, and median lumbricals and the sensation to the first through third fingers and radial aspect of the fourth finger, sparing the sensation over the thenar eminence. In pregnancy, however, the syndrome commonly is too mild and short-lived to cause these findings. Clinical diagnosis is usually adequate; however, more severe cases can be confirmed by nerve conduction studies and electromyography (EMG), which may show delayed distal latencies, slowing of conduction velocity across the wrist, a relative delay in the median component of the palmar mixed study, and, ultimately, reduced compound muscle action potentials and EMG evidence of acute and chronic denervation in the abductor pollicis brevis and opponens pollicis. Treatment includes removal of any offending activities that may promote compression, such as repetitive hand work. When the symptoms are mild, night-time splinting of the wrist in a neutral position may afford adequate relief. When they are more severe, intermittent use of splints during the day can be added. Continuous use risks compromise of full range of motion. When splinting is inadequate, local injection with corticosteroids usually provides relief. In the large majority of cases, the symptoms will subside after delivery. Cases progressing to axonal loss may require surgical decompression, but this is rarely necessary in cases complicating pregnancy.

## Femoral Neuropathy

The femoral nerve is formed in the lumbar plexus from the L2–L4 roots. It gives motor supply to the iliopsoas (hip flexion) and quadriceps group (knee extension and knee jerk) and sensory supply to the intermediate and medial femoral cutaneous nerves innervating part of the anterior and medial thigh, and terminates as the saphenous nerve providing sensory innervation of the skin of the anteromedial lower leg. The same roots supply the obturator nerve that innervates the thigh adductors, which should be spared in patients with isolated femoral neuropathy. The nerve gives off motor twigs to the iliopsoas and then passes through the pelvis to emerge beneath the inguinal ligament. It is vulnerable to compression by the head of the infant during delivery, and a postpartum compressive femoral neuropathy is common. Patients complain of weakness of the leg, especially buckling of the knee, which may lead to falls. Variable degrees of motor, reflex, and sensory deficit may be noted on examination, especially weakness of knee extension and hypesthesia on the anterior and medial thigh and anteromedial lower leg. Because the compression occurs distally to the iliopsoas motor branches, hip flexion is typically spared. Sparing of the obturator functions distinguishes this neuropathy from L2–L4 radiculopathy. The typical clinical picture is adequate for diagnosis in most cases. When there is doubt, nerve conduction and EMG can demonstrate the femoral neuropathy. The major competing considerations in a postpartum syndrome are radiculopathy resulting from lumbar disc disease and retroperitoneal hematoma or laceration of femoral twigs after intrapelvic surgery. The prognosis is good for full recovery. Because the lesions are caused by short-term compression, most are neurapraxic (demyelinating) and resolve completely in the 6–8 weeks after delivery. Less commonly, axonotmesis (axonal injury) results, and slower recovery by axonal regeneration can be expected. Electrophysiologic studies delayed by at least 2 weeks can determine the presence or absence of denervation and allow prediction of the functional outcome. Physical therapy to strengthen and recondition the involved muscles and occupational therapy to teach proper compensation are helpful in severe and enduring cases.

## Obturator Neuropathy

The obturator nerve is formed in the lumbar plexus from the L2–L4 roots. It runs along the lateral wall of the pelvis to emerge through the obturator foramen. It gives motor supply to the hip adductors and sensory supply to a small area of the medial thigh. Its course through the pelvis renders it vulnerable to compression during delivery. Symptoms are usually paresthesias and hypesthesia involving the medial thigh, occasionally extending well below the knee. Weakness of hip adduction may be found. By a logic analogous to that used to assess femoral neuropathy, a lesion of the L2–L4 roots can be ruled out by the sparing of the functions of the femoral nerve. When both obturator and femoral deficits are found, a lesion of the plexus or roots should be sought. Prognosis and treatment are as for femoral neuropathy.

### Guillain-Barré Syndrome

Guillain-Barré syndrome (GBS) is rare in pregnancy. Roughly 40 cases have been described in the literature. Pregnancy does not appear to affect the course of GBS, and termination of pregnancy is not generally recommended. When mild, GBS does not significantly affect pregnancy. However, when severe, it increases the risk to both mother and fetus. The need for mechanical ventilation especially increases this risk. Many patients have now received therapeutic plasma exchange for severe GBS in pregnancy with favorable outcome. Therefore, it is recommended that pregnancy not influence the decision to proceed aggressively with plasma exchange in an effort to prevent the need for mechanical ventilation [76]. Although some women presenting at term with acute GBS have been reported to do well after cesarean section, in general surgical delivery is not recommended unless demanded by obstetric considerations.

### Low Back Pain and Lumbosacral Radiculopathies

Low back pain is a common complication of pregnancy. Most cases appear to arise from skeletal strain, and symptoms and signs suggest a mechanical mechanism. Degenerative disc disease may also be exacerbated by pregnancy, and disc herniation with radiculopathies may occur. Because lumbar epidural anesthesia is commonly used at the time of delivery, it is often suspected as the cause of low back and leg pain after delivery. Although this procedure is safe, and the connection is usually unwarranted, occasionally lumbar radiculopathies and rarely myelopathies may occur as sequelae. Lumbar spinal stenosis predisposes to complications. This suggests that the introduction of fluid into the already compromised space or edema in this space may contribute to compression of roots of the cauda equina or, perhaps, that pre-existing stenosis predisposes to the neurotoxic effect of the anesthetic medications [77]. Other possible mechanisms of injury include direct needle injury of roots, inadvertent injection into the subarachnoid space of the higher doses of anesthetic medication intended for the epidural space, lumbar epidural hematoma or abscess, and arachnoiditis. When there is a significant neurologic deficit or back or leg pain after epidural anesthesia, MRI scanning is indicated to look for hematoma or abscess. Gadolinium contrast increases sensitivity in this situation. In cases where no such lesion is found, the prognosis is good, especially in the young and healthy obstetric population.

# MUSCLE AND NEUROMUSCULAR JUNCTION DISORDERS IN PREGNANCY

## Myasthenia Gravis

One incidence peak of myasthenia gravis occurs in young women. Pregnancy does not predictably affect the course of myasthenia gravis [78]. In a literature review, Plauché reported that among 322 pregnancies in 225 mothers, 41% had exacerbations, 29% had remissions, and 32% had no clinical change during pregnancy. Thirty percent had postpartum exacerbations. He noted that postpartum exacerbations were inclined to be severe and sudden, with frequent respiratory failure. Some evidence suggests that AFP has a protective effect by binding to maternal acetylcholine receptor antibodies and that the occurrence of exacerbations is greatest early in pregnancy, when AFP levels are not yet high, and in the puerperium, when they fall rapidly [79]. Myasthenia gravis increases the risk of prematurity, congenital arthrogryposis, and neonatal myasthenia with a significant increase in perinatal mortality [80].

Diagnosis is as for all cases of myasthenia gravis. Patients typically complain of fluctuating symptoms exacerbated by activity. Involvement of the eyelid, ocular, and pharyngeal muscles is common. Clear improvement after edrophonium injection is strongly suggestive. EMG with repetitive stimulation at 2–3 Hz shows a decremental response, and single-fiber EMG shows jitter. Most patients with generalized myasthenia have antibodies to the acetylcholine receptor, a highly specific test.

The principles of treatment are the same in pregnant and nonpregnant patients. Most patients can be managed with anticholinesterase medications alone. However, nausea and vomiting, erratic intestinal absorption, and changing renal clearance may make frequent dosage adjustments necessary. Corticosteroids should be given when needed because of an inadequate response to anticholinesterase medication. Patients should know, however, that fetal exposure does confer a small increase in risk of cleft lip and palate, fetal virilization, and adrenal suppression [81]. When a woman becomes pregnant while taking corticosteroids, withdrawal risks exacerbation, and the lowest effective dosage should be continued, preferably in an alternate-day regimen. In those with myasthenia who desire pregnancy, a steroid-induced remission may be the safest time to attempt pregnancy. Thymectomy has been reported during pregnancy. However, because remissions after thymectomy are delayed and major complications can accompany the surgery in severe cases, this therapy should be deferred until after delivery. Therapeutic plasma exchange has been successfully used during pregnancy, and it should be used when myasthenic crisis demands aggressive intervention. General measures are recommended to minimize the risk of exacerbations. Adequate rest and sleep should be ensured during the pregnancy and puerperium. Infections should be promptly treated, and screening and therapy for asymptomatic bacteriuria should be included. Aminoglycosides and certain other antibiotics should be avoided, because they impair neuromuscular transmission (Table 23.7).

During labor and delivery, the woman should be observed closely for respiratory compromise. Parenteral anticholinesterase inhibitors should be given to circumvent problems with absorption of orally administered medications

*Table 23.7*   Drugs that may impair neuromuscular transmission

---

Antibiotics
   Aminoglycosides, tetracycline, polymyxin B
Quinine and related drugs
   Quinidine, procainamide, lidocaine, antimalarials
Psychotropics
   Benzodiazepines, phenothiazines, monoamine oxidase inhibitors, lithium carbonate
Beta blockers
Antiepileptics
   Phenytoin, diazepam
D-Penicillamine
Acetazolamide
Morphine

---

(Table 23.8). Magnesium sulfate impairs neuromuscular transmission and should be avoided during labor [82]. The uterine smooth muscle does not contract under the influence of myoneural junctions and is unaffected by the myasthenic process. Voluntary muscle recruited in the second stage of labor may be affected, and the obstetrician may need to assist with forceps or vacuum extraction when the patient tires [79]. If weakness emerges during delivery, care should be taken to follow vital capacity or peak pressures to forestall respiratory decompensation, which may otherwise progress unnoticed. Plauché recommends epidural anesthesia when respiration is not compromised. This decreases the need for systemic medication and provides good anesthesia for forceps delivery. Surgical delivery imposes increased risks on the mother caused by the stress of surgery, anesthesia, and the postoperative recovery, and should be avoided except in cases where obstetric considerations demand it. When surgical delivery is necessary in cases of ocular or mild generalized myasthenia without involvement of respiratory muscles, spinal or epidural anesthesia may be used. Where there is bulbar and respiratory involvement, endotracheal anesthesia is recommended for maximum control [83].

Neonatal myasthenia occurs as a result of the exposure of the newborn to the maternal IgG antibodies that have crossed the placenta, rather than from intrinsic disease of the newborn. Caretakers should survey all infants of myasthenic mothers for this syndrome of weakness, poor feeding, and respiratory distress, which usually begins after a latency of 12–48 hours. This delay may be the result of a temporary effect of anticholinesterase medication also trans-

*Table 23.8*   Enteral/parenteral dose equivalencies of acetylcholinesterase inhibitors

| *Medication* | *PO dose* | *IM/SQ dose* |
|---|---|---|
| Pyridostigmine bromide (Mestinon) | 60 mg | 2 mg |
| Neostigmine bromide (Prostigmin) | 15 mg | 0.5 mg |

ferred from the mother or to initially high AFP levels, which fall rapidly after birth. In a series review, Plauché found that 52 of 276 newborns (19%) were affected [79]. The condition is self-limiting and resolves over several weeks of supportive therapy. It is serious, however, and contributes to the fivefold increase in risk of newborn mortality among infants of myasthenic mothers. IgG acetylcholine receptor antibodies enter breast milk and may exacerbate neonatal myasthenia. Anticholinesterase medications also enter breast milk and may cause gastrointestinal hypermotility in newborns. Mothers in remission with low antibody titers receiving low medication dosages can safely breast-feed [79].

## Inflammatory Myopathy

Pregnancy may occur in a patient with pre-existing polymyositis or dermatomyositis, or myositis may begin during pregnancy or the postpartum period. Both situations are rare. Only a handful of cases have been reported [84–86]. In these few cases, the disease has usually been severe, sometimes with extreme elevations of creatine kinase. Steroid resistance or relapse has occurred in many. The incidence of fetal loss has been high, occurring in about half of the cases beginning during pregnancy. It has been hypothesized that reactivation of a latent viral infection in response to the immunosuppression of pregnancy is responsible for the association of dermatomyositis and polymyositis with pregnancy, but other mechanisms may pertain [85]. Because of the potential severity of the maternal disease and high fetal risk, it is recommended that corticosteroids be given as they would in the nonpregnant patient.

## Myotonic Dystrophy

Myotonic dystrophy is a disorder of the muscle membrane characterized by an irritable muscle membrane and spontaneous muscle discharges, called *myotonic discharges*. The lesion on chromosome 19 has been identified as a CTG triplet repeat expansion in a noncoding region of the gene for *myotonin*, a protein kinase. The mode of inheritance is autosomal dominant with variable penetrance. As with other triplet repeat disorders, anticipation occurs with progressive severity in successive generations corresponding to increased length of the triplet expansion. It is important to recognize myotonic dystrophy in parents, because this will facilitate early detection and diagnosis of weakness of the newborn. Also, maternal myotonia may predispose the mother to complications related to underlying cardiac disease. Myotonia can sometimes be demonstrated on examination by observing that patients have difficulty relaxing a handshake grip or opening the eyelids after forced closure. Percussion myotonia may be demonstrated as a sustained contraction when the thenar eminence is tapped gently with a reflex hammer. Patients may have a characteristic facies with a receding hairline, temporal wasting, ptosis, and bifacial weakness that creates a straight smile. Other features include distal weakness and atrophy, mild mental retardation, and cardiac arrhythmias, especially atrial fibrillation.

## CHOREA GRAVIDARUM

Chorea gravidarum is chorea beginning during pregnancy. The largest series of cases was reported by Willson and Preece in 1932 [87]. The majority of their cases had a history of rheumatic fever with or without Sydenham's chorea. This observation and the declining incidence of chorea gravidarum suggest that it results somehow from an effect of pregnancy on a brain predisposed to chorea by prior damage. A similar isolated movement disorder can be precipitated by oral contraceptives, which indicates a possible role for female sex hormones in the pathogenesis. Estrogen and progesterone may sensitize dopamine receptors, or they may act as weak dopamine agonists, thereby inducing chorea in patients made vulnerable by an acquired striatal lesion [88]. Despite these observations, the pathogenesis of chorea gravidarum remains poorly understood. The characteristic involuntary movements are often severe and asymmetric, with one side predominant. Patients who have chorea during pregnancy or while taking oral contraceptives should undergo an evaluation for the various causes of chorea, including rheumatic fever, systemic lupus erythematosus, thyrotoxicosis, polycythemia vera, adverse reactions to various drugs, and the antiphospholipid antibody syndrome (recurrent midterm abortions, thrombotic events, thrombocytopenia, migraine-like headaches). Contraceptive use should be stopped. Family history of Huntington's disease should be sought. Helpful laboratory tests include throat culture for *Streptococcus*, serologic tests for prior streptococcal infection, thyroid function studies, complete blood count, and chemistry profile. Laboratory studies when systemic lupus erythematosus is suspected should include testing for antinuclear, anti-DNA, and anti-Sm antibodies, as well as serologic testing for syphilis, anemia, leukopenia, and thrombocytopenia. Laboratory tests confirm the diagnosis of the antiphospholipid antibody syndrome, either through a positive lupus anticoagulant test (Russell's viper venom, kaolin clotting time, a modified partial thromboplastin time, or platelet neutralization test) or an elevated enzyme-linked immunosorbent assay for anticardiolipin antibodies of significant titer. In most cases, the chorea is self-limiting and will resolve after delivery or discontinuance of oral contraceptives. When treatment of the movement disorder is needed, haloperidol is effective. Some patients with evidence of autoimmunity have benefited from administration of corticosteroids. Patients with other features of the antiphospholipid antibody syndrome may be treated with low dosages of aspirin, anticoagulants (heparin while pregnant), or corticosteroids.

## NEUROLOGIC MANIFESTATIONS OF TUMORS IN OBSTETRICS AND GYNECOLOGY

### Neurologic Manifestations of Gynecologic Tumors

Gynecologic malignancies may present with paraneoplastic neurologic syndromes. These may occur well before the tumor is found, so that recognition of the characteristic syndromes may lead to a search that culminates in diagnosis of the tumor.

## Subacute Cerebellar Degeneration

Subacute cerebellar degeneration is a syndrome characterized by truncal and appendicular ataxia, dysarthria, and nystagmus, especially downbeat nystagmus, that progresses over weeks. Histopathology reveals loss of Purkinje cells, sometimes proliferation of Bergmann's astrocytes and microglia, and loss of granule cells [89]. Although paraneoplastic cerebellar degeneration may develop in men or women with several cancers, including small-cell lung carcinomas, a subset of the women with this clinical syndrome have a cytoplasmic antineuronal antibody, designated anti-Yo and associated with gynecologic tumors. Structural cerebellar lesions should be ruled out by MRI. In paraneoplastic cerebellar degeneration, scanning is normal early but will later reveal cerebellar atrophy. Familial cerebellar degeneration can be distinguished by the family history and slower rate of progression. Serum and cerebrospinal fluid should be tested for anti-Yo antibodies. Seropositive patients usually harbor a gynecologic tumor. Ovarian, uterine, fallopian tube, or breast tumors have been found in almost all patients. Only a rare patient has had a nongynecologic tumor [90]. If anti-Yo antibodies are found, a careful search for such a tumor, including exploratory laparotomy, is indicated. Because the neurologic syndrome has been reported to occur up to 4 years before tumor diagnosis, an aggressive diagnostic search may lead to early diagnosis at a stage when the malignancy is treatable. Patients with anti-Purkinje cell antibodies have been noted to have a lesser burden of metastatic disease, suggesting an antitumor effect [91]. In most cases, a severe deficit develops and then stabilizes within weeks. Treatment of the neurologic syndrome with plasma exchange and immunosuppressive agents has been disappointing.

## Opsoclonus-Myoclonus with Breast Cancer

Opsoclonus is a chaotic, conjugate, rapid, spontaneous myoclonic movement of the eyes. Polymyoclonus is a random rapid movement of the body. Opsoclonus-myoclonus may occur as a paraneoplastic syndrome in the context of various tumors. Although it is not as coherent a syndrome as the subacute cerebellar degeneration with anti-Yo antibodies, some women with opsoclonus-myoclonus and breast cancer have an antineuronal antibody, designated anti-Ri, in their serum and cerebrospinal fluid. In Luque's report of eight cases, seven patients had cancer—five had breast cancer, one had adenocarcinoma in an axillary node, and one had a carcinoma of the fallopian tube [92]. Therefore, adults who present with opsoclonus-myoclonus should have serum and cerebrospinal fluid assays for anti-Ri antibodies, breast and gynecologic examination, and mammography.

## Effects of Pregnancy, Breast Cancer, and Oral Contraceptive Pills on Nongynecologic Tumors

### Meningioma

Meningiomas occur with a female predominance of about 2 to 1 in mature adults. They express estrogen and progesterone receptors as well as receptors for androgens, glucocorticoids, somatostatin, and dopamine. Hormones and growth factors appear to play a major role in their proliferation. These tumors may make their first symptomatic appearance during pregnancy and regress after delivery. Symptoms may also fluctuate with the menstrual cycle. They have been found to occur in a disproportionate number of women with breast cancer. Tumors most likely to behave in this way are those near critical neurologic structures, such as sphenoid wing or sella region meningiomas. The emergence of symptoms may occur as a result of vascular engorgement or, more likely, rapid growth under hormonal influence. Therefore, when focal neurologic symptoms emerge during pregnancy or in the context of breast cancer, meningioma should be considered. Also, women with unexcised meningiomas who become pregnant should be observed for evidence of rapid tumor growth.

## Pituitary Adenomas

Patients with prolactin-secreting pituitary adenomas may come to the neurologist's attention when they present with visual symptoms due to mass effect or headache. Hyperprolactinemia is one of the commonest causes of infertility. Treatment with bromocriptine and surgery can restore fertility in many cases and allow these women to become pregnant. They may then come to the neurologist for follow-up during the pregnancy. When a patient with hyperprolactinemia desires pregnancy, it is important to differentiate idiopathic hyperprolactinemia and microadenomas (<10 mm) from macroadenomas (≥10 mm). Pregnancy stimulates growth of prolactinomas, and pregnant women with untreated macroadenomas have a rate of complications requiring intervention of 15–36%. Those with untreated microadenomas have a rate of symptomatic complications of about 1.6% [93]. Therefore, it is recommended that those with macroadenomas undergo transphenoidal resection before conception. This procedure will lower the symptomatic complication rate to 4.3%. In patients with microadenomas or some small macroadenomas limited to the sella, the tumors should be controlled with bromocriptine to restore ability to conceive. When pregnancy is diagnosed, the bromocriptine can be discontinued. There is no evidence of adverse effects on the pregnancy or newborn with this approach [94]. In either case, the patient should be followed for clinical symptoms and signs of tumor enlargement. Typically, headache precedes the occurrence of visual field defects and loss of acuity caused by compression. If symptoms emerge, use of bromocriptine should be reinstituted during the pregnancy with close follow-up. If deficits progress despite administration of bromocriptine, the woman should undergo transphenoidal resection during pregnancy or early delivery, when appropriate. With this approach, most women with hyperprolactinemia can be carried through multiple pregnancies. Follow-up ophthalmologic examination, imaging, and prolactin level testing should be done to establish a new baseline 6–8 weeks after delivery. Prolactin levels have not been found to be higher than prepregnancy levels in breast-feeding mothers, and breast-feeding is encouraged [95]. If the woman does not wish to breast-feed, use of bromocriptine should be reinstituted.

## Choriocarcinoma and Molar Pregnancy

Choriocarcinomas are rare tumors of trophoblastic origin with potential neurologic complications. Most tumors arise from placenta, although rarely they arise within the ovary in nonpregnant women. They occur in approximately 1 in 20,000–50,000 term pregnancies and 1 in 30 molar pregnancies [96,97]. Cerebral metastases are the most common neurologic complication and occur in 10–20% of cases [97]. The tumor infiltrates vessels and can cause cerebral infarcts and neoplastic intracranial aneurysms, leading to intracerebral hemorrhage within the tumor and subarachnoid hemorrhage [97]. Local extension from the pelvis may also invade the lumbosacral plexus and lumbosacral epidural space to compress spinal roots of the cauda equina. Presentation may be delayed until several years after pregnancy. Beta human chorionic gonadotropin is elevated with these tumors as well as with normal and molar pregnancy, and is most useful as a marker of response to therapy. Treatment with chemotherapy and whole-brain irradiation may confer a survival rate of 80–90% [97]. Surgery is usually reserved for therapy of hemorrhagic complications or when single residual tumor deposits remain after nonsurgical treatments.

## MISCELLANEOUS DISORDERS INFLUENCED BY PREGNANCY

### Porphyria

Porphyria is a disorder of porphyrin metabolism caused by a genetic lesion leading to reduced production of one of the enzymes in the pathway of hemoglobin formation. It has a dominant mode of inheritance. The commonest form, acute intermittent porphyria, is a result of reduced activity of porphobilinogen (PBG) deaminase. The genetic lesion is present in 5–10 per 100,000 patients; however, expression of the clinical features of the disease is much less common and intermittent, occurring in about 10% of those with the genetic lesion. Anything that induces alpha-aminolevulinic acid (ALA) synthase, the rate-limiting enzyme in heme synthesis, can precipitate a clinical attack. Precipitants include various medications, especially phenobarbital; menstruation and pregnancy (a fact that accounts at least in part for the female predominance of expression); and other stresses, such as fasting and infection. Attacks are characterized by abdominal pain; acute polyneuropathy; mental changes, including psychiatric symptoms or confusion; and hypermetabolic symptoms and signs, such as fever, tachycardia, and sweating. Diagnosis is made by identification of the abnormal products of metabolism. These are the metabolites proximal to the site of the metabolic block. In the case of acute intermittent porphyria, these products include ALA and PBG. Levels of these compounds are elevated during attacks and can be assayed in the urine and serum. During remissions, serum levels of these products will usually return to normal. In this state, the erythrocytes can be tested for PBG deaminase activity, which should be reduced by 50% in heterozygotes. Therapy includes the administration of adequate glucose and hematin. The latter feeds back negatively on ALA synthase to reduce production of the downstream metabolites.

## Fibrous Dysplasia

Fibrous dysplasia is caused by the production of an abnormal G-protein that leads to a gain of function and overproduction of a vascular fibrous tissue that replaces normal bone. The germ line mutation in the gene coding for this G-protein is likely lethal, and the disease is typically expressed in a mosaic pattern after a postmitotic somatic mutation [98]. This leads to a patchy distribution of focal bony lesions, most commonly in the long bones and face. The bone lesions have been shown to contain estrogen and progesterone receptors, and they tend to increase in size during puberty. They may also grow at an increased rate during pregnancy. Growth of lesions can lead to fracture of long bones. Patients with this disease may come to the neurologist's attention when lesions involve the frontal or sphenoid bones of the skull, where they may compromise the optic canal and impair vision. When they involve the temporal bone, they may impair hearing. Pregnant patients with fibrous dysplasia involving the facial bones should be followed closely for evidence of progression. Surgical decompression of the optic canal should be considered when there is progressive vision loss.

## REFERENCES

1. Somerville BW. The role of estradiol withdrawal in the etiology of menstrual migraine. Neurology 1972;22:355–365.
2. deLignières B, Vincens M, Mauvais-Jarvis P, et al. Prevention of menstrual migraine by percutaneous oestradiol. BMJ 1986;293:1540.
3. Magos AL, Zilkha KJ, Studd JWW. Treatment of menstrual migraine by oestradiol implants. J Neurol Neurosurg Psychiatry 1983;46:1044–1046.
4. Sarno AP Jr, Miller EJ Jr, Lundblad EG. Premenstrual syndrome: beneficial effects of periodic, low-dose danazol. Obstet Gynecol 1987;70:33–36.
5. Powles TJ. Prevention of migrainous headaches by tamoxifen. Lancet 1986;2:1344.
6. Callaghan N. The migraine syndrome in pregnancy. Neurology 1968;18:197–199.
7. Somerville BW. A study of migraine in pregnancy. Neurology 1972;22:824–828.
8. Lance JW, Anthony M. Some clinical aspects of migraine: a prospective survey of 500 patients. Arch Neurol 1966;15:356–361.
9. Reik L. Headaches in pregnancy. Semin Neurol 1988;8:187–192.
10. Somerville BW. A study of migraine in pregnancy. Neurology 1972;22:824–828.
11. Briggs GG, Freeman RK, Yaffe SJ. Drugs in Pregnancy and Lactation. Baltimore: Williams & Wilkins, 1990.
12. Redmond GP. Propranolol and fetal growth retardation. Semin Perinatol 1982;6:142–147.
13. Ryan RE. A controlled study of the effect of oral contraceptives on migraine. Headache 1978;17:250–252.
14. Digre KB, Varner MW, Corbett JJ. Pseudotumor cerebri and pregnancy. Neurology 1984;34:721–729.
15. Commission on Genetics, Pregnancy, and the Child, International League Against Epilepsy. Guidelines for the care of epileptic women of childbearing age. Epilepsia 1989;30:409–410.
16. Delgado-Escueta AV, Janz D. Consensus guidelines: preconception counseling, management, and care of the pregnant woman with epilepsy. Neurology 1992;42(suppl 5):149–160.
17. Hanson JW, Smith DW. The fetal hydantoin syndrome. J Pediatr 1975;87:285–290.
18. Lindhout D, Meinardi H, Meijer JWA, et al. Antiepileptic drugs and teratogenesis in two consecutive cohorts: changes in prescription policy paralleled by changes in pattern of malformations. Neurology 1992;42(suppl 5):94–110.
19. Lindhout D, Meinardi H. Spina bifida and in-utero exposure to valproate. Lancet 1984;2:396.
20. Lindhout D, Julliette GC, Omtzigt JGC, et al. Spectrum of neural-tube defects in 34 infants prenatally exposed to antiepileptic drugs. Neurology 1992;42(suppl 5):111–118.

21. Rosa FW. Spina bifida in infants of women treated with carbamazepine during pregnancy. N Engl J Med 1991;324:674–677.
22. Lindhout D, Höppener RJEA, Meinardi H. Teratogenicity of antiepileptic drug combinations with special emphasis on epoxidation (of carbamazepine). Epilepsia 1984;25:77–83.
23. Feldman GL. Weaver DD. Lovrien EW. The fetal trimethadione syndrome: report of an additional family and further delineation of this syndrome. Am J Dis Child 1977;131:1389–1392.
24. Kaneko S, Otani K, Kondo T, et al. Malformation in infants of mothers with epilepsy receiving antiepileptic drugs. Neurology 1992;42(suppl 5):68–74.
25. Khoshbin S, Harvey EA, Holmes LB. Adverse outcomes among infants of mothers on anticonvulsants. Neurology 1994;44(suppl 2):A187.
26. Gaily E, Granström M-L, Hiilesmaa V, Bardy A. Minor anomalies in offspring of epileptic mothers. J Pediatr 1988;112:520–529.
27. Koch S, Lösche G, Jager-Romän E, et al. Major and minor birth malformations and antiepileptic drugs. Neurology 1992;42(suppl 5):83–88.
28. Ashwal S. Congenital Structural Defects. In KF Swaiman (ed), Pediatric Neurology: Principles and Practice (2nd ed). St. Louis: Mosby, 1994.
29. Gaily E, Granström M-L. A transient retardation of early postnatal growth in drug-exposed children of epileptic mothers. Epilepsy Res 1989;4:147–155.
30. Dansky LV, Rosenblatt DS, Andermann E. Mechanisms of teratogenesis: folic acid and antiepileptic therapy. Neurology 1992;42(suppl 5):32–42.
31. Wegner C, Nau H. Alteration of embryonic folate metabolism by valproic acid during organogenesis: implications for mechanisms of teratogenesis. Neurology 1992;42(suppl 5):17–24.
32. MRC Vitamin Study Research Group. Prevention of neural-tube defects: results of the Medical Research Council Vitamin Study. Lancet 1991;338:131–137.
33. Bleyer WA, Skinner AL. Fatal neonatal hemorrhage after maternal anticonvulsant therapy. JAMA 1976;235:626–627.
34. Mountain KR, Hirsch J, Gallus AS. Neonatal coagulation defect due to anticonvulsant drug treatment in pregnancy. Lancet 1970;1:265–268.
35. Yerby MS. Problems and management of the pregnant woman with epilepsy. Epilepsia 1987; 28(suppl 3):S29–S36.
36. Leppik IE, Rask CA. Pharmacokinetics of antiepileptic drugs during pregnancy. Semin Neurol 1988;8:240–246.
37. Nadel AS, Green JK, Holmes LB, et al. Absence of need for amniocentesis in patients with elevated levels of maternal serum alpha-fetoprotein and normal ultrasonographic examination. N Engl J Med 1990;323:557–561.
38. Lindhout D, Meinardi H, Meijer JWA, et al. Antiepileptic drugs and teratogenesis in two consecutive cohorts: changes in prescription policy paralleled by changes in pattern of malformations. Neurology 1992;42(suppl 5):94–110.
39. McCrae KR, Samuels P, Schreiber AD. Pregnancy-associated thrombocytopenia: pathogenesis and management. Blood 1992;80:2697–2714.
40. Kaplan PW, Repke JT. Eclampsia. Neurol Clin 1994;12:565–582.
41. Dinsdale HB. Does magnesium sulfate treat eclamptic seizures? Yes. Arch Neurol 1988;45:1360–1361.
42. Kaplan PW, Lesser RP, Fisher RS, et al. No, magnesium sulfate should not be used in treating eclamptic seizures. Arch Neurol 1988;45:1361–1364.
43. Kaplan PW, Lesser RP, Fisher RS, et al. A continuing controversy: magnesium sulfate in the treatment of eclamptic seizures. Arch Neurol 1990;47:1031–1032.
44. The Eclampsia Trial Cooperative Group. Which anticonvulsant for women with eclampsia? Evidence from the Collaborative Eclampsia Trial. Lancet 1995;345:1455–1463.
45. Lucas MJ, Leveno KJ, Cunningham G. A comparison of magnesium sulfate with phenytoin for the prevention of eclampsia. N Engl J Med 1995;333:201–205.
46. Lipton SA, Rosenberg PA. Excitatory amino acids as a final common pathway for neurologic disorders. N Engl J Med 1994;330:613–622.
47. Mantello MT, Schwartz RB, Jones KM, et al. Imaging of neurologic complications associated with pregnancy. Am J Roentgenol 1993;160:843–847.
48. Greer IA. Haemostasis and Thrombosis in Pregnancy. In AL Bloom, CD Forbes, DP Thomas, EGD Tuddenham (eds), Haemostasis and Thrombosis (3rd ed). Edinburgh: Churchill Livingstone, 1994;987–1015.
49. Bremme K, Östlund E, Almqvist I, et al. Enhanced thrombin generation and fibrinolytic activity in normal pregnancy and the puerperium. Obstet Gynecol 1992;80:132–137.
50. Wiebers DO. Ischemic cerebrovascular complications of pregnancy. Arch Neurol 1985;42:1106–1113.

51. Cross JN, Castro PO, Jennett WB. Cerebral strokes associated with pregnancy and the puerperium. Br Med J 1968;3:214–218.
52. Wiebers DO, Whisnant JP. The incidence of stroke among pregnant women in Rochester, Minn., 1955 through 1979. JAMA 1985;254:3055–3057.
53. Sharshar T, Lamy C, Mas JL. Incidence and causes of strokes associated with pregnancy and puerperium: a study in public hospitals of Ile de France. Stroke 1995;26:930–936.
54. Kittner SJ, Stern BJ, Feeser BR, et al. Pregnancy and the risk of stroke. N Engl J Med 1996;335:768–774.
55. Imperiale TF, Petrulis AS. A meta-analysis of low-dose aspirin for the prevention of pregnancy-induced hypertensive disease. JAMA 1991;266:260–264.
56. Ginsberg JS, Hirsh J. Use of antithrombotic agents during pregnancy. Chest 1992;102(suppl):385S–390S.
57. Hull RD, Raskob GE, Rosenbloom D, et al. Optimal therapeutic level of heparin therapy in patients with venous thrombosis. Arch Intern Med 1992;152:1589–1595.
58. Einhäupl KM, Villringer A, Meister W, et al. Heparin treatment in sinus venous thrombosis. Lancet 1991;338:597–600.
59. Toglia MR, Weg JG. Venous thromboembolism during pregnancy. N Engl J Med 1996;335:108–114.
60. Dias MS, Sekhar LN. Intracranial hemorrhage from aneurysms and arteriovenous malformations during pregnancy and the puerperium. Neurosurgery 1990;27:855–866.
61. Weir B, Macdonald RL. Management of Intracranial Aneurysms and Arteriovenous Malformations during Pregnancy. In RH Wilkins, SS Rengachary (eds), Neurosurgery. New York: McGraw-Hill, 1996;2421–2427.
62. Monga M, Creasy RK. Cardiovascular and Renal Adaptation to Pregnancy. In RK Creasy, R Resnik (eds), Maternal-Fetal Medicine: Principles and Practice. Philadelphia: Saunders, 1994;758–760.
63. Horton JC, Chambers WA, Lyons SL, et al. Pregnancy and the risk of hemorrhage from cerebral arteriovenous malformations. Neurosurgery 1990;27:867–872.
64. Robinson JL, Hall CS, Sedzimir CB. Arteriovenous malformations, aneurysms, and pregnancy. J Neurosurg 1974;41:63–70.
65. Lidegaard Ø. Oral contraception and risk of a cerebral thromboembolic attack: results of a case-control study. Br Med J 1993;306:956–963.
66. Birk K, Rudick R. Pregnancy and multiple sclerosis. Arch Neurol 1986;43:719–726.
67. Davis RK, Maslow AS. Multiple sclerosis in pregnancy: a review. Obstet Gynecol Surv 1992;47:290–296.
68. Birk K, Ford C, Smeltzer S, et al. The clinical course of multiple sclerosis during pregnancy and the puerperium. Arch Neurol 1990;47:738–742.
69. Sadovnick AD, Eisen K, Hashimoto SA, et al. Pregnancy and multiple sclerosis: a prospective study. Arch Neurol 1994;51:1120–1124.
70. Poser S, Poser W. Multiple sclerosis and gestation. Neurology 1983;33:1422–1427.
71. Adour KK. The bell tolls for decompression. N Engl J Med 1975;292:248–250.
72. Austin JR, Peskind SP, Austin SG, Rice DH. Idiopathic facial nerve paralysis: a randomized double blind controlled study of placebo versus prednisone. Laryngoscope 1993;103:1326–1332.
73. Adour KK. Diagnosis and management of facial paralysis. N Engl J Med 1982;307:348–351.
74. Murakami S, Mizobuchi M, Nakashiro Y, et al. Bell palsy and herpes simplex virus: identification of viral DNA in endoneural fluid and muscle. Ann Intern Med 1996;124(1, pt 1):27–30.
75. Dawson DM, Hallet M, Millender LH. Entrapment Neuropathies. Boston: Little, Brown, 1990;51.
76. Hurley TJ, Brunson AD, Archer RL, et al. Landry-Guillain-Barré-Strohl syndrome in pregnancy: report of three cases treated with plasmapheresis. Obstet Gynecol 1991;78:482–485.
77. Yuen EC, Layzer RB, Weitz SR, Olney RK. Neurologic complications of lumbar epidural anesthesia and analgesia. Neurology 1995;45:1795–1801.
78. Varner MW. Autoimmune disorders and pregnancy. Semin Perinatol 1991;15:238–250.
79. Plauché WC. Myasthenia gravis in mothers and their newborns. Clin Obstet Gynecol 1991;34:82–99.
80. Plauché WC. Myasthenia gravis. Clin Obstet Gynecol 1983;26:592–604.
81. Pitkin RM. Drugs in Pregnancy. In EJ Quilligan, N Dretchmer (eds), Fetal and Maternal Medicine. New York: Wiley, 1989;396.
82. Cohen BA, London RS, Goldstein PJ. Myasthenia gravis and preeclampsia. Obstet Gynecol 1976;48(suppl):35s–37s.
83. Roblin SH, Levinson G, Shnider SM, Wright RG. Anesthetic consideration for myasthenia gravis and pregnancy. Anesth Analg 1978;57:441–447.
84. Pinheiro GRC, Goldenberg J, Atra E, et al. Juvenile dermatomyositis and pregnancy: report and literature review. J Rheumatol 1992;19:1798–1801.
85. Satoh M, Ajmani AK, Hirakata M, et al. Onset of polymyositis with autoantibodies to threonyl-tRNA synthetase during pregnancy. J Rheumatol 1994;21:1564–1566.

86. Rosenbaum RB, Donaldson JO. Peripheral nerve and neuromuscular disorders. Neurol Clin 1994;12:461–478.
87. Willson P, Preece AA. Chorea gravidarum. Arch Intern Med 1932;49:471–533, 671–697.
88. Nausieda PA, Koller WC, Weiner WJ, Klawans HL. Modification of postsynaptic dopaminergic sensitivity by female sex hormones. Life Sci 1979;25:521–526.
89. Anderson NE, Rosenblum MK, Posner JB. Paraneoplastic cerebellar degeneration: clinical-immunological correlations. Ann Neurol 1988;24:559–567.
90. Posner JB. Paraneoplastic syndromes. Neurol Clin 1991;9:919–936.
91. Hetzel DJ, Stanhope CR, O'Neill BP, Lennon VA. Gynecologic cancer in patients with subacute cerebellar degeneration predicted by anti-Purkinje cell antibodies and limited in metastatic volume. Mayo Clin Proc 1990;65:1558–1563.
92. Luque FA, Furneaux HM, Ferziger R, et al. Anti-Ri: an antibody associated with paraneoplastic opsoclonus and breast cancer. Ann Neurol 1991;29:241–251.
93. Molitch ME. Pregnancy and the hyperprolactinemic woman. N Engl J Med 1985;312:1364–1370.
94. Turkalj I, Braun P, Krupp P. Surveillance of bromocriptine in pregnancy. JAMA 1982;247:1589–1591.
95. Zarate A, Canales, ES, Alger M. The effect of pregnancy and lactation on pituitary prolactin secreting tumours. Acta Endocrinol 1979;92:407–412.
96. Athanassiou A, Begent RHJ, Newlands ES, et al. Central nervous system metastases of choriocarcinoma. Cancer 1983;52:1728–1735.
97. Seigle JM, Caputy AJ, Manz HJ, et al. Multiple oncotic intracranial aneurysms and cardiac metastasis from choriocarcinoma: case report and review of the literature. Neurosurg 1987;20:39–42.
98. Weinstein LS, Shenker A, Gejman PV, et al. Activating mutations of the stimulatory G-protein in the McCune-Albright syndrome. N Engl J Med 1991;325:1688–1695.

# 24
# Orthopedic Surgery

Kenneth K. Nakano

Few training programs prepare the orthopedic surgeon for evaluating patients complaining of pain, paresis, or paresthesias. Clearly defined syndromes are in the minority, and often orthopedists treat patients on the basis of their prejudices, convinced that time and supportive therapy will allow most unrecognized conditions to improve spontaneously. Even common conditions such as back pain or neck pain are treated empirically in widely different fashions. Explanations for certain forms of therapy are difficult to understand and often conflict with each other. Orthopedic surgeons frequently choose particular treatments because they are satisfied that they "work" in most patients. When they do not, patients are referred to or sent to other physicians who use different approaches. The neurologist sees many of these patients in consultation with orthopedic colleagues, and often the orthopedist, limited in neurologic background and approach, has failed to define a situation adequately in terms of its anatomy and physiology. The lack of breadth of background in these basic science disciplines has created a chasm between neurologists and others who often care for patients with problems affecting the nervous system.

This chapter discusses certain situations in which the orthopedic surgeon requests a neurologist to see a patient in a hospital situation; namely, to evaluate patients with neck and back pain, neuropathies (e.g., entrapments, systemic disorders), perioperative nerve lesions and trauma, compartment syndromes, reflex sympathetic dystrophy, spinal cord disorders, and connective tissue and rheumatologic diseases with neurologic complications; to conduct electrodiagnostic studies (electromyography and nerve conduction studies); and to give "neurologic clearance" for an upcoming surgical procedure.

## NECK PAIN

### Clinical Evaluation

The essential means of diagnosis and management of neck pain include taking the history and performing the physical and neurologic examinations (Table 24.1) [1,2]. The most common symptom of cervical spine disorders is pain; cervical nerve root irritation causes a well-localized area of pain, whereas poorly defined areas of pain arise from deep connective tissue structures, muscle, joint, bone, or disk (Table 24.2). The patient's description of the pain gives the neurologist essential clues to diagnosis. Stiffness with consequent limitation of motion of neck, shoulder, elbow, wrist, and even fingers may occur after earlier injury response, articular involvement, nerve root irritation, or reflex sympathetic dystrophy (RSD). Tenosynovitis and tendinitis often accompany syndromes of the cervical spine and may involve the rotator cuff or tendons around the wrist or hand, with stenosis or fibrosis of tendon sheaths and palmar fascia. Numbness and tingling follow the segmental distribution of the nerve roots in cervical spine disorders; however, this condition occurs frequently without demonstrable sensory change. Muscular weakness and fasciculation indicate a lower motor neuron (LMN) disorder secondary to a radiculopathy. Pain and guarding produce functional weakness. Head pain is common and is characteristic of cervical spine disorders. It results from nerve root compression, vertebral artery pressure, compression of sympathetic nerves, and posterior occipital muscle spasm, as well as osteoarthritic changes of the apophyseal joints of the upper three cervical vertebrae. A lesion of C6 and C7 may produce neuralgic or myalgic tenderness in the precordium or scapular region, and may be confused with angina pectoris.

Systematic physical and neurologic examination of patients with neck pain includes examination of the head, neck, upper thoracic spine, shoulders, arms, forearms, wrists, and hands with the patient fully undressed. The physician observes the patient's posture, movements, facial expression, and gait and observes the patient in various positions (sitting, standing, supine). As the patient walks into the office, the physician observes the head position and how naturally and rhythmically the head and neck move with body movement. There is a large range of motion of the cervical spine, which, in turn, provides a wide scope of vision and is essential to the sense of balance. The basic movements of the neck include flexion, extension, lateral flexion to the right and left, and rotation to the right and left. A decrease in specific motion may occur with blocking at a joint, pain, fibrous contracture, bony ankylosis, muscle spasm, or mechanical alteration in joint and skeletal structure, or with tension and uncooperativeness on the part of the patient. Other causes of muscle spasm include injury to muscle, involuntary splinting over painful joints or skeletal structure, and irritation or compression of nerve roots of the spinal cord. Reflexes indicate the state of the nervous system and its afferent pathways. Certain abnormal reflexes appear only with spasticity and paralysis; these indicate injury to the corticospinal tract. The primary deep tendon reflexes and plantar responses should be routinely examined in every patient complaining of neck pain.

*Table 24.1*   Cervical spine syndromes

*Localized neck disorders*
    Osteoarthritis (apophyseal joints, C1–C2–C3 levels most often)
    Rheumatoid arthritis (atlantoaxial)
    Juvenile rheumatoid arthritis
    Sternocleidomastoid tendinitis
    Acute posterior cervical strain
    Pharyngeal infections
    Cervical lymphadenitis
    Osteomyelitis (staphylococcal infection, tuberculosis)
    Meningitis
    Ankylosing spondylitis
    Paget's disease
    Torticollis (congenital, spasmodic, hysterical)
    Neoplasms (primary or metastatic)
    Occipital neuralgia (greater and lesser occipital nerves)
    Diffuse idiopathic skeletal hyperostosis
    Rheumatic fever (infrequently)
    Gout (infrequently)
*Lesions producing neck and shoulder pain*
    Postural disorders
    Rheumatoid arthritis
    Fibrositis syndromes
    Musculoligamentous injuries to neck and shoulder
    Osteoarthritis (apophyseal and joints of Luschka)
    Cervical spondylosis
    Intervertebral osteoarthritis
    Thoracic outlet syndromes
    Nerve injuries (serratus anterior, C3–C4 nerve root, long thoracic nerve)
*Lesions producing predominantly shoulder pain*
    Rotator cuff tears and tendinitis
    Calcareous tendinitis
    Subacromial bursitis
    Bicipital tendinitis
    Adhesive capsulitis
    Reflex sympathetic dystrophy
    Frozen shoulder syndromes
    Acromioclavicular secondary osteoarthritis
    Glenohumeral arthritis
    Septic arthritis
    Tumors of the shoulder
*Lesions producing neck and head pain with radiation*
    Cervical spondylosis
    Rheumatoid arthritis
    Intervertebral disk protrusion
    Osteoarthritis (apophyseal and joints of Luschka; intervertebral disk osteoarthritis)
    Spinal cord tumors
    Cervical neurovascular syndromes
    Thoracic outlet and associated syndromes

Source: Reprinted with permission from KK Nakano. Neck and Back Pain. In J Stein (ed), Internal Medicine (5th ed). St. Louis: Mosby–Year Book, 1998;969.

*Table 24.2*   Structures and conditions causing neck pain

Acromioclavicular joint
Heart and coronary artery disease
Apex of lung, Pancoast's tumor, bronchogenic cancer (C3, C4, C5 nerve roots in common)
Diaphragm muscle (C3, C4, C5 innervation)
Gallbladder
Spinal cord tumor
Temporomandibular joint
Fibrositis and fibromyositis syndromes (upper thoracic spine, proximal arm, and shoulder)
Aorta
Pancreas
Disorders of any somatic or visceral structure (produce cervical nerve root irritation)
Peripheral nerves
Central nervous system (posterior fossa lesions)
Hiatus hernia (C3, C4, C5)
Gastric ulcer

Source: Reprinted with permission from KK Nakano. Neck and Back Pain. In J Stein (ed), Internal Medicine (5th ed). St. Louis: Mosby–Year Book, 1998;968.

## Differential Diagnosis

Several medical conditions arising outside the cervical spine but perceived in or around the neck area mimic cervical nerve root irritation, muscle spasm, ligament strain, bone disease, and joint disorder (see Table 24.2). A peripheral neuropathy may produce pain, both proximal and distal to the irritative site. Spinal cord tumors produce a poorly localized and ill-defined neck pain, hyper-reflexia, and spasticity; immobilization does not relieve the pain, and deep tenderness and local muscle spasms are absent. Cerebral or subarachnoid hemorrhage, meningitis, head and neck trauma, and a central tumor produce neck pain that mimics cervical spine syndromes. In these instances, clinical examinations, magnetic resonance imaging (MRI), computed tomographic (CT) scans, and spinal fluid evaluation may be used to differentiate the various conditions. An important clinical fact in the differential diagnosis of neck pain is that compression or irritation of cervical nerve roots with radiation of pain is associated with deep tenderness at the site of pain. Segmental areas of deep tenderness that are not painful until palpated indicate nerve root involvement. A 1% injection of lidocaine into the painful area results in transient reproduction of the radicular pain, followed by relief of pain for days or weeks in the patient with nerve root involvement. If local anesthetic injection fails to reproduce (and relieve) the pain, potential visceral or somatic structures that have the same segmental neural supply should then be examined. Neck pain occurs in malingerers, depressed persons, people seeking compensation, and hysterical and psychoneurotic individuals. These patients possess no concomitant nerve root irritation and derive no relief from local anesthetic injections. Furthermore, absence of muscle spasm and an antalgic position and feigning of limitation of neck motion should arouse the physician's suspicion. Skilled elicitation of historic data and the physical and neurologic examinations constitute the principal reproducible means of making a differential diagnosis (Figure 24.1).

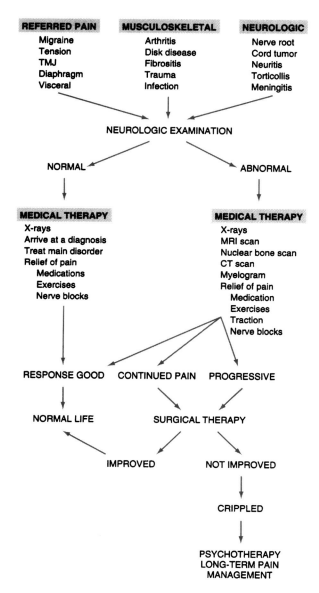

*Figure 24.1* Algorithm in the evaluation and treatment of neck pain. (TMJ = temporomandibular joint; MRI = magnetic resonance imaging; CT = computed tomography.) (Reprinted with permission from KK Nakano. Neck and Back Pain. In JH Stein [ed], Internal Medicine [5th ed]. St. Louis: Mosby–Year Book, 1998;963–971.)

## Diagnostic Evaluation

The clinical investigation of patients experiencing neck pain is constructed to evaluate the origin of the symptoms and signs, the extent of the lesion, and the need for medical or surgical treatment. Components of the investigation are radiographic (including neuroimaging), neurophysiologic, and laboratory studies. If the clinical history or general physical and neurologic examinations suggest an abnormality, then appropriate laboratory studies, electrodiagnostic evaluation (electromyography [EMG], nerve conduction study [NCS], measurement of somatosensory evoked response [SER]), and neuroimaging assessment (MRI, CT myelography) may be required for an accurate diagnosis and appropriate therapy (see Figure 24.1).

When ordering cervical spine radiography, the physician should not rely solely on the radiologist. The bones should be specifically examined for osteoporosis. The joints might reveal osteophytes with or without foraminal encroachment or even the erosions of systemic arthritis. The physician should look for congenital abnormalities such as vertebral fusion. Ligamentous calcification might indicate degeneration, trauma, ankylosing spondylosis, or diffuse idiopathic skeletal hyperostosis. Instability in the action views might be due to trauma (e.g., an athletic injury or automobile crash) but is far more often due to constitutional ligament laxity in a person who is not physically fit. Signs of previous surgery might give clues as to the nature of the clinical problem.

Neuroimaging studies include MRI, CT myelography, and radionuclide bone scans. MRI combines the best features of these conventional techniques; it can display vertebrae, intervertebral disks, the thecal space, neural elements, blood vessels, and paraspinal structures without requiring the use of radiographic or intravenous or intrathecal contrast agents or both. Furthermore, MRI is the preferred modality for the evaluation of suspected cervical radiculopathy, spinal stenosis, congenital anomalies (particularly Chiari malformations), syringomyelia, spinal cord neoplasm, multiple sclerosis, and early disk degeneration. Radioisotope bone scans are best used for the evaluation of possible inflammatory joint disease or metabolic disorder of the bone. At times it is helpful to do a full-body bone scan in these cases and to take radiographs (and at times CT scans) of those areas of increased uptake that might help in the overall assessment. Three-phase bone scans and single photon emission CT techniques can be helpful in the diagnosis and follow-up of RSD and other inflammatory conditions.

Neurophysiologic studies can be used to distinguish sensory and motor dysfunction of the peripheral nerves, and they can be used to distinguish between a lesion in the periphery and a central lesion. EMG with NCS can be used to differentiate a nerve disorder from a muscle disorder.

The clinical laboratory offers some assistance in the diagnosis and management of neck pain in specific diseases (e.g., rheumatoid arthritis [RA], hyperparathyroidism, infection with human immunodeficiency virus [HIV], multiple myeloma, ankylosing spondylosis, and certain metastatic malignant cancers). Cerebrospinal fluid evaluation should be performed in patients with neck pain who are suspected of having infection (meningitis) or subarachnoid hemorrhage; in the latter conditions, the cerebrospinal fluid becomes diagnostic.

**Treatment**

In establishing a treatment regimen for neck pain, the physician considers the following: (1) the severity of the symptoms, (2) the presence or absence of neurologic findings, and (3) the severity of the condition as indicated by radiologic/neuroimaging and electrodiagnostic studies. Medical therapy aims at the relief of pain and stiffness in the neck and upper limbs. Early mobilization exercises in patients with acute sprains often improve outcome. For relief of pain, nonsteroidal anti-inflammatory drugs (NSAIDs) and muscle relaxant medications suffice. Most acute neck pain subsides within 7–10 days. When the pain subsides, the patient may commence therapeutic and rehabilitative exercises. Traction, either continuous or intermittent, should be considered when rest fails. Continuous cervical traction should be reserved for more severe cases with symptoms of nerve root compression. However, traction is unsuitable for patients with gross changes of the cervical spine visible on radiograph because of the danger of spinal cord compression or pressure on the vertebral arteries. Occasionally side effects of traction are seen, and rarely hemianopic visual field defects develop. Cervical collars may prove helpful, in part because they also help correct posture faults. These should fit well and maintain the neck in the most comfortable position. Collars should not be worn continuously for more than 2 months, to prevent weakness and wasting of neck muscles. Physical therapy benefits most patients with neck pain. Various modalities, including cryotherapy, heat, mechanical therapy (e.g., therapeutic massage), electrotherapy, and transcutaneous nerve stimulation, may be beneficial. Some patients may respond to biofeedback and relaxation techniques.

Surgery appears appropriate for two groups of patients: the first group is patients whose symptoms relate principally to the nerve roots emerging from the cervical spine and whose condition is manifested as either neck or arm pain; the second group is patients with a slowly progressive spinal cord syndrome that involves first the legs and then the arms. One of the primary factors in the pathogenesis of radiculopathy and myelopathy is compression. Treatment is aimed at the elimination of this pressure. The most definitive indication for surgery is the presence of a neurologic deficit related to compression that is unrelieved by medical treatment. Many orthopedic surgeons have advocated an anterior approach, and the results have been excellent in over 80% of cases. Success is especially likely in cases of a centrally herniated disk. In cases of myelopathy, the surgical approach may be either anterior or posterior. However, surgical repair of cervical myelopathies is less effective than repair of acute radiculopathy, with approximately 60–70% of treated patients remaining stable or improving. In patients with a cervical bony canal diameter of 11 mm or less at several levels, a long posterior decompression may be necessary. When there is a diffuse bulging disk or an osteophytic ridge, and when the bony elements are normal (or slightly small), the site of compression and approach may be anterior (several levels may be operated on at the same time). In patients with a large, centrally herniated cervical disk, the orthopedic surgeon may have difficulty deciding on the appropriate approach. It should be emphasized that opinions differ as to the optimal surgical technique in these cases.

## LOW BACK PAIN

### Clinical Evaluation

Many disorders cause low back pain (Table 24.3); as a result, various modes of diagnosis and treatment challenge one's clinical acumen [3,4]. Medical management can be complicated by the absence of consistent, commonly accepted diagnostic terminology and variation in the use of diagnostic procedures and therapies among clinicians from various specialties. A precise anatomic explanation of the patient's low back pain can be objectively identified in less than one-fourth of cases. Only 1–2% of individuals with low back pain have lumbar disk herniation with a radiculopathy. However, frequently the clinical evaluation and the patient's concerns focus on a possible disk rupture and nerve involvement. Documentation of the history becomes a vital aspect of the examination.

### Differential Diagnosis

Three clinical features assist in directing the medical diagnosis and management of back pain: (1) duration of the symptoms, (2) distribution of the pain, and (3) age of the patient. Low back pain can be classified according to its duration. Acute low back pain can be defined as pain beginning less than 4 weeks previously; subacute pain as that beginning 5–12 weeks earlier; and chronic pain as that beginning more than 12 weeks previously. The duration of the low back pain has implications for diagnosis and prognosis. The majority of acute low back pain resolves quickly with little medical intervention. At least 60% of patients suffering with acute low back pain return to work within 1 month, and 90% return within 3 months. In the early diagnostic evaluation of a patient with low back pain, the physician should focus on recognizing the rare individual with a visceral or inflammatory cause of the pain. If symptoms fail to resolve as expected, the physician should re-evaluate the patient and identify complicating issues (e.g., nonorganic or psychosocial factors) that may be delaying recovery. In the clinical evaluation of a patient with low back pain, the distribution of the pain (i.e., the ratio of back pain to leg pain) is important in establishing the differential diagnosis. Leg pain as a primary symptom, especially pain below the knee and involving the foot, is characteristic of true sciatica. Absence of leg pain raises a different set of possibilities. Sciatica has several causes, the most common being lumbar disk herniation with nerve root involvement (Table 24.4). Greater than 95% of lumbar disk herniations occur at the L4–L5 or L5–S1 levels, producing an L5 or S1 radiculopathy, respectively. Typically, the leg pain extends below the knee and into the foot; this finding is useful for discriminating sciatica from other nonsciatic entities. An additional clinical feature of sciatica is greater pain when the patient is seated, when intradiskal pressure is highest. Pain is often relieved when the patient is in the supine position. Pain increases with coughing or the Valsalva maneuver. Over 80% of patients with L5 or S1 radiculopathy who have disk herniation show a positive straight-leg-raising (SLR) test (sciatic pain when the straight leg is passively raised between 30 degrees and 60 degrees while the patient is supine) [5]; a positive SLR test

*Table 24.3*   Classification of disorders causing low back pain

Lumbar disk syndromes
    L4 nerve root compression
    L5 nerve root compression
    S1 nerve root compression
    Large midline disk herniation
Congenital abnormalities
    Facet asymmetry
    Transitional vertebral (Bertolotti's syndrome)
    Spondylolisthesis and spondylolysis
    Scheuermann's disease
    Achondroplasia
Arthritic conditions
    Hypertrophic arthritis
    Osteoarthritis
    Ankylosing spondylitis
    Rheumatoid arthritis
    Osteitis condensans ilii
Infections
    Acute bacterial disk space infection
    Tuberculosis spondylitis
    Sacroiliac infection
Tumors
    Benign
        Meningioma or neurinoma
        Osteoid osteoma
        Osteoblastoma
    Malignant
        Metastatic cancer (breast, lung, prostate, etc.)
        Primary neural tumors
        Myelogenous diseases
            Multiple myeloma
            Hodgkin's disease
            Lymphoma
            Eosinophilic granuloma
            Hand-Schüller-Christian syndrome
Metabolic disease
    Osteoporosis
    Ochronosis
    Paget's disease
    Sickle cell disease
Trauma
    Lumbar strain
    Compression fracture
    Subluxation of facet joint
Nonskeletal disorders
    Myofascial pain
    Pelvic disorders (pelvic inflammatory disease, uterine fibroids, tumors)
    Ectopic pregnancy
    Retroperitoneal tumors or hematoma
    Prostatitis
    Abdominal aortic aneurysm

*Table 24.3*   (continued)

Kidney stones
Pyelonephritis
Pancreatitis
Peptic ulcer
Large-bowel obstruction

Source: Reprinted with permission from KK Nakano. Neck and Back Pain. In J Stein (ed), *Internal Medicine* (5th ed). St. Louis: Mosby–Year Book, 1998;965.

*Table 24.4*   Differential diagnosis of true sciatica versus pseudosciatica

*Pseudosciatica*
Meralgia paresthetica
Hip disease (e.g., osteoarthritis)
Trochanteric bursitis
Diabetic amyotrophy
Vascular claudication
*True sciatica*
Herniated disk (nucleus pulposus)
Lateral and/or femoral stenosis
Intraspinal infection
Intraspinal tumor
Piriformis syndrome
Lumbar canal stenosis

is more common in lumbar disk herniation than in spinal stenosis. The piriformis syndrome is characterized by buttock and leg pain, and low back pain and difficulty sitting and walking occur in over half of patients. The piriformis muscle arises from the inside of the pelvis over the sacrum and courses laterally through the sciatic notch. Trauma to the piriformis muscle with spasm and inflammation may produce sciatic nerve impingement. Patients with the piriformis syndrome show muscle tenderness, which may require a rectal examination to demonstrate. In patients with lumbar spinal stenosis, the patient complains of pseudoclaudication characterized by buttock, thigh, or leg pain, paresthesia, or weakness on standing or walking; pain is relieved with spinal flexion. The majority of patients with spinal stenosis complain of bilateral symptoms, while the symptoms of lumbar disk herniation and sciatica are unilateral. Lateral recess or foraminal stenosis may cause more unilateral symptoms but they are unlike those of sciatica related to lumbar disk herniation. Symptoms are not relieved by lying down, and sciatic pain on the SLR test is less common. Individuals over age 50 are at greater risk for serious nonmechanical sources of subacute and chronic low back pain (e.g., malignancy or infections). In addition, degenerative disk and joint disease, often at multiple levels, is another frequent cause of low back pain in this age group. The peak age for lumbar disk herniation and sciatica is 30–50 years; fibromyalgia is also more common in patients younger than age 50. Subacute or chronic low back pain in younger patients should make the clinician suspicious of a spondyloarthropathy such as ankylosing spondylitis or Reiter's syndrome.

## Diagnostic Evaluation

The physical examination is aimed at determining whether systemic or vascular disease is present. The neurologic evaluation seeks to determine whether there is nerve root compression, whether there is instability, and whether there is any indication of a nonmusculoskeletal origin of the symptoms. Because most patients with lumbar disk herniation and sciatica improve with nonoperative care, and the results of imaging studies do not affect initial management in most cases, imaging should be considered only in cases of diagnostic uncertainty, failure of nonoperative care (symptoms persisting 6–12 weeks), or suspected cauda equina syndrome (the usual presentation of which is the triad of saddle anesthesia, leg weakness, and loss of bowel and bladder control) (Figure 24.2). Electrodiagnostic studies have the greatest diagnostic value in cases of atypical sciatic syndromes (e.g., piriformis syndrome) or in patients who have had prior lumbosacral surgery. The purpose of EMG and NCS is to define the nerve roots or peripheral nerves involved (as well as the level—paraspinal or distal) in the pain syndrome. MRI and CT myelography possess comparable sensitivity and specificity in identifying disk herniation. Gadolinium contrast enhancement allows MRI to distinguish scar formation from disk material as the source of radicular symptoms. Approximately 20% of people under age 60 without symptoms are found to have herniated disks on MRI or CT scan [4]. In addition, spinal stenosis or lumbar disk degeneration is frequently found in asymptomatic persons, particularly after age 60. These imaging findings must be integrated with the clinical picture for appropriate interpretation.

## Treatment

Non-narcotic or nonsteroidal anti-inflammatory drugs often ease the acute low back pain, and muscle relaxants can curtail the spasm, with the goal of permitting the patient to resume normal physical activity. In cases of severe acute low back pain, narcotic drugs may be necessary; however, these should be used only on a short-term basis to minimize the possibility of addiction. Passive modalities such as ultrasound, massage, or heat therapy may be used briefly for early symptomatic relief. Most patients with acute low back pain improve by 4–6 weeks. If the patient does not show the expected improvement, the clinician should consider three questions: (1) Was the initial diagnosis accurate? (2) Do psychophysiologic or social factors hinder recovery? (3) Was the original therapy appropriate? In addressing the first question, if a patient with acute low back pain fails to improve within 6 weeks, the examiner should expand the differential diagnosis and order additional diagnostic studies such as neuroimaging. With regard to the second question, a clinical history and physical findings assist in identifying patients for whom nonorganic factors are present (e.g., compensation claims, job dissatisfaction, anxiety and depression, substance abuse, nonanatomic distribution of pain

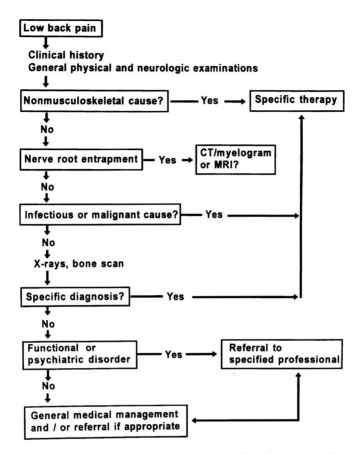

*Figure 24.2*   Algorithm in the evaluation and treatment of low back pain. (CT = computed tomography; MRI = magnetic resonance imaging.) (Reprinted with permission from KK Nakano. Neck and Back Pain. In JH Stein [ed]. Internal Medicine [5th ed]. St. Louis: Mosby–Year Book, 1998;967.)

symptoms and sensory reports). To answer the third question, the physician must ascertain whether the therapy was too passive for too long, resulting in deconditioning, depression, pain behavior, and anxiety of reinjury. In this situation, aggressive physical rehabilitation and exercise should be used that emphasize functional restoration to a normal level. Conservative regimens should not be used in the following circumstances: (1) if the patient has loss of bowel or bladder function, and (2) if the patient has another major or progressive neurologic deficit, or such intractable pain that adequate analgesia becomes impossible. In the above clinical situations, prompt diagnosis and surgery may become necessary. Most patients—even those with minor neurologic changes such as a reflex abnormality, radicular sensory change, or discernible but unimportant weakness—should initially be placed on a conservative, noninterventional medical regimen with close and careful clinical monitoring. In populations of patients complaining of low back and leg pain, only 1–2% suffer from a significant disk herniation that requires low back surgery.

## ENTRAPMENT NEUROPATHIES

The term *peripheral entrapment* describes the mechanical irritation by which a specific peripheral nerve becomes locally injured at a vulnerable anatomic site (Table 24.5) [6,7]. Peripheral nerve entrapment may result from a number of mechanisms, including pressure (compression), stretch, friction, and angulation. The pathophysiology of the nerve entrapment syndromes differs because of this variety in mechanism. Additional clinical circumstances, including the patient's age and the presence of underlying systematic disease (e.g., diabetes mellitus, rheumatologic disease), influence these disorders. Compression on the nerve within a closed space can occur wherever a peripheral nerve passes through an opening in fibrous tissue or through an osseofibrous canal (e.g., cubital tunnel), soft tissue swelling (as in RA), an anomalous or hypertrophied muscle (as in the pronator teres syndrome), a constricting scar or ligament, a bony deformity, or a mass (e.g., benign or malignant tumor, ganglion, synovial cyst) (see Table 24.5). Damage to a peripheral nerve may result from high pressure exerted for a short time (as in acute radial palsy) or from moderate or low pressure exerted for long periods of time or intermittently (as in tardy ulnar palsy).

In addition to the clinical examination, the evaluation of patients with peripheral nerve entrapments should include various electrophysiologic studies (EMG, NCS, SER) [8,9]. These electrodiagnostic procedures are valuable under four circumstances: (1) when the clinical diagnosis is uncertain; (2) to follow patients with entrapment neuropathies who are being treated conservatively; (3) to detect or exclude coexisting conditions, such as a radiculopathy or subclinical polyneuropathy; and (4) before a surgical procedure. Computerized neuroimaging technology in the form of CT, MRI, and ultrasonography has assisted in diagnosis and planning of surgical approaches to certain peripheral entrapment syndromes. Orthopedic surgeons deal with peripheral nerve entrapments on a regular basis. Entrapment neuropathies occur commonly, and the clinician must have a method of evaluating, assessing, and treating patients with these syndromes (Figure 24.3). Peripheral nerve entrapments produce focal disturbances of nerve function. The differential diagnosis of peripheral nerve entrapments therefore revolves around other conditions that may damage nerves in a focal manner. These disorders include degenerative diseases, hereditary disorders (i.e., hereditary neuropathy with liability to pressure palsies, or HNLPPs), vascular disorders, inflammatory diseases, and metabolic diseases. The physician must be alert to the possibilities of diagnostic confusion. The following conditions may resemble entrapment neuropathies: polyneuropathies (symmetric, asymmetric, demyelinating), brachial plexopathy, radiculopathy, amyotrophic lateral sclerosis, and connective tissue and vasospastic conditions (Raynaud's phenomenon, peripheral neuropathies with vasomotor changes, RSD).

The different entrapment neuropathies are discussed here according to the peripheral nerves that they involve.

*Table 24.5*   Peripheral entrapment neuropathies

| Nerve | Entrapment syndrome |
| --- | --- |
| **Upper limbs** | |
| Median | Carpal tunnel |
| | Pseudo–carpal tunnel (sublimis) |
| | Digital nerve |
| | Anterior interosseous nerve |
| | Pronator teres |
| | Ligament of Struthers |
| | Double crush |
| Ulnar | Guyon's canal |
| | Digital nerve |
| | Cubital canal |
| | Tardy ulnar palsy |
| | Double crush |
| Radial | Saturday night palsy |
| | Posterior interosseous nerve |
| | Tennis elbow |
| Musculocutaneous | Coracobrachialis |
| Suprascapular | Suprascapular foramen |
| | Infraspinatus branch |
| Dorsal scapular | Scalenus medius |
| Brachial plexus | Thoracic outlet |
| | Scalenus anticus |
| | Costoclavicular |
| | Hyperabduction |
| **Lower limbs** | |
| Sciatic | Piriformis |
| | Popliteal (Baker's) cyst |
| Common peroneal | Hereditary compression neuropathy |
| | Ganglion |
| | Leprosy |
| | Popliteal (Baker's) cyst |
| Posterior tibial | Popliteal (Baker's) cyst |
| | Tarsal tunnel |
| | Medial and lateral plantar nerve |
| | Interdigital nerve |
| Femoral | Pressure by space-limiting process |
| Saphenous | Subsartorial (Hunter's) canal |
| Lateral femoral cutaneous | Meralgia paresthetica |
| Obturator | Obturator canal |
| | Osteitis pubis |
| Ilioinguinal | Anterior superior iliac spine |
| Genitofemoral | Adhesions after surgery |

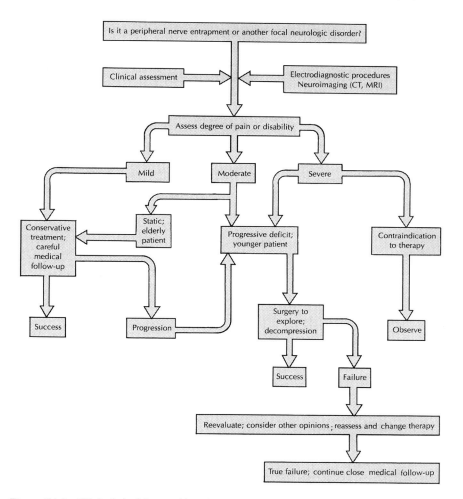

*Figure 24.3* Clinical decision making for patients with entrapment neuropathies. (CT = computed tomography; MRI = magnetic resonance imaging.) (Reprinted with permission from KK Nakano. Entrapment Neuropathies and Related Disorders. In WN Kelley, ED Harris Jr, S Ruddy, CB Sledge [eds], Textbook of Rheumatology [5th ed]. Philadelphia: Saunders, 1998;570.)

## Upper Limbs

Median Nerve

*Carpal Tunnel Syndrome*

**Clinical Evaluation.**   The most common entrapment neuropathy occurs in the carpal tunnel of the hand, at the point where the median nerve passes in company with the flexor tendons of the fingers. In the majority of cases of carpal tunnel syndrome (CTS), the clinical symptoms and the physical findings are specific. Patients affected with CTS report numbness, tingling, and pain in the hand, which often worsens at night or after use of the hand. Some individuals complain of pain that radiates proximally into the forearm and arm. In the early stages of CTS, examination frequently reveals no abnormality; with greater severity of median nerve compression, the patient experiences sensory loss over some or all of the digits innervated by the median nerve and weakness of thumb abduction. Clinical assessment includes evaluation for Tinel's sign (paresthesia in the median territory elicited by gentle tapping over the carpal tunnel) and positive response to Phalen's maneuver (appearance or worsening of paresthesias with maximal passive wrist flexion for 1 minute). Reverse Phalen testing (passive wrist and finger extension for 1 minute) may yield higher intracarpal canal hydrostatic pressure and result in prolonged sensory latencies and altered amplitudes when compared with the response with traditional or modified Phalen's maneuvers.

The following disorders may be associated with CTS: diabetes, RA, hypothyroidism, gout, acromegaly, pregnancy and lactation, renal failure with chronic hemodialysis, lipoma of the flexor digitorum superficialis, fascia of the flexor digitorum superficialis, ganglion cysts, gonococcal tenosynovitis, pigmented villonodular synovitis, Lyme borreliosis, arterial anomalies (including aneurysms of the median nerve), trauma (including those due to automobile accident and sports), and other previously known inflammatory reactions involving tendons and connective tissues of the wrist. CTS may also arise in paraplegic patients as a result of daily activities or athletic pursuits.

**Differential Diagnosis.**   In the differential diagnosis of CTS, the clinician must exclude a cervical radiculopathy, which often can be identified by the occurrence of proximal radiation of pain above the shoulder, paresthesias with coughing or sneezing, or a pattern of motor or sensory disturbances beyond the territory of the median nerve. Occasionally, thoracic outlet syndrome (TOS) may be of concern. Transient ischemic attacks and pure sensory strokes (e.g., from a lesion of the medial lemniscus of the mid-lower pons) may present with confusing symptoms, but usually pain is absent during an episode of numbness. Because no more than half of the patients with CTS can reliably report the location of their paresthesias, and because of the anomalous anatomy of peripheral nerves, ulnar neuropathies must be considered in certain clinical presentations. In an occupational setting, the overuse syndrome (OS) may become a common diagnostic problem. In OS or cumulative trauma syndrome, the patient experiences muscle pain or ache, tendinitis, fibrositis, and epicondylitis; psychological problems may contribute to the symptoms. OS has accounted for over one-half of all occupational illnesses in the United States since 1989. Automation and specialization in the workplace, with concentration of the workload on a few smaller groups of muscles, are thought to explain the higher prevalence of OS in certain occupational environments. Overall, CTS accounts for a minority of cases of OS; however, the frequency of both CTS and OS appears to increase in parallel in workers who are at risk.

**Diagnostic Evaluation.**   Electrodiagnostic testing is important for the accurate diagnosis of CTS. The sensitivity of sensory nerve conduction testing improves with sequential measurements at short distances over the course of the nerve in the palm. Caution should be taken in performing electrodiagnostic studies, because approximately one-half of patients with CTS possess abnormalities of the contralateral median nerve; therefore, NCS values in patients should be compared with reference data for normal individuals as well as with the involved patient's own contralateral median and ipsilateral ulnar and radial latency values. In addition, the electromyographer must take into consideration the data of normal control subjects, limb temperature, age, and body mass index, and consider forearm mixed median NCS. EMG of the limb muscles as well as the paraspinal cervical muscles should usually be performed in order to consider in the differential diagnosis the presence of coexisting disease (such as radiculopathy due to cervical spine disease, diffuse peripheral neuropathy, proximal nerve lesions). In patients with CTS, no tests provide higher diagnostic accuracy than EMG and NCS. However, false-positive and false-negative results do occur; many of the apparent false-positive results occur in patients who have measurable abnormalities on NCS but no symptoms (e.g., there is a high rate of abnormalities in the contralateral hands of patients with CTS). On the other hand, rarely patients who have typical symptoms of CTS have normal EMG and NCS studies, yet respond to carpal tunnel surgical release.

**Treatment.** Early diagnosis and treatment are important, because delay can result in irreversible median nerve damage with persistent symptoms and permanent disability. Nonsurgical treatment would be advised for patients with mild symptoms, intermittent symptoms, or an acute flare-up of CTS from a specific injury. Five types of nonsurgical therapy include: (1) patient avoidance of the activities that precipitate the condition, (2) splinting of the wrist firmly in the neutral position for night and day use, (3) local steroid injection by an experienced clinician, (4) administration of a brief course of either oral steroids or NSAIDs, and (5) a trial of diuretics, particularly when the CTS symptoms appear premenstrually. For mild nighttime CTS symptoms, a removable volar wrist splint that holds the wrist in a neutral position can often alleviate all symptoms. If symptoms persist or recur, additional treatment is indicated. Local steroid injections or a trial of oral medication are recommended for patients with mild persistent symptoms or for patients who complain of pain from the CTS and are elderly or are poor surgical risks. Local steroid injections often relieve the pain but may not change the other symptoms of CTS. Patients with thenar atrophy or muscle weakness or those with advanced sensory loss should not receive local steroid injections. Surgical treatment of CTS demands care and skill and is one of the most successful operations that can be performed on the hand. Furthermore, such surgery is reliably good and may now be performed with low morbidity by means of a variety of minimally invasive techniques that use limited incisions involving less extensive exposure than the classic open procedure. These include flexor tenosynovectomy without transverse carpal ligament (TCL) division, endoscopic release of the TCL, and subcutaneous TCL division with a two-incision technique. Complications of CTS surgery and poor results are usually related to poor surgical technique. Indications for surgical therapy of CTS include: (1) failure of nonoperative treatment or clinical evidence of thenar atrophy, (2) persistent sensory loss, and (3) re-exploration when the patient fails to respond to CTS release or when recurrent CTS is present. Surgery with $CO_2$ laser may offer an alternative technique in treatment of some patients with CTS; however, some recent reports indicate that the use of lasers may affect nerve conduction.

## Anterior Interosseous Nerve Syndromes

**Clinical Evaluation.**   The anterior interosseous nerve (AIN) is a purely motor branch of the nerve that arises from the median nerve 5–8 cm distal to the lateral epicondyle and supplies the flexor pollicis longus (FPL), the pronator quadratus (PQ), and the flexor digitorum profundus (FDP) of the index and middle fingers. It contains no fibers of superficial sensation but does supply deep pain and proprioception to some deep tissues, including the wrist joint.

**Differential Diagnosis.**   Either trauma, inflammation, or anatomic variations may cause AIN paralysis; acute localized neuritis may be more common than trauma or compression. In the AIN syndromes, patients often complain of a nonspecific pain in the forearm or elbow and frequently demonstrate weakness of the FPL, PQ, FDP1, and FDP2 on examination. Sometimes only the FPL or FDP1 is involved; in the latter situation, one must rule out tendon ruptures of the FPL or the FDP1, which occasionally develop in RA.

**Diagnostic Evaluation.**   In the AIN syndromes, routine motor and sensory NCS of the radial, median, and ulnar nerves are normal; however, the latency and duration of the evoked action potential from elbow to PQ are prolonged, and EMG demonstrates denervation in the PQ, FPL, and the FDP1 and FDP2 muscles.

**Treatment.**   Therapy depends on the cause. Penetrating wounds require immediate exploration and surgical repair. Impending Volkmann's contracture demands immediate surgical decompression. In spontaneous AIN syndrome cases, the initial steps in management include avoiding activity that exacerbates the symptoms, resting the affected upper limb, and taking NSAIDs. If no improvement occurs within 8–12 weeks, surgical exploration by an experienced hand surgeon should be considered. In cases of partial lesions of the AIN, a longer trial of nonsurgical therapy may be warranted.

## Pronator Teres Syndrome

**Clinical Evaluation.**   In the pronator teres syndrome (PTS), entrapment of the median nerve occurs at the level of the pronator teres muscle, producing pain and tenderness of the proximal forearm as well as paresthesias of the hand. PTS is relatively rare. Patients with PTS demonstrate weakness in the FPL and the abductor pollicis brevis, and pronation of the forearm remains normal. Causes of PTS include trauma, fracture, muscle hypertrophy, and abnormal vascular structures.

**Differential Diagnosis.**   Rarely, median neuralgia can be caused by a brachial pseudoaneurysm as a neurovascular complication of an antebrachial arteriovenous fistula or complication of blood donation. Other instances in which the median nerve can be involved are when entrapment occurs beneath the bicipital aponeurosis, an anomalous muscle causes pressure in the distal half of the arm, after physeal fractures of the distal radius, after operative treatment of intra-articular distal humerus fracture with intact supracondylar process, and when compression occurs in the proximal forearm.

**Diagnostic Evaluation.**   NCSs reveal median nerve slowing in the proximal forearm but normal distal motor latencies and sensory action potentials at the wrist. EMG abnormalities are found in the median innervated muscles below the level of the pronator teres muscle, and the pronator teres muscle shows normal electrical activity.

**Treatment.**   Nonsurgical treatment is indicated in cases of PTS with mild, intermittent symptoms associated with strenuous use of the involved limb (especially repeated elbow flexion and pronation). Use of NSAIDs and splints on the elbow and wrist often prove beneficial in conjunction with avoidance of exacerbating activities. Surgical therapy is indicated in those PTS cases with persistent or progressive symptoms and signs of nerve dysfunction. Adequate exploration and decompression both distally and proximally are required.

## *Ligament of Struthers Entrapment*

**Clinical Evaluation.**   On rare occasions, the median nerve may become entrapped by a ligament of Struthers (LS), a fibrous band from a supratrochlear spur or supracondylar process at the distal anteromedial humerus. This structure encloses a foramen, the other boundaries of which are the median intermuscular septum and the distal and anterior surface of the medial humeral condyle. The median nerve and brachial artery pass through this foramen.

**Differential Diagnosis.**   Entrapment of the median nerve by an LS occurs in the upper arm area and simulates a PTS. In a true PTS, the innervation to the pronator teres muscle is often spared, and entrapment above the elbow weakens the pronator teres muscle.

**Diagnostic Evaluation.**   In an LS entrapment, palpation and routine radiographs demonstrate a spur about 5 cm above the median epicondyle. Careful EMG of the pronator teres and of more distal median-innervated muscles, as well as NCS from above and below the elbow and from elbow to wrist, can localize the deficit as proximal to the pronator teres muscle. Because the brachial artery has been entrapped along with the median nerve, the radial pulse often decreases or disappears when the forearm is fully extended or supinated.

**Treatment.**   Surgery appears to benefit those patients in whom focal entrapment by a fibrous band produces a proximal median neuropathy.

## *Entrapment of Digital Nerves in the Hand*

**Clinical Evaluation.**   Prolongations of the median nerve end as interdigital nerves, which provide sensation to the index fingers and to part of the middle fingers. An anastomosis between the median and ulnar nerves forms the interdigital nerve to the middle and ring fingers. An entrapment of the interdigital nerve may occur in the intermetacarpal tunnel of the hand region if trauma or a mass (tumor, osteophyte, cyst) obstructs the passageway. When the finger is hyperextended and spread laterally, the interdigital nerve draws tightly against the edge of the deep transverse metacarpal ligament.

**Differential Diagnosis.**   Direct trauma, phalangeal fracture, and tenosynovitis may also produce this entrapment. Alteration in the flexor tendon sheath complex or in the lumbrical muscle can result from arthritis, from an inflammatory response of the metacarpophalangeal joint, or infrequently, from a tumor. Patients with an interdigital neuropathy complain of pain in one or two fingers. Clinical examination reveals hyperpathia or anesthesia, secondary vasomotor changes, and acute tenderness of the interdigital nerve upon palpation at the palmar surface of the interdigital web between the metacarpal heads.

**Diagnostic Evaluation.**   Spreading the involved finger away from the affected web space in hyperextension is painful for the patient. Local infiltration of steroids may assist in diagnosis, and repeated injections may relieve the entrapment.

**Treatment.**   Neurolysis should be considered in patients with a cyst or tumor and in those with severe neuropathy who fail to respond to other measures. In addition, chronic trauma to the hands, as seen in woodchoppers, musicians, laborers, and staplers, should be avoided if possible.

### Palmar Cutaneous Nerve Entrapment

**Clinical Evaluation.**   Isolated entrapment of the palmar cutaneous branch of the median nerve can be caused by a ganglion compressing the nerve within its tunnel.

**Differential Diagnosis.**   Neuroma of the palmar cutaneous nerve (PCN) can cause pain after CTS surgery with secondary diminished wrist range of motion and reduced grip.

**Diagnostic Evaluation.**   Careful clinical examination and sensory NCS help localize the patient's symptoms to the PCN.

**Treatment.**   When a ganglion is the cause of the PCN entrapment, decompression and excision of the ganglion relieve the symptoms. Resection and implantation of the PCN have been shown to reduce pain and allow patients to return to their jobs in cases where neuromas arise as a complication of CTS surgery.

### Ulnar Nerve

### Entrapment of the Ulnar Nerve in the Region of the Elbow

**Clinical Evaluation.**   Ulnar nerve entrapment in the region of the elbow is the second most frequent upper limb compression neuropathy. As the ulnar nerve passes through the ulnar groove in the vicinity of the medial epicondyle of the elbow, it is subject to several types of compressive injury. Causes of ulnar nerve entrapment at the elbow, in approximate order of frequency, include cubital tunnel syndrome (CUBTS), external compression, previous fracture and scarring, recurrent subluxation of the ulnar nerve, and entrapment. A CUBTS can occur where the ulnar nerve passes the aponeurosis of origin of the flexor carpi ulnaris (FCU) muscle. In certain individuals, the aponeurosis is drawn taut over the ulnar nerve, particularly with elbow flexion; the point of constriction lies 1.5–3.5 cm distal to the medial epicondyle. External compression results from repeated resting of the elbow on a flat surface, especially if the ulnar groove is shallow. Persons subjected to immobility (e.g., in anesthesia, coma, restrained positions) appear at risk for prolonged pressure on the ulnar nerve.

**Differential Diagnosis.**   Previous fracture may damage the elbow, and scarring can compromise the ulnar nerve. Recurrent subluxation of the ulnar nerve, which can roll anteriorly over the medial epicondyle, may contribute to ulnar neuropathies, especially in an athlete who throws. Compression of the ulnar nerve at the elbow can occur in association with synovial cysts. Rarely a CUBTS is caused by an abnormal insertion of the medial head of the triceps muscle of the arm onto the medial epicondyle of the elbow. Also, a high ulnar nerve palsy may be caused by the arcade of Struthers, or entrapments may occur distal to the cubital tunnel (more than 4 cm beyond the medial epicondyle) in the flexor-pronator aponeurosis. Clinically, patients with a CUBTS experience onset of or increase in one or more of the following symptoms: pain, numbness, or tingling with the elbow flexion test (full elbow flexion with full extension of the wrists for 3 minutes). If weakness occurs, it affects functions of the hand, including finger abduction, thumb abduction, pinching of the thumb and forefinger, and, eventually, power grip. Athletes and performing artists who require very fine control of the fingers may note a decline in performance with minimal ulnar nerve compression. Cervical radiculopathy of the C8 nerve root can cause radiating paresthesias in the hand. Rarely a brachial plexus lesion (e.g., metastatic tumor) or a TOS can mimic symptoms of an ulnar neuropathy. The ulnar nerve can be constricted at the wrist rather than the elbow by repeat trauma to the palm or by a mass (tumor or ganglion).

**Diagnostic Evaluation.**   Electrodiagnostic testing includes both motor and sensory NCS. The site of the abnormality is located by sequentially assessing ulnar nerve conduction across the elbow segment. EMG should test the intrinsic muscles of the hand as well as forearm, arm, and paraspinal muscles to verify that no other condition exists, because other disorders can present with numbness of the little finger and motor weakness.

**Treatment.**   Therapy depends on the cause and severity of the ulnar nerve compression, and on the length of time the symptoms have been present. Nonsurgical therapy appears to be indicated for the patient with intermittent symptoms, acute or chronic mild neuropathy, or mild neuropathy associated with an occupational cause. Treatment entails avoiding repetitive flexion and extension of the elbow, resting the elbow, or splinting the elbow in extension. For intermittent symptoms associated with repetitive flexion-extension, change of activity may alleviate the condition. For a mild neuropathy produced by a blow or chronic pressure, splinting the elbow in an extended position may prove helpful. A bivalved long-arm cast can be fabricated for use for a more prolonged period. Splinting may be continued for 2–3 months, especially if the symptoms remain intermittent or show improvement. As long as symptoms or signs do not progress, and particularly as long as there is no motor involvement or objective sensory loss, surgical intervention is not necessary. Careful clinical follow-up is important, and the patient should be checked for development of motor deficit, atrophy, or weakness, because development of any of these findings calls for a change in the therapeutic program. Surgical techniques for the treatment of ulnar neuropathies at the elbow remain controversial; however, the best results of surgery occur in patients with mild signs and symptoms, and poor results are seen for patients with severe atrophy. Medial epicondylectomy for ulnar neuropathy at the elbow may provide symptomatic improvement, but the outlook for improved motor strength is less optimistic. In patients with an ulnar neuropathy at the elbow and an associated epitrochleoanconeus muscle, surgical treatment with excision of the epitrochleoanconeus and cubital tunnel release without anterior transposition of the ulnar nerve has been successful.

*Ulnar Nerve Entrapments at the Wrist*

**Clinical Evaluation.**    Ulnar nerve entrapment occurs less frequently at the wrist in Guyon's canal than at the elbow. Tendons pass through Guyon's canal, and no tenosynovium should entrap the nerve. In rare instances, however, the tenosynovium within the carpal tunnel bulges and compresses the ulnar nerve proximal to the canal, thereby producing symptoms that clinically simulate an ulnar neuropathy at the elbow. On examination, however, one finds normal motor function of the FCU and of the FDP to the ring and little fingers. In addition, the sensory loss is confined to the palmar branch, while the dorsum of the hand has normal sensation (the dorsal cutaneous branch lies proximal to the wrist).

**Differential Diagnosis.**    A ganglion is the most likely cause of entrapment in Guyon's canal; however, trauma, RA, long-distance bicycling (as in "handlebar palsy"), masses (including rarely a tuberculoma), anomalies, or inflammation can produce similar clinical symptoms.

**Diagnostic Evaluation.**    The diagnosis is confirmed if prolonged motor and sensory terminal latencies are demonstrable in the ulnar nerve of the affected hand.

**Treatment.**    Treatment of ulnar nerve compression at the wrist depends on the origin and duration of the condition responsible. For mild compressions associated either with a single traumatic event or with chronic trauma, conservative treatment should initially be prescribed. Avoidance of the trauma, with or without splinting, often results in complete return of function. In cases that do not respond to nonsurgical care, surgical exploration, decompression, and neurolysis should be performed. If the hook of the hamate bone is fractured, it should be excised, and decompression and neurolysis of the nerve should be performed. Ganglia and other soft tissue masses should be removed.

## Dorsal Sensory Branch Compression

**Clinical Evaluation.**   Isolated neuropathy of the dorsal sensory branch of the ulnar nerve is associated with either blunt trauma, laceration, or tight restraints.

**Differential Diagnosis.**   Tightly applied handcuffs may produce a neuropathy of the dorsal ulnar cutaneous nerve.

**Diagnostic Evaluation.**   The clinical neurologic examination and sensory NCS confirm the diagnosis.

**Treatment.**   Treatment in most cases of blunt trauma includes protecting the area of injury; symptoms subside within weeks. When painful neuromas occur after laceration, surgical exploration may be considered. If the involved nerve is entrapped in scar tissue, neurolysis may prove beneficial.

## Digital Ulnar Nerve Entrapment

**Clinical Evaluation.**   The interdigital nerves to the ring and little fingers arise as prolongations of the ulnar nerve; the nerves to the middle and ring fingers are formed by an anastomosis between the median and ulnar nerve.

**Differential Diagnosis.**   Mechanisms and causes for ulnar digital entrapment syndromes are similar to those for median digital neuropathies.

**Diagnostic Evaluation.**   Clinical examination demonstrates the characteristic pattern of sensory loss and pain.

**Treatment.**   Therapy is similar to that for other interdigital entrapments.

Radial Nerve

## High Radial Nerve Compression

**Clinical Evaluation.**   High radial nerve compressions occur proximal to the elbow prior to the division of the posterior interosseous branch and the sensory branch.

**Differential Diagnosis.**   Most of these radial nerve lesions are traumatic (e.g., due to shoulder dislocations, humeral neck fractures) or secondary to pressure (e.g., due to the use of crutches). A lesion localized to the region of the spiral groove may produce an acute retrohumeral radial neuropathy, and a high radial nerve palsy may follow strenuous muscular activity (the radial nerve becomes constricted by the lateral head of the triceps muscle). Furthermore, rarely a compressive radial nerve palsy can appear after military training (e.g., after shooting a rifle for many hours).

**Diagnostic Evaluation.**   EMG and NCS help localize the site of, and assess the extent of, radial nerve compression or injury.

**Treatment.**   Treatment of traumatic radial nerve compression is generally conservative, because most patients with radial nerve paresis secondary to compression recover spontaneously. Treatment of a compression lesion of a high radial nerve should include a cockup splint made of plaster or plastic for the wrist joint. This splint should be applied if the paresis lasts longer than 1 week. When there is long-lasting weakness, a spring-loaded extensor brace for the fingers may be used. In cases of humeral fracture requiring surgical exploration, the radial nerve should also be explored at the time of surgery. When there is displaced fracture of the distal part of the humerus, early exploration is necessary because of the high incidence of radial nerve entrapment between the fracture fragments.

### Posterior Interosseous Nerve Syndrome

**Clinical Evaluation.**   Posterior interosseous nerve syndrome (PINS) is an entrapment of the deep branch of the radial nerve just distal to the elbow joint. Motor weakness of the extensors of the wrist and fingers is seen; the extensor carpi radialis longus (ECRL) and extensor carpi radialis brevis (ECRB) are spared.

**Differential Diagnosis.**   Infrequently, PINS occurs after excision of the radial head, as an isolated paralysis of the descending branch, or in association with congenital hemihypertrophy; rarely, it occurs secondary to vasculitis or a myxoma. The patient with PINS shows pain, limitation of movement, and elbow spasm; in patients with RA, evidence of elbow synovitis is also present. A positive tenodesis effect is noted with PIN paralysis. When the wrist is passively flexed, the metacarpophalangeal joints extend; this extension demonstrates that the extensor tendons are intact. In patients with ruptured extensor tendons, the ends of the tendons are distal to the wrist, and therefore no tenodesis is seen. The most important physical finding is radial deviation of the wrist on dorsiflexion, due to noninvolvement of the ECRL and ECRB, with paralysis of the extensor carpi ulnaris (ECU). Even with partial paralysis, the digits that extend show marked weakness.

**Diagnostic Evaluation.**   EMG confirms the diagnosis, because denervation changes are present in the muscles supplied by the PIN, including the extensor digitorum communis, ECU, extensor digiti minimi, extensor indicis proprius, abductor pollicis longus, extensor pollicis brevis, and extensor pollicis longus.

**Treatment.**   In most cases of PINS, treatment is surgical. Ganglia, tumors, and lipomas should be removed surgically, and the PIN should be freed from any compressive bands or other constricting structures. When the PIN is entrapped and mimics lateral epicondylitis in resistant tennis elbow, treatment includes surgical exploration with release of the ECR tendon origin and removal of any constricting vascular or fibrous band.

## Superficial Radial Nerve Entrapment

**Clinical Evaluation.** The superficial radial nerve can be damaged by lacerations or compression around the wrist because of its superficial position.

**Differential Diagnosis.** Infrequently, the superficial radial nerve can be compressed by handcuffs, a tightly fitting wristwatch, or other straps and bandages around the wrist. Wartenberg's disease is entrapment of the superficial radial nerve in the forearm; de Quervain's disease can be found in association in 50% of these cases [10].

**Diagnostic Evaluation.** The clinical examination as well as sensory NCS provide a diagnosis.

**Treatment.** Both conservative and surgical treatments for Wartenberg's disease yield good results. It is important to identify Wartenberg's disease before operating on tenosynovitis in order to avoid postoperative complications.

## Radial Digital Nerve Entrapment

**Clinical Evaluation.** Infrequently, a palmar ganglion produces diminished sensation in the distribution of the radial digital nerve of the thumb.

**Differential Diagnosis.** Occasionally, a C6 sensory radiculopathy may be confused with a radial digital nerve disorder.

**Diagnostic Evaluation.** Selective sensory NCS and MRI techniques may be useful in certain cases.

**Treatment.** Surgical excision using an extensile incision has been successful in treating this condition.

## Brachial Plexus: Thoracic Outlet Syndrome

### Clinical Evaluation

Bony, fascial, and muscular structures can interfere with functions of the neurovascular bundle located in the thoracic outlet. Neurogenic TOS is caused by abnormal bands that cross the brachial plexus, often inserting on the rudimentary cervical rib; paresthesias commonly precede the development of persistent pain, atrophy, or muscle weakness. The anatomic territories affected include those of the ulnar nerve and the medial cutaneous nerve of the forearm.

## Differential Diagnosis

The pathophysiology of reversible, positionally dependent paresthesias remains unknown. A change in pulse with arm abduction is not a reliable indicator of TOS, because a change is found in 15% of normal persons. Moreover, a pseudoneurogenic TOS may occur with multifocal right cerebral infarctions and present with focal atrophy and weakness secondary to the central lesion, thus simulating TOS. Brachial plexus lesions result more often from birth injuries or trauma during anesthesia and surgical and medical procedures.

## Diagnostic Evaluation

Electrodiagnostic testing shows no abnormalities in patients with the more common reversible paresthesias; however, in true neurogenic TOS, the following findings are seen: (1) low amplitude of the median nerve motor response, (2) low or relatively low amplitude of the ulnar sensory action potential, (3) normal low or normal amplitude of the ulnar motor response, and (4) normal amplitude of the median sensory action potential. MRI may be a useful diagnostic tool in certain disorders of the brachial plexus.

## Treatment

Two types of nonsurgical therapy for TOS are (1) use of a corset and restraints to prevent elevation of the arms or hands that are placed behind the head, and (2) prescription of a set of exercises designed to correct slumping shoulder posture, increase the range of motion of the neck and shoulders, strengthen the rhomboid and trapezius muscles, and provide behavior modification [11]. Surgical treatment of TOS carries some risk and should be reserved for the rare patient with documented worsening of neurologic functions. The clinician should consider the following criteria: (1) signs of muscle wasting in the involved hand, (2) replacement of intermittent paresthesias by sensory loss, and (3) incapacitating pain. First-rib resection through the transaxillary approach has been commonly used. Alternatively, exploration from above, usually with removal of the anterior scalene muscle and exploration of the thoracic outlet, has been used. This latter supraclavicular procedure has the advantage that a cervical rib, if present, is directly within the field of operation. In addition, constricting bands may be found passing from the rudimentary rib, or from the transverse process of C7, to attach to the first rib. Disadvantages to the supraclavicular approach include the following: (1) the surgical scar is cosmetically less acceptable than that in a transaxillary approach, (2) there may be temporary damage to the phrenic nerve or to the long thoracic nerve from retraction during the extensive dissection, and (3) more surgical dissection may be required with this procedure.

Suprascapular Nerve

*Clinical Evaluation*

The suprascapular nerve is a purely motor nerve and arises from the upper trunk of the brachial plexus, which is formed from the roots of C5 and C6; suprascapular nerve entrapment occurs when the nerve's passage through the suprascapular foramen is compromised and produces pain and weakness or atrophy of the supraspinatus and infraspinatus muscles.

*Differential Diagnosis*

Suprascapular nerve syndromes may result from exertion during sports activities (e.g., volleyball, baseball) or Latin dancing; from work exertion, especially the lifting of heavy objects overhead; from masses (e.g., ganglions, sarcomas, metastatic cancer, hematoma); as a complication of certain surgeries when the patient is put in predisposing surgical positions; from certain exercises; from an arthrodetic shoulder; or from primary shoulder dislocations and humeral fractures.

*Diagnostic Evaluation*

Electrodiagnostic procedures are helpful in the diagnosis of the lesion or entrapment. MRI has been useful in the evaluation of patients with suprascapular entrapments.

*Treatment*

Observation and conservative care are indicated in cases of acute blunt trauma with or without scapular fracture. When a severe comminuted fracture of the scapula is present with obvious involvement of the scapular notch, earlier surgical exploration should be considered. In patients who experience repetitive minor trauma, avoiding the trauma generally corrects the problem. Whenever persistent signs and symptoms occur, or when spontaneous onset occurs without known cause, surgical exploration may be indicated.

Dorsal Scapular Nerve

*Clinical Evaluation*

The dorsal scapular nerve arises primarily from spinal segment C5 and innervates the levator scapulae and the rhomboids.

*Differential Diagnosis*

Following trauma and in rare entrapments, weakness of the rhomboideus major and minor and the levator scapulae occurs as well as a tendency of the vertebral border of the scapula (particularly the lower portion) to be displaced dorsally. This displacement forms a prominence under the skin, and the scapula shifts laterally.

### Diagnostic Evaluation

The neurologic examination and EMG localize the problem to the dorsal scapular nerve distribution.

### Treatment

Because this syndrome is often secondary to scalene hyperactivity caused by inadequacy of the spinal stabilization system, treatment should be directed toward the cervical spine and includes sedation, use of muscle relaxants and analgesics, and physical therapy. In severe cases, surgical neurolysis may be considered.

## Long Thoracic Nerve

### Clinical Evaluation

The long thoracic nerve originates from the undivided anterior primary rami of C5, C6, and C7 after they emerge from the intervertebral foramina; it traverses the neck behind the cords of the brachial plexus, enters the medial aspect of the axilla, and continues downward on the lateral wall of the thorax to reach the serratus muscle. The long thoracic nerve follows a straight course and becomes fixed by the scalene and muscle slips of the serratus anterior; in this condition, the shoulder girdle displaces slightly backward, and the lower scapula demonstrates undue winging.

### Differential Diagnosis

Because of the straight anatomic course and fixation of the long thoracic nerve, it can be stretched; this stretching occurs most often with heavy labor or after direct trauma.

### Diagnostic Evaluation

The clinical examination and EMG and NCS localize the findings to the long thoracic nerve.

### Treatment

Recovery from this syndrome usually occurs within 6 months of the original stretch injury in the large majority of patients.

## Musculocutaneous Nerve

*Clinical Evaluation*

Rarely an injury affects the musculocutaneous nerve (MCN) in the vicinity of the lateral cord of the upper trunk of the brachial plexus. In MCN injuries, flexion of the forearm at the elbow is weakened because of biceps and brachialis involvement; however, the disability is not severe, because the brachioradialis and pronator teres muscles take part in producing this movement. With the forearm in pronation, flexion at the elbow becomes impossible; sensation is reduced along the lateral border of the forearm.

*Differential Diagnosis*

Very occasionally, the MCN may become entrapped by the coracobrachial muscle, or it may even be ruptured by violent extension of the forearm.

*Diagnostic Evaluation*

The neurologic examination and electrodiagnostic studies localize the clinical problem to the MCN.

*Treatment*

Surgical exploration may be necessary to differentiate a nerve entrapment from a nerve rupture. If coracoid mobilization becomes necessary during surgery, the MCN and its branches should be identified and protected; the variations in anatomy and the level of penetration should be kept in mind.

## Axillary Nerve

*Clinical Evaluation*

Most lesions of the axillary nerve are due to trauma (e.g., a blow on the tip of the shoulder after motor vehicle accidents, football injuries, anterior dislocations of the shoulder).

*Differential Diagnosis*

The quadrilateral space syndrome occurs secondary to compression of the axillary nerve by fibrous bands in the quadrilateral space and is a cause of shoulder pain.

*Diagnostic Evaluation*

Electrodiagnosis localizes the clinical problem to the axillary nerve; in the case of quadrilateral space syndrome, MRI confirms atrophy of the teres minor muscle.

*Treatment*

The treatment of an axillary nerve injury depends on the cause. There is a poor prognosis for full recovery from stretch injuries of the distal portions of the brachial plexus, and the shoulder sags with deltoid atrophy.

## Lower Limbs

Sciatic Nerve

*Clinical Evaluation*

The sciatic nerve originates from undivided primary rami at L4, L5, S1, S2, and S3 and can be divided into component parts: tibial nerve, common peroneal nerve, and the nerve to the hamstring muscles.

*Differential Diagnosis*

Sciatic nerve entrapments are uncommon; most patients complaining of symptoms traceable to the sciatic nerve suffer from effects of trauma, fracture, or arthroplasty, or have disease of the lumbosacral spine (e.g., spinal stenosis, degenerative disease, RA, osteoarthritis, ankylosing spondylitis, intravertebral tumor, metastatic disease). Rarely, sciatic neuropathies appear during correction of knee flexion deformities, as a complication of a prolonged position during surgical procedures, and secondary to a pelvis mass (namely, *cyclic sciatica*). At times a high sciatic lesion can mimic a peroneal neuropathy at the fibular head. A variation in the course of the sciatic nerve involves its passage between parts of the piriformis muscle (the division of the nerve that becomes the peroneal trunk is usually the one that deviates). True compression of the sciatic nerve may occur from the piriformis muscle, from a myofascial band in the distal portion of the thigh between the biceps femoris and the adductor magnus, from Baker's cyst, secondary to a traumatic gluteal compartment syndrome, from muscle fibrosis after intramuscular injections, as a complication of anticoagulant therapy, and after trauma (e.g., hip operation, needle biopsy, or sitting on hard surfaces).

*Diagnostic Evaluation*

The clinical assessment as well as careful EMG and NCS often define and localize the sciatic neuropathy.

*Treatment*

In the case of piriformis syndrome, surgery includes removal of one of the heads of origin of the muscle and release of any constriction. Other causes of slowly progressive sciatic palsy should be treated in accordance with the condition that caused the symptoms (e.g., withholding anticoagulants when bleeding has contributed to the neuropathy).

Peroneal Nerve

*Compression Neuropathy*

**Clinical Evaluation.**    The most vulnerable spot for compression of the peroneal nerve is where the nerve winds around the neck of the fibula near its division into the deep and superficial peroneal nerves. The mechanism of damage to the peroneal nerve at the head of the fibula is a compression causing a neuropraxic lesion.

**Differential Diagnosis.**    Palsy of the common, deep, or superficial peroneal nerves secondary to trauma or undue pressure can be seen in either medical patients (e.g., those with leprosy, HNLPP) or surgical patients (e.g., those with fractures and perioperative complications); it is seen infrequently as an obstetric complication during childbirth. Compressive causes of peroneal nerve damage include improperly applied plaster casts, tight bandages, tight stockings, other constrictive garments, and rarely cysts. Unconsciousness from drug overdose, anesthesia, or acute illness with stupor or coma can render patients susceptible to a peroneal compressive neuropathy.

**Diagnostic Evaluation.**    The careful use of electrodiagnostic studies and clinical correlation generally leads to the correct diagnosis.

**Treatment.**    In the majority of cases of peroneal neuropathy, treatment is nonsurgical. With motor disturbance, bracing with a plastic orthosis molded to the posterior calf and projecting into the shoe on the plantar surface of the foot provides stability. When this type of brace is used, a compressive lesion of the peroneal nerve can be monitored for several months before a surgical approach need be considered. Surgical therapy should be considered in those patients with a slowly progressive disturbance of peroneal nerve function in whom there is pain and progressive motor and sensory loss, entrapment neuropathy, or ganglion, cyst, or other tumor. In such conditions relatively early exploration is indicated, because little would be gained by further delay and a simple entrapment is unlikely.

*Anterior Tarsal Tunnel Syndrome*

**Clinical Evaluation.**    Anterior tarsal tunnel syndrome (ATTS) is a rarely reported entrapment neuropathy of the deep peroneal nerve under the extensor retinaculum at the ankle. The roof of the tunnel is the inferior extensor retinaculum; the floor is the fascia overlying the talus and navicular bone. Within the tunnel are four tendons, an artery, a vein, and the deep peroneal nerve.

**Differential Diagnosis.**   Patients with a peroneal or sciatic neuropathy or an L5 radiculopathy may present with similar symptoms. Rarely a pyramidal tract lesion may also mimic limited symptoms into the foot.

**Diagnostic Evaluation.**   Patients with an ATTS present with foot pain and dysesthesias. NCS shows prolonged peroneal distal latencies with reduced amplitude from the extensor digitorum brevis (EDB) muscle. EMG abnormalities are confined to the EDB; however, the electrodiagnostician must be aware of the possibility of an accessory peroneal nerve that does not go through the tunnel (thus masking the EMG findings in the EDB), fibrillation potentials that can appear in the EDB secondary to shoe wear or other localized trauma, and prolongation of peroneal latencies in cool limbs.

**Treatment.**   Nonsurgical therapy includes assuring a comfortable foot position by splint, rest, or a combination of both. Surgical release of the entrapment may be needed. In such cases it is necessary to trace the nerve far enough proximally to exclude a lesion in the ankle under the extensor retinaculum.

Posterior Tibial Nerve

*Posterior Tarsal Tunnel Syndrome*

**Clinical Evaluation.**   In posterior tarsal tunnel syndrome (PTTS), the posterior tibial nerve becomes entrapped at the level of the medial malleolus, the point from which the nerve supplies sensory innervation to the sole of the foot and motor innervation to the intrinsic muscles of the foot. Pain in the sole of the foot is the primary symptom of PTTS.

**Differential Diagnosis.**   A posterior tibial or sciatic neuropathy, an S1 radiculopathy, and rarely a pyramidal tract lesion may present with symptoms similar to those seen in PTTS.

**Diagnostic Evaluation.**   EMG and NCS localize the site of the posterior tibial nerve entrapment to the tarsal tunnel.

**Treatment.**   Nonsurgical therapy begins with removal of any irritating process and bracing of the foot with a medial arch support. NSAIDs work against local phlebitis or tenosynovitis. Surgery may be needed in as many as 60% of cases of PTTS. The surgical approach involves a curved incision below the medial malleolus, extending beyond the distal limit of the retinaculum. The lacinate ligament and the retinaculum are opened, and the nerve is freed. The release and dissection of the nerve must be carried as far distally as possible, typically to the level of its bifurcation into the plantar nerve.

## *Medial and Lateral Plantar Nerve Syndromes*

**Clinical Evaluation.** A partial PTTS (either a medial or a lateral plantar nerve deficit in the foot) alerts the clinician to the possibility of a process distal to the flexor retinaculum. Symptoms include weakness and burning of the feet.

**Differential Diagnosis.** Conditions similar to those listed in the differential diagnosis of PTTS as well as a systemic polyneuropathy should be borne in mind when evaluating patients with either a medial or lateral plantar nerve syndrome.

**Diagnostic Evaluation.** Selective NCS localizes the level of entrapment of the plantar nerve involved in the entrapment.

**Treatment.** Conservative measures, including rest and local steroid injections into the appropriate area, should be considered initially. Surgery should be considered if the symptoms or signs progress, or if the exact level of compression is uncertain in a symptomatic individual.

## *Interdigital Nerve Disorders*

**Clinical Evaluation.** The medial and lateral plantar nerves terminate as the interdigital nerves.

**Differential Diagnosis.** Morton's neuroma may occur at the region of the interdigital nerve in the third and fourth interspaces of the foot and become a source of lower limb pain.

**Diagnostic Evaluation.** The clinical evaluation usually localizes the problem to the interdigital nerves of the foot. Occasionally, selective nerve blocks may be used to localize the source of symptoms.

**Treatment** Initial conservative management consists of padding the metatarsal head of the foot or changing to shoes that cause less lateral pinching. Occasionally, a surgical excision of the nerve is required. This is done by an incision over the web space between the toes; the branch of the nerve is identified and tracked proximally until the branch point at which the two digital nerves are formed from the proper interdigital nerve.

## Sural Nerve

### *Clinical Evaluation*

The sural nerve originates from an anastomotic branch of the tibial nerve; this branch joins the peroneal anastomotic nerve and extends down the back of the leg to the outer side of the foot.

## Differential Diagnosis

The sural nerve is subject to laceration or compressive lesions primarily at the level of its exit through fascia; subsequent paresthesias radiate into the lateral part of the foot. Because the sural nerve can be a site for nerve biopsy, clinical symptoms similar to lacerations and compressive lesions may occur after such a biopsy.

## Diagnostic Evaluation

Antidromic sural sensory NCS is useful in assessment of a sural lesion. Because this is a purely sensory nerve, EMG is of no clinical utility in this instance.

## Treatment

If avoidance of continued irritation and rest of the affected area do not produce resolution of the symptoms, surgical exploration may be considered.

## Lateral Femoral Cutaneous Nerve

### Clinical Evaluation

The lateral femoral cutaneous nerve (LFCN) is derived from the L2 and L3 nerve roots and emerges from the lateral border of the psoas major muscle to cross the iliacus muscle; it goes forward to the lateral end of the inguinal ligament and at first lies under the iliacus fascia. It then enters in and runs between the fascial layers just before going through a tunnel in the lateral attachment of the inguinal ligament to the anterior superior iliac spine. Beyond its opening in the inguinal ligament, the nerve is beneath the deep fascia of the upper thigh for a short portion of its course, piercing it to reach its final subcutaneous and intracutaneous position. About 12.5 cm below the anterior superior iliac spine, the nerve divides into anterior and lateral aspects of the thigh as far as the knee. The posterior branch innervates the skin over the lateral and posterior portions of the thigh from the trochanteric region to the middle of the thigh.

## Differential Diagnosis

*Meralgia paresthetica* is the term used for the condition caused by entrapment of the LFCN as it passes underneath or through the inguinal ligament at its origin on the anterior iliac spine. Other causes of LFCN dysfunction include leprosy and tumor of the psoas, and it can also occur as a complication of laparoscopic procedures and surgery.

## Diagnostic Evaluation

The characteristic sensory symptoms and findings on examination as well as changes noted in the sensory nerve action potentials of the LFCN are diagnostic.

*Treatment*

Nonsurgical therapy consists of avoiding any new or recently started exercises and removing constricting binders, corsets, or tight belts. If pregnancy or weight gain appears to be a provocative factor, the passage of time or weight reduction improves symptoms. In certain conditions, the use of local nerve blocks may be beneficial. Surgical procedures should be considered if the symptoms are relatively long-lasting or very painful. Surgery consists of release of the entrapment at the level of the nerve's exit under the inguinal ligament. If the LFCN is severed, unpleasant paresthesias will increase.

Femoral Nerve

*Clinical Evaluation*

The femoral nerve arises from the L2, L3, and L4 nerve roots; it traverses the psoas muscle in a lateral direction and then, in the pelvis, makes its way in the fossa between the psoas and iliacus muscles. Immediately under Poupart's ligament, the femoral nerve reaches the extensor side of the thigh, where, a few centimeters below, it divides into motor and sensory terminal branches. The motor branches of the femoral nerve innervate the quadriceps, sartorius, and pectineus muscles. Sensory branches divide as the anterior femoral cutaneous nerve (which supplies the anterior aspect of the thigh), the medial femoral cutaneous nerve (which supplies part of the medial aspect of the thigh), and the long saphenous nerve (which, along with the infrapatellar branch, supplies the medial tibial surface of the leg, reaching to the medial malleolus and medial edge of the foot). Femoral nerve lesions produce weakness and atrophy of the quadriceps muscle, reduction in the knee reflex on the affected side, and a sensory loss over the anterior thigh and medial calf.

*Differential Diagnosis*

Entrapments of the femoral nerve occur rarely. More common causes of a femoral neuropathy include trauma (penetrating, blunt, and stretch injuries), diabetes mellitus, and vascular disease; infrequently a femoral neuropathy occurs during surgical procedures, after renal transplantation, as a complication of cardiac catheterization, or as a result of malignancies, infections, or hemorrhage in either the psoas or iliacus compartments.

*Diagnostic Evaluation*

EMG and NCS document a femoral neuropathy, and MRI may be useful in eliminating the various causes noted above.

*Treatment*

Treatment of femoral entrapment usually does not require surgery; most pelvic lesions in the femoral triangle at the region of the inguinal ligament are treated by waiting if a vascular process is suspected, or by medical management if a tumor or other mass lesion is the cause. Treatment of a femoral neuropathy may require use of a long leg brace, including a spring-loaded knee assist to produce knee extension so the patient may walk safely. Alternatively, if the lesion is expected to be of short duration, assistance with a crutch often suffices.

## Saphenous Nerve

### *Clinical Evaluation*

The saphenous nerve is one of three sensory branches of the femoral nerve. It has a long course through the adductor canal, penetrating fascia above the level of the knee and supplying the medial calf, the medial malleolus, and a small portion of the medial part of the arch of the foot.

### *Differential Diagnosis*

Entrapments, trauma, or surgical procedures may produce a saphenous neuropathy.

### *Diagnostic Evaluation*

A careful sensory examination on neurologic assessment as well as sensory evoked responses over the saphenous nerve are useful in arriving at a diagnosis.

### *Treatment*

Symptomatic treatment in the form of rest, use of NSAIDs, and physical therapy are effective in the majority of cases.

## Ilioinguinal Nerve

### *Clinical Evaluation*

The point of entrapment of the ilioinguinal nerve is located slightly medial to the anterior iliac spine near its exit from the superficial inguinal ring, where it lies almost directly superior to the pelvic tubercle. Clinically the patient complains of burning pain over the lower abdomen that radiates down into the inner portion of the upper thigh and into the scrotum or labia majora.

### *Differential Diagnosis*

Causes of an ilioinguinal nerve syndrome include trauma (blow to the abdominal wall), a surgical incision or procedure, or a scar; rarely this entrapment can occur with scleroderma.

*Diagnostic Evaluation*

The characteristic symptoms and clinical anatomic localization allow the clinician to arrive at a diagnosis.

*Treatment*

Neurolysis is indicated in severely affected patients who experience persistent pain.

## Genitofemoral Nerve

*Clinical Evaluation*

The genitofemoral nerve supplies the skin over the upper thigh below the femoral triangle and the lower lateral scrotum or labia, and descends through the pelvis over the iliac muscle near the obturator nerve.

*Differential Diagnosis*

In retroperitoneal processes, such as tumor, infection and, rarely, during laparoscopic varicocelectomy, the genitofemoral nerve may be involved.

*Diagnostic Evaluation*

The patient's description of the symptoms and the findings localized to the distribution of the nerve provide a diagnosis.

*Treatment*

In cases where adhesions entrap the nerve, relief of symptoms can be provided by surgery.

## Obturator Nerve

*Clinical Evaluation*

The clinical symptoms of obturator neuropathy are sensory, including paresthesias, sensory loss, and radiating pain in the medial thigh.

*Differential Diagnosis*

Most obturator nerve lesions are traumatic and result from pelvic and acetabular fractures, gunshot wounds, or pelvic laparoscopic procedures and may be produced during extracorporeal shock-wave lithotripsy. Also, a benign schwannoma of the retroperitoneal space as well as pelvic cancers can rarely produce an obturator neuropathy.

*Diagnostic Evaluation*

Symptoms of an obturator neuropathy are characteristic, and the sensory loss follows the anatomy of the nerve. When a retroperitoneal mass is suspected, MRI or CT may be used.

*Treatment*

Initial therapy includes rest and administration of appropriate analgesics and NSAIDs. Rarely, surgical exploration and epineural repair may be necessary.

Pudendal Nerve

*Clinical Evaluation*

In the Alcock syndrome, temporary penile insensitivity occurs due to compression of the pudendal nerve within the Alcock canal [12].

*Differential Diagnosis*

Other causes of pudendal palsy include a complication of intramedullary nailing of the femur during surgery and induction by fracture table.

*Diagnostic Evaluation*

The clinical symptoms and findings on examination assist the clinician in arriving at a diagnosis.

*Treatment*

When compression is the cause, surgical relief is necessary. During surgical procedures, care should be taken to avoid trauma to the pudendal nerve.

## Miscellaneous Entrapment Syndromes

Double Crush Syndromes

*Clinical Evaluation*

The double crush hypothesis attempts to explain the clinical observation that patients with distal compression neuropathies also frequently have signs of a more proximal nerve injury. The double crush hypothesis suggests that serial constraints to axoplasmic flow, each of which is insufficient to cause changes in function by itself, can be additive in causing ultimate dysfunction of the nerve.

## Differential Diagnosis

Degenerative cervical spine disease, with variable degrees of spondylosis, is a common clinical condition. When a patient becomes symptomatic from the cervical spine disorder and develops a concomitant entrapment neuropathy (especially CTS and ulnar neuropathies), confusion may arise not only with regard to diagnosis but with regard to therapy as well. An expansion of the double crush concept suggests increased vulnerability of the nerve to compression when predisposed by a metabolic injury to nerve fibers (the metabolic insult, such as diabetes mellitus, is one of the "crushes"). Moreover, *reverse double crush* describes the circumstance in which a pre-existing distal lesion predisposes to the development of symptoms following proximal injury.

## Diagnostic Evaluation

Comparing the results of neurologic examination and testing at rest with those after provocation of the patient's symptoms may allow the clinician to quantify an abnormality that corresponds to the patient's symptoms. These syndromes can often be discerned using electrodiagnostic studies and MRI techniques.

## Treatment

Usually the patient with a double crush syndrome responds when treatment is directed toward both processes (i.e., the cervical spine syndrome as well as the more distal entrapment neuropathy). When the causative factor appears work related, it would be prudent to modify the patient's work habits and consider job modifications.

## Rectus Abdominis Syndrome

### Clinical Evaluation

Any of the branches of the intercostal nerves T7 to T12 may rarely be entrapped within the substance of the rectus muscle. Such entrapment leads to localized pain in the abdominal wall that becomes exaggerated by pressure over the rectus muscle or by elevation of one leg while the patient is in a supine position.

### Differential Diagnosis

Disease or syndromes affecting the thoracic spine and abdominal disorders are important to diagnose and exclude in patients suspected of having the infrequent rectus abdominis syndrome.

*Diagnostic Evaluation*

MRI and CT studies can assist in excluding thoracic spine and abdominal diseases.

*Treatment*

Conservative measures, including local steroid injections, often provide relief of symptoms.

## Pseudoradicular Syndromes

*Clinical Evaluation*

In cases of undiagnosed persistent leg pain, a pseudoradicular syndrome may be considered.

*Differential Diagnosis*

Disorders to consider in the differential diagnosis include peripheral nerve entrapments (saphenous nerve entrapments about the knee, peroneal nerve entrapments at or above the popliteal fossa, tibial nerve entrapments in the popliteal space).

*Diagnostic Evaluation*

The diagnosis can be made on the basis of selective spinal and nerve blocks as well as electrodiagnostic tests.

*Treatment*

In certain suspected cases, surgical exploration and external neurolysis (peroneal, tibial, saphenous and femoral nerve lesions) may be performed. Peripheral nerve lesions should be ruled out prior to lumbar spine surgery in patients with leg symptoms.

## Compartment Syndromes

*Clinical Evaluation*

Compartment syndromes (CS) occur in specific clinical situations as a serious potential complication of trauma to the extremities. Buildup of intracompartmental tissue pressure results from increases in fluid pressure plus the contribution of cells, fibers, gel, and matrix material; the result is increased venous pressure that reduces the arteriovenous pressure gradient and leads to reduced blood flow and neuromuscular function [13]. The frequency of CS correlates with the prevalence of limb trauma, drug and alcohol abuse, limb surgery, limb ischemia, use of the lithotomy position, and physical exertion of the muscles in sports or forced exertion (e.g., in military drills and training). Factors that reduce the tolerance of limbs for increased tissue pressure include hypotension, hemorrhage, arterial occlusion, and limb elevation.

*Differential Diagnosis*

Rarely, CS can appear as a complication of HIV disease, leukemia, hypothyroidism, medication with gemfibrozil in chronic renal failure, polyarteritis nodosa, hemophilia, or theophylline toxicity with rhabdomyolysis, or can occur secondary to the use of pressure-monitoring devices or infusion pumps, diabetes insipidus, and popliteal artery entrapment. Other medical conditions that may be confused with CS include (1) infection or inflammation, (2) arterial occlusion, and (3) primary nerve injury or entrapment (or both).

*Diagnostic Evaluation*

The clinical features of CS include (1) tense compartment envelope, (2) severe pain in excess of that clinically expected for the specific condition, (3) pain on passive stretch of the muscles in the compartment, (4) muscle weakness within the compartment, and (5) altered sensation in the distribution of the nerves coursing through the compartment. Anatomic locations within the body in which the CS may occur include (1) leg (anterior, lateral, and posterior—deep and superficial), (2) thigh (quadriceps muscle), (3) buttock (gluteal muscles), (4) hand (interosseous muscles), (5) forearm (dorsal and volar), (6) arm (deltoid, biceps, and triceps), (7) foot, and (8) scapula.

Careful clinical examination, tissue pressure measurements, direct nerve stimulation, electrodiagnostic studies, Doppler sonography, arteriography, venography, and MRI assist in differentiating between these conditions and the various true CS (Figure 24.4).

*Treatment*

Treatment of CS aims to minimize neurologic deficits by promptly restoring local blood flow and avoiding compression. Nonsurgical measures include eliminating external envelopes and maintaining local arterial pressures and preserving peripheral nerve function. The objective of surgery is to decompress limiting envelopes and débride nonviable tissue.

## REPETITIVE STRAIN DISORDER, OCCUPATIONAL SYNDROMES, AND NEUROMUSCULAR DISORDERS RELATED TO THE PERFORMING ARTS

Patients with repetitive strain disorder, occupational syndromes, and neuromuscular disorders can be placed into three categories. The first category includes patients for whom the diagnosis of repetitive strain disorder is beyond doubt, such as those with peritendinitis crepitans (de Quervain's disease), a tender swelling

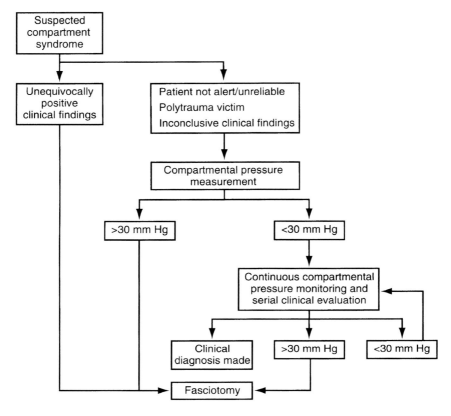

*Figure 24.4*   Algorithm used in the diagnosis and treatment of an acute compartment syndrome of the lower leg. (Reprinted with permission from KK Nakano. Entrapment Neuropathies and Related Disorders. In WN Kelley, ED Harris Jr, S Ruddy, CB Sledge [eds], Textbook of Rheumatology [5th ed]. Philadelphia: Saunders, 1998;584.)

where the radial wrist extensors cross under the abductor pollicis longus and extensor pollicis brevis that was first described in washerwomen in England [14]. Also included in this group, but with less defined pathophysiology, are musicians [15], dancers, keyboard operators, and avid athletes (e.g., joggers, cross-country skiers, sailboarders, rock climbers, and those participating in other sport activities). When the pain arises in the arm and shoulder in this last group of individuals, it is best conceptualized as a form of fatigue. In the second category of patients are those who have genuine problems that are mistakenly believed to be caused by their employment but that are just part of many of the natural processes that affect the human body. In fact, some forms of usage can exacerbate the symptoms of some regional musculoskeletal illnesses (namely, CTS). Apparently, sociopolitical phenomena allow some of these patients to attribute the symptoms to their work. The third, and evidently the smallest category includes those who realize that their symptoms, if indeed they exist, are not caused by their work but hope to establish such a relationship in order to gain financial or other reward. An optimal clinical approach to the treatment of repetitive strain disorders combines physical and psychological techniques.

## Overuse Syndromes

### Clinical Evaluation

OSs are symptom complexes defined as injuries caused by the cumulative effects on tissues of repetitive physical stresses that exceed physiologic limits. Among musicians and dancers, OSs originate in the constant repetition of intense practice of a musical instrument or dancing, respectively. This situation most commonly affects the muscle-tendon units. The usual symptom is pain while playing the instrument or dancing and, not long thereafter, disability. In the initial stages, the pain subsides when the activity stops. During later advanced stages (after severe or prolonged injury to the muscle-tendon unit) pain persists, and if injury continues accurate performance may become impossible.

Musicians using keyboard instruments must repeat movements of extension, flexion, and rotation of their fingers. Overuse (or misuse) problems with the extensors of the fingers and wrist, the lumbrical muscles, and the interosseous muscles of the dominant hand can easily develop. Viola and violin players can develop problems in the fingers, hands, and wrists that are compounded by the awkward position in which the instrument must be held. Rotation of the neck to the left and abduction and external rotation of the left shoulder predispose the cervical spine and the left shoulder to pain at these points. Viola and cello players may have the same digital and manual difficulties, and they have the added risk of developing paresthesias in the legs. Wind instrument players may suffer overuse that affects the embouchure (position of the lips), the soft palate, and the muscles of the pharynx and leads to inadequate volume, imperfect control, and, at times, inaccuracy of intonation. It appears that overuse leads to muscle-fiber injury. Muscle biopsy studies from players with OS show glycogen depletion and acute degenerative changes in muscle fibers and edema of the perimysium as well as leukocytes around arterioles. Additional changes include hypertrophy of type 2 muscle fibers, increase in the number of central nuclei, and mitochondrial abnormalities.

### Differential Diagnosis

OSs and peripheral nerve entrapments may overlap, because hypertrophy of small muscle groups can cause compression of nerves at various anatomic sites. An important clinical difference between entrapment neuropathies and OSs is that the former produce weakness, sensory changes, or both in addition to discomfort, pain, and loss of ability to play or dance accurately. Among the entrapment syndromes, CTS is the one most often seen in musicians, even though subjective symptoms of a TOS may be a more common complaint. Other rare entrapment syndromes include entrapment of the median nerve in the arm (PTS) or in the forearm (AIN syndrome). The ulnar nerve can be entrapped at the elbow or wrist (especially in flute players). Rarely will the radial nerve become involved among musicians.

## Diagnostic Evaluation

The characteristic symptoms among patients in susceptible professions as well as selective electrodiagnostic studies assist in the diagnosis of these conditions.

## Treatment

Most authorities recommend rest for the OSs. Use of NSAIDs and limited physical therapy may be beneficial in these conditions.

## Dystonias

### Clinical Evaluation

Dystonia has been defined as a movement disorder characterized by sustained muscle contractions, which frequently cause repetitive movements, twisting, or abnormal postures. A classical example of dystonia is "writer's cramp." As many as 15% of instrumental performers experience focal dystonias in one form or another. These individuals initially report loss of coordination while playing an instrument, often accompanied by curling or extension of the fingers during passages that require rapid and forceful finger movements. Once the disorder develops, the loss of motor control progresses slowly over years and is not accompanied by sensory symptoms.

### Differential Diagnosis

No firm evidence exists that relates focal dystonias to an overuse injury preceding the dystonia. When a physician is confronted by a painless hand problem suggesting some features of an entrapment syndrome, focal dystonia should be considered when loss of motor function is characterized by some loss of voluntary motor control. A diagnosis of hysteria should be excluded in these patients [16].

### Diagnostic Evaluation

Electrodiagnostic studies have demonstrated abnormalities of muscle control, with concurrent contraction of both agonist and antagonist muscle groups, and abnormalities in the normal reflex inhibition of antagonist muscles in cases of dystonia.

### Treatment

Some symptomatic relief has been achieved with benzodiazepine medications and relaxation techniques. More recently, botulinum toxin injections have been shown to provide temporary benefit.

## PERIOPERATIVE NERVE LESIONS

Perioperative nerve lesions refer to focal neuropathies that are the result of acute trauma during surgical procedures [17]. In the differential diagnosis, events that are only indirectly related to a medical procedure as well as others that are only coincidental are included. No specific pattern of pathophysiologic mechanisms in perioperative nerve lesions seems to exist. The syndromes are discussed according to the clinical setting in which they occur.

### Brachial Plexus

Clinical Evaluation

The brachial plexus appears to be the most susceptible of all nerve groups to damage from poor positioning during anesthesia. Stretching appears to be the usual cause of injury. The plexus has a relatively long course, traveling from the vertebral foramina to the axilla, and lies in proximity to a number of mobile bony structures.

Differential Diagnosis

Open-heart surgery by a median sternotomy approach can give rise to a brachial plexus palsy. In this clinical situation, it is not clear that improper positioning always produces the palsy. Serious neurologic complications can develop from a surgical procedure for TOS; patients may develop causalgia with relatively few neurologic deficits on clinical examination.

Diagnostic Evaluation

MRI evaluation may provide clinical information regarding distal as well as proximal lesions of the brachial plexus and assist in defining both the nature and the extent of injury. EMG, NCS, and SER studies often prove helpful in localizing the clinical problem to the brachial plexus.

Treatment

Surgery is not indicated in most cases. Some studies suggest improvement in motor function after certain types of brachial plexus injury. In brachial plexus stretch injuries, most patients recover within 3 months; however, recovery may be prolonged for more than a year.

### Ulnar Nerve

Clinical Evaluation

Among the most common focal peripheral neuropathies are those involving the ulnar nerve; intraoperative damage to the ulnar nerve in anatomic variants due to surgical position has been reported. Other cases occur during the postoperative period, or symptoms that previously had been mild or transient may abruptly become obvious and disabling.

## Differential Diagnosis

Because ulnar nerve disorders are often heterogenous—with some reflecting long-standing trauma and some entrapment in the cubital tunnel—it appears that various factors play a role in postoperative ulnar neuropathies. The occurrence of ulnar nerve lesions during surgical procedures may reflect the additive effects of positioning as well as a subclinical compression associated with pre-existing neuropathy at the cubital tunnel. Furthermore, diabetic patients may be more susceptible to compressive neuropathies.

## Diagnostic Evaluation

NCS and EMG are helpful in localizing the site of ulnar trauma or injury.

## Treatment

In cases of increased mobility of the ulnar nerve at the elbow, it is recommended that the arm be placed in supination, with the elbow extended and carefully padded, at the time of surgical procedures.

## Peroneal Nerve

Peroneal nerve palsies can occur with knee arthroplasties. This complication appears most commonly in those with prior severe knee deformities. Surgical positioning or use of certain appliances may also produce a peroneal neuropathy.

## Sciatic Nerve, Obturator Nerve, and Femoral Nerve

Sciatic, obturator, or femoral nerve injury may occur after cardiac surgery or cardiac catheterization, or with total hip arthroplasty; rarely, patients have had one or more nerves embedded in methacrylate during surgery. Sciatic nerve palsy may occur more often with surgical procedures in diabetic patients. Hematoma formation may be a potential source of femoral neuropathy during renal transplantation.

## Lateral Femoral Cutaneous Nerve

Meralgia paresthetica may occur after iliac bone grafting, as a complication of a groin flap procedure, and after laparoscopic procedures and surgery. In these instances, injury to the LFCN seems to occur where it passes close by the iliac crest.

### Iliohypogastric Nerve, Ilioinguinal Nerve, and Genitofemoral Nerve

Hernia repairs, lower abdominal surgery, or gynecologic surgery may injure the iliohypogastric nerve, ilioinguinal nerve, and genitofemoral nerve as they traverse the lower abdominal wall. In patients suffering long-standing pain and paresthesias as a result of injury to one of these nerves of the lower abdomen, a surgical exploration may be warranted.

## NEURALGIC PAIN IN THE LIMBS AFTER INJURY: CAUSALGIA AND REFLEX SYMPATHETIC DYSTROPHY

### Clinical Evaluation

Causalgia is an uncommon complication of peripheral nerve injury; the onset of pain varies from days to several weeks after injury. The pain, which is usually described as burning (hence the name causalgia), appears within a few days of injury. In most patients the injury affects the median or sciatic nerve, either alone or in combination with other nerves. Causalgia is usually associated with an incomplete lesion of a peripheral nerve. Even though functional loss is complete, partial or complete continuity of the nerve may be preserved. Usually the pain is limited to the skin distribution of the affected nerve, but it may spread to involve the distal part of the limb or the entire extremity. When more than one nerve is injured, the pain is often in the distribution of only one of the affected nerves. In injuries to the brachial plexus, the pain is present in the palm, fingertips, and entire hand or arm, rather than in a peripheral nerve or nerve root distribution. The pathogenesis of the causalgic pain has been attributed to the sympathetic fibers in the nerve trunks. When the pain is severe enough to prevent use of the limb, rapid development of trophic changes in the skin and nails and periarticular fibrosis occurs; these changes are referred to as *RSD*.

### Differential Diagnosis

Causalgia may develop after an injury to any of the sensory or mixed nerves or damage to the brachial and lumbar plexuses, with or without damage to the major arteries of the limbs. Operations such as neurolysis, removal of neuromas, sectioning, and resuturing of the nerve have not relieved the causalgic pain in patients; this fact supports the concept that the pathogenesis relates to injury to the sympathetic fibers in nerve trunks.

### Diagnostic Evaluation

Considerable variation in the severity of the pain is present; in some cases it is so extreme that the patient is completely incapacitated. In these cases the affected limb is constantly protected from movement or external stimuli. Examination of the affected limb may be strenuously resisted by the patient. In other patients the pain is described as severe, but the affected limb can be used (minor causalgia). Examination of motor and sensory function in the affected limb is carried out with difficulty in severe cases, because any stimulation causes an exacerbation of the pain. In the majority of patients, extreme vasodilatation occurs, and the limb is pink, warm, and velvety to palpation. Perspiration may be decreased or increased. RSD refers to the local tissue swelling and bony changes that accompany causalgia. Similar changes may be encountered after minor trauma or arthritis of the wrist. In the shoulder-hand syndrome, inflammatory arthritis of the shoulder joint may be followed by painful swelling of the hand, with local vascular changes, disuse, and atrophy of muscle and bone.

## Treatment

The course of causalgia is variable. In mild cases, the pain may disappear spontaneously after a few weeks or months without the development of any trophic changes in the affected limb. Spontaneous remission is less common among severe cases, and permanent contractures may result unless the condition is relieved by therapy. Operative procedures on the peripheral nerve rarely relieve the symptoms. The most successful form of treatment has been sympathectomy or sympathetic block. Preganglionic denervation of the limb appears to be more effective than postganglionic denervation or paravertebral sympathetic block.

## REFERRALS FOR ELECTRODIAGNOSTIC STUDIES

On many occasions, orthopedic surgeons request electrodiagnostic studies from neurologists in search of a clinical diagnosis when the patient's complaints include muscular weakness. Weakness may be secondary to disease involving the muscle, nerve, neuromuscular junction, upper motor neuron (UMN) and spinal cord, or cerebrum. In such a case, the orthopedic surgeon is actually asking for a clinical consultation and is under the impression that the EMG and NCS will provide a diagnosis. The specific need for more definitive treatment, including surgery, can be established only when the physician is aware of the cause, extent, and prognosis of the weakness. Therefore, a clinical assessment including history taking as well as a general physical and neurologic examination, coupled with evaluation of the electrical activity of muscle tissue and of muscle response to nerve stimulation, is necessary to solve the clinical problem. At other times the orthopedic surgeon asks for specific studies to document an entrapment neuropathy (e.g., CTS) or radiculopathy (e.g., of the L5 root) in order to confirm a diagnosis and plans a surgical procedure. Various EMG and NCS patterns help differentiate the normal from a diffuse polyneuropathy, focal entrapment neuropathy, radiculopathy, myopathy, disorder of the neuromuscular junction, or anterior horn cell disease (Table 24.6). No one feature of EMG (except true myotonia) provides a diagnosis; rather, the clinician uses summated information from the electrodiagnostic studies to evaluate the patient.

*Table 24.6*   Summary of the electromyographic and nerve conduction velocity findings by location of disease in the motor unit

| Study | Spinal cord: anterior horn cell | Nerve root | | | | | |
|---|---|---|---|---|---|---|---|
| | | Anterior motor root | Predorsal ganglion | Postdorsal ganglion | Peripheral nerve | Neuro-muscular junction | Muscle |
| MNCV | N | N | N | N | + | N | N |
| SNAP | N | N | N | ± | + | N | N |
| EMG | + | + | N | N | + | ± | + |
| Repetitive stimulation | ± | N | N | N | ± | + | N |
| F wave | + | + | N | N | + | N | N |
| H reflex | + | + | + | + | + | N | N |
| SER | N | N | + | + | + | N | N |

MNCV = motor nerve conduction velocity; N = normal; + = abnormal; SNAP = sensory nerve action potential; ± = occasionally abnormal; EMG = electromyography; SER = somatosensory evoked response.

Source: Reprinted with permission from KK Nakano. Entrapment Neuropathies and Related Disorders. In WN Kelley, ED Harris Jr, S Ruddy, CB Sledge (eds). Textbook of Rheumatology (5th ed). Philadelphia: Saunders, 1997;567.

# SPINAL CORD LESIONS

## Clinical Evaluation

Spinal cord and nerve root lesions may be extradural or intradural. If the lesion is intradural, it may be extramedullary or intramedullary. Clinical clues are useful in the localization of the lesion. Extramedullary lesions often produce unilateral signs. Intradural lesions usually show slower progression than extradural lesions. Intramedullary lesions include slow-growing gliomas. Occasionally, intramedullary metastatic cancer occurs, but the epidural space more frequently is involved in metastatic tumors and inflammatory processes.

## Differential Diagnosis

Neurologic localization involves differentiating lesions involving the spinal cord, nerve, root, plexus, and peripheral nerve. The differential diagnosis between nerve compression and peripheral entrapment neuropathies is the most difficult. Each dorsal root innervates a unique area that differs from that of any peripheral nerve. Likewise, the muscle innervated by each ventral root differs from those supplied by any peripheral nerve. Purely sensory loss may result from dorsal root lesions; however, this occurs uncommonly in peripheral nerve disorders unless a terminal cutaneous branch becomes involved. The sensory deficit from a peripheral nerve lesion shows a sharper boundary than

*Table 24.7*   Clinical features differentiating upper and lower motor neuron weakness

| Clinical feature | Upper motor neuron weakness | Lower motor neuron weakness |
|---|---|---|
| Weakness | Greater in extensors of upper limbs and in flexors of lower limbs (pyramidal distribution); usually involves one side of body, but may also produce paraparesis, quadriparesis, or (rarely) monoparesis; usually does not produce weakness in one muscle group or bilateral cranial nerve weakness | Nonpyramidal distribution; may be present in one muscle group; paraparesis, quadriparesis, and bilateral cranial nerve weakness also seen |
| Deep tendon reflexes | Usually increased, but acutely may be decreased; also may be decreased with parietal and cerebellar lesions | Decreased |
| Tone to passive motion | Increased; may be decreased with cerebellar and parietal lesions | Decreased |
| Pathologic reflexes | Babinski's and others | Absent |
| Associated symptoms | Defect of cortical association areas; front-release signs; defect of sensation; cerebellar defects; cranial nerve defects | Cranial nerve signs; sensory signs |

Source: Reprinted with permission from KK Nakano. Neurology of Musculoskeletal and Rheumatic Disorders. Boston: Houghton Mifflin, 1979;27.

is seen in most nerve root disorders. When a nerve root is compressed at the intervertebral foramen (e.g., secondary to a herniated disk), coughing or straining frequently causes radiation of pain into the affected dermatomal area. This phenomenon does not occur with peripheral nerve deficits.

If the patient demonstrates weakness, the clinician must distinguish between a UMN lesion and a LMN lesion (Table 24.7). LMN signs may be secondary to lesions at any site from the anterior horn cells of the spinal cord out to the most distal branches of the spinal nerve. If the LMN signs arise from involvement of the anterior horn neurons in the spinal cord, neighboring structures such as the long corticospinal tract are usually involved. Central lesions rarely confine themselves to the anterior horn grey matter of the spinal cord. LMN and spinal cord deficits usually limit themselves to a segment or to the segments affected by the lesion, and some type of sensory involvement should be seen at the injured site.

When the lesion involves the ventral roots, it may or may not be large enough to compress the spinal cord. In a ventral root lesion the weakness affects the muscles of a single myotome, a distribution that differs from that of a peripheral nerve problem. Complete paralysis of limb or girdle muscles never results from lesions of single ventral roots, because each muscle receives contributions from more than one ventral root. Peripheral nerve lesions, on the other hand, frequently cause complete weakness because all the axons from the various ventral roots must travel through the nerve to reach a specific muscle.

Several principles are used to differentiate peripheral nerve from spinal cord or nerve root involvement. If sensory and motor losses are confined to the distribution of the dorsal or ventral root or to a single segment of the spinal cord, the lesion is central or radicular. With a central lesion, such as a lesion within the spinal cord, long-tract signs should be present. Caudal to the lesion UMN signs appear, and an altered sensory level is present for one or more modalities at the site of the involvement. If the lesion occurs at the intervertebral foramen, both the dorsal and ventral roots of the segment are affected; the patient complains of pain in the root distribution when he or she strains. A sharp border of sensory loss in an extremity suggests peripheral nerve rather than nerve root involvement. With involvement of single dorsal roots, the border of the loss is vague, and frequently little or no loss can be demonstrated, although pain in the involved segment may be severe.

## Diagnostic Evaluation

Suspicion of any spinal cord lesion should prompt the examiner to investigate the patient's skin and skeleton, in addition to taking a complete history and performing a detailed neurologic examination. Neurocutaneous lesions such as café-au-lait spots may suggest a neurofibroma or a meningioma. An abnormal amount of hair or other skin defects over the vertebral column suggests congenital anomaly of the spinal cord. Cutaneous angiomas should be investigated, and if they are suspected, the patient should be asked to perform a Valsalva maneuver to visualize an occult angioma over the back. Skeletal abnormalities such as a short, immobile neck suggest Klippel-Feil syndrome. Scoliosis is associated with spinal cord tumors, as well as degenerative neuromuscular diseases. Pes cavus occurs with spinocerebellar degeneration and also can be seen with caudal tumors of the spinal cord. Careful palpation of the spinous processes of the vertebrae may reveal a spina bifida.

Diagnosis of spinal cord lesions has been facilitated by MRI and CT myelography. SER studies can be useful in identifying UMN lesions, while EMG and NCS are useful in delineating LMN disease.

## Treatment

Because many disorders of the spinal cord require specific therapy, a diagnosis must be determined before irreversible damage is done.

## RHEUMATOLOGIC AND CONNECTIVE TISSUE DISEASES

### Clinical Evaluation

A rheumatologic or connective tissue disease (CTD) may present as a neurologic disorder, with the primary diagnosis of an underlying disease or condition being made during the course of the neurologic assessment [18]. The possibility of a CTD or rheumatologic condition—including systemic lupus erythematosus, antiphospholipid antibody syndrome, RA, Takayasu's arteritis, granulomatous

*Table 24.8*   Neuropathies associated with connective tissue disease

| |
|---|
| Distal axonal polyneuropathy (not clearly vasculitic) |
| Compression neuropathy (e.g., carpal tunnel syndrome, cubital tunnel syndrome) |
| Sensory neuropathy |
| Trigeminal sensory neuropathy |
| Vasculitic neuropathy |
|     Mononeuropathy multiplex, or overtly multifocal mononeuropathies |
|     Asymmetrical polyneuropathy, or multiple mononeuropathies with partial confluence |
|     Distal symmetric polyneuropathy, or confluent multifocal mononeuropathies |
| Other neuropathies that may be associated with connective tissue disease |
|     Acute demyelinating polyneuropathy |
|     Chronic demyelinating polyneuropathy |
|     Brachial plexus neuropathy |

giant cell arteritis, periarteritis nodosa, Wegener's granulomatosis, polymyositis, dermatomyositis, polymyalgia rheumatica, scleroderma (spinal stenosis–systemic sclerosis), Sjögren's syndrome, mixed connective tissue syndrome, and temporal arteritis— should be kept in mind when a new onset of neurologic symptoms or signs occurs in young individuals, particularly women.

**Differential Diagnosis**

The symptoms and signs resulting from these disorders include those resulting from systemic reaction to the disease and involvement of the viscera. Disorders of the peripheral nerves that develop in association with CTD are a medical challenge (Table 24.8). First of all, a patient with known CTS may have more than one type of peripheral neuropathy. Second, certain types of peripheral neuropathy may represent the initial manifestation of an undiagnosed CTD.

Vasculitis can be defined as inflammation of blood vessels; it is associated with necrosis and causes compromise of vessel lumen and secondary ischemia in involved tissues. Consequently, vasculitis appears often in the differential diagnosis of nearly all neurologic disorders, because it can closely mimic most central nervous system (CNS) and peripheral nervous system (PNS) diseases. However, certain clinical symptoms and signs, alone or in combination, can be suggestive of a vasculitic disorder. Three types of peripheral neuropathy appear when vasculitis affects the PNS: (1) mononeuritis multiplex, (2) distal symmetric "stocking-glove" sensorimotor peripheral neuropathy, and (3) overlapping, extensive mononeuritis multiplex. Regardless of the type of peripheral neuropathy seen in the vasculitic syndromes, the symptoms include a severe, burning paresthesia in the distribution of the involved nerve or nerves.

When skeletal muscle becomes involved in vasculitis, patients demonstrate symmetric proximal muscle weakness that appears clinically indistinguishable from that seen in polymyositis or dermatomyositis. In patients with an underlying CTD (such as systemic lupus erythematosus, RA, Sjögren's syndrome, spinal stenosis), the skeletal muscle involvement is often caused by a primary inflammatory involvement of the muscle itself, rather than by vasculitis.

Two primary patterns of clinical involvement occur for CNS vasculitis, depending on whether the vasculitis is predominantly diffuse or focal. With diffuse involvement the patient complains of acute or subacute headache, psychiatric impairment (personality, behavioral, and affective disturbances), and cognitive deficits (memory and mental status changes). Generalized seizures may occur in association with an encephalopathy. On the other hand, focal CNS vasculitis causes focal cerebral deficits. Any stroke-like event, especially in a young person without risk factors for stroke, should alert the clinician to the possibility of a vasculitis. Furthermore, single or multiple cranial nerve palsies (vision loss, diplopia, facial paresthesias or weakness, vertigo, tinnitus, dysphagia) can be manifestations of focal CNS vasculitis. Less commonly, focal CNS vasculitis causes intracerebral or subarachnoid hemorrhage, movement disorder (e.g., chorea), and an isolated myelopathy (e.g., isolated granulomatous angiitis). Overlap in the symptoms of these two patterns occurs because all of the vasculitides can produce either diffuse or focal CNS disease.

## Diagnostic Evaluation

Because CTDs are multiple-system diseases, an interdisciplinary medical team approach should be used in the assessment and management of these patients. Often evaluation of these patients requires multiple laboratory studies; when neurologic complications occur, neuroimaging techniques (in cases of CNS involvement) or electrodiagnostic studies (in cases of PNS involvement) are necessary.

## Treatment

It is important to note that most of the vasculitic syndromes can produce disease in both the CNS and PNS, often simultaneously. Atypical cases that do not fit neatly into any of the diagnostic categories occur frequently and suggest that the clinical syndromes overlap some (e.g., systemic lupus erythematosus and RA). The initiation of therapy (including immunosuppressive therapy) can alter the natural history of many forms of vasculitis that were previously untreatable and often fatal. Therefore, it is vital that the clinician arrives at an early diagnosis and classification to prevent the development of progression of CNS and PNS manifestations of the CTD.

## RHEUMATOID ARTHRITIS

When RA becomes recurrent or is sustained over the years, increasingly serious and permanent disturbance in joint function develops. Neurologic complications

*Table 24.9*   Neurologic manifestations of rheumatoid arthritis

*Articular involvement, cervical spine disease*
  Cervical subluxations (four types)
      Movement of C1 anteriorly on C2
      Movement of C1 posteriorly on C2
      Vertical subluxation of odontoid
      "Staircase" or multiple lower-level subluxations
  Radiologic findings, often with clinical symptoms
      Double crush syndrome
      Narrowed disk spaces above C5
  Radiologic findings without clinical symptoms
      Vertebral plate erosion
      Apophyseal joint erosion
      Basilar impression of the skull
*Extra-articular manifestations*
  Peripheral neuropathies
      Compression leading to entrapment
      Mild sensory neuropathy with a good prognosis
      Diffuse sensorimotor neuropathy
      Fulminant sensorimotor neuropathy
  Diffuse myopathy and focal myositis
  Polymyositis and dermatomyositis
  Vasculitis, often with other connective tissue disorders
      Mononeuritis complex
      "Cerebral vasculitis," often with lupus erythematosus and rheumatoid arthritis
  Dural rheumatoid nodules causing brain and spinal cord compression
  Progressive multifocal leukoencephalopathy

Source: Reprinted with permission from KK Nakano. Neurorheumatology. In J Stein (ed), Internal Medicine (5th ed). St. Louis: Mosby–Year Book, 1998;1094.

manifest themselves with moderate and severe forms of the disease and can be divided into articular and extra-articular disorders (Table 24.9) [19,20].

## Articular Involvement

### Clinical Evaluation

Approximately 30–40% of all patients with chronic RA and severe peripheral joint disease who are hospitalized have radiologic evidence of cervical spine subluxation. Often, these radiographic findings are not associated with neurologic symptoms. However, in 2–5% of all patients with significant cervical subluxation, pyramidal tract signs or vague subjective sensory findings are evident on neurologic examination. Usually, RA affects the upper levels of the cervical spine and produces different clinical features at different ages. In children with RA, growth is deficient and apophyseal joints often fuse, with a resulting limitation in neck movement. In adults, the main change in the cervical spine is subluxation, which can take four forms: (1) anterior movement of C1 on C2 (this form is the most common and results from insufficiency of the transverse ligament or from ero-

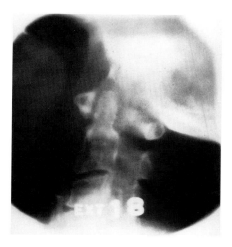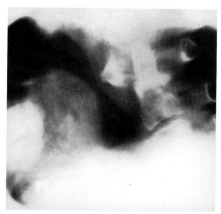

*Figure 24.5* C1–C2 cervical subluxation in a patient with advanced rheumatoid arthritis. (Reprinted with permission from KK Nakano. Neurology of Musculoskeletal and Rheumatic Disorders. Boston: Houghton Mifflin, 1979;363.)

sion or fracture of the odontoid) (Figure 24.5); (2) posterior movement of C1 on C2 (this form results from severe erosion or fracture of the odontoid); (3) vertical subluxation of the odontoid and body of C2 (which results from destruction of the lateral atlantoaxial joints or of the bone around the foramen magnum and is the rarest form of cervical subluxation in RA); and (4) "staircase" subluxation of one vertebra on another, often involving multiple vertebrae and occurring below the C2 level (this form is the second most common cervical subluxation in RA and results from destruction of the apophyseal joints rather than loss of ligamentous connections).

## Differential Diagnosis

Characteristic neuritic pain radiating up to the occiput is frequently present in patients with RA. Crepitation and instability of the cervical spine can cause alarm. Paresthesias can be caused by head or neck movement, and Lhermitte's sign may be elicited by sudden flexion of the neck. Rarely, the complaints reflect transient ischemic attacks in the posterior cerebral circulation (signaled by transient visual disturbances, such as diplopia, vertigo, paresthesias, or paresis). Early spinal cord compression or ischemia may produce subtle spastic quadriparesis and hyperreflexia, which may be especially unwelcome when a patient is already debilitated. Pyramidal tract signs (increased reflexes and Babinski's responses) or early proprioceptive loss in the hands represent early signs of impending spinal cord compression. The classic spinal cord compression picture—including an altered sensory level to all modalities, bladder and bowel dysfunction, and flaccid quadriplegia—is a late development.

## Diagnostic Evaluation

To make a clinical diagnosis of cervical subluxation in RA, radiologic confirmation is necessary. Lateral views of the cervical spine, in extension and flexion to open the gap between the odontoid and the arch of C1, are indicated. Tomography, CT scans, and MRI may be necessary for detailed anatomic study and precise measurement of the spinal cord and canal.

## Treatment

Treatment for less severe and neurologically asymptomatic cases of cervical subluxation includes the use of firm cervical collars aimed at improving stability and easing pain. Neurosurgical and orthopedic surgical immobilization of the neck and halo traction should be considered in the patient with progressive spinal cord signs. Stabilization is most useful before permanent neurologic or vascular damage occurs to the spinal cord. If surgery is considered, it should be done before the patient has suffered permanent cord injury and at a center experienced in treating chronic RA patients and familiar with techniques of cervical and occipitocervical fusion.

## Extra-Articular Manifestations

### Clinical Evaluation

**Peripheral Neuropathies.**   Various types of neuropathy occur with RA: compression leading to entrapment (e.g., CTS, ulnar nerve entrapment at the elbow, PINS, PTTS), mild sensory neuropathies with a good prognosis, diffuse sensorimotor polyneuropathy, and a fulminant sensorimotor disorder often related to a generalized vasculitis. The neuropathy most commonly encountered is a mild sensory one, primarily of the feet and legs. Patients often complain of varying degrees of paresthesia, dysesthesia, or "burning feet" for varying periods of time. A more severe sensorimotor polyneuropathy, in which the patient has some objective weakness in addition to the sensory symptoms, can be seen occasionally in patients with acute joint disease.

**Myopathy and Focal Myositis.**   Approximately 70–80% of patients with chronic and recurrent RA have some muscle weakness, usually around the areas of joint involvement. These patients report diminished proximal strength and peripheral joint disability. Although a combination of muscle and joint inflammation is present, the prognosis depends more on the joint disease than on the muscle involvement.

**Vasculitis.**   Generalized RA vasculitis is rare and occurs in severe cases of RA with multiple neurologic findings that suggest CNS involvement or a mononeuritis complex.

**Dural Rheumatoid Nodules.**   In rare cases, RA patients who have severe subcutaneous nodules go on to develop dural nodules, which can compress the brain or spinal cord.

**Progressive Multifocal Leukoencephalopathy.**  Progressive multifocal leukoencephalopathy, a rare complication of RA, is an asymmetrically diffuse CNS disorder evidenced by multifocal areas of demyelination. It is an infection by the papovaviruses that overwhelms an immunologically suppressed host.

*Differential Diagnosis*

**Peripheral Neuropathies.**  Often those RA patients with a severe sensorimotor polyneuropathy have neglected their RA, or an acute recurrence of the disease has occurred. Other conditions such as diabetes mellitus, alcohol abuse, and effects of toxins or drugs should be excluded as a cause of the neuropathy. In a small percentage of cases, malignant rheumatoid vasculitis presents with a fulminant sensorimotor disorder, often with a mononeuritic component. Often these patients have been treated with steroids or their disease has followed an unremitting course. Evidence of vasculitis is seen on the skin, and the neurologic picture can be similar to that of periarteritis. These patients may have a concomitant CTD, or their symptoms may represent a spectrum of diseases (e.g., a patient can have RA and features of systemic lupus erythematosus).

**Myopathy and Focal Myositis.**  RA myopathy is independent of steroid therapy, and patients with this condition do not progress to diffuse and severe muscle necrosis if their RA remains controlled.

*Diagnostic Evaluation*

**Peripheral Neuropathies, Myopathy, and Focal Myositis.**  Careful electrodiagnostic studies allow categorization of the neuropathy and documentation of the myopathy.

**Vasculitis.**  In cases of vasculitis, EEG, MRI, and cerebrospinal fluid examination may be necessary.

**Dural Rheumatoid Nodules.**  Dural nodules cannot be clinically separated from other disorders causing compression of either the brain or spinal cord (such as subdural hematoma, metastatic cancer, or neurofibroma). When a compressive lesion within the CNS is suspected on clinical grounds, MRI of the brain and spine should be performed to make a diagnosis.

*Treatment*

**Peripheral Neuropathies.**  The aim of therapy should be to effect remission of the RA. Subjective relief of pain can be achieved with carbamazepine, amitriptyline hydrochloride, or clonazepine medications. Generally, the patient recovers most of the neurologic function independent of therapy, and the neuropathy improves. A small number of patients may be left with a chronic neuropathy, as evidenced by neurologic examination and NCS.

**Myopathy and Focal Myositis.**   RA myopathy is independent of steroid therapy, and patients with this condition do not progress to diffuse and severe muscle necrosis if the RA remains controlled with medications and physical therapy.

**Vasculitis.**   Medical therapy should be directed at control of the vasculitis and the RA. Short-term steroid therapy or treatment with immunosuppressive drugs may be indicated in the acute condition. Even with optimal therapy, most of these patients are left with severe neuropathies.

**Dural Rheumatoid Nodules.**   If these produce compression signs and symptoms involving the CNS, surgical intervention should be considered.

**Progressive Multifocal Leukoencephalopathy.**   No known therapy exists, and the patient's course is rapidly fatal.

Ankylosing Spondylitis

*Clinical Evaluation*

Ankylosing spondylitis represents a chronic progressive form of arthritis involving the sacroiliac joints, the spinal apophyseal (synovial) joints, and the paravertebral soft tissues. Characteristically, ankylosing spondylitis produces ossification of the annulus fibrosus of the intervertebral disks and of the connective tissue immediately adjacent to the annulus, and changes in the intervertebral diarthrodial joints similar to those occurring in RA. Over a period of 10–20 years, the patient with ankylosing spondylitis develops the poker-type deformity or the cervicodorsal kyphosis. Both atlantoaxial and atlantooccipital subluxations can occur.

*Differential Diagnosis*

Other neurologic involvement in ankylosing spondylitis includes the cauda equina syndrome, vertebrobasilar insufficiency, and peripheral nerve lesions.

*Diagnostic Evaluation*

Because other medical disorders can produce similar clinical pictures, appropriate laboratory studies as well as electrodiagnostic and neuroimaging studies often are necessary to arrive at the specific diagnosis.

*Treatment*

External bracing may provide relief of bulbar symptoms from vascular ischemia in cases of atlantoaxial and atlanto-occipital subluxations. Therapy should be directed at controlling the ankylosing spondylitis. When the cauda equina syndrome occurs, neurosurgical or orthopedic decompression of the lower spine may be necessary.

## NEUROLOGIC CONSULTATION TO CLEAR A PATIENT FOR AN ORTHOPEDIC PROCEDURE OR SURGERY

Orthopedic surgeons often ask the neurologist to "clear" a patient for an upcoming procedure or surgery. A systematic approach to evaluating each patient with symptoms suggesting disease of the nervous system is an essential preliminary to accurate diagnosis. The initial question concerns the location of the lesion or systemic process responsible for the symptoms and signs. Is the disease extracerebral or within the cerebrum, brain stem, or cerebellum? If the clinical findings indicate, for example, a disorder of the spinal cord or of the LMN, is the lesion in the spinal column, meninges, spinal cord, spinal roots, plexuses, peripheral nerves, motor end plates, or muscles? In each of these situations, the clinician should consider whether the condition is traumatic, inflammatory, neoplastic, degenerative, metabolic, or congenital. What influences and constitutional factors play a role in its genesis? Is disease present in the lungs, heart, vessels, or other organs that could be responsible for the patient's symptoms and signs? Are psychological or emotional factors responsible for any part of the patient's symptoms or disability? Although in many cases the answers to the above questions are self-evident, it is good that they be asked, for only such a comprehensive approach to evaluating patients with neurologic conditions leads to an accurate diagnosis. An accurate diagnosis, in turn, provides a foundation on which to assess the patient's medical treatment and ability to withstand certain therapies and procedures, including orthopedic surgery.

## SUMMARY

Orthopedic surgeons and neurologists must deal with the medical diseases and syndromes discussed in this chapter on a regular basis. These conditions account for the symptoms of many patients who present with pain, numbness, tingling, or weakness in an extremity and must be considered in the differential diagnosis of many other disorders. An occupational history may be an important clue to the diagnosis of an entrapment syndrome or a repetitive strain or OS. Certain entrapment syndromes are caused by friction, pressure, or traction on nerves from chronic occupational or athletic use.

Several general treatment considerations apply to all the entrapment neuropathies as well as to the other conditions mentioned in this chapter. Nonsurgical therapies are important to consider before proceeding to surgery. For many mild entrapment neuropathies as well as neck and back pain syndromes a change in occupation, hobby, or repetitive activity can make a difference. Surgical therapy is advisable for peripheral nerve entrapments and cervical and lumbar radiculopathies when the diagnosis is definite and when nonsurgical therapy has failed or is known to be ineffective. In some instances a definite structure must be removed, such as a tumor, a ganglion, an aberrant muscle or artery, or a thickened fascia or muscle origin. Poor surgical results are often the result of scarring or fibrosis.

New basic information has been coming forth in the field of peripheral neuropathy, spine disorders, and the connective tissue diseases. The electrophysiologic study of patients has also advanced, and EMG, NCS, and SER techniques are widely available to contribute to patient care. Moreover, computerized imaging in the form of CT scans and MRI has revolutionized diagnostic potential. Yet the evaluation of patients with the various disorders discussed in this chapter remains a clinical discipline for which laboratory, electrophysiologic, and computerized neuroimaging cannot substitute. The emphasis therefore is on the clinical features and evaluation of the different diseases and syndromes, their differential diagnosis, and the results expected from currently accepted treatments.

## REFERENCES

1. Nakano KK. Neck Pain. In WN Kelley, ED Harris Jr, S Ruddy, CB Sledge (eds), Textbook of Rheumatology (5th ed). Philadelphia: Saunders, 1998;395.
2. Nakano KK. Neurology of Musculoskeletal and Rheumatic Disorders. Boston: Houghton Mifflin, 1979;297.
3. Frymoyer JD. Back pain and sciatica. N Engl J Med 1988;318:291.
4. Frymoyer JW. Quality: an international challenge to the diagnosis and treatment of the lumbar spine. Spine 1993;18:2147.
5. Jonsson B, Stromqvist B. The straight leg raising test and the severity of symptoms in lumbar disk herniation: a preoperative and postoperative evaluation. Spine 1995;20:27.
6. Nakano KK. Entrapment neuropathies. Muscle Nerve 1978;1:264.
7. Dawson DM, Hallet M, Millender LH. Entrapment Neuropathies (2nd ed). Boston: Little, Brown, 1990.
8. Iyer VG. Understanding nerve conduction and electromyographic studies. Hand Clin 1993;9:2373.
9. Levin KH. Common focal mononeuropathies and their electrodiagnosis. J Clin Neurophysiol 1993;10:181.
10. Lanzetta M, Foucher G. Entrapment of the superficial branch of the radial nerve (Wartenberg's syndrome): a report of 52 cases. Int Orthop 1993;17:342.
11. Walsh MT. Therapist management of thoracic outlet syndrome. J Hand Ther 1994;7:131.
12. Oberpenning F, Roth S, Leusmann DB, et al. The Alcock syndrome: temporary penile insensitivity due to compression of the pudendal nerve within the Alcock canal. J Urol 1994;151:423.
13. Mabee JR, Bostwick TL. Pathophysiology and mechanisms of compartment syndromes. Orthop Rev 1993;22:175.
14. Barton N. Repetitive strain disorder. BMJ 1989;299:405.
15. Lockwood AH. Medical problems of musicians. N Engl J Med 1989;320:221.
16. Fry H, Hallet M. Focal dystonia (occupational cramp) masquerading as nerve entrapment or hysteria. Plast Reconstr Surg 1988;82:989.
17. Dawson DM, Krarup C. Perioperative nerve lesions. Arch Neurol 1989;46:1355.
18. Nakano KK. Neurorheumatology. In J Stein (ed), Internal Medicine (4th ed). St. Louis: Mosby–Year Book, 1994;1188.
19. Nakano KK. The neurological complications of rheumatoid arthritis. Orthop Clin North Am 1975;6:861.
20. Bathon JM, Moreland LW, Dibartolomeo AG. Inflammatory central nervous system involvement in rheumatoid arthritis. Semin Arthritis Rheum 1989;18:258.

# 25
# Urology

Steven Mandel, Michael B. Chancellor,
Ramon Mañon-Espaillat, and David A. Rivas

The Thomas Jefferson University Hospital, a university hospital with a large volume of neurologically impaired patients, is fortunate to have two urologists with fellowship training in both neurourology and female urology who are highly interested in, and work closely together with, neurologists in the assessment and treatment of patients afflicted with neurogenic lower urinary tract dysfunction. Despite our extensive experience with neurourology, we are unaware of a comprehensive textbook chapter written specifically for the neurologist who has been consulted by a urologist to ascertain the cause of a given patient's voiding dysfunction. We have taken a practical approach in this chapter, describing the most common situations in which neurologic consultation is required for the patient with urologic dysfunction.

## URINARY VOIDING DYSFUNCTION AND ITS NEUROLOGIC IMPLICATIONS

### Urinary Incontinence

Urinary incontinence may be caused by intrinsic factors—such as pathologic, anatomic, or physiologic factors that directly affect the urinary tract structures—as well as by extrinsic factors that do not cause abnormalities of the urinary tract per se but that significantly affect lower urinary tract function. The effects of many of these factors are reversible, and their treatment brings about the resolution of symptomatology. Reversible causes of lower urinary tract dysfunction include microbial infection, atrophic vaginitis, acute confusional states, restrictions in mobility, fecal impaction, pharmacologic side effects, and medical conditions that cause polyuria or nocturia.

*Table 25.1*   Common neurologic causes of urinary incontinence

Upper motor neuron lesions
   Cerebral lesions
      Cerebrovascular disease
      Dementia
      Hydrocephalus
      Infections
      Multiple sclerosis
      Tumors
      Traumatic encephalopathy
   Spinal cord lesions
      Cord compression
      Ischemia
      Multiple sclerosis
      Trauma
Lower motor neuron lesions
   Conus medullaris
      Degenerative disease
      Ischemia
      Multisystem atrophy
      Multiple sclerosis
      Spinal dysraphism
   Cauda equina lesions
      Ankylosing spondylitis
      Lumbosacral trauma
      Herniated intervertebral disk
      Lumbar canal stenosis
   Peripheral nerve lesions
      Autonomic neuropathy
      Childbirth-associated pelvic floor nerve injuries
      Diabetic neuropathy
      Pelvic lesions (tumors, abscess, endometriosis)
      Pelvic surgery injury (hysterectomy, colon resection)
      Pudendal/perineal nerve stretch injury

Urinary incontinence is a common manifestation of many neurologic disease states (Table 25.1). Therefore, the diagnosis and treatment of both the primary neurologic disease and its secondary urologic complications are intimately related. It must be remembered that the principal objective of the treatment of neurogenic lower urinary tract dysfunction is to preserve renal function while establishing urinary continence. In order to accomplish this goal, a balance must be found between maximizing urinary bladder storage capability and maximizing urethral sphincter control. In cases of patients with a new onset of urinary incontinence and signs of neurologic impairment, a neurology consultation is mandatory.

## Neurologic Causes of Incontinence

Urinary incontinence may occur as a result of a disease process affecting the central and peripheral nervous systems. In addition, anatomic stress urinary incontinence may also have a neurogenic etiology, as in cases where damage has occurred to the innervation of the pelvic floor sphincter muscles. Urinary and fecal incontinence may often occur concurrently. For example, senile dementia is often accompanied by fecal impaction, which ultimately results in overflow incontinence of both feces and urine. A second example is that of patients with diabetes mellitus, in whom autonomic and sensorimotor neuropathy produces incontinence of both urine and feces.

## Central Nervous System Lesions

Lesions in the central nervous system may induce incontinence by the interruption of ascending and descending pathways influencing bladder and sphincter control. Voluntary control of the bladder originates in the neurons of the cerebral cortex. The bladder is represented on the medial surfaces of the cerebral hemispheres; the motor and sensory representations are situated adjacent to each other across the rolandic fissure of the brain. Frontal lobe lesions, particularly of the inferior and medial surfaces, are well-known causes of urinary incontinence. With such lesions, incontinence occurs as a result of inappropriate micturition, rather than as a result of involuntary detrusor contraction. In essence, the patient simply voids at a socially unacceptable time and place. This loss of socially acceptable micturition, characteristic of frontal lobe lesions, is a common manifestation of dementia, post-traumatic encephalopathy, and some cerebrovascular diseases.

Incontinence may also be associated with hydrocephalus. Although no evidence exists of functional disturbance of cortical function, the incontinence is believed to result from damage to the descending pathways between the control centers in the cortex itself and the brain stem. This damage may result either from a direct pressure effect, because these pathways project through the corticospinal pathway around the lateral side of the distended lateral ventricles, or from a stretch injury at this site. The corticomotor pathway, from the medial surface of the hemisphere, is more likely to be deformed by expansion of the lateral ventricle than are the motor fibers that take origin from the lateral surface of the hemisphere. The latter project to motor neurons innervating the upper limb and bulbar muscles. Therefore, an association exists between the development of incontinence and slowly progressive spastic paraplegia, without involvement of the upper limbs, as the hydrocephalus advances. Thus, the typical clinical features of occult hydrocephalus consist of incontinence, extensor plantar responses, and spastic paraparesis associated with a shuffling, apractic gait.

In brain stem vascular disease, supranuclear control of the sacral centers for micturition is lost. In the absence of bladder outlet obstruction, an automatic pattern of bladder emptying may be established. If the lesion disrupts the pontine centers of micturition, however, urinary retention may occur, and there may be progression to the development of "overflow" incontinence. Most lesions in this region of the brain produce relatively extensive and complex functional disturbances, often with sensory impairment. As the normal appreciation of bladder filling becomes impaired, bladder overfilling, distension, and the loss of locally mediated reflexes in the bladder and bowel wall occur. Thus, the normal viscoelasticity of the wall of the bladder becomes compromised, and not only the characteristic smooth-muscle tone but also the expected storage function of this organ is adversely affected. In cases of spinal cord lesions, these pathways may

*Table 25.2*   Segmental innervation of the genitourinary system

| Location | Nerve |
| --- | --- |
| Testis (well established) | T8 |
| Penile sensations and reflex erections (most likely) | S2 |
| Rectum and anal contraction (Brindley's studies indicate that strong stimulation of any of these roots will increase rectal pressure and contraction of the anal sphincter.) | S3–S4 |
| Bladder (predominantly S3) | S2–S4 |
| External urethral sphincter (predominantly S3) | S2–S3 |
| Reflexes | |
| Bulbocavernosus reflex | S2–S3 |
| Anal reflex | S3 |
| Other peripheral muscles that can be tested and are innervated by sacral roots | |
| Gluteus maximus | S1–S2 |
| Gastrocnemius | S1–S2 |
| Flexor digitorum brevis | S1–S2 |

be disrupted; the result is separation of the pontine detrusor and storage mechanisms from the effector organs.

## Peripheral Nervous System Lesions

Damage to the somatic afferent and efferent nervous pathways to the bladder and urethral sphincter results from lesions in the lumbosacral spine (Table 25.2). Examples of such lesions include those resulting from lumbosacral spondylosis, tumors, sacral meningomyelocele, and trauma. Abnormal neural impulse conduction may also occur with intrapelvic disease involving the sacral plexus, especially metastatic deposits or traumatic fracture of the bony pelvis. Peripheral neuropathy, such as diabetic proximal neuropathy, mononeuropathies involving the pudendal or perineal nerves, and even polyarteritis nodosa may produce a similar functional disturbance. More commonly, these nerves may be affected at least temporarily during childbirth via vaginal delivery.

Symptoms arising from peripheral pelvic nerve injury are often vague. The patient, who may have a history of previous lumbosacral surgery, may describe low back or pelvic pain, which is often induced by movement or by certain postures. There may be associated complaints of diminished perineal sensation or a diminished sensation of bladder filling. Urinary retention and fecal incontinence may develop in established cases. In patients with lumbosacral spondylosis and spinal stenosis, micturition may be possible only with the spine held in an exaggerated or maximally extended posture. Of additional concern, men may develop erectile and ejaculatory dysfunction. Physical examination reveals impaired sensation in the perineal and perianal region that extends forward into the anterior perineum and involves the vulva or scrotum. The anal, cremasteric, and bulbo-cavernosus reflexes are classically absent, and anal sphincter contraction may not even accompany coughing. Marked perineal descent occurs with Valsalva maneuvers, as muscular tone of the entire perineum is impaired. Although full, the bladder is usually not painful during palpation and compression. Urodynamic evaluation reveals an essentially acontractile bladder, while sphincter electromyography (EMG) reveals denervation potentials, polyphasic motor units, and decreased recruitment in the perianal muscles. Electrophysiologic investigation can be useful in confirming the diagnosis by demonstrating abnormal conduction in the cauda equina nerve roots between the T12 and L1 levels. Magnetic resonance imaging (MRI) or computerized tomographic scanning and myelography are required to determine the cause of the neural deficit and establish the definitive diagnosis for these patients.

Urge Incontinence

Urge incontinence is defined as the involuntary loss of urine associated with an abrupt and strong desire to urinate. Urge incontinence is usually, although not without exception, associated with the urodynamic finding of involuntary detrusor contractions, referred to as *detrusor overactivity*. Involuntary detrusor contractions occur not only in patients with neurologic disorders but also in individuals who are neurologically normal. When no associated neurologic disorder is present, the occurrence of uninhibited detrusor contractions during urodynamic testing is referred to as *detrusor instability*. When uninhibited detrusor contractions occur in conjunction with a neurologic deficit, the urodynamic diagnosis is that of *detrusor hyperreflexia*. Cerebrovascular accidents and multiple sclerosis are commonly associated with detrusor hyperreflexia. In patients with suprasacral spinal cord lesions, detrusor hyper-reflexia may occur in conjunction with external sphincter dyssynergia. These patients may develop some degree of urinary retention, vesicoureteral reflux, and ultimately, renal damage.

Urethral instability, the involuntary relaxation of the urethral sphincter mechanism, may also account for some cases of urge incontinence; it may or may not be associated with involuntary detrusor contraction. The existence of urethral instability as an independent entity, however, is still controversial. Another urodynamic finding associated with the symptom of urge incontinence in frail, elderly patients is detrusor hyperactivity with impaired bladder contractility (DHIC). These patients suffer from involuntary detrusor contractions, yet the magnitude of detrusor activity is inadequate to achieve normal voiding. Commonly, patients with DHIC must strain to assist micturition and are unable to completely empty the bladder. Clinically, patients with DHIC generally describe not only symptoms of urge incontinence but also symptoms of obstruction, stress incontinence, or overflow incontinence. Detrusor hyperactivity with impaired detrusor contractility represents a significant clinical entity because it can mimic other causes of urinary incontinence and result in inappropriate treatment. Because DHIC can only be diagnosed urodynamically, those with significant symptomatology should not be treated empirically but should instead be evaluated with formal urodynamic study.

Overflow Incontinence

The involuntary loss of urine occurring as a result of overdistension of the urinary bladder is referred to as *overflow incontinence*. Such incontinence may vary in its presentation. Although patients classically complain of frequent or constant dribbling, urge or stress incontinence symptoms may predominate. Although overflow incontinence may be caused by an underactive or acontractile detrusor, bladder outlet or urethral obstruction may also be responsible for bladder overdistension and overflow.

A decrease in detrusor activity or contractility may not only result from idiopathic, iatrogenic, or reversible causes, such as pharmacologic therapy or fecal impaction, but also from permanent or progressive neurologic conditions. These include diabetic neuropathy, low-level spinal cord injury, or pelvic plexus neuropathy following radical surgery.

In men, overflow incontinence associated with obstruction is commonly due to benign prostatic hyperplasia and less frequently due to either adenocarcinoma of the prostate or urethral stricture disease. Although outlet obstruction is rare in women, it can develop from severe pelvic prolapse in which the organ involved protrudes to or beyond the vaginal orifice (e.g., prolapsing cystocele, uterine prolapse) or as a complication of anti-incontinence surgery.

Other Causes of Incontinence

Urinary incontinence may result not only from dysfunction of the lower urinary tract but also from factors extrinsic to the detrusor and sphincter, such as chronic impairments of physical and cognitive functioning. Such a condition is termed *functional incontinence*. This diagnosis, however, should be one of exclusion. Even though many functionally incontinent patients are either immobile, cognitively impaired, or both, each should be evaluated individually, because a treatable cause of incontinence may be partially responsible. Urinary incontinence can often be dramatically improved, or even cured, simply by improving the patient's functional status, treating other medical conditions, discontinuing certain types of medication, adjusting the hydration status, or reducing environmental barriers, despite the presence of intrinsic lower urinary tract dysfunction.

It is not unusual for patients to complain of mixed urinary incontinence, characterized by a combination of urge and stress incontinence symptoms. Alternatively, many frail, elderly patients exhibit mixed incontinence consisting of urge and functional components. The identification of the individual components of a mixed incontinence presentation is essential in determining the most appropriate therapy.

Urinary loss may occur in some patients who have no overt neurologic dysfunction in the absence of sensory awareness, as may be experienced by paraplegics. Other presentations of urinary incontinence include dribbling, which may be described as either postmicturitional or continuous dribbling. *Nocturnal enuresis* represents a voiding disorder in which incontinence occurs during sleep. At times, the characterization of a patient's incontinence may be difficult, especially when the incontinence occurs only in unusual circumstances.

An abnormal bladder condition, diagnosed urodynamically and associated with urinary incontinence, is that of *decreased bladder compliance*. It may result from bladder injury after pelvic radiation, as in radiation cystitis; from inflammatory bladder conditions, such as chemical cystitis or interstitial cystitis; and from some neurogenic lower urinary tract disorders, such as those caused by radical pelvic surgery or congenital defects such as myelomeningocele. Many patients with a nonneurogenic cause for their decreased bladder compliance, such as chemical cystitis or radiation cystitis, suffer with severe urgency and bladder hypersensitivity without demonstrable detrusor overactivity. This condition is termed *sensory urgency*. The loss of bladder wall elasticity and poor bladder accommodation produce a steep rise in intravesical pressure during bladder filling but without detrusor contraction. In patients in whom the urethral sphincter mechanism may already be compromised by the primary condition that impaired the bladder's compliance (radiation, neurologic dysfunction, etc.), the abnormal increase in intravesical pressure may exceed urethral sphincter pressure and result in urinary incontinence. Of major concern in patients with a poorly compliant bladder, especially in those who are neurologically impaired, is persistently elevated intravesical pressure, which will predispose to the development of hydronephrosis, vesicoureteric reflux, and a deterioration of renal function.

## Urinary Retention and Dysfunctional Voiding

A *functional* voiding disorder is characterized by symptoms referable to the genitourinary organs, although organic or neurologic pathology is demonstrably absent. The severity of voiding symptomatology often varies in proportion to the intensity of psychosocial disturbance. A functional voiding disorder, in general, results in either idiopathic urinary retention or idiopathic urinary urgency and frequency. An emotional or psychiatric basis has historically been suspected for idiopathic retention, whereas urinary urgency and frequency correlate less frequently with psychosomatic dysfunction. Functional urinary retention afflicts women more commonly than men. The incidence of acute urinary retention in a group of women is approximately 7 per 100,000 per year. Men are much more likely than women to develop acute urinary retention; the ratio of men to women developing acute urinary retention is 13 to 1. This fact can most easily be explained by the prevalence of benign prostatic hyperplasia causing bladder outlet obstruction in men and the rarity of urethral obstruction in women.

The relationship between organic urologic or neurologic diseases, psychological disturbances, and voiding symptoms is currently poorly defined. Noted, however, is the analogy between irritable bowel syndrome and chronic constipation in the field of gastroenterology, and urinary urgency and retention in urology. Perhaps the incomplete understanding of functional voiding disorders is due in part to the fact that many different mechanisms can act to produce similar symptoms in the urinary tract. Irreversible and destructive surgery, such as cystectomy and prostatectomy, should be avoided as treatment of functional voiding disorders. It has been well documented in the literature that some patients, despite the removal of the genitourinary structure (prostate and bladder) to which intractable symptoms were attributed, have received no appreciable improvement in their symptom complex from the surgery.

## Underlying Neurologic Disease

A variety of organic etiologies demand consideration in the evaluation of a patient afflicted with unexplained urinary retention. In the past, the cause of retention was most commonly considered psychogenic, because often no objective evidence of organic disease was present to account for the inability to void. With the availability of urodynamic evaluation and MRI, many factors that may contribute to the development of acute urinary retention can now be more readily diagnosed. These different causes should be excluded before the diagnosis of psychogenic retention can be applied. Even if a patient manifests clear signs of hysteria, it is important to exclude organic pathology, such as an occult neurologic disease, that may contribute to voiding symptoms.

## Transient Retention

Causes of transient acute urinary retention include acute bacterial lower urinary tract infection, immobility, fecal impaction, hypothyroidism, and medications. Viral infections, including herpes zoster and herpes simplex, have also been reported to induce the development of acute urinary retention by producing inflammation of the sacral nerve roots. Other diseases with neurologic sequelae, such as Lyme disease, can also present with acute urinary retention as their initial clinical manifestation. Fecal impaction has been implicated as a causal factor due to both direct compression and a reflex detrusor inhibition produced by a distended rectum.

Medications usually cause acute urinary retention either by inhibiting detrusor contractility or by increasing outlet resistance at the bladder neck. Antiparkinsonian and antipsychotic medications—such as benztropine mesylate, chlorpromazine hydrochloride, and some of the tricyclic antidepressants—have potent anticholinergic effects, as do antihistamines, such as diphenhydramine hydrochloride. Because acetylcholine is the chief neurotransmitter responsible for initiating detrusor contraction, inhibition by these agents will significantly reduce detrusor contractility. Alpha-adrenergic receptors, located in the musculature of the area of the bladder neck, are in part responsible for passive urinary continence. Alpha-adrenergic agonists, then, can cause urinary retention due to sympathetic stimulation of the bladder neck and internal sphincter mechanism. Examples of these agents include phenylpropanolamine hydrochloride and related ingredients in over-the-counter appetite suppressants, as well as pseudoephedrine hydrochloride and related nasal decongestants.

The combination of medications with anticholinergic effects, pain that triggers sympathetic neurotransmission, analgesic medications that blunt sensory awareness or partially interrupt the sacral reflex arc, and postoperative immobility predisposes to the development of urinary retention after surgery. Under such circumstances, the mechanism for retention seems to be an initial sensory loss, followed by bladder overdistention, detrusor decompensation, and ultimately, the inability to urinate. A classic example of this phenomenon is that of the woman who shortly after normal vaginal delivery is unable to urinate because of epidural anesthesia. Organic causes, such as diabetes mellitus, pernicious anemia, hypothyroidism, and tabes dorsalis, can lead to urinary retention by affecting the sacral nerves; the result is a weak or acontractile bladder. Surgical causes of urinary retention include injury to the parasympathetic nerves during radical pelvic surgery, such as may occur during abdominoperineal resection of the rectum or radical hysterectomy.

## Evaluation of Urinary Retention

For those with idiopathic urinary retention, both neurologic and urologic consultations are recommended. The urologic evaluation should include a medical history and physical examination, renal ultrasonography, urine analysis, and urodynamic evaluation. The neurologic evaluation could possibly involve cerebrospinal fluid analysis, MRI of the head and lumbosacral spine, and serum testing for a Lyme titer in areas where Lyme disease is endemic. Physical examination of the patient with urinary retention must include the careful evaluation of pinprick sensation of the saddle area, anal sphincter tone, and the bulbocavernosus reflex. Abnormalities in one or more of these areas are indicative of an organic neurologic lesion and indicate that further testing is required. For example, distortion of the cauda equina, as occurs with the tethered cord syndrome, may be responsible for lower urinary tract dysfunction.

As mentioned, the patient who develops acute urinary retention should be evaluated with formal urodynamic testing to establish whether impaired detrusor contractility or bladder outlet obstruction is chiefly responsible for the inability to void. The cystometry portion of the urodynamic evaluation of patients with retention has revealed a consistent pattern of detrusor areflexia, whereas EMG evaluation may indicate a failure of complete relaxation of the pelvic floor and urethral sphincter musculature during attempts at urination.

Although psychiatric consultation should be obtained for those with idiopathic urinary retention, many patients are offended by the suggestion of an underlying psychological condition unless thorough neurologic and urologic evaluations are first completed. Patients often consult multiple physicians in search of an elusive neurologic cause for their symptoms.

## Sphincter Electromyography

Spontaneous myotonic-like sphincter EMG activity has been proposed as a cause of urinary retention. Such EMG activity is composed of complex, repetitive discharges with pronounced "decelerating bursts." The sound produced by a decelerating burst is highly reminiscent of myotonic discharges and has therefore been called *pseudomyotonic*. This activity mimics the EMG activity of the urethral sphincter noted with other voiding dysfunctions. The spontaneous sphincter activity is associated with poor relaxation of the striated urethral sphincter, which results in increased bladder outlet resistance and, ultimately, impaired urinary flow. Interestingly, many women who develop idiopathic urinary retention have been found to have polycystic ovaries. It has been suggested that endocrine abnormalities, such as progesterone deficiency, may be associated with abnormal sphincter EMG activity.

## NEUROLOGIC DISEASE WITH PRIMARILY UROLOGIC COMPLAINTS

### Infectious Neurologic Diseases

One of the most common reasons for emergent admission to the hospital by a urologist is acute urinary retention. Although the condition is potentially caused by intrinsic pathology of the lower urinary tract, it is important for the urologist to consider the possibility of an underlying neurologic condition in cases of acute urinary retention. For example, several infectious diseases that primarily affect neurologic function can cause the patient to present with acute urinary retention. Although only a few publications have objectively evaluated the urologic dysfunction associated with infectious processes of the central and peripheral nervous system, including the sexually transmitted diseases, it appears that patients with these disease entities can indeed present with urologic dysfunction. When a neurogenic cause for voiding dysfunction is suspected, infectious neurologic processes should be considered by the neurology consultant.

### Acquired Immunodeficiency Syndrome

Acquired immunodeficiency syndrome (AIDS) is commonly associated with neurologic dysfunction. Such dysfunction occurs in as many as 40% of patients with AIDS and may involve both the central and peripheral nervous systems. The neurologic sequelae of AIDS may result from a direct infection of the nervous system, secondary opportunistic infections, immunologic injury and inflammatory demyelination, or the tumors associated with AIDS and their effect on central and peripheral nerves.

Urinary retention as a result of detrusor areflexia is probably the most common presenting symptom in patients with AIDS. Toxoplasmosis of the brain has been reported to be the predominant lesion, affecting one-third of the AIDS patients with retention in one study. As mentioned previously, urodynamic evaluation is quite valuable in the evaluation and proper management of AIDS patients with voiding dysfunction.

### Neurosyphilis (Tabes Dorsalis)

Neurosyphilis has long been recognized as causing abnormal central and peripheral nerve function. Voiding dysfunction related to neurosyphilis was quite common in the era prior to penicillin availability. With the advent of penicillin and better diagnostic tools, the complications of syphilis have been dramatically reduced. Only rarely is urologic impairment associated with neurosyphilis reported. In general, it is found in conjunction with serious central nervous system abnormalities.

Parenchymatous neurosyphilis includes the syndromes known as tabes dorsalis and general paresis of the insane. Tabes dorsalis is a demyelinating atrophy of the dorsal spinal cord, which results in the loss of bladder sensation and increased residual urine. The most common urodynamic finding in neurosyphilis is that of detrusor areflexia. Because the corticospinal tracts are not involved in the disorder, sphincteric EMG activity is generally normal. This entity is best treated by administering antimicrobial agents for the underlying disease and performing clean intermittent catheterization as management for secondary urinary retention. Because the voiding dysfunction and other symptoms of neurosyphilis are multifocal and mimic many diseases, examination of the cerebrospinal fluid is crucial to establish the diagnosis with certainty.

## Tropical Spastic Paraparesis

Urinary symptoms are reported in up to 60% of cases of tropical spastic paraparesis. Classically, these symptoms include hesitancy, urgency, and incontinence. Urodynamic findings in patients with tropical spastic paraparesis include detrusor hyperreflexia with or without external sphincter dyssynergia. A patient afflicted with tropical spastic paraparesis must be differentiated from one with multiple sclerosis. It must be remembered that multiple sclerosis is the most common cause of chronic spastic myelopathy during middle age in the temperate regions. Because of the frequent finding of detrusor and external sphincter dyssynergia, it is prudent to evaluate and treat aggressively patients with tropical spastic paraparesis who have urinary symptoms.

## Herpes Zoster and Herpes Simplex

When viral invasion of the lumbosacral dorsal roots does occur, visible skin vesicles may appear along the corresponding dermatome; cystoscopy may reveal a similar grouping of vesicles along the urethral and bladder mucosa. The early stages of lower urinary tract involvement with herpes are manifested by symptomatic detrusor instability accompanied by urinary frequency and urgency. The later stages evolve with a decreased sensation of filling, increasing postvoid residual urinary volume, and, ultimately, urinary retention. Fortunately, the inability to urinate associated with herpes infection is self-limited and usually resolves spontaneously over several months.

## Guillain-Barré Syndrome

As with other inflammatory processes, Guillain-Barré syndrome may involve the afferent sensory neurons and produce a loss of sensation of both proprioception and vibration. This occurrence may explain the findings of both detrusor motor and sensory deficits associated with Guillain-Barré syndrome. Although the retention of urine may occur in the early stages and require either intermittent or long-term bladder catheterization to assure urinary drainage, it is transient, and irreversible urologic dysfunction is uncommon.

## Lyme Disease

Lyme disease, caused by the spirochete *Borrelia burgdorferi*, is associated with a variety of neurologic sequelae and may affect all ages of both sexes. The urologic manifestations of Lyme disease may be either the primary or a late manifestation of the disease. Renal involvement in Lyme disease has been described by Steere and associates in 18 of 314 patients (6%) with an erythema chronicum migrans rash (1983). Although the serum creatinine level remained normal in these patients, transient microscopic hematuria and mild proteinuria of 1–2 weeks' duration were noted. Transient testicular pain has also been described but without definite explanation or pathology.

The lower urinary tract may be involved in two different ways in the course of Lyme disease. The spirochete may directly invade the structures of the urinary tract and lead to voiding symptoms. Alternatively, a truly neurogenic voiding dysfunction may develop as part of neuroborreliosis. We recently described seven patients with neuroborreliosis with concurrent lower urinary tract dysfunction (Chancellor et al., 1992). Urinary urgency, nocturia, and urge incontinence were the most common urologic symptoms in our series. Urodynamic evaluation revealed detrusor hyper-reflexia in five patients and detrusor areflexia in two patients. EMG failed to reveal detrusor and external sphincter dyssynergia in any patient. Six of seven patients were afflicted with neurogenic voiding dysfunction, analogous to the voiding dysfunction caused by other neurologic diseases such as multiple sclerosis.

Only one patient, who had an unusual case of Lyme disease that presented with a fulminant course and multisystem involvement, suffered direct bladder invasion by the spirochete. In this case, it was unclear whether the patient's urologic dysfunction resulted from neuroborreliosis or Lyme cystitis. This patient's course of Lyme disease was marked by relapse, prolonged recovery, and persistent neurologic deficits. Up to one-half of the patients who receive antibiotic therapy thought to be appropriate for their stage of disease may still have progression of their illness. A possible reason for relapse is failure to eradicate the spirochete completely with a 2-week course of intravenous ceftriaxone sodium therapy. An additional consideration is that those patients who do not improve may have already suffered irreversible nervous system damage.

In endemic areas, Lyme disease must be included in the differential diagnosis of voiding dysfunction. Lyme disease—like the previous great imitator, syphilis—can be manifested in the most unexpected fashion. Conservative bladder management, guided by thorough urodynamic evaluation, is recommended because our understanding of the disease and its outcome continues to be somewhat limited.

## Parkinson's Disease

Another example of a neurologic disease with manifestations of severe urologic complications is Parkinson's disease, one of the most common neurologic entities causing voiding dysfunction. Bladder overactivity and sphincter bradykinesia, an impairment of relaxation of the striated external urinary sphincter musculature, are commonly documented as contributing to the voiding dysfunction seen in patients with Parkinson's disease. Therapy should be based on a carefully performed urodynamic investigation, which forms the basis for a rational urologic treatment plan for patients with Parkinson's disease. Most important in the management of lower urinary tract dysfunction of Parkinson's disease is ensuring that the parkinsonian patient is receiving optimal neurologic evaluation and treatment.

The treatment of the urologic symptoms of patients afflicted with Parkinson's disease has been largely empiric and notoriously ineffective. Rational therapy requires not only a clear understanding of the underlying functional disorder but also an assessment of the patient's emotional, psychological, and physical limitations. Because of the poor correlation between a patient's symptom complex and treatment outcome, urodynamic evaluation is crucial in the evaluation of any patient with neurologic disease and voiding symptoms. The primary treatment goal in parkinsonian patients is to achieve not only continence but also periodic complete bladder emptying. To accomplish this goal, the two most effective primary tools that the clinician may use are the anticholinergic agents and a program of intermittent self-catheterization.

The patient with documented hyper-reflexia and incomplete emptying usually benefits from combination therapy including both anticholinergic medication and intermittent catheterization. A patient with a postvoid residual bladder urine volume greater than 150 ml should be evaluated and counseled regarding the institution of a program of intermittent catheterization. Commonly, simply ensuring a regular program of complete bladder emptying is sufficient to provide relief from the symptoms of frequency and urgency for a number of hours. In most of these patients, however, involuntary detrusor contractions eventually occur as bladder volume increases with urine production, mandating the use of anticholinergic medication.

## UROLOGIC CANCER WITH NEUROLOGIC SEQUELAE

Renal adenocarcinoma is the fifth or sixth most common cause of spinal metastatic cancer in both men and women. In men, prostate adenocarcinoma is the second most common malignancy, after lung cancer, with neurologic sequelae. Spinal cord compression develops in up to 10% of men with adenocarcinoma of the prostate. It usually involves the thoracic spine, with such cases accounting for nearly three-fourths of all cases.

### Pathophysiology

In cases of metastatic prostate cancer, the epidural space is involved secondarily by extension from an eroded vertebral body or spinous process. An element of cord compression may develop because of the vertebral body collapse and displacement of bony elements. Alternatively, though the dura is an effective barrier to tumor invasion of the cord (intradural metastases are rare), metastatic tumor may exert an additional neuropathic effect by compromising the blood supply to the cord from the epidural space.

### Evaluation and Findings

Back pain is a common and worrisome symptom in men with prostate cancer. Patients with prostatic carcinoma may develop pain because of skeletal and soft tissue metastases, compression and infiltration of nervous structures, local tumor in the prostate with or without infiltration into surrounding tissues (i.e., bladder or colon), and visceral and retroperitoneal metastases. Fortunately, most prostatic cancer patients with back pain secondary to spinal metastatic disease never develop clinically evident cord compression.

Back pain, however, is the most common clinical manifestation of vertebral body and paraspinous metastatic disease and occurs in 75–92% of such patients. A careful neurologic examination of prostate cancer patients with back pain, and thus early diagnosis of incipient spinal cord compression, is crucial to avoid permanent neurologic deficit. Other indications of spinal metastasis include weakness, autonomic dysfunction, and sensory loss. The degree of muscular weakness correlates directly with the chance of treatment success and neurologic recovery in preserving or restoring ambulation. Post-treatment ambulation rates for patients who were ambulatory, paraparetic, and paraplegic prior to treatment are 70%, 44%, and 22%, respectively. Those with long-standing paralysis are not likely to recover neurologically.

Although autonomic dysfunction—with symptoms of urinary retention, overflow urinary incontinence, and severe constipation—is rarely the first symptom appreciated, it may affect 50% of patients by the time the diagnosis of metastatic disease is established. The loss of sensation, recognizable by complaints of numbness or tingling in the toes, is also rarely recognized at first but can occur in up to 50% of patients with metastatic disease. In addition, a loss of proprioception can be present, while compression of the cauda equina characteristically produces a saddle anesthesia and loss of sphincter control.

### Diagnostic Evaluation

Traditionally, myelography has been essential for the diagnosis of spinal cord compression. The imaging modality of choice in patients with suspected spinal cord compression, however, is MRI. It is noninvasive and has a sensitivity and specificity similar to those of the more invasive myelography. The neurologic status and rate of neurologic change influence the timing of diagnostic studies. Even though plain radiographs of the entire spine are helpful in the diagnostic evaluation of suspected spinal metastases, radionuclide bone scanning is more sensitive in detecting bony metastases than plain radiography. Although the bone scan is probably the most useful tool to the urologist for overall treatment planning and subsequent follow-up, bone scintigraphy is ineffective in establishing the extent of spinal cord compression. Bony abnormalities, such as erosion or the collapse of vertebral bodies, paraspinal soft-tissue masses, and osteoblastic changes may be confirmed as caused by metastatic disease through biopsy with a needle technique.

### Management

Spinal cord or cauda equina compression caused by malignancy of urologic origin represents a medical emergency. The close correlation between pretreatment neurologic status and treatment outcome underscores the importance of immediate treatment when indicated. Most, if not all, of the patients who present before the onset of paraparesis caused by metastatic genitourinary carcinoma are ambulatory after treatment, whereas less than one-third of those who present with paraparesis ultimately are not ambulatory after treatment. Full-dose external-beam radiation therapy is the treatment of choice for spinal cord compression resulting from metastatic disease. Decompressive laminectomy is reserved for selected patients who have recurrence at a previously irradiated site, who show canal stenosis secondary to osteoblastic metastases, who have not responded to radiation, or who suffer from an acute onset of paraplegia.

No uniform recommendations have been established for the treatment of spinal cord compression caused by metastatic genitourinary cancer. Treatment options include high-dose steroid therapy, androgen deprivation therapy, radiation to the involved spine, and surgical decompression. The immediate administration of high doses of exogenous steroids coupled with immediate androgen deprivation therapy is universally recommended. The role of immediate surgical decompression versus radiation is more controversial. Research has shown that most men with spinal metastasis of prostate cancer who were ambulatory preoperatively remained so after laminectomy. However, only about one-half of men who were nonambulatory preoperatively recovered the ability to walk after surgical spinal decompression. In another study series by Smith and associates (1993), a cord compression treatment included not only radiation therapy but also androgen deprivation therapy and laminectomy decompression. Twelve of 35 patients who were ambulatory at presentation remained ambulatory. Of 12 patients who were paraparetic at presentation, 10 regained the ability to ambulate after treatment. However, two of the 10 patients who regained ambulation subsequently developed recurrent cord compression and became permanently paraplegic. Overall, seven patients developed recurrent spinal cord compression. Of five patients who either presented with paraplegia or in whom paraplegia developed secondary to recurrent spinal cord compression, four remained paraplegic despite treatment. The average survival of these five patients after treatment was 3.9 months, versus 18 months for the group as a whole.

External-beam radiation therapy to the spinal and paraspinal areas plays an important role in the treatment of spinal compression caused by metastatic cancer. Increasing the ratio of ports from one to two vertebral bodies above and below the lesion has resulted in a decrease in local recurrences. In addition, prophylactic irradiation to incidentally discovered subclinical spinal compressive lesions may be a suitable palliative treatment option. Patients with recurrences at previously irradiated sites must be considered for surgical decompression.

Patients who have paraplegia often do not recover function when treated with radiation, steroids, and androgen deprivation. In these patients, laminectomy may be a suitable alternative. However, enthusiasm for a decision to proceed with surgery must be tempered in light of the poor prognosis and less than 6 months' life expectancy of those who are in such an advanced stage of malignancy. Patients with metastatic genitourinary carcinoma often suffer from significant, chronic pain. Higher dosages of oral and parenteral pain medications may be required to alleviate discomfort than for subjects without malignancy. Neurosurgery, including percutaneous cordotomy or neurectomy with rhizotomy, may be especially useful in attempts to ameliorate the pain of metastatic urologic malignancy when peripheral and spinal cord lesions become symptomatic and are poorly controlled with oral medications. Percutaneous cordotomy should be reserved for those patients with unilateral pain and a short life expectancy, generally not more than 1 year.

## Syndrome of Inappropriate Antidiuretic Hormone Secretion

The syndrome of inappropriate antidiuretic hormone secretion (SIADH) is a common cause of hyponatremia and results from the ectopic production or inappropriate release of antidiuretic hormone from the neurohypophysis. The most common cause of ectopic antidiuretic hormone production is malignancy, with oat cell carcinoma of the bronchus being the most frequent cause. Urologic malignancies, including renal and prostatic adenocarcinoma, may induce the development of SIADH. Hormonal ablation therapy has proven effective in the treatment of SIADH caused by adenocarcinoma of the prostate; SIADH caused by renal cancer is more difficult to control.

## MYELODYSPLASIA

Major myelodysplasia centers are becoming increasingly aggressive in early urologic assessment and treatment. Such timely urologic intervention was stimulated not only by the findings that urodynamic evaluation may detect early the signs of progressive denervation and cord tethering, but also by the fact that urodynamic evaluation can identify children at risk of upper urinary tract deterioration before renal insufficiency and failure occur.

The type of neurogenic bladder disorder that results from a myelodysplastic event is not predictable by neurologic examination. Indeed, urodynamic evaluation is necessary in order to effectively characterize the neurologic dysfunction of the lower urinary tract in cases of myelodysplasia. The neurologic lesion in myelodysplasia is a dynamic pathologic process, in which changes that occur during growth may influence neurologic control over the bladder. In addition, secondary problems, such as tethering of the cord, syrinx development, increased intracranial pressure, or partial herniation of the brain stem and cerebellum, may also profoundly affect the neurologic control of the lower urinary tract. Manifestation of such secondary neurologic developments may be reflected by the worsening of urinary incontinence or a new onset of voiding symptoms or pyelonephritis. Alterations in the voiding symptoms or the development of febrile urinary tract infection in a patient with myelodysplasia should prompt the urologist to obtain neurologic consultation.

## Changing Urodynamic Pattern in Myelomeningocele

Roach and colleagues studied 43 infants with myelodysplasia to determine whether bladder behavior altered with development. Two groups of patients were categorized based on favorable versus unfavorable prognosis. Only 55% of the initial urodynamic studies were found to be predictive of future clinical course.

The patients who worsened generally did so in the first 6 months of life. Of the patients who had been given an unfavorable prognosis initially, 86% improved or stabilized with therapy. One-third of the patients who initially were believed to have a favorable prognosis demonstrated deterioration at the 6-month evaluation. This study demonstrated the importance of serial neurourologic examination of all infants afflicted with myelodysplasia.

## Urologic Management

The proper management of the child with myelomeningocele requires individualized attention. Not only the level of the vertebral bony defect but also the degree of involvement of the spinal cord, the peripheral nerve roots, and the brain and brain stem (due to the Arnold-Chiari malformation) will vary. Differences may exist in the neurologic deficit on opposing sides of the spinal cord, even at the same level.

Intervention to improve upper or lower urinary tract drainage is generally undertaken at the first sign of hydroureteronephrosis, bladder enlargement, or vesicoureteral reflux. As a result of the findings on urodynamic assessment in newborns and older children, and the high degree of predictability for urinary tract deterioration, early intervention has been advocated for children with detrusor and external sphincter incoordination and outflow obstruction and has led to an improvement in the ability to preserve renal function.

In older children, urodynamic testing may be performed only if initial attempts at achieving continence are unsuccessful or if upper urinary tract deterioration has been documented. Persistent incontinence despite a regularly timed intermittent catheterization or Credé's maneuver may indicate elevated bladder-filling pressure, uninhibited detrusor contractions, low urethral resistance, or excessive intravesical volume. Except for the last condition, which results in overflow incontinence, the specific cause of incontinence can be determined only by urodynamic testing. Appropriate therapy with anticholinergic drugs such as oxybutynin chloride or propantheline bromide, which decreases detrusor tone and contractility, and alpha sympathomimetic agents such as phenylpropanolamine hydrochloride or pseudoephedrine, which raise urethral resistance, may be necessary to improve continence between emptying. Urinary volumes should be quantified easily each time the child is catheterized. If fluid intake, and therefore urinary output, is excessive, mild fluid restriction may further help achieve continence.

## SYRINX

An increasingly common reason for neurology consultation in a neurologically impaired patient with voiding dysfunction is the identification of a syrinx on spinal CT or MRI. Classically, these spinal cord injury or spinal cord surgery patients, with documented neurogenic lower urinary tract dysfunction, develop a change in voiding symptoms with syrinx formation. A common example is a man who injured his neck in a motor vehicle accident and required a cervical laminectomy and diskectomy. Such a patient might be left with neurogenic voiding symptoms of urgency, frequency, and nocturia of two episodes per night. The development of several episodes of urge incontinence and increased frequency of nocturia to four episodes per night should prompt a neurologic consultation. Sometimes a careful neurologic examination can uncover a subtly diminished sensation and motor weakness, although the greatest sensitivity would be obtained with a spinal imaging with MRI to demonstrate a spinal cord syrinx.

After this evaluation, the neurologist is left with the difficult evaluation as to not only whether the syrinx is newly formed, but also whether the presence of the syrinx can account for the worsening voiding symptoms and, most importantly, whether surgery could potentially improve the urologic symptoms. Unfortunately, unless serial spinal imaging and urodynamic evaluations exist, no aspect of the urologic examination can accurately predict which patients can potentially benefit from the surgical treatment of a syrinx.

## MEDICAL-LEGAL ISSUES

With increasing frequency, neurologic consultation is sought by the patient who complains of voiding or erectile dysfunction after neurologic trauma or surgery. A common example is a woman who complains of new-onset urinary frequency and urge incontinence after a cervical laminectomy, or a man who complains of straining to urinate and erectile impotence after hurting his back lifting heavy objects at work and whose MRI demonstrates a small to moderate herniation of a lumbar intervertebral disk. These cases are likely to be involved in workers' compensation and medical-legal proceedings for a protracted period. It is essential that the urologist consult his or her neurologic colleague for a thorough evaluation of such patients. For the neurologist-consultant, documenting the patient's complaints and performing objective studies such as spinal CT scan, MRI, myelography, and EMG are important to aid in confirming the presence or absence of a bona fide neurologic impairment. For the urologist, urodynamic evaluation is essential for a complete evaluation of lower urinary tract dysfunction.

The objective testing and evaluation of erectile dysfunction are more difficult because of the wide spectrum of normality in sexual function. Measurement of serum testosterone and prolactin levels is important to rule out a hormonal basis for decreased erectile activity. Nocturnal penile tumescence (NPT) studies can be helpful in differentiating organic, as opposed to psychogenic, impotence. NPT equipment continuously measures the diameter and rigidity of the phallus during three normal nights of sleep. Neurologically intact men generally achieve four episodes of spontaneous erection during rapid eye movement phases of sleep. NPT can therefore help to corroborate or refute complaints of erectile impotence depending on whether spontaneous erectile function can be elicited; true neurogenic erectile dysfunction would result in absolute impotence. Penile intracorporeal pharmacologic injection testing using prostaglandin $E_1$ ($PGE_1$) may also be helpful in discriminating between vasculogenetic and neurogenic impotence. On injection of $PGE_1$ into the corpora of the penis, normal men and men with neurogenic impotence most likely achieve an erection within 10–15 minutes. In cases of impotence due to poor arterial inflow to the penis, no erection may be achieved. In cases of venous leak erectile dysfunction, although an erection may be achieved, it will not be maintained after pharmacologic penile injection.

As with the cases of neurogenic bladder and erectile dysfunction, groin and genital pain are also problems for which neurologic consultations are sometimes requested in litigious cases in which the patients have suffered lower back or pelvic injury. The main issue is that of differentiating between orchitis or epididymitis as the cause of orchialgia, and prostatitis as the cause of pelvic or perineal pain, versus cauda equina or pelvic plexus injury as the primary cause of chronic pain. Close communication between the neurologist and urologist is important in these often difficult cases.

## SUGGESTED READING

### Urologic Cancer

Bridwell KH. Treatment of prostate cancer of the spine. Urol Clin North Am 1991;18:153–159.

Flynn DF, Shipley WU. Management of spinal cord compression secondary to metastatic prostatic carcinoma. Urol Clin North Am 1991;18:145–152.

Gasparine ME, Broderick GA, Narayan P. The syndrome of inappropriate antidiuretic hormone secretion in a patient with adenocarcinoma of the prostate. J Urol 1993;150:978–980.

Ghandur-Mnaymneh L, Satterfield S, Block NL. Small cell carcinoma of the prostate gland with inappropriate antidiuretic hormone secretion: morphological, immunohistochemical and clinical expressions. J Urol 1986;135:1263–1266.

Kuban DA, Schellhammer PF, el-Mahdi AM. Hemibody irradiation in advanced prostatic carcinoma. Urol Clin North Am 1991;18:131–137.

Smith EM, Hampel N, Ruff RL, et al. Spinal cord compression secondary to prostate carcinoma: treatment and prognosis. J Urol 1993;149:330–333.

### Myelodysplasia

Bauer SB. Neurogenic Vesical Dysfunction in Children. In PC Walsh, AB Retik, TA Stamey (eds), Campbell's Urology (6th ed). Philadelphia: Saunders, 1992;1634–1668.

Bauer SB, Hallett M, Khoshbin S, et al. The predictive value of urodynamic evaluation in the newborn with myelodysplasia. JAMA 1984;252:650–652.

Dator DP, Hatchett L, Dyro FM, et al. Urodynamic dysfunction in walking myelodysplastic children. J Urol 1992;148:362–365.

McGuire EJ, Woodside JR, Borden TA, Weiss RM. The prognostic value of urodynamic testing in myelodysplastic patients. J Urol 1981;126:205–209.

Roach MB, Switters DM, Stone AR. The changing urodynamic pattern in infants with myelomeningocele. J Urol 1993;150:944–947.

Salzman AA, Elder JS, Mapstone TB. Urologic consequences of myelodysplasia and other congenital abnormalities of the spinal cord. Urol Clin North Am 1993;20:485–504.

Shenot PJ, Rivas DA, Mandel S, et al. Urological manifestations of reflex sympathetic dystrophy versus interstitial cystitis. J Urol 1994;151:282A.

### Urinary Incontinence

International Continence Society Committee for the Standardization of Terminology of the Lower Urinary Tract Function. Br J Obstet Gynaecol 1990;6:1–16.

Nathan PW, Smith MC. The centrifugal pathway for micturition within the spinal cord. J Neurol Neurosurg Psychiatry 1958;21:177–189.

Resnick NM, Yalla SV. Detrusor hyperactivity with impaired contractile function: an unrecognized but common cause of incontinence in elderly patients. JAMA 1987;257:3076–3081.

Snooks SJ, Swash M, Setchell M, Henry MM. Injury to innervation of pelvic floor sphincter musculature in childbirth. Lancet 1984;ii:546–550.

Urinary Incontinence Guideline Panel. Urinary Incontinence in Adults: Clinical Practice Guideline. Rockville, MD: Agency for Health Care Policy and Research, Public Health Service, U.S. Department of Health and Human Services, March 1992. AHCPR Pub. No. 92-0038.

# Urinary Retention

Chancellor MB, McGinnis DE, Shenot PJ, et al. Lyme cystitis and neurogenic bladder dysfunction secondary to Lyme disease. Lancet 1992;339:1237–1238.

Egley CC, Fox JS. Vaginal myxoma presenting as acute urinary retention. Obstet Gynecol 1989;73(2):883–892.

Fidas A, MacDonald HL, Elton RA, et al. Neurological defects of the voiding reflex arcs in chronic urinary retention and their relation to spina bifida occulta. Br J Urol 1989;63:16–20.

Fontanarosa PB, Roush WR. Acute urinary retention. Emerg Med Clin North Am 1988;6:419–437.

Fowler CJ, Christmas TJ, Chapple CR, et al. Abnormal electromyographic activity of the urethral sphincter, voiding dysfunction, and polycystic ovaries: a new syndrome? Br Med J 1988;297:1436–1438.

Klarskov P, Anderson JT, Asmussen CF, et al. Acute urinary retention in women: a prospective study of 18 cases. Scand J Urol Nephrol 1987;21:1:29–31.

Patel BR, Rivner MH. Herpes zoster causing acute urinary retention. South Med J 1988;81:929–930.

Smith AY, Woodside JR. Urodynamic evaluation of patients with spinal stenosis. Urology 1988;32:472–477.

# Infection

Chancellor MB, McGinnis DE, Shenot PJ, et al. Lyme cystitis and neurogenic bladder dysfunction. Lancet 1992;339:1237–1238.

Chancellor MB, McGinnis DE, Shenot PJ, et al. Urinary dysfunction in Lyme disease. J Urol 1992;149:26–30.

Hattori T, Yasuda K, Kita K, Hirayama K. Disorders of micturition in tabes dorsalis. Brit J Urol 1990;65:497–499.

Kahn Z, Singh VK, Yang WE. Neurogenic bladder in acquired immune deficiency syndrome (AIDS). Urology 1992;40:289–291.

Steere AC, Grodzicki RL, Kornblatt AN, et al. The spirochetal etiology of Lyme disease. N Engl J Med 1983;308:733–735.

Walton GW, Kaplan SA. Urinary dysfunction in tropical spastic paraparesis: preliminary urodynamic survey. J Urol 1993;150:930–932.

Wheeler JS Jr, Culkin DJ, O'Hara RJ, Canning JR. Bladder dysfunction and neurosyphilis. J Urol 1986;136:903–905.

Wheeler JS Jr, et al. The urodynamic aspects of the Guillain-Barré syndrome. J Urol 1987;137:197–200.

# Parkinson's Disease

Berger Y, Blaivas JG, DeLaRocha ER, Salinas J. Urodynamic findings on Parkinson's disease. J Urol 1987;138:836–838.

Berger Y, Salinas JN, Blaivas JG. Urodynamic differentiation of Parkinson disease and the Shy-Drager syndrome (SD). Neurourol Urodyn 1990;9:117–121.

Chancellor MB, Blaivas JG. Incontinence associated with neurologic disorders. Compr Ther 1991;17:37–43.

Eardley I, Quinn NP, Fowler CJ, et al. The value of urethral sphincter electromyography in the differential diagnosis of Parkinsonism. Br J Urol 1989;64:360–362.

# III
## PSYCHIATRY

# 26
# Neurology's Interface with Psychiatry

Bruce H. Price

> Men ought to know that from nothing else but the brain comes joys, delights, laughter, and sports, and sorrows, griefs, despondency, and lamentations. And by this, in an especial way, we acquire wisdom and knowledge, and see and hear and know what are foul and what are fair, what sweet and what unsavory.

> —Hippocrates (470–370 BC)

This chapter is a summation of the author's experience as the chief of neurology at McLean Hospital, a 160-bed inpatient psychiatric facility. During this challenging experience, with a background practicing behavioral neurology at a large general hospital, a paradigm shift was necessary from lesion-based behavioral neurology to neurologically based psychiatry. My aim is to present clinical phenomena as I have observed and studied them along with relevant pathophysiologic changes. My hope is to convince the reader that this approach has utility in hospital-based neurologic consultations regarding patients with salient psychiatric features.

Mental disorders pose a number of special problems not ordinarily encountered in other fields of medicine. Such wide variations in personality, character, and behavior are present that the line demarcating where normality ends and abnormality begins is often obscure. Psychiatric diagnosis is difficult in general because it is based on symptoms more than on signs. Symptoms of mental illness are expressed in behavior, cognition, and subjective feelings. They are considerably more difficult to quantify than pulse, temperature, and blood pressure. Patients' awareness of their own deficits and ability to describe symptoms varies widely. Their subjective descriptions rely on metaphors and therefore draw on their intelligence, education, culture, personality, and cognitive status. Patients are often not consistent; their symptoms can be paradoxical, tend to fluctuate over time, and may change according to different circumstances. Two psychiatric disorders, such as depression and anxiety, often co-occur in the same patient. Primary psychiatric diseases are for the most part not verifiable by laboratory tests or postmortem examinations. Diagnoses are largely syndromic, relying on the clinician's ability to recognize a constellation of defining symptoms and signs that coalesce to provide a recognizable entity with predictive value regarding intervention and outcome.

The neurologic approach assumes that all clinical manifestations of nervous system disorders have a neuronal basis. The standard procedures of history taking and physical examination are supplemented by biochemical, physiologic, and cognitive tests. Clinical manifestations are interpretable in terms of neuroanatomy, neurophysiology, and neuropsychology. Neuropathologic examination usually provides the final confirmation of diagnosis. Historically, diseases presenting with salient behavioral and cognitive symptoms that have demonstrable pathology include Alzheimer's disease, Pick's disease, Huntington's disease, multiple sclerosis (MS), tertiary neurosyphilis, and viral encephalitides, particularly the encephalitis lethargica epidemic of 1917–1926.

The psychological approach assumes that some mental disorders are best understood in the context of previous or present life circumstances. It postulates that psychological trauma can induce temporary or permanent changes in behavior. A major premise is that the purpose of the mammalian brain is to learn and change, that normal learning in response to pathologic surroundings can lead to adjustment difficulties, and that insight and relearning can lead to better adaptation. The lack of consistent biological markers and postmortem neuropathology in affective, thought, addictive, and personality disorders and their positive response to psychotherapy have bolstered this view. However, the neuroscientist retorts, these diseases probably involve more subtle structural and molecular changes still waiting to be defined.

Both the neurologic and psychological approaches have tended to foster myopic and mutually exclusive views that can lead to incorrect diagnoses and treatment. Hence, a young woman with difficulty swallowing may be incorrectly diagnosed as suffering from globus hystericus instead of myasthenia gravis. An elderly man with apparent intellectual decline may be wrongly diagnosed with probable Alzheimer's disease instead of major depression.

Our increasingly sophisticated understanding of mind-brain interactions is eroding these narrow views. The approach is no longer "either psychological or neurologic"; instead, there is recognition of the complex interplay between biological phenomena and environmental influences that shapes human behavior and gives rise to mental health and illness. For instance, it is now widely accepted that emotional stress may exacerbate underlying seizures or MS. Conversely, environmental deprivation in infancy can alter normal brain organization. In patients with obsessive-compulsive disease, those responding to either cognitive therapy alone or pharmacologic intervention alone demonstrate similar reductions in post-treatment versus pretreatment caudate activity on metabolic scans. Anyone who investigates human behavior and mental abnormalities should do so with a completely open mind and be prepared to review critically any reasonable neurologic or psychological hypothesis as to cause.

## DEFINITIONS OF PSYCHIATRIC TERMS

Winston Churchill once remarked that the English and American people "are separated by a common language." The same observation can be made about neurologists and psychiatrists, regardless of nationality. Common definitions are essential to link our two increasingly related specialties. The following simplified glossary of descriptive terms is a starting point:

*Abulia* is the state of reduced impulse to act and think associated with indifference about consequences of action.

*Anxiety* is the feeling of apprehension caused by anticipation of danger that may be internal or external.

*Apathy* is dulled emotional tone associated with detachment or indifference.

*Catatonia* is a range of qualitative psychomotor and volitional disturbances including stereotypies, mannerisms, automatic obedience, catalepsy, echokinesis, echopraxia, mutism, negativism, automatisms, and impulsive acts. These phenomena may occur against a background of hyperkinesia, hypokinesia, or akinesia.

*Compulsion* is the pathologic need to act on an impulse that, if resisted, produces anxiety. The action has no true end in itself other than to prevent something from occurring in the future.

*Confusion* is the inability to maintain a coherent stream of thought due to impaired attention and vigilance. Secondary deficits in language, memory, and visual spatial skills are common.

*Delusion* is a false, unshakable conviction or judgment that is out of keeping with reality and with socially shared beliefs of the individual's background and culture.

*Dementia* is the insidious onset of progressive mental decline that gradually interferes with activities of daily living appropriate for age and background.

*Depression* is a psychopathologic feeling of sadness often accompanied by a variety of associated symptoms, particularly anxiety, agitation, feelings of unworthiness, suicidal ideas, abulia, psychomotor retardation, and various somatic symptoms and physiologic dysfunctions and complaints.

*Dissociation* is the subjective sense of feeling unreal, strange, or unfamiliar to oneself or one's environment.

*Hallucination* is a sensory misperception in any modality occurring in the absence of the appropriate external stimulus.

*Mania* is a disorder in which mood is elevated out of keeping with the individual's circumstances. It may vary from irritability to carefree joviality to almost uncontrollable excitement. Elation is accompanied by increased energy, difficulties sustaining attention, and marked distractibility. Self-esteem is often inflated with grandiose ideas. Flight of ideas, pressure of speech, delusions (usually grandiose), and hallucinations may occur.

*Obsession* is the pathologic persistence of an irresistible thought or feeling that cannot be eliminated from consciousness by logical effort despite the individual's knowledge that it is not true. It is associated with anxiety and rumination.

*Paranoia* is a descriptive term designating either morbid dominant ideas or delusions of self-reference concerning one or more of several themes, most commonly persecution, love, hate, envy, jealousy, honor, litigation, grandeur, or the supernatural.

*Psychosis* is a gross disorder of perception and thought rendering the patient mentally incompetent. It is the misapprehension of the nature of reality.

*Schizophrenia* is a disorder characterized in general by fundamental and characteristic distortions of thinking and perception accompanied by an affect that is inappropriate or blunted. Clear consciousness and intellectual capacity are usually maintained. Although no strictly pathognomonic symptoms can be identified, the most important positive psychopathologic phenomena include thought echo, insertion, withdrawal, or broadcasting; delusions of control, influence, or passivity; perceptions of hallucinatory voices commenting on or discussing the patient in the third person; disorders in the train of thought; and catatonia. Negative symptoms include poverty in quantity or content of speech, impairment of attention, psychomotor slowing, affective blunting, apathy, social withdrawal, poor nonverbal communication, poor self-care, and poor social performance.

## PRINCIPLES OF DIFFERENTIAL DIAGNOSIS

The neurologic investigation of psychiatric symptoms requires a shift in traditional neurologic thinking. It presents challenges not ordinarily encountered in other neurologic consultations. The following principles guide my approach (Table 26.1).

   1. Depression, mania, delusions, hallucinations, obsessions and compulsions, dissociation, and personality alterations are etiologically nonspecific symptoms (Table 26.2). They are common in both primary neurologic and psychiatric dis-

*Table 26.1*   Principles of differential diagnosis

Depression, mania, delusions, hallucinations, obsessions and compulsions, dissociation, and personality alterations are etiologically nonspecific symptoms. They are common in both primary neurologic and psychiatric disease.

Persistent behavioral sequelae may be more disabling than elemental or cognitive neurologic deficits.

Atypical presentations of neuropsychiatric syndromes are common.

A patient's decompensated behavior may be concordant with their past psychiatric profile, but this concordance does not necessarily imply that the decompensation is psychogenic.

A detailed assessment of mental status or elemental neurologic examination may be impossible in the setting of agitation or psychosis.

Normal findings from elemental examination, routine laboratory testing, brain imaging, electroencephalography, and cerebrospinal fluid analysis do not exclude diseases of neurologic origin.

Psychopharmacologic medications often complicate the neurologic picture.

Beneficial responses to neuroleptics, antidepressants, or even electroconvulsive therapy do not necessarily point to a specific disease or narrow the differential diagnosis.

Disturbances of the frontal, temporal, limbic, and striatal regions are most likely to produce psychiatric manifestations.

No simple rules exist. No single feature is common to all forms of brain disease with behavioral disorders.

*Table 26.2*  Neurologic differential diagnosis of psychiatric symptoms

| Symptom | Disease |
|---|---|
| Mania/hypomania | Stroke (primarily right hemisphere) |
| | Huntington's disease |
| | Head trauma |
| | Multiple sclerosis |
| | Seizures (peri-ictal) |
| | Frontal-temporal dementia/Pick's disease |
| | Basal ganglia calcifications (Fahr's disease) |
| | Parkinson's disease/diffuse Lewy body disease |
| | Human immunodeficiency virus (HIV) encephalitis |
| | Tertiary neurosyphilis |
| | Metachromatic leukodystrophy |
| | Tay-Sachs disease |
| Delusions | Degenerative and vascular dementias |
| | Huntington's disease |
| | Seizure (primarily complex partial) |
| | Head trauma |
| | Stroke |
| | Parkinson's disease/diffuse Lewy body disease |
| | Encephalitis |
| | Multiple sclerosis |
| | Brain tumor |
| | Mental retardation |
| | Vitamin $B_{12}$ deficiency |
| | Metachromatic leukodystrophy |
| | Tay-Sachs disease |
| Visual hallucinations | Cataracts |
| | Enucleation |
| | Macular degeneration |
| | Toxic or metabolic encephalopathies |
| | Drug intoxication or withdrawal |
| | Optic nerve ischemia |
| | Degenerative dementias |
| | Stroke |
| | Tumor |
| | Migraine headache |
| | Complex partial seizure |
| | Multiple sclerosis |
| | Parkinson's disease/diffuse Lewy body disease |
| | Narcolepsy |
| | Metachromatic leukodystrophy |
| | Tay-Sachs disease |
| Auditory hallucinations | Bilateral hearing loss |
| | Complex partial seizure |
| | Stroke |
| | Tumor |
| Obsessive-compulsive behavior | Frontal-temporal dementia |
| | Pick's disease |
| | Huntington's disease |
| | Parkinson's disease |
| | Progressive supranuclear palsy |

*Table 26.2*    (continued)

| Symptom | Disease |
| --- | --- |
| Dissociative states | Tourette's syndrome |
| | Anoxic/ischemic encephalopathy |
| | Sydenham's chorea |
| | Magnesium and carbon monoxide poisoning |
| | Complex partial seizure |
| | Migraine headache |
| | Postconcussive syndromes |
| | Toxic or metabolic encephalopathy |
| | Encephalitis |
| Personality alterations | Stroke |
| | Tumor |
| | Head trauma |
| | Complex partial seizure |
| | Huntington's disease |
| | Vitamin $B_{12}$ deficiency |
| | HIV encephalitis |
| | Neurodegenerative disease |

ease. Regardless of etiology, prodromes may be similar, core symptoms may be indistinguishable, and symptoms may fluctuate over time. A multidimensional pathway or final common pathway is implied.

It is clear that single neurologic diseases can be associated with multiple, overlapping psychiatric features. The incidence of known brain disease in all patients with depression, mania, delusions, hallucinations, obsessions, compulsions, and dissociation is probably low. Other contributing factors such as premorbid psychological and genetic predispositions remain largely unknown to date. Psychiatric symptoms of neurologic disease are usually not seen in isolation and are recognized by the neurologist using history, clinical context, mental status, elementary neurologic examinations, and diagnostic tests.

2.  Persistent behavioral sequelae may be more disabling than elemental or cognitive neurologic deficits, preventing a return to normal baseline activities. More often than not, behavioral features associated with traumatic brain injury, hypoxic encephalopathy, and dementia syndromes are the most salient, disruptive, and exhausting features for caregivers and families. They are the primary determinants of institutionalization.

3.  Atypical presentations of neuropsychiatric syndromes are common. By the time a neurologic evaluation is requested, common presentations have already been detected and treated by other medical disciplines. Hence, psychosis in the context of a multiorgan systemic lupus erythematosus (SLE) flare-up or a brain tumor with seizures and lateralized findings has already become self-evident. SLE-related psychosis outside of the context of multisystem disease or isolated cognitive and behavioral changes due to primary brain tumors are more unusual presentations that require a higher degree of neurologic suspicion.

4. A patient's decompensated behavior may be concordant with his or her past psychiatric profile, but this fact does not necessarily imply that the decompensation is psychogenic. An elderly schizophrenic patient with sudden exacerbation of symptoms may have an underlying stroke or tumor. Psychiatric diseases provide no immunity from coexistent medical or neurologic diseases.

5. A detailed assessment of mental status or elemental neurologic examination may be impossible in the setting of agitation or psychosis. Agitated psychosis or profound depression does not usually allow the patient cooperation required.

6. Normal findings from elemental examination, routine laboratory testing, brain imaging, electroencephalography (EEG), and cerebrospinal fluid (CSF) analysis do not exclude diseases of neurologic origin. Neuropsychiatric changes in Huntington's disease, Parkinson's disease, Lewy body disease, and Alzheimer's disease, as well as lysosomal storage diseases, may precede all other syndromic symptoms or signs by months or years. Clinical judgment remains paramount.

7. Psychopharmacologic medications often obscure the neurologic picture. An ever-expanding array of psychiatric medications is available, both typical and novel, with either idiosyncratic or toxic neurologic side effects. Many of them can induce behavioral, cognitive, and neurologic reactions that may mimic primary brain disease. Behavioral and cognitive changes include apathy, sedation, impaired attention and memory, word searching, and stuttering. Abnormal movements include extrapyramidal syndromes, tardive dystonias and dyskinesias, dysarthria, tremors, glabellar reflex, choreoathetosis, myoclonus, and asterixis. For example, gabapentin and clozapine, new drugs with neurologic and psychiatric indications, may induce choreoathetosis and asterixis, respectively, in therapeutic doses. Other adverse reactions include seizures, ataxia, disturbed temperature regulation, and neuroleptic malignant syndrome. The treating physician must always consider the possibility of these medication-induced changes. Physicians should consult recent psychopharmacologic texts and journals to remain current.

8. Positive responses to neuroleptics, antidepressants, or even electroconvulsive therapy (ECT) do not necessarily point to a specific disease or narrow the differential diagnosis. For instance, depression embedded in the context of Huntington's disease or Parkinson's disease is usually responsive to ECT. Intravenous benzodiazepines often relieve catatonic symptoms regardless of underlying cause.

9. The underlying anatomic site of a lesion, pathology, size of the lesion, and rate of lesion growth remain important syndromic predictors. Although localization is not as exquisite as with single strokes, right-left, front-back, and cortical-subcortical deductions can often be made. Disturbances of frontal, temporal, limbic, and striatal regions are most likely to produce psychiatric manifestations.

10. No simple rules exist. No single feature is common to all forms of brain disease with behavioral disorders. No two patients are identical, even when they have a similar diagnosis. The clinical spectrum is broad, and rigid classifications often do not conform to reality. The importance of a thorough history, detailed examination, and focused investigations cannot be underestimated. The enlightened clinician must be knowledgeable and suspicious. Recognition of the clinical context and natural course of different syndromes is essential.

## PATHOPHYSIOLOGY OF PSYCHOTIC SYMPTOMS

The brain is not only the organ of cognition, perception, and action but also of affect and thought. The proper equilibrium between thought, experience, and affect is indispensable to mental health. It is not surprising that certain brain lesions can disrupt this balance in a way that may lead to severe behavioral disturbances. Inferences drawn from neurologic diseases offer important insights into the biological substrates of human behavior. However, the pathophysiology of psychotic symptoms remains largely unknown.

The cytoarchitecture of brain organization is helpful in understanding complex behaviors. From a behavioral viewpoint, the cerebral hemispheres can be divided into four major components: primary sensory cortex, primary motor cortex, association cortex, and the limbic system. The primary motor and sensory cortices have no known major role in complex mentation. The association cortex can be subdivided into unimodal and heteromodal regions. Each major sensory modality (visual, auditory, olfactory, somesthetic, and gustatory) has an area of primary cortex dedicated to the reception of signals from that sensory system. Within unimodal sensory cortex, sensory stimuli are processed through stages of quantitative and qualitative discriminations, differentiated from simultaneously received stimuli, and compared with previous experiences of a similar nature. This process results in a composite realization of the currently perceived stimulus as related to previously experienced stimuli. Disruption at any step within this matrix, from the source of stimulation to the unimodal association cortex, can lead to a single-modality misperception or hallucinatory experience.

Multimodal sensory integration and elaboration occur in the heteromodal association cortex. When these multiple sensory perceptions are matched against prior memories and merged with the limbic system, which regulates emotion, drive, and affect, complex behaviors such as thought, language, self-awareness, attention, mood, and judgment are formed. The association cortex and limbic regions provide the neural bridge that mediates between the individual's inner drives and the necessities framed by the extrapersonal world. Within this framework, it appears that the right hemisphere is more dominant for emotional mediation, misperceptions, hallucinations, delusions, and the sense of recognition and familiarity.

Neurologic models of hallucinations are instructive. Ictal hallucinations in complex partial seizures are produced by abnormal neuronal discharges involving temporal-limbic regions. They are brief and stereotyped and may manifest as visual, auditory, olfactory, gustatory, or somesthetic hallucinations. Another model for hallucinations is exemplified by peduncular hallucinosis. These release hallucinations are dreamlike states of isolated visual hallucinations in which small people, animals, or objects carry out activities. They are associated with a variety of nonepileptic, primarily ischemic disorders affecting the upper midbrain region.

Metabolic scans of psychotic patients are in agreement with neuroanatomic postulates. Positron emission tomography of schizophrenic patients with active auditory or visual hallucinations suggests activation of subcortical nuclei (thalamic and striatal), limbic structures (especially hippocampus), paralimbic/association cingulate gyrus, and orbitofrontal cortex. Auditory hallucinations also activate auditory-linguistic association cortex, specialized for speech perception, while visual hallucinations are associated with additional activity in visual association cortex, specialized for higher-order visual perception.

Large-scale neural networks may also offer a parsimonious explanation of psychotic symptoms. Cortical-subcortical circuitry involving prefrontal cortex, striatum, thalamus, cerebellum, and brain stem is most likely dysfunctional in schizophrenia and other psychoses. This circuitry represents various meeting points at which internal and affective data are coordinated with current and past sensory representations. Disinhibition of these intermediary circuits may lead to the pathologic release of behaviors and experiences during psychotic episodes. A neurologic model of disordered reality supporting this paradigm is frequently seen after the acute phase of Wernicke's encephalopathy due to thiamine deficiency. Wernicke-Korsakoff syndrome presents with underlying disturbances of anterograde and retrograde memory and is often associated with the denial of memory loss and euphoria. Confabulation is common and consists of fabricated verbal responses concerning the patient's memory of recent experiences. It sometimes occurs spontaneously but is most often induced by the examiner's questions. The patient's narrative is largely implausible or fictional. Superficial analysis of information and impaired temporal and contextual ordering of events is a plausible explanation for confabulation. However, the term *psychosis* is inappropriate, given the lack of hallucinations, delusions, or paranoia. The neuropathologic lesions are always bilateral and symmetric and involve subcortical structures. Mammillary body lesions are uniformly present, whereas thalamic lesions of the dorsomedial and pulvinar nuclei are seen in most but not all patients. Disruption of pathways involving the amygdala, thalamic nuclei, and orbitofrontal cortex is the postulated mechanism.

Prefrontal cortex plays a role in internal governance, self-correction, concern, awareness, motivation, and mental sequencing, as well as conflict resolution and confabulation. Neuronal dysfunction in this area may cause difficulties in information processing and conflict resolution, and delusions, paranoia, disturbed reality testing, or apathy may emerge. Hallucinations may arise due to impaired self-modulation when internally generated material such as thoughts, language, or visions are incorrectly perceived as coming from an external source. A crucial factor in the persistence of delusions and paranoia may be the length of time the perceptual distortion continues with the patient's inability to correct the misperception on the basis of new information. Hence, some psychotic symptoms may be attributable to a failure of reasoning or possible subtle memory dysfunction that lend themselves to distortions.

## SPECIAL CLINICAL CONSIDERATIONS

In the author's experience, three clinical considerations deserve special neurologic attention. These considerations include the high frequency of depression in some neurologic disorders, the neurologic possibilities underlying acute or subacute personality changes, and the neurologic and medical differential diagnosis of catatonia.

### Depression in Neurologic Diseases

Depression is the most common major neuropsychiatric complication of brain disease. It has been linked to a wide variety of brain diseases, listed in Table

*Table 26.3*   Estimated frequency of depression in neurologic disorders

| | |
|---|---|
| Stroke | 30–60% |
| Parkinson's disease | 40–60% |
| Huntington's disease | 30–40% |
| Alzheimer's disease | 30–40% |
| Multiple sclerosis | 20–60% |
| Human immunodeficiency virus infection | 25–50% |
| Head trauma | 25–50% |
| Vascular dementia | 25–60% |
| Epilepsy | 10–50% |

26.3. Diseases affecting the frontal and temporal lobes as well as the basal ganglia are most vulnerable to accompanying depressive syndromes. This specificity for certain brain regions and high comorbid frequency in some neurologic diseases suggests that mood disorders are intrinsically related to the underlying neuropathology. It is less likely that they represent primary adjustment disorders to chronic disease. The neuropsychiatric aspects of these diseases will be addressed separately in this chapter. Given the availability of successful treatments with an 80% response rate, depression should be correctly diagnosed and aggressively treated.

## Personality Alterations

Subacute and acute personality changes deserve special mention. Personality alterations such as apathy are most often seen with bilateral medial frontal, basal ganglia, or thalamic lesions. Vascular lesions, traumatic encephalopathy, human immunodeficiency virus (HIV) encephalitis, and vitamin $B_{12}$ deficiency are common settings. Disinhibition often occurs in the wake of orbitofrontal and caudate lesions as a result of degenerative diseases, strokes, brain tumors, or head trauma. Irritable and explosive behaviors are common with bilateral orbitofrontal lesions, usually due to strokes, head trauma, or Huntington's disease. Indifference, placidity, and impaired judgment and insight are hallmarks of frontal-temporal dementia or Pick's disease. As Alzheimer's disease progresses, this profile can also emerge.

## Catatonia

Although catatonia is uncommon, the author has been confronted with six patients in catatonic states over the past 2 years. The majority of patients suffer from a primary psychosis. Catatonia is more common in affective disease than in schizophrenia. However, an estimated 10–20% of patients with catatonic signs have underlying neurologic and medical contributions. Table 26.4 lists neurologic and medical diseases associated with catatonia, although the association does not necessarily imply a causal relationship.

*Table 26.4*   Neurologic and medical diseases associated with catatonic features

Akinetic mutism with or without aphasia
Lesions of thalamus and globus pallidus
Strokes
Central nervous system tumors
Cerebral anoxia
Subdural hematoma
Closed-head trauma
Encephalitides
    Human immunodeficiency virus encephalopathy
    Viral infection, especially herpes simplex
    Bacterial infection, tertiary neurosyphilis
Multiple sclerosis
Progressive multifocal leukoencephalopathy
Systemic lupus erythematosus with cerebritis
Nonconvulsive seizures/status
Acute intermittent porphyria
Paraneoplastic limbic encephalitis
Wernicke's encephalopathy
Hyperthyroidism
Hyperparathyroidism
Addison's disease
Cushing's disease
Diabetic ketoacidosis
Hepatic/metabolic encephalopathies
Drug-related conditions
Neuroleptic malignant syndrome
Idiopathic conditions

    The majority of cases have multifactorial causes. Catatonia has also been asso-
ciated with the use of neuroleptics, antidepressants, anticonvulsants, disulfiram,
lithium, hallucinogens, and stimulants. Meta-analysis favors neurologic disorders
as the single contributing factor more often than drugs or toxic or metabolic conditions. Although diencephalic or supplementary motor lesions are probable, the
anatomy and pathophysiologic mechanisms underlying catatonia remain uncertain. Although catatonia has multiple causes, treatment with intravenous benzodiazepines and ECT is usually beneficial, at times producing dramatic relief.

## BEHAVIORAL AND COGNITIVE ASPECTS OF NEUROLOGIC DISEASES

Because psychiatric symptoms are common in both primary neurologic and psychiatric disease, the neurologist should understand the disease patterns of those
neurologic syndromes that are particularly prone to psychiatric presentations. The
possibility of stroke, brain tumor, and history of traumatic brain injury should be
considered in all psychiatric patients. Elderly patients deserve special attention
when they present with late-onset psychiatric symptoms.

When the clinician understands the incidence and prevalence of such syndromes and how these differ with race, age, sex, inheritance patterns, and associated medical and neurologic abnormalities, the differential diagnosis is more focused and less overwhelming. The following sections review neurologic diseases that may present with neuropsychiatric features. The list is necessarily incomplete and does not address medical illnesses that can also present in similar ways.

## Stroke

Over 50% of the cortex is composed of association and limbic regions. These regions are supplied by the anterior, middle, and posterior cerebral arteries. Strokes in these areas are not necessarily accompanied by primary motor, sensory, visual, or brain stem symptoms. Alterations of mood, personality, and comportment may arise as the sole or most salient feature of focal brain disease in frontal, temporal, or parietal cortex. Poststroke depression occurs in approximately 50% of patients. The majority demonstrate major depression. The closer the lesion is to the left frontal pole, the more frequent and severe is the depression.

Table 26.5 lists other behavioral disorders associated with nonhemiplegic stroke syndromes. The sudden onset of apathy or abulia can be seen with prefrontal insults in either or both hemispheres, more commonly in the left. Wernicke's aphasia is notable for language fluency, lack of appropriate awareness or concern, and occurrence of neologisms with diminished comprehension. The lack of bizarre thought content, a right superior temporal visual field cut, and left upper-extremity apraxia help differentiate this disorder from schizophrenia in an acute setting. Paranoia may develop several days after the onset. Broca's aphasia is usually more apparent due to nonfluent language, associated right homonymous hemianopsia, and right-sided hemiparesis. Pure word deafness is an isolated loss of the ability to comprehend and therefore repeat spoken language. It usually implies left or bilateral auditory association cortex lesions and is typically embolic in origin. Onset of agitation and paranoia may be immediate.

Visual hallucinations can be caused by retinal or optic nerve ischemia, macular degeneration, or defects in any portion of the visual system from the retina through temporal and parietal cortices. Thalamic or midbrain strokes may also be accompanied by visual hallucinations. Visual hallucinations and delusions occur more frequently in right hemisphere strokes. Mania occurs primarily in right hemisphere strokes involving inferior frontal, caudate, thalamic, or basal temporal regions.

Amnesia can occur when the posterior cerebral artery supply to either left, right, or both hippocampal regions is disrupted. Confusional states with or without agitation can be produced by occlusion of right middle cerebral artery flow to parietal-temporal regions. Posterior cerebral artery ischemia to either left, right, or both mesial temporal-occipital areas may also present in this manner.

Right hemisphere lesions can result in diminished expression or comprehension of prosody—the affective component of spoken language involving melodic intonation. A right posterior inferior frontal stroke may induce poor expression of emotional prosody and gesturing, with intact comprehension. Although the expressions of such patients are monotone, they deny feelings of depression.

*Table 26.5*   Behavioral disorders associated with nonhemiplegic stroke syndromes

| Clinical feature | Vascular territory | Anatomic location | Lateralization | | | |
|---|---|---|---|---|---|---|
| | | | Right | Left | Either | Both |
| Apathy, abulia | Anterior cerebral artery | Frontal/ thalamic | | | | + |
| Paranoia/ Wernicke's aphasia | Middle cerebral artery | Temporal | | + | | + |
| Paranoia/ pure word deafness | Middle cerebral artery | Auditory association cortex | | + | | + |
| Paranoia, agitation | Middle cerebral artery | Temporal | | | + | + |
| Visual hallucinations | Posterior cerebral artery | Thalamic/ peduncular | | | + + | + + |
| Mania | Anterior, middle, or posterior cerebral arteries | Inferior frontal/ caudate/ thalamic/ basal temporal | + + + + | | | |
| Delusions, hallucinations | Middle cerebral artery | Frontal/ temporal/ parietal | + + + | | | |
| Amnesia | Posterior cerebral artery | Mesiotemporal | | | + | + |
| Confusional state | Middle cerebral artery | Parietal- temporal | + | | | |
| | Posterior cerebral artery | Mesiotemporal/ occipital | + | | | |
| Expressive aprosody | Middle cerebral artery | Posterior inferior frontal | + | | | |
| Receptive aprosody | Middle cerebral artery | Posterior inferior parietal | + | | | |

Right posterior inferior parietal or posterior superior temporal strokes may yield impaired prosodic comprehension and gesturing, intact expression, and difficulties empathizing with others.

## Head Trauma

Traumatic brain injury strikes 200–400 persons in 100,000 per year in the United States. Peak incidence occurs between the second and third decades of life; incidence peaks again in the sixth decade. Men are more commonly injured than women.

Psychiatric sequelae and personality changes are common after moderate to severe brain trauma. The primary mechanism of injury is mechanical stretching and shearing of nerve axons. Orbitofrontal and anterior temporal regions are particularly susceptible to contusions, hematomas, and intracerebral hemorrhages. Diffuse white matter injury may disrupt frontal connections with other cortical and subcortical regions, including the limbic system.

Self-regulation deficits involving attention, emotions, reasoning, initiation, and planning are typical. Personality changes such as slowness, apathy, indifference, and loss of initiative most often occur with dorsal lateral frontal convexity damage. Orbitofrontal lesions typically give rise to diminished impulse control, irritability, and hyperkinesis. Anxiety, depression, disinhibition, and anger are also common. Deficits vary from patient to patient and often fluctuate within the same patient. Estimated rates of occurrence of psychotic features range up to 20% and include paranoia, mania, and auditory or visual hallucinations.

The neuropsychiatric consequences of traumatic brain injury are usually the most disabling, preventing a return to baseline functioning. Among patients with mild head injury, forgetfulness is reported in approximately 40%, depression in 40%, anxiety in 40%, anger in 35%, and impulsivity in 25%. These complaints may become chronic. Two years after severe head injury, forgetfulness is reported in approximately 50%, irritability in 40%, depression in 35%, and anxiety in 30%.

Magnetic resonance imaging (MRI) usually documents gliosis in the appropriate regions. Neuropsychological testing is the most sensitive instrument but is not necessarily specific. The complications of complex partial seizures and hydrocephalus should also be considered.

## Brain Tumors and Paraneoplasia

A substantial proportion of brain tumors are associated with psychiatric symptoms and cognitive deficits. These may be the initial and most salient features depending on tumor location, rate of growth, size, and age of patient. Among patients given a primary psychiatric diagnosis, 1–2% actually have an undiagnosed brain tumor. This figure is significantly higher than the prevalence of brain tumors in the general population. However, much of our knowledge in this field is based on retrospective, uncontrolled small series.

The spectrum of behavioral changes may run the gamut from personality changes to affective and thought disorders with psychotic features. Biological mechanisms include disconnection of network pathways, complex partial seizures, raised intracranial pressure, and diaschisis.

Several general guidelines can be used. Supratentorial tumors present with behavioral and cognitive changes more frequently than infratentorial tumors. Tumors involving the frontal and temporal areas produce behavioral changes more commonly than those in parietal and occipital areas. Anatomic localization may not be as helpful as in stroke syndromes, given tumors' different rates of growth, size, and lack of respect for vascular distribution.

Meningiomas arising from the floor of the anterior cranial fossa, pituitary tumors, craniopharyngiomas with suprasellar extension, and hypothalamic gliomas often lead to orbitofrontal dysfunction with behavioral changes. These include depression, apathy, and abulia. Meningiomas arising from the middle sphenoidal wings and gliomas or metastases with temporal lobe compression may give rise to psychosis, anxiety, and atypical mood disorders with euphoria and hypomania. Increased frequency of behavioral symptoms occurs in patients with multiple tumor foci. Rapidly growing tumors tend to present with psychosis, while slow-growing tumors typically manifest as personality changes, depression, or apathy. Older patients are more likely to manifest cognitive difficulties as the presenting symptom. Any patient with the new onset of marked behavioral changes accompanied by seizures, headaches, sensory changes, or focal neurologic signs and symptoms should be investigated for the possibility of a brain tumor.

Paraneoplastic complications occur in approximately 7% of all patients with tumors. They are rarely seen in patients under 40 years of age. Middle-aged men and women appear equally affected. Common tumor associations include small-cell carcinoma of the lung and ovarian, stomach, breast, and colon cancer. Paraneoplastic disorders usually occur before the tumor is diagnosed but may appear any time after the diagnosis as well. The course is subacute and progressive with injury to specific neuron groups. In the case of limbic encephalitis, anxiety and depression are common, early signs. Schizophrenic features may occur as well. As the disease progresses, amnesia, depression, and personality changes ensue. Complex partial seizures and major motor seizures are common. Most patients show brain stem, cerebellar, spinal cord, or peripheral nerve signs as well. A purely psychiatric presentation is uncommon.

No clinical features or routine laboratory tests clearly mark paraneoplastic encephalomyelitis. Computed tomographic (CT) scan or MRI is usually normal but may demonstrate mesial temporal changes. CSF analysis usually reveals mild lymphocytosis and increased protein. Anti-Hu antibodies may be detected and are associated with small-cell carcinoma of the lung. If this antibody is detected and no primary tumor is known, CT scan of the chest and bronchoscopy should be performed. If these are negative, the search for other carcinomas should be pursued. Close neurologic follow-up is important. At times the behavioral and cognitive deficits of paraneoplastic limbic encephalitis may stabilize or burn out. More usual is rapid progression to dementia and death. Dramatic, even complete reversals of paraneoplastic neurologic conditions have been reported with successful treatment of the primary cancer.

## Confusion

Although aging is associated with increased susceptibility to dementia, confusion, and depression, major cognitive or behavioral decline is not the natural course of old age. Normal cognitive and behavioral aging, even into the ninth decade, is compatible with independent living. The elderly are particularly prone to confusion secondary to toxic or metabolic insults. Additional risk factors include pre-existing brain disease, polypharmacy, and abrupt medication withdrawal. The diagnosis of confusional state (or delirium) is made when the patient's primary deficit involves the inability to maintain a coherent stream of thought or action due to impaired attention and vigilance. Secondary deficits in memory, naming, visuospatial skills, and gait are common. A routine EEG typically demonstrates background slowing and disorganization. With proper treatment, recovery may occur gradually over weeks to months. It is particularly gratifying when the simple withdrawal of medications or treatment of an infection returns the patient to his or her normal baseline.

## Sensory Deprivation

The onset of visual or auditory hallucinations and paranoia in the elderly deserves special attention. Ocular conditions such as macular degeneration, cataracts, enucleation, and ischemia or compression of the optic nerve must be included in the differential diagnosis. Auditory hallucinations can occur with acquired deafness. Musical hallucinations are particularly common in elderly individuals with progressive bilateral sensorineural hearing loss. Suspicion with paranoid ideation can occur in the context of severe hearing or vision loss. Treatment of vision and hearing loss can have dramatic effects.

## Depression

Depression misdiagnosed as a degenerative dementia occurs in 8–15% of patients referred for assessment of cognitive decline. Depressed patients may exhibit poor attention and memory, apathy, social withdrawal, and even mutism and incontinence. Particularly in patients 60 years or older, sadness may not be openly expressed. Somatic concerns and excessive fatigue may displace neurovegetative features. The differentiation between depression and dementia can be challenging. The problem is compounded by the coexistence of depression in 25–60% of patients with degenerative or vascular dementias. Helpful clues that suggest either primary or coexistent depression include a history of depression in the patient or family, onset over days to several weeks, marked agitation with pacing and persecutory delusions, precipitation by a serious life event, and persistent complaints of memory difficulties. In a minority of patients, depression may be the initial feature heralding the subsequent development of Alzheimer's disease. In general, the more advanced the dementia, the less frequent the comorbid diagnosis of depression.

## Alzheimer's Disease

Alzheimer's disease typically begins with the insidious onset of progressive amnesia over months to years, accompanied by fluent aphasia, inattention, diminished awareness and concern, visual-spatial difficulties, and a normal elementary neurologic examination. In contrast, a previously fastidious person who over months to years suffers progressive decline in personal hygiene, personality, comportment, and planning with relative sparing of recent memory and language in the context of a normal elementary neurologic examination is more likely to have Pick's disease or nonspecific neuronal loss as seen in frontal-temporal dementia. Given the wide array of behavioral presentations in Pick's disease and frontal-temporal dementia, including apathy, inappropriate behavior, delusions, and misperceptions, the diagnosis may not be apparent on initial examination. Blunted awareness, concern, insight, and judgment are usually striking.

Of patients with probable Alzheimer's disease, 30–60% have neuropsychiatric manifestations. These include delusions, hallucinations, anxiety, restlessness, agitation, and aggression. Verbal outbursts are associated with delusions; physically aggressive behaviors may be driven by hallucinations and restlessness. There is no clear relationship between these features and the severity of dementia, coexistent depression, education, sex, or age. Negative symptoms include disturbances of initiation, motivation, and concern as well as social and emotional withdrawal. These also appear to be independent of depression, medications, co-morbid systemic illness, and severity of dementia. In the author's experience, patients with an underlying dementia are most often admitted to inpatient geriatric services because of behavioral dyscontrol. Sudden deterioration after gradual decline suggests a "beclouded dementia," a dementia worsened by superimposed toxic-metabolic or systemic insults.

## Multi-Infarct Dementia

Ischemic lesions of the frontal, temporal, or parietal lobes may produce restricted cognitive deficits that mimic dementia. Aphasia, dyscalculia, amnesia, and inattention may occur. Usually only one major area of cognition is disordered; other intellectual activities are spared. Sudden or stepwise course, accompanying neurologic deficits, and focal EEG and neuroimaging abnormalities help in the differential diagnosis of multi-infarct dementia. Pseudobulbar affect, gait abnormalities, visual field cuts, hemiparesis, and hemineglect are most consistent with cortical or subcortical infarcts. Sudden agitation, delusions, and hallucinations can occur. Pure multi-infarct dementia may be overdiagnosed, particularly in those patients with nonfocal elemental examinations. In these patients, post-mortem examination usually reveals a mixed picture of multiple infarcts and Alzheimer's pathology.

## Parkinson's Disease

Cognitive deficits seen in subcortical diseases such as Parkinson's disease include slowed and inefficient cognitive processing and alterations in personality, mood, or behavior. Approximately 50% of patients develop a concomitant depression; half of these suffer from severe unipolar disease. The occurrence of depression has a bimodal distribution, with one peak occurring early after onset unassociated with impaired motor or cognitive skills, and the other occurring late in the disease associated with motor and cognitive decline. Depression may be the earliest symptomatic marker of ensuing Parkinson's disease. Clinical evaluation of the patient's affect may be perplexing due to the paucity of facial emotion, motor retardation, and cognitive slowing. Withdrawal and apathy may be secondary to motoric worsening, medication, depression, and cognitive decline. Suicide is relatively rare. Over the disease's course, approximately 50% of patients with Parkinson's disease develop concomitant Alzheimer's disease. A variant of

Parkinson's disease, diffuse Lewy body disease, is characterized by relative lack of tremors; early behavioral manifestations such as agitation, hallucinations, and other psychotic features; relative unresponsiveness to dopamine agonists; and early diffuse EEG slowing.

## Huntington's Disease

Huntington's disease is a progressive neurodegenerative disorder with an autosomal dominant mode of inheritance that is characterized by involuntary movements of the limbs or facial muscles, dementia, and neuropsychiatric disturbances. Age of onset is typically in the third to fifth decade, although onset in childhood and after 65 years of age may occur. Of interest is the fact that onset of Huntington's disease in patients over age 60 is not necessarily accompanied by choreiform movements. The Huntington's disease gene was isolated in 1993; genetic linkage analysis can now confirm the clinical diagnosis of Huntington's disease and, after appropriate counseling, evaluate at-risk presymptomatic individuals with a confirmed or suspected family history of Huntington's disease. It should be remembered that up to 3% of Huntington's disease cases are the result of new mutations. Thus, the absence of a family history does not entirely rule out the possibility that an individual carries the Huntington's disease gene. There are emerging reports of elderly patients with the Huntington's disease gene whose only manifestations are abnormal movements.

Psychiatric symptoms may precede the movement disorder of Huntington's disease by up to 10 years. Symptoms include affective disorders in 30–40% of cases and a high incidence of attempted and completed suicide, in addition to apathy, irritability, disinhibition, aggression, and social and functional deterioration. Up to 30% of patients with the disease develop a schizophrenia-like psychosis marked by delusions and hallucinations. A small subset of patients with Huntington's disease develop a self-limited bipolar-like disorder. It is not uncommon to diagnose previously unrecognized Huntington's disease in a young psychiatric population. The behavioral manifestations of such patients often lead to intermittent psychiatric hospitalizations for improved control. Incidence of attempted and completed suicide is significant.

## Wilson's Disease

Although Wilson's disease is rare, the possibility of the disease is frequently raised in psychiatric patients. The disease is an autosomal recessive disorder of copper metabolism with a prevalence of 1 in 30,000. It has been identified in every ethnic and geographic population that has been studied. Median age of onset is 16.2 years; range of onset is from age 5 through the sixth decade. Approximately one-third of patients present with liver involvement such as hepatitis or cirrhosis. Among offspring of parents with Wilson's disease, 1 in every 200 is at risk of developing the disease. Although 1 in every 200 people carries this abnormal gene as heterozygotes, these carriers remain asymptomatic.

Neurologic signs and symptoms are highly variable. Extrapyramidal symptoms usually predominate, with tremors of any type, dystonias, rigidity, dysarthria, or postural instability. Cerebellar symptoms may be most salient. Two-thirds of patients with Wilson's disease develop neuropsychiatric features. One-third of patients with the eventual diagnosis initially receive a diagnosis of primary psychiatric disorder. Personality changes are common and include lability, irritability, impulsive action, sexual preoccupations, and diminished sexual inhibitions. Some 10–20% of patients with Wilson's disease initially present with psychotic syndromes indistinguishable from schizophrenia or bipolar disease. Many of their bizarre behaviors defy classification. Intellectual deterioration may occur as well. Lesions in the caudate and putamen most likely account for the behavioral disturbances.

The neurologic examination usually reveals a fixed smile and Kayser-Fleischer rings of copper deposition that begin in the superior quadrants, migrate over time to the inferior quadrants, and then form a complete arc in the limbus of the cornea. If a patient does not have Kayser-Fleischer rings when examined by a trained observer with a slit lamp, the diagnosis can be nearly excluded. The delay between disease onset and time of correct diagnosis is usually 1–5 years. This lag is particularly disturbing because favorable outcome depends on early diagnosis and treatment. Chelation therapy is usually helpful and may result in dramatic improvement over the course of 1–2 years. However, it usually fails to entirely eliminate all neuropsychiatric features. Liver transplant may be curative.

The usual context is a patient under 40 years with personality or psychotic changes who has an unexplained disorder of the central nervous system (CNS), signs and symptoms suggestive of hepatitis or extrapyramidal disease, and an immediate relative who has a similar disease.

## Epilepsy

Approximately 0.5–2.0% of the U.S. population suffers from an active seizure disorder. The prevalence is greatest in areas of the world that have a high incidence of brain disease due to high rates of infection, poor perinatal care, or frequent head trauma. It can occur at any age throughout the life span. Complex partial seizures are the most common form of seizure acquired in adulthood. Transient ictal events commonly include psychiatric features such as olfactory, auditory, and visual hallucinations, dissociative states, mania, and delusions.

Although controversy exists regarding the relationship between seizures and psychosis, their co-occurrence is probably not just the mere coincidence of two relatively common diseases. Among epileptics, a schizophrenia-like syndrome occurs more commonly than chance would predict. This condition is not clearly distinguishable from idiopathic schizophrenia on phenomenologic grounds. Preservation of affect and a paucity of some negative schizophrenic features may occur. Complex partial epilepsy is overrepresented in this subgroup.

A family history of schizophrenia does not occur more often in patients with complex partial epilepsy who develop a schizophrenia-like picture than in the normal population. In contrast, idiopathic schizophrenia tends to demonstrate a pattern of familial transmission. The onset of seizures almost invariably precedes the development of psychotic symptoms, usually by several years. The schizophrenia-like syndrome is usually associated with a dominant hemisphere seizure focus. The highest risk profile is that of a left-handed woman with abnormal tissue in the left hemisphere and onset of complex partial seizures during pubescence. Mesial temporal lesions are identified in greater than 50% of these patients on MRI. Because psychotic features do not usually respond to traditional anticonvulsants, neuroleptics are typically necessary.

Although patients with seizures have an increased incidence of mood disorder, a similar predisposition does not seem to exist for the development of affective psychosis. Postictal psychosis can occur within 1 week after the ictal event. This picture usually emerges in those patients with a long-standing seizure disorder and may be heralded by the increased frequency of secondarily generalized events. It may endure from days to a month or more, during which time hallucinations, delusions, and affective symptoms develop with or without a confusional state.

## Dementia and Encephalitis Resulting from Infection with Human Immunodeficiency Virus

Acquired immunodeficiency syndrome (AIDS) dementia is the AIDS-defining illness in approximately 10% of patients with HIV infection. Clinically significant AIDS dementia complex eventually develops in approximately 60% of patients. Ninety percent of patients show histologic evidence of subacute encephalitis at autopsy. Most commonly it develops and progresses in parallel with the later stages of AIDS. Early involvement of subcortical regions such as the thalamus and basal ganglia most likely explains the early behavioral changes. The development of AIDS dementia is usually an ominous prognostic event.

Acute psychosis can be the initial and sole presenting symptom of HIV encephalitis. Mania, delusions, paranoia, hallucinations, depression, and catatonia may occur. Affective symptoms often precede other cognitive and behavioral changes. Neuropsychological tests usually reveal a subcortical dementia profile with apathy, inattention, slowed mentation, and secondary recent memory difficulties.

HIV encephalitis most often occurs in an HIV patient when the CD4 lymphocyte count is below 200/ml and a concurrent constitutional illness is present. CSF analysis and MRI with gadolinium help exclude opportunistic infections and neoplasms, which occur in 33% of AIDS patients. In HIV encephalitis, CSF analysis reveals mononuclear pleocytosis in 20% of patients. Increased CSF protein occurs with or without symptoms of HIV encephalitis in 60% of patients. Polymerase chain reaction (PCR) testing is the most sensitive diagnostic tool. However, no correlation exists between the presence of HIV in the CSF and the clinical presence of AIDS dementia. MRI may reveal atrophy, enlarged ventricles, and white matter changes, but these can also be seen in asymptomatic patients. EEG abnormalities are documented in 30% of patients and consist of slowed background rhythms in the delta and theta ranges. Seizures occur in approximately 30% of patients.

The usual clinical context is that of a homosexual man between 20 and 40 years of age with known HIV infection, a CD4 lymphocyte count of less than 200/ml with a concurrent HIV-related illness, and a manic or hypomanic presentation. No major therapeutic interventions are available other than palliative treatment and administration of medications to control the behavioral manifestations.

Other encephalitides may present with an agitated psychotic state. Herpes encephalitis has no seasonal predilection and typically presents with fever, aphasia, amnesia, and agitation. A field cut is usually present. Clinical context demands CSF analysis, brain imaging, and PCR identification. Early intervention with antiviral drugs is essential, because their introduction usually leads to recovery. Occasional cases of encephalitis lethargica with neuropsychiatric presentations have been reported. It is important to note that, whereas neuropsychiatric complications of Lyme disease may be common, psychotic presentations are exceedingly rare.

## Neurosyphilis

The populations at highest risk for the contraction of primary syphilis have changed. The current epidemic is now occurring predominantly among African-American and Hispanic heterosexual men and women in large urban population centers. It is more prevalent among men than among women and more prevalent among homosexual and bisexual men than among heterosexual men. The prevalence of syphilis is a barometer of a nation's public health measures and is directly related to poverty, illiteracy, lack of public screening, and access to medical care. Current cases of neurosyphilis are now more likely to be variants of classic syndromes. The reasons are most probably the use of antimicrobials for other diseases, the emergence of penicillin-resistant strains, and incidental partial treatment with penicillin. Centuries before the description of MS, Lyme disease, and HIV, neurosyphilis was known as the great neurologic mimic because of its protean presentations.

Ten days to 10 weeks after exposure to primary syphilis, a chancre develops. With or without treatment, it heals within 1 month, and only 50% of individuals remain actively infected. Secondary syphilis presents with a rash over the palms and soles in addition to joint symptoms. Approximately 25% of individuals develop mild meningitis with meningismus. Most cases of syphilitic meningitis subside without treatment. Over time, 50% of these cases spontaneously remit without further recurrence. After an incubation period of 5–20 years, the remaining 50% develop tertiary neurosyphilis by CNS infiltration via Virchow-Robin spaces. Therefore, only 6.5% of all patients infected with syphilis will eventually develop tertiary neurosyphilis. Currently, it occurs in a ratio of four to seven men for every woman. Meningovascular neurosyphilis may involve cranial nerves, particularly CN VII and CN VIII, vascular occlusions with arteritis and subsequent symptoms, and hydrocephalus. Tabetic neurosyphilis presents with lightning-like pains, primarily in the lower extremities. Patients may have Argyll Robertson pupils (bilateral small, irregular pupils that respond to accommodation effort but do not react to light), ataxia, diminished proprioception, bladder hypotonia with overflow incontinence, absent deep tendon reflexes, and positive Romberg's sign.

The third form, general paresis of the insane, may present as virtually any psychiatric disorder. Delusions, grandiosity, irritability, emotional lability, depression, and diminished comportment are typical features. Argyll Robertson pupils are uncommonly seen. Expressionless facies and increased deep tendon reflexes are common. Intention tremors of the face, tongue, and extremities may occur. Cranial nerve palsies and optic atrophy are uncommon. If treated properly, the disease can be arrested. Mental symptoms may improve over time.

Because VDRL tests may be negative in patients with late neurosyphilis, fluorescent treponemal antibody absorption (FTA/ABS) tests must be performed before neurosyphilis can be reasonably excluded. Fewer than 10% of patients with treated or current neurosyphilis have negative FTA/ABS results. Definitive diagnosis is made by CSF analysis. It is nearly always abnormal with positive VDRL test results, increased protein, and increased white blood cells, primarily lymphocytes. CT scan or MRI may show selective frontal atrophy and thickened arachnoid spaces.

In the United States, first admissions to mental hospitals due to syphilitic psychosis peaked in 1940 at 7,694 patients. In large part because of effective treatment with penicillin, syphilitic psychosis admissions had declined to 154 by 1968. This is the last year figures were made available. Unfortunately, in large part due to deficient public health measures and the emergence of penicillin-resistant strains, neurosyphilis is making a comeback in both HIV and non-HIV population groups. Its re-emergence must be recognized.

## Systemic Lupus Erythematosus

There are 15–50 reported cases of SLE per 100,000 persons in the United States every year. Ninety percent of cases are in women, usually women of childbearing age. The disease is three times more common among African-Americans and Asian Americans than among American whites. Some Native American tribes may have a higher incidence than African-Americans. Arthralgias are the single most common manifestation. The majority of patients have fatigue, fever, and weight loss at the time of diagnosis.

One of the more frequent reasons for neurologic referrals in the psychiatric population is the possibility of SLE. The disease involves the CNS more than the peripheral nervous system. Psychosis as the initial feature of SLE is uncommon. However, neuropsychiatric signs and symptoms occur in up to two-thirds of all patients over their disease course. Personality disturbances are reported in 50% of patients. Psychotic features, including depression, paranoia, mania, and schizophrenia, are noted in 20%. Seizures occur in approximately 20%. Strokes, peripheral neuropathy, migraine headache, or movement disorders are seen in 10% or fewer of patients with SLE.

No consistent relationship exists between neuropsychiatric symptoms and other symptoms of SLE. Initial presentation may not allow a definitive diagnosis. No specific marker for CNS SLE is currently available. An antinuclear antibody test is the screening method of choice. More than 95% of patients with SLE have positive results on this test. However, many patients with both unrelated and related diseases may also have positive results. An occasional patient with SLE has negative antinuclear antibody test results. Erythrocyte sedimentation rate is usually but not invariably elevated during active disease. Nonspecific EEG abnormalities with diffuse or focal slowing are reported in approximately 70% of cases. Protein elevation and mononuclear cells in the CSF are frequent findings. MRI may demonstrate atrophy, periventricular white matter changes, or focal lesions that may enhance, primarily in the frontal region. However, these lesions do not distinguish between those with and without active SLE cerebritis. The diagnosis and treatment of the neuropsychiatric aspects of SLE remain a clinical challenge. Close alliance with an expert rheumatologist is essential.

The typical patient is a black woman of childbearing age with more than one neurologic symptom whose psychosis occurs in the setting of an SLE flare-up with the presence of CSF abnormalities. Treatment with steroids, immunosuppressants, and neuroleptics offers its own set of neuropsychiatric challenges.

## Multiple Sclerosis

The prevalence of MS in the northern United States, Canada, and northern Europe is approximately 60 cases per 100,000 persons. It occurs in women more than in men. Although onset is unusual before adolescence, onset has been reported from age 2 to age 74. The incidence steadily increases from adolescence to age 35 and declines gradually thereafter.

Earlier literature on personality disturbances in MS emphasized euphoria as common. Although euphoria can be seen in conjunction with cognitive dysfunction, more recent studies have emphasized the higher rate of depression, both unipolar and bipolar, in patients with MS. Reported frequencies range from 20–60%. There is little relation to the extent of neurologic dysfunction. Emotional incontinence, marked by pathologic crying or laughing, can be mistaken for depression.

Psychosis, including mania, paranoia, and visual hallucinations, occurs in approximately 10% of patients over the disease course. However, psychosis is almost always preceded by or accompanied by other neurologic features.

Although bedside mental status examinations suggest that fewer than 5% of MS patients are cognitively impaired, formal neuropsychological studies estimate the overall prevalence of mild to moderate cognitive dysfunction at approximately 40%. A subcortical dementia profile is characteristic, with salient deficits seen on measures of sustained attention, information-processing speed, mental flexibility, conceptual and abstract reasoning, and recent memory retrieval. Immediate attention span, language, and general intellectual functions remain relatively well preserved. Over a 3-year period, approximately 20% of patients endure further cognitive decline. The deterioration does not correlate with severity of physical disability but may correspond to the volume of pathologic lesions seen on MRI. It is unclear whether interventions such as administration of steroids, immunosuppressants, or interferon are associated with significant cognitive or behavioral improvement. These interventions raise their own neuropsychiatric challenges.

## Acute Intermittent Porphyria

Acute intermittent porphyria (AIP) is the most common type of hepatic porphyria in the United States. It is caused by a defect in the gene for porphobilinogen (PBG) deaminase. Although it is a rare autosomal dominant disorder with variable expression, the possibility of AIP is often raised in younger psychiatric patients. The disease occurs with an estimated prevalence of two cases per 100,000 persons in all ethnic groups studied. The prevalence is especially high in northern Sweden (100 per 100,000). Most heterozygotes remain clinically asymptomatic unless exposed to factors that increase the production of porphyrias. Symptom onset rarely occurs before puberty and most commonly begins in the third decade. More women than men become symptomatic. It is a relapsing, remitting disorder that occurs in attacks lasting from 48 hours to weeks or months. An attack is usually heralded by restlessness and irritability and develops rapidly. Attacks may be precipitated by a number of porphyrinogenic drugs, such as anticonvulsants, including phenobarbital, phenytoin, valproate sodium, and carbamazepine; tricyclic antidepressants; birth-control pills; steroids; methyldopa; alcohol; and sulfonamides. Anesthesia with halothane may be lethal. Additional precipitants include infection, first trimester pregnancy, childbirth, fasting, and smoking. Attacks are associated with increased urinary excretion of the porphyrin precursors delta-aminolevulinic acid ($\delta$-ALA) and PBG. These sediments may turn the urine wine-colored or brown during attacks.

The usual clinical triad includes abdominal pain, peripheral neuropathy, and neuropsychiatric symptoms. Abdominal pain is the most common feature. Gastrointestinal symptoms include ileus with distention, constipation, or diarrhea. Acute abdomen occurs secondary to autonomic dysfunction and is often accompanied by nausea or vomiting, constipation, tachycardia, and hypertension. No evidence exists for inflammation, fever, or leukocytosis. Diagnosis is often delayed because symptoms are nonspecific and physical findings may be minimal. Abdominal surgical scars from past negative explorations suggest the diagnosis. Primary motor peripheral neuropathy does not develop in all patients with acute AIP attacks even when abdominal symptoms are severe. Weakness usually begins proximally, more commonly in the upper than in the lower extremities, and can be asymmetric. Deep tendon reflexes may be unchanged or slightly increased during early stages. They usually decrease or are absent with advanced neuropathy.

Approximately 40% of patients have mental status changes during the attacks. Anxiety, depression, hallucinations, delusions, confusion, and paranoia may be especially severe during acute attacks. Underlying depression may be chronic. In the minority of cases, neuropsychiatric symptoms precede abdominal symptoms and may not be accompanied by motor neuropathy. In rare instances, neuropsychiatric symptoms present without abdominal or neuropathic symptoms. The prevalence of AIP in patients with chronic psychiatric disorders in the United States has been estimated at 210 in 100,000, forty times greater than in the normal population.

Additional neurologic signs may include bilateral ptosis, unilateral pupillary dilation, and nystagmus. Approximately 20% of patients have seizures. Treatment of seizures in patients with AIP is problematic because most anticonvulsants, except for bromides, can exacerbate AIP. Clonazepam may be less likely to exacerbate AIP than phenytoin, phenobarbital, valproate sodium, or carbamazepine. Because gabapentin and lamotrigine do not induce hepatic oxidation, they may be useful in this context.

Although no strict correlation exists between the levels of urinary $\delta$-ALA and PBG and severity of attack, elevated plasma levels of $\delta$-ALA and PBG occur only in the acute attack. Confirmation of the diagnosis, between and during attacks, is based on the detection of 50% reduction of PBG deaminase in erythrocytes, fibroblasts, or mitogen-stimulated lymphocytes. The EEG is frequently abnormal but nonspecific. Brain images are unremarkable, as is CSF. Treatment with intravenous hematin, which reduces $\delta$-ALA and PBG levels, usually leads to rapid recovery within 48–72 hours. Recovery from severe motor neuropathy may continue for months to years.

The usual clinical presentation of AIP is that of an irritable young woman with severe abdominal complaints and evidence of surgical scars. History typically reveals a porphyrinogenic precipitant. Her history includes paresthesias, paroxysmal episodic psychosis, and dark urine during the attacks.

## Lysosomal Storage Diseases (Adult Onset)

Although lysosomal storage diseases are rare, the author has diagnosed and observed these diseases in the adult psychiatric population. Given the possibility that genetically engineered enzyme replacement therapies will be available in the near future, early diagnosis is becoming important.

Adult-onset metachromatic leukodystrophy has both dominant and recessive forms. Although metachromatic leukodystrophy is rare, with an estimated incidence of 1 in 40,000, in approximately 50% of patients the disease first presents sometime from the second through the fifth decade of life. Psychosis with auditory hallucinations and delusions is the most common presentation in the adult-onset form. The diagnosis is often overlooked. A history of psychiatric hospitalizations is common. Peripheral neuropathy, decreased deep tendon reflexes, and a history of cholecystitis are also characteristic. The deficiency in arylsulfatase A leads to demyelination, predominantly in the frontal and parietal subcortical regions. MRI usually confirms demyelination and atrophy, which may involve the cerebellum as well. Interventions are currently being studied. Bone marrow transplantation may play a therapeutic role in the future.

Tay-Sachs disease is a $GM_2$ gangliosidosis resulting from a deficiency of beta-hexosaminidase A. This condition has several late-onset variants. People of Eastern European Jewish or French Canadian heritage may have a risk more than 100 times higher than the risk for other populations. Any patient from one of these groups who is 20 years or older and presents with an atypical, intractable psychosis or bipolar disease with accompanying cerebellar signs should be screened for this disease. Cerebellar features include dysmetria and impaired tandem gait. Vertical gaze paresis may be present. Two heterozygotic parents will have a 1 in 4 chance of producing offspring with this disease. The incidence of Tay-Sachs disease has been considerably reduced by screening of couples at risk and by prenatal diagnosis.

Kufs' adult type of neuronal ceroid lipofuscinosis is a disease involving abnormal storage of a complex lipopigment yet to be enzymatically characterized. It is a rare disorder that starts as late as the third or fourth decade. Both autosomal dominant and recessive modes of inheritance have been reported. Neuropsychiatric complications are common. Patients usually develop myoclonus, seizures, and dementia. Amblyopia and retinal changes do not occur. The diagnosis is made by demonstrating accumulated storage product in buffy coat or skin biopsies, which show curvilinear bodies or a fingerprint pattern on electron microscopy.

Hepatosplenomegaly is prominent in all types of Niemann-Pick disease due to sphingomyelin accumulation. A history of hepatitis is also suggestive. Type C, which has an unknown primary defect but a secondary defect in cholesterol esterification, can present with neuropsychiatric symptoms. Clinical symptoms may not appear until adolescence or adulthood. Myoclonic or akinetic seizures, vertical supranuclear gaze paralysis, ataxia, and the presence of macular cherry-red spots are common.

## INDICATIONS FOR NEUROLOGIC CONSULTATION

Given the wide array of neurologic possibilities in the differential diagnosis of psychiatric symptoms, the question for neurologists and psychiatrists is when to

*Table 26.6*   When to suspect neurologic disease in patients with psychiatric symptoms

1. Patient has no psychiatric history, symptoms have subacute or abrupt onset, major psychosocial stressors are absent.
2. Patient has atypical psychiatric features:
   Cognitive decline
   Diminished comportment
   Intractability or failure to respond
   Progression
3. Patient has past or present history that includes
   Significant head trauma
   Seizures
   Movement disorders
   Hepatitis or cirrhosis
   Cholecystitis
   Abdominal crises (without known cause), surgical scars
   Peripheral neuropathy
   Increased size of liver, spleen
4. Patient has new onset of
   Headache
   Neuroendocrine changes
   Inattention
   Somnolence
   Incontinence
   Anorexia
5. Patient has significant cerebrovascular risk factors:
   Age of 55 years or more
   Past strokes or ischemic events
   Hypertension
   Coronary artery disease
   Atrial fibrillation
   Diabetes mellitus
6. Patient has abnormal or unexplained elemental neurologic findings.
7. Patient has unexplained laboratory results:
   Abnormal screening results
   Abnormal electroencephalogram
   Abnormal magnetic resonance image
   Abnormal cerebrospinal protein level
8. Patient has two or more first-degree relatives with similar diseases.
9. Young catatonic patient has no preceding major idiopathic psychiatric disorder.

suspect underlying neurologic disease. Table 26.6 details the circumstances in which neurologic disease should be suspected. The table should serve as a review of previously described neurologic syndromes.

In contrast, psychiatric patients at lowest risk for neurologic disease include those age 55 or younger with normal vital signs, intact cognition, no active polysubstance abuse, and no new onset of psychiatric symptoms. The following are indications for psychiatric consultation by the neurologist: (1) Psychiatric symptoms have no apparent neurologic explanation; (2) the history suggests significant premorbid psychiatric problems; (3) masked depression or coexistent anxiety is

*Table 26.7*   Clinical signs suggesting psychiatric manifestations
of underlying neurologic diseases

| Sign | Disease |
| --- | --- |
| Fever | Human immunodeficiency virus (HIV) or herpes infection |
| Abdominal scars (condition unexplained) | Acute intermittent porphyria |
| Skin lesions | Systemic lupus erythematosus (SLE), syphilis |
| Seizures/myoclonus | SLE, masses, paraneoplasia, HIV, stroke, Kufs' disease |
| Hepatitis/cirrhosis | Wilson's disease, Niemann-Pick disease |
| Cholecystitis | Metachromatic leukodystrophy |
| Increased size of liver or spleen | Niemann-Pick disease |

suspected; (4) chronic pain or fatigue is present; (5) behavioral and psychopharmacologic management of psychiatric symptoms is required; and (6) individual or family adjustment difficulties exist.

## SUSPICIOUS CLINICAL SIGNS

Table 26.7 lists clinical signs suggesting underlying neurologic diseases that may give rise to psychiatric symptoms.

## THE NEUROLOGIC EXAMINATION AND DISEASE ASSOCIATIONS

Table 26.8 reviews neurologic examination abnormalities and associated diseases that may cause psychosis. It recapitulates diseases previously described in the context of the elemental neurologic examination. When examining a psychiatric patient, the neurologist should pay particular attention to these details of the elemental neurologic examination.

## DIAGNOSTIC TESTS IN THE EVALUATION OF PSYCHIATRIC SYMPTOMS

### Computed Tomography and Magnetic Resonance Imaging of the Brain

The following criteria may be used as indications for brain imaging in the evaluation of patients with salient psychiatric symptoms:

1. First episode of psychosis regardless of age that is not associated with a known precipitant such as intoxication.

*Table 26.8*   Neurologic examination abnormalities and associated diseases
that may cause psychiatric symptoms

| Examination type | Disease associations |
|---|---|
| **Cranial Nerve** | |
| Visual field cuts (may be accompanied by aphasia, hemiparesis, hemisensory deficits) | Strokes<br>Masses<br>Systemic lupus erythematosus<br>Herpes infection<br>Paraneoplasia<br>Tertiary neurosyphilis |
| Pupils | |
| Argyll Robertson | Tertiary neurosyphilis |
| Unilateral dilation | Acute intermittent porphyria |
| Limbus/cornea | |
| Kayser-Fleischer rings | Wilson's disease |
| Fundi | |
| Papilledema | Masses<br>Systemic lupus erythematosus |
| Macular cherry-red spots | Tay-Sachs disease<br>Niemann-Pick disease |
| Optic pallor | Multiple sclerosis<br>Other demyelinating diseases<br>Tay-Sachs disease<br>Acute intermittent porphyria |
| Bilateral ptosis | |
| Cranial nerve dysfunction | Systemic lupus erythematosus<br>Paraneoplasia<br>Tertiary neurosyphilis |
| Vertical gaze paresis | Tay-Sachs disease<br>Niemann-Pick disease |
| **Extrapyramidal** | |
| Tremors/rigidity/chorea/athetosis | Parkinson's disease<br>Huntington's disease<br>Wilson's disease<br>Systemic lupus erythematosus<br>Acute intermittent porphyria<br>Tertiary neurosyphilis |
| Fixed smile | Wilson's disease |
| Expressionless face | Parkinson's disease<br>Tertiary neurosyphilis |
| **Peripheral nerve** | |
| Primary motor neuropathy (usually symmetric) | Acute intermittent porphyria<br>Paraneoplasia<br>Metachromatic leukodystrophy |
| Mononeuritis multiplex | Systemic lupus erythematosus |
| **Cerebellar** | |
| Dysarthria/ataxia | Wilson's disease<br>Systemic lupus erythematosus<br>Tay-Sachs disease<br>Acute intermittent porphyria<br>Multiple sclerosis |

**Deep tendon reflex**

| | |
|---|---|
| Absent | Acute intermittent porphyria |
| Increased or decreased | Metachromatic leukodystrophy |
| | Tertiary neurosyphilis |

2. First episode of a major affective disorder in a patient over 40 years of age.
3. Any psychiatric syndrome accompanied by unexplained neurologic deficits, including movement disorders, cognitive deterioration, or focal signs and symptoms.
4. Anorexia nervosa, particularly in men.
5. A psychotic or major affective disorder that has atypical features or that is refractory to standard pharmacotherapy.

Normal imaging does not exclude the possibility of underlying neurologic disease, however. EEGs, lumbar CSF analysis, neuropsychological tests, or even brain biopsies may be necessary as guided by clinical judgment. MRI has the advantage of higher resolution and better distinction of grey and white matter than CT scanning. MRI is superior for imaging almost all forms of brain pathology. However, it may fail to differentiate hemorrhages, tumors, and abscesses from edema. CT scanning may be preferable because it takes less time than MRI and induces less claustrophobia. CT scanning is also superior for studying skull, spine, and calcified lesions. MRI is contraindicated for patients who have ferrous-containing cardiac pacemakers, neurostimulators, and aneurysm clips; metallic implants, prostheses, pumps, or cardiac valves; or metal fragments in the body or eyes. Claustrophobic reactions or any condition that prevents the patient from holding still for 30 minutes may lead to technical difficulties.

Atrophy affecting primarily the frontal-temporal regions suggests Pick's disease, whereas more generalized atrophy (and in particular selective hippocampal atrophy) favors Alzheimer's disease. Multiple vascular lesions documented on T1 and T2 pulse sequences, when located in the appropriate anatomic sites, point toward a multi-infarct dementia. Multiple small infarcts suggest the possibility of SLE. Selective caudate atrophy points toward the possibility of Huntington's disease. Mild generalized atrophy, if not a normal variant, suggests HIV infection, SLE, idiopathic schizophrenia, or Alzheimer's disease. Periventricular white matter T2 densities that are excessive for the patient's age favor a diagnosis of MS or another demyelinating disorder. Mesial temporal sclerosis, seen best in coronal views, may point to the focal origin of complex partial seizures. Brain imaging is usually less helpful in the differential diagnosis of movement disorders. Imaging techniques cannot currently differentiate Parkinson's disease from related syndromes such as progressive supranuclear palsy or diffuse Lewy body disease.

## Electroencephalography

Epileptiform activity may occur in epilepsy, but it also occurs in some patients with nonepileptic cerebral disorders. Serial studies indicate that only 33% of patients with epilepsy consistently exhibit discharges in the interictal, waking state. Approximately 17% never do so. In the remaining 50% of patients, the EEG profile varies, and a 1 in 3 probability exists of capturing epileptiform activity in any given 30-minute record during waking. The most important recent development in epileptology has been long-term EEG and video monitoring. The EEG can be sampled over days, and this record is useful when a patient has an episodic clinical event. If this event is accompanied by simultaneous epileptic EEG discharges, then the causal mechanism has been identified.

A normal EEG is compatible with any dementia, especially early in the course. In Alzheimer's disease, an early decrease in alpha frequency and amplitude can occur. Later, generalized irregular slow activity appears, with a frontal emphasis. Focal EEG changes, with or without generalized slowing, suggest either multi-infarct dementia or normal-pressure hydrocephalus. Clinically significant changes in the EEG are uncommon in Huntington's disease, Pick's disease, and alcoholic dementia. In the course of Creutzfeldt-Jakob disease, diffuse or focal slowing develops with characteristic stereotyped, bilaterally synchronous sharp waves. In the advanced stages, regular slow triphasic bursts occur on a slow background.

Although they are nonspecific, EEG abnormalities have an increased incidence in bipolar affective disorder and schizophrenia. However, EEG abnormalities of positive diagnostic value are confined to those psychiatric syndromes with an overtly organic basis. In neurologically based confusional states, the EEG typically shows background disorganization and slowing. A routine EEG is especially helpful in the confused patient for distinguishing between organic causes, such as toxic or metabolic encephalopathies or nonconvulsive status epilepticus, and primary psychiatric diseases.

**Neuropsychological Assessment**

Neuropsychological assessment involves the administration and interpretation of cognitive tests that are quantitative, standardized, reliable, and valid. It can indirectly measure a patient's premorbid cognitive skills. It can evaluate a patient's present cognitive state, including general intellectual level, alertness and attention, executive skills, language, memory, and academic, visual, and spatial perceptual abilities. Neuropsychological assessment can suggest possible neuroanatomic and neuropathologic correlates. It can help distinguish between early dementia, anxiety, mood disorders, and normal aging. Repeat assessments over time can provide information regarding rate of cognitive decline, which can help patients and their families plan for their care. It can also be used to assess the benefits of various interventions.

**CONCLUSION**

Neurologic diseases that cause mental disturbances are increasingly relevant and common in the differential diagnosis of psychiatric symptoms. The associated clinical syndromes offer important insights into the biological substrates of human behavior. They also underscore the complex interplay between the forces of nature and nurture in determining mental function. The well-informed neurologist can play an important role in the evaluation of patients with psychiatric symptoms.

This is an exciting time to be involved in neurology and psychiatry. Neurobiology is beginning to be able to address disorders of thinking and emotion. Progress in neuroscience, neurology, and psychiatry is inevitably drawing our specialties closer together. With better scientific understanding, more definitive approaches toward prevention, early intervention, and symptom control are within reach. Patient and family education and support remain essential. Clearly, multiple disciplines are needed to understand and treat complex human behavioral and cognitive disorders. Hippocrates continues to urge us forward.

## SUGGESTED READING

Adams RD, Victor M. Principles of Neurology (6th ed). New York: McGraw-Hill, 1997.

Fogel BS, Schiffer RB, Rao SM. Neuropsychiatry. Baltimore: Williams & Wilkins, 1996.

Heilman KM, Valenstein E. Clinical Neuropsychology (3rd ed). New York: Oxford University Press, 1993.

Lishman WA. Organic Psychiatry (2nd ed). Oxford: Blackwell, 1987.

Shader RI. Manual of Psychiatric Therapeutics (2nd ed). Boston: Little, Brown, 1994.

Yudofsky SC, Hales RE. The American Psychiatric Press Textbook of Neuropsychiatry (3rd ed). Washington, DC: American Psychiatric Press, 1997.

# IV
## Pediatrics

# 27
# Neonatal Seizures

Kalpathy S. Krishnamoorthy

Seizures in the newborn usually occur as a symptom of a significant underlying neurologic disorder. Their occurrence is a common reason for neurologic consultation in the newborn intensive care unit. The clinical events recognizable as neonatal seizures are listed in Table 27.1. Their classification, diagnosis, and management are controversial. The first and foremost role of a neurologic consultant is to confirm that the events noted are indeed seizures, because in the newborn infant, some of the motor and atypical paroxysms are mistaken for convulsive events. Taking a detailed history to probe the events is very important. A review of high-risk perinatal events such as perinatal asphyxia and maternal or fetal complications during late gestation, labor, and delivery often supports the suspicion. Most neurologic consultants still rely on the direct observations made by the nursing staff or neonatologists to consider the diagnosis of neonatal seizures, and this reliance is a most pragmatic approach.

The development of synchronized video electroencephalographic (EEG) bedside monitoring has allowed more precise diagnosis of neonatal seizures. Some clinically observed seizures may not have EEG correlates [1,2]. In contrast, EEG abnormalities may be noted without clinical signs. In their study, Scher and Painter found that more than 50% of neonates with electrographic signs of seizures had no clinical accompaniments. Both clinical and electrographic signs of seizure were noted in only 45% of 62 preterm and 53% of 33 full-term neonates [2]. Clancy and colleagues found that approximately 80% of 393 electrographic events were not accompanied by clinical seizures [3]. Because prolonged video telemetry is not easily available to most clinicians, high reliance on clinical diagnosis is reasonable. In practical terms, bedside video telemetry is very useful when seizure diagnosis is difficult or cannot be established on clinical grounds alone.

*Table 27.1*   Clinical events recognizable as neonatal seizures

| |
|---|
| Clonic motor movements: Focal, multifocal |
| Tonic posturing: Focal, generalized |
| Myoclonic jerks |
| Subtle: Staring, nystagmus, blinking, tonic eye deviation, sucking of saliva or tongue protrusion, bicycling, swimming, autonomic signs, episodic heart rate changes, hypertension, apnea, pupillary changes |

Sources: Adapted with permission from EM Mizrahi. Consensus and controversy in the clinical management of neonatal seizures. Clin Perinatol 1989;16:485–500; and JJ Volpe. Neonatal seizures: current concepts and revised classification. Pediatrics 1989;84:422–428.

## CLASSIFICATION

The revised classification of neonatal seizures proposed by Volpe [4] is highly practical. This classification takes into consideration both clinical and EEG signs and draws on studies that conducted prolonged bedside EEG monitoring [1,2,3]. The clinical characteristics of the seizure types in this classification are described below.

### Subtle Seizures

Prolonged video telemetry has shown that many subtle clinical events previously called subtle seizures have poor correlation with EEG events; yet subtle seizures may occur without simultaneous EEG changes. Therefore, it is useful to inquire about any signs noted in careful bedside observation, such as brisk nystagmoid eye movements, tonic eye deviation, tonic extremity stiffening, cyanosis, or apnea. A constellation of these manifestations, rather than isolated features, strongly supports the diagnosis of subtle seizures. The presence of autonomic alterations while these events occur, such as oxygen desaturation spells, tachycardia or bradycardia, and blood pressure elevations, may often be seen in subtle seizures. When one is unable to observe clinical manifestations of seizures in a pharmacologically paralyzed infant, abrupt autonomic changes may be highly suggestive of seizure activity. Subtle seizures appear to occur more commonly in preterm than in full-term infants [4]. Clinical inspection alone may underestimate subtle seizure activity. The presence of subtle seizures coincident with electrographic discharges as shown by bedside EEG study may be helpful. Seizures manifesting solely as recurrent apneic spells are seen especially in the full-term neonate. Unexplained apneic spells that require vigorous bag-mask resuscitation should raise a strong suspicion of seizures. Some apneic seizures may be accompanied by eye, motor, or orobuccal movements; however, in some cases sudden, unprovoked apneic spells with oxygen desaturation may be the sole manifestation. In these cases, EEG telemetry may offer more diagnostic information during these spells; the EEG record is usually characterized by paroxysmal rhythmic sharp or rhythmic high-voltage slow-wave activity, especially from the temporal regions, that is indicative of seizure.

## Clonic Seizures

Both focal and multifocal clonic seizures are easily recognizable on clinical grounds alone. They also have a high correlation with electrographic events [1,2,4]. Clonic seizures occur from diverse causes, the most common of which are hypoxic-ischemic encephalopathy and intracranial hemorrhage. In the newborn, focal clonic seizures may be noted even in acute metabolic encephalopathy (hypocalcemia and hypoglycemia). An underlying focal structural lesion such as an arterial infarct should always be considered in cases in which there are consistent focal clonic seizures.

## Tonic Seizures

Most generalized tonic episodes that resemble seizures are not associated with electrographic discharges [1,2,4]. Many of these tonic episodes are believed to be a form of "brain stem release phenomenon" and therefore might mimic decerebrate posturing. However, sustained and repetitive asymmetric focal tonic movements of a limb have been associated with EEG discharges and therefore are regarded as tonic seizures [1,2,4]. Diagnosis of generalized tonic seizures should be determined in the context of the clinical picture.

## Myoclonic Seizures

Myoclonic movements are rapid and jerky and are seen particularly in flexor muscle groups. When myoclonic movements are focal or fragmentary, they have a poor correlation with time-synchronized EEG discharges [1–3]. However, brisk symmetric generalized myoclonus (often mistaken for infantile spasms) has a high correlation with EEG discharges and, therefore, should be regarded as a seizure manifestation. Benign sleep myoclonus should be considered in the differential diagnosis when multifocal myoclonic movements occur with drowsiness or during sleep in an otherwise normal infant who has a normal EEG study.

Some studies have been helpful in the reclassification and characterization of neonatal seizures [1–4]. Absence of EEG seizure activity may not always rule out the diagnosis of seizures, because specific types of clinical seizures in the human newborn may originate from the deep cerebral structures (limbic regions). These discharges may not be detectable with surface EEG electrodes. The clinical distinctions between an epileptic and a nonepileptic phenomenon are provided in Table 27.2. Some of the common phenomena confused with neonatal seizures include jitteriness, multifocal myoclonus, sleep myoclonus, decerebrate posturing, and rapid eye movement (REM) sleep in neonates. Rarely, neonatal hyperexplexia may be mistaken for neonatal seizures or the two may coexist [5].

*Table 27.2*   Clinical distinctions between seizures and nonseizures

| Clinical feature | Seizure | Nonseizure |
|---|---|---|
| Increase with physical stimulation | No | Yes |
| Rhythmic tremorlike movements | No | Yes |
| Arrhythmic amplitude with clonic movements | Yes | No |
| Diminution with restraint | No | Yes |
| Autonomic accompaniments (tachycardia or bradycardia, apnea, desaturation) | Yes | No |
| Paroxysmal, orobuccal, tongue, or eye abnormalities with motor movements | Yes | No |

## ETIOLOGY

A list of the most common etiologic factors, type of seizure, and time of onset of these seizures is provided in Table 27.3. By far the most common cause of neonatal seizures is perinatal encephalopathy [6,7]. It is important, however, to diagnose the exact cause in order to determine long-term prognosis and formulate treatment plans. Methodical investigations (see Table 27.3) assist in arriving at a specific diagnosis in more than 85% of cases of neonatal seizure.

A rapid workup for seizures should include a complete history, blood chemistries, blood gases, cerebrospinal fluid examination, and an EEG. Cranial ultrasonography alone is not sufficient to evaluate a newborn with seizures, and therefore a computed tomographic (CT) scan should be obtained. Both standard-protocol magnetic resonance imaging scan and diffusion-weighted imaging are very useful for further delineation in cases of hypoxic-ischemic encephalopathy, stroke, and venous sinus disease in the newborn. An in-depth metabolic workup to look for inborn errors of metabolism is not routinely necessary but should be ordered on a selective basis. More than 90% of neonatal seizures are controlled by adequate therapy. When one is faced with a case of neonatal status epilepticus, further studies should be undertaken to search for possible causes.

## APPROACH

An accurate diagnosis is essential for appropriate treatment. Historical details pertinent to various causes of neonatal seizures, including family history of neonatal seizures, should be obtained. A complete general physical examination and a neonatal neurologic examination should be performed. It is helpful initially to take a standard EEG to arrive at a diagnosis and to offer therapeutic intervention. Epileptic seizures should be stopped to prevent further brain injury from repetitive seizures [7]. When the diagnosis is in doubt, or when the events are suggestive of nonepileptic paroxysms, treatment with anticonvulsants may be withheld pending further observation in the newborn intensive care unit. If the

*Table 27.3*  Neonatal seizures: common etiology, seizure type, and workup

| Cause | Time of onset | Common seizure type | Useful additional workup |
|---|---|---|---|
| Hypoxic-ischemic encephalopathy (peri-natal encephalopathy) | 0 hrs–2 days | Subtle (apnea), focal, multifocal, or tonic | Magnetic resonance imaging (MRI) with diffusion-weighted imaging (DWI), electroencephalography (EEG) |
| Intracranial bleeds | 1–2 days | Focal or multifocal | Computed tomographic (CT) scan, cranial ultra-sound, MRI |
| Acute metabolic derangements | 0 hrs–3 days | Apnea, focal, or multifocal | Measurement of electrolytes, glucose, calcium, phospho-rus, magnesium |
| Inborn error of metabolism | 3–15 days | Apnea, focal, multifocal, or tonic | Measurement of blood amino acids, ammonia, blood gases, urine organic acids and amino acids; vitamin $B_6$ infusion trial (100 mg IV × 2) |
| Intracranial infection | 3–15 days | Multifocal or focal | Toxoplasmosis, rubella, cytomegalovirus, herpes titers; cerebrospinal fluid analysis; herpes simplex virus polymerase chain reaction; CT scan; MRI; ophthalmologic examina-tion; brain stem auditory response |
| Cerebrovascular lesions (strokes) | 1–3 days | Focal or multifocal | CT scan, MRI, stroke profile (blood) |
| Venous sinus thrombosis | 3–7 days | Focal or multifocal | CT scan, stroke profile (blood), MRI with DWI, magnetic resonance venography |
| Central nervous system malformations | 2–15 days | Multifocal or myoclonic | CT scan, MRI, chromo-some testing |
| Drug withdrawal | 2–15 days | Multifocal or myoclonic | Blood and urine testing, toxic screen |
| Neonatal epileptic encephalopathy | 7–15 days | Multifocal, myoclonic, or tonic | EEG, MRI |
| Neurodegenerative disorder | 7–15 days | Multifocal, myoclonic, or tonic | EEG, lysosomal studies, peroxisomal workup, serum lactate level, pyruvate level, measurement of ammonia, skin biopsy, muscle biopsy, neuro-ophthalmologic examination |

*Table 27.3*   (continued)

| Cause | Time of onset | Common seizure type | Useful additional workup |
|---|---|---|---|
| Benign familial neonatal seizures and benign idiopathic neonatal seizures | 3–15 days | Focal, multifocal, apneic spells, or tonic | EEG, family history |

Most infants with neonatal seizures should undergo the following basic workup:
  Hemogram
  Electrolyte levels
  Calcium, phosphorus, magnesium levels
  Lumbar puncture—cerebrospinal fluid analysis/culture
  Cranial ultrasonography
  CT brain scan
  Blood culture

equipment required to perform prolonged bedside EEG video telemetry is available, it should be used as a part of complete evaluation in complex cases.

Typically, perinatal hypoxic-ischemic encephalopathy with seizures has its onset from several hours to 48 hours after birth. Apneic spells may herald full-blown seizures, while multifocal clonic and stiffening spells are the most common. In full-term infants, intracranial hemorrhage of various types—including intraventricular, posterior fossa, subdural, or tentorial bleeds or subarachnoid hemorrhage—is manifested by multifocal clonic or focal tonic seizures. Acute metabolic derangements such as hypoglycemic and hypocalcemic seizures present within the first 48 hours after birth with focal or multifocal clonic seizures, jitteriness, or apnea. In some infants, sepsis—even without meningoencephalitis—may herald itself with seizures. A severe encephalopathy with frequent clonic and tonic seizures should always raise the possibility of viral meningoencephalitis; an inborn error of metabolism, especially a urea-cycle disorder with hyperammonemia, encephalopathy, and organic acidurias. Benign familial neonatal convulsions may present with recurrent apneic attacks accompanied by multifocal clonic seizures and typical EEG changes [7]. Brisk myoclonic generalized seizures often indicate diffuse encephalopathy, neurodegenerative disorders, or mitochondrial or peroxisomal disorders. Infants with perinatal middle cerebral artery strokes often present with focal clonic seizures within the first 72 hours after birth.

Seizures in very-low-birth-weight preterm infants may appear as brisk multifocal clonic movements associated with hypoxic encephalopathy, sepsis, or meningoencephalitis. Associated autonomic changes are frequently seen in these instances. Orobuccal automatisms, multifocal twitching, and eye deviations may be seen during the onset of normal REM sleep and may easily be mistaken for subtle seizures. Tonic seizures are characteristic of large intraventricular hemorrhage in the preterm newborn, whereas multifocal clonic or tonic seizures often may be the initial presentation of intracranial hemorrhage in the full-term infant.

## DRUG THERAPY

It is a reasonable goal to attempt to eliminate all clinical seizure activity. Yet electrographic seizure activity in the absence of clinical change poses a difficult therapeutic problem. Mizrahi et al. [1] have shown that the administration of phenobarbital often leads to cessation of clinical seizures despite persistence of EEG seizures. However, by attempting to eliminate all electrographic seizures, the neonate's ventilatory and cardiovascular status may be jeopardized [4]. Furthermore, it appears that, with adequate blood levels of standard anticonvulsants, most electrographic seizure discharges subside in due course [4]. Therefore, clinical seizure control rather than electrographic seizure control is the goal in most cases. Our recommendation, similar to that of Volpe [4,7], is not to attempt overzealously to eliminate all electrographic seizure discharges. For pharmacologically paralyzed infants who show seizures on EEG, it is reasonable to administer appropriate anticonvulsant medications guided by therapeutic blood levels. When these paralyzed infants exhibit an unclear cluster of autonomic changes, such as spells of oxygen desaturation, tachycardia or bradycardia, or blood pressure elevation, re-evaluation by bedside EEG monitoring is appropriate, and administration of additional anticonvulsants to control electrographic seizures is reasonable.

The drugs of choice and dosages are provided in Table 27.4. Phenobarbital and phenytoin remain the mainstay of anticonvulsant therapy. Lorazepam may be used as needed to stop breakthrough seizures. Experience with fosphenytoin sodium in neonates is limited. Occasionally, rectal or oral valproic acid may be used, or rectal paraldehyde, to control intractable seizures. If there is poor seizure control despite high therapeutic levels, it is important to consider an inborn error of metabolism, pyridoxine-dependency seizures, or a severe epileptic disorder.

Duration of therapy is based upon the underlying cause, normal or abnormal neurologic status, and normal or abnormal EEG [4,7]. The risk of recurrence, both immediate and long term, is less than 20% for all cases of neonatal seizures collectively. In most infants meeting the normal criteria, the anticonvulsants can

*Table 27.4*   Neonatal seizure therapy

---

*Immediate therapy*
Phenobarbital, loading dose 20 mg/kg in two divided doses, may give up to 40 mg/kg total; phenytoin/fosphenytoin sodium, loading dose 20 mg/kg in two divided doses, may give additional 5 mg/kg if required; lorazepam, loading dose 0.05–0.10 mg/kg, may repeat two to three more doses if required
*Maintenance therapy*
Maintain on phenobarbital, 2.5 mg/kg twice daily. Discontinue phenytoin as soon as IV line access is not available or good seizure control is achieved for 5 days.
*Short-term goal*
Discontinue phenobarbital in 4 wks provided neurologic evaluation is normal and normal EEG is documented. If EEG remains significantly abnormal, continue phenobarbital for 3–6 mos. Repeat EEG and consider stopping phenobarbital between 3 and 6 mos.

---

*Note:* For intractable seizures, a trial of IV vitamin $B_6$ infusion (100–200 mg) is indicated.

be discontinued within the first 4 weeks of life. Long-term anticonvulsant therapy beyond 4 weeks is recommended for those infants with a significantly abnormal EEG or for those with a significantly abnormal neurologic examination. In most of even these infants, the anticonvulsant therapy may be discontinued by 3–6 months. However, it is important to recognize that this group of infants has a high risk of recurrence of seizures in later life. We generally advocate a follow-up EEG on all infants before discontinuation of anticonvulsant therapy.

## ELECTROENCEPHALOGRAPHY

EEG data are helpful in the assessment of neonatal seizures and neurologic outcome, especially in infants with encephalopathy. It is essential to evaluate voltage, synchrony, and symmetry as appropriate for gestational age. Certain age-related patterns such as delta brushes and frontal sharp transients are to be distinguished from paroxysmal activity. Background activity helps in assessment of an infant's level of encephalopathy. The presence of frequent focal sharp or multifocal sharp discharges and rhythmic runs of paroxysmal activity are all significant for the diagnosis of electrographic seizures. Markedly abnormal isoelectric background, severe burst suppression, and excessive discontinuity all indicate an unfavorable prognosis. Many abnormal neonatal EEG patterns improve with time; therefore, prognostication should be based on the findings of an early EEG measured during acute encephalopathy when there are maximal changes in the background [8].

## INTRACTABLE NEONATAL SEIZURES

A certain number of neonates experience intractable seizures, although the occurrence is not common. Usually, the difficulty in seizure control is temporary and can be overcome with appropriate anticonvulsant therapy. Some of the common causes of intractable neonatal seizures are outlined in Table 27.5. Severe hypoxic-ischemic injury is one of the most common causes. Infants with this condition have a diffusely abnormal EEG (burst suppression) and a grossly abnormal CT

*Table 27.5*   Causes of intractable neonatal seizures

Severe hypoxic-ischemic perinatal encephalopathy, especially with cortical necrosis
Meningoencephalitis, especially due to herpesvirus
Inborn errors of metabolism, especially urea-cycle disorder with hyperammonemia, encephalopathy, and organic acidurias
Pyridoxine-dependency (vitamin $B_6$–dependency) seizures
Early-onset epileptic encephalopathic syndromes
Mitochondrial disorders
Peroxisomal disorders
Central nervous system malformations

scan showing poor gray-white differentiation and prominent central gray nuclei. They later demonstrate cortical necrosis and multicystic encephalomalacia on neuroimaging studies. Other important causes of intractable seizures are viral meningoencephalitis, inborn error of organic acid metabolism, urea-cycle disorder with hyperammonemic encephalopathy, nonketotic hyperglycinemia, and pyridoxine-dependency seizures. In addition to performing appropriate laboratory studies to uncover the cause, administration of multiple doses of phenobarbital in boluses of 5 mg/kg up to a total of 40 mg/kg to achieve levels greater than 40 mg/liter and administration of phenytoin to reach a level of up to 20 mg/liter may be required. Repeated boluses (three or four) of lorazepam given intravenously are often helpful in terminating neonatal status epilepticus. At all times, vital cardiovascular and respiratory functions should be carefully monitored. The use of rectal paraldehyde or valproic acid is sometimes helpful. There is limited experience with continuous intravenous infusion of midazolam hydrochloride or pentobarbital sodium in the therapy of neonatal status epilepticus.

A strong suspicion of vitamin $B_6$–dependency epilepsy is raised when there are recurrent multifocal clonic and tonic seizures with very early onset. Clinical events that raise suspicion of intrauterine seizures may be another clue to this diagnosis. In these infants, the condition may be mistaken for encephalopathy related to perinatal asphyxia. A trial of 100–200 mg intravenous pyridoxine during EEG monitoring is indicated whenever the neonate fails to stop seizing despite adequate standard anticonvulsant therapy or when there is no clearcut cause for the seizures.

## REFERENCES

1. Mizrahi EM. Consensus and controversy in the clinical management of neonatal seizures. Clin Perinatol 1989;16:485–500.
2. Scher MS, Painter MJ. Electrographic Diagnosis of Neonatal Seizures: Issues of Diagnostic Accuracy, Clinical Correlation and Survival. In C Wasterlain, P Vert (eds), Neonatal Seizures. New York: Raven Press, 1990;15–25.
3. Clancy RR, Legido A, Lewis D. Occult neonatal seizures. Epilepsia 1988;29:256–261.
4. Volpe JJ. Neonatal seizures: current concepts and revised classification. Pediatrics 1989;84:422–428.
5. Nigro AN, Lim HCN. Hyperexplexia and sudden neonatal death. Pediatr Neurol 1992;8:221–225.
6. Bernes SM, Kaplan AM. Evolution of neonatal seizures. Pediatr Clin North Am 1994;41:1069–1104.
7. Volpe JJ. Neurology of the Newborn (3rd ed). Philadelphia: Saunders, 1995.
8. Wical BS. Neonatal seizures and electrographic analysis: evaluation and outcomes. Pediatr Neurol 1994;10:271–275.

# 28
# Status Epilepticus in Children

Kalpathy S. Krishnamoorthy

Status epilepticus (SE) is an important medical emergency that requires prompt recognition and treatment. The definition of SE varies, but the most common criterion for diagnosis has been based on the absolute duration of seizure activity; previously, a minimum duration of 30 minutes was the time most frequently used. A trend in the treatment of SE eliminates the requirement for a specific time duration in making the diagnosis. For example, the Epilepsy Foundation of America defines SE as including "two or more sequential seizures without full recovery of consciousness between seizures" [1]. In 1991, the American Epilepsy Society recommended that therapeutic intervention be initiated if a seizure or series of seizures persists for more than 10 minutes [2]. Thus, the trend is toward requiring a shorter duration and fewer number of seizures for the diagnosis of SE.

## CLASSIFICATION

SE can be classified as follows:

1. Generalized SE
   a. Convulsive tonic-clonic
   b. Nonconvulsive (absence; petit mal)
2. Partial SE
   a. Simple partial (epilepsia partialis continua)
   b. Complex partial

The division of SE into either convulsive or nonconvulsive SE may be too simplistic in certain instances. Nonconvulsive SE may occur when convulsive SE has been prolonged. The term *subtle generalized convulsive SE* is sometimes used to describe the condition of patients who show only partial or subtle clinical signs of convulsive activity despite a marked impairment of consciousness and bilateral ictal discharges on electroencephalogram (EEG) [3]. This condition may also result from unsuccessful treatment of prolonged convulsive SE. Generalized tonic-clonic convulsive SE usually manifests as overt seizure activity. However, in subtle generalized SE, the patient is in a state of stupor or coma and exhibits repetitive rhythmic subtle motor convulsions in association with bilateral ictal activity on EEG. In the management of convulsive states, one should not overlook this subtle tonic-clonic epileptic state. The fundamental reason to treat acute or frequent seizures is to avoid further brain damage resulting from altered cerebral metabolism and neuronal damage as well as secondary effects from hypoxemia, lactic acidosis, and hypercapnia. This chapter focuses on generalized tonic-clonic convulsive SE.

## INCIDENCE

The greatest number of cases of SE occurs either in very young children or in persons older than 60 years. Between 4% and 16% of patients with epilepsy experience at least one episode of SE [4]. For a large number (70%) of patients less than 1 year of age who later develop epilepsy, SE is the initial manifestation [4].

## PATHOPHYSIOLOGY

The pathophysiology of SE has been well described by Lothman in a comprehensive review [5]. As the seizure activity becomes recurrent and prolonged (about 30 minutes in duration), the EEG reflects continuous epileptiform discharges. Associated tachycardia, hypertension, hyperglycemia, and lactic acidosis contribute to a state of metabolic acidosis. In the brain, a marked increase occurs in cerebral blood flow, with an associated increase in oxygen and glucose utilization. After 30 minutes of SE, decompensation may start to occur. Blood pressure normalizes or falls, serum glucose may be normal or low, and hyperthermia occurs. Respiratory failure may be impending at this time. In the brain, oxygen and glucose delivery diminishes, although oxygen and glucose utilization remains high; a potential discrepancy is thus created between substrate supply and demand. At this point, irreversible brain injury may ensue. At the biochemical level, a cascade of events leads to the propagation of neuronal injury. These events include excitatory amino acid toxicity, free-radical production, membrane phospholipid hydrolysis, and alteration in calcium homeostasis. Prolonged SE can lead to rhabdomyolysis and myoglobinuria, resulting in renal failure. Cardiac arrhythmias, pulmonary edema, and pulmonary aspiration are all potential complications in patients with SE. Meldrum's studies using bicuculline (a gamma-aminobutyric-acid inhibitor) to induce electrographic SE in paralyzed and ventilated baboons have shown that neuronal loss can occur in the neocortex and hippocampus despite adequate oxygenation and ventilation [6]. These findings have long implied that treatment should control electrographic seizure activity in SE in addition to halting the clinical seizure activity.

# ETIOLOGY

SE is broadly considered either symptomatic or cryptogenic. Symptomatic SE is commonly the result of an acute brain injury (acute symptomatic) or related to chronic encephalopathy (remote symptomatic). Febrile SE alone is considered one of the common manifestations of cryptogenic SE in children below the age of 2. Approximately 5% of children with febrile seizures experience febrile SE [4]. The incidence of various causes of SE in children varies. Intracranial infections, head trauma, metabolic conditions (especially hyponatremia in infancy), cerebral anoxia, epilepsy, drug intoxications, cerebral malformation, and anticonvulsant withdrawal are all common causes of SE in children younger than 16 years. In three large series [7–9] of pediatric cases of SE, the idiopathic category accounted for 16–24% of all cases. An acute and treatable cause was identified in 23–41% of cases in the study group. Febrile SE was represented in 24–29% of all cases. Therefore, an underlying cause must be sought to appropriately manage the patient.

# MANAGEMENT

## General Measures

The goal of management is to stop the seizure activity and to prevent metabolic complications such as hypoxemia, hypercarbia, lactic acidosis, hypoglycemia, and hyperthemia, all of which may cause myocardial depression and hypotension that result in decreased cerebral blood flow. Most important, one must evaluate the patient's cardiorespiratory status and provide supportive care as soon as possible. The use of airway adjuncts, such as oral and nasal airways, can be lifesaving and may obviate the need for tracheal intubation. A constant re-evaluation of airway, breathing, and circulation must occur to ensure adequate oxygenation and prevention of secondary organ dysfunction. There should be a low threshold for performing tracheal intubation, because respiratory function often deteriorates as seizure duration lengthens. Anticonvulsant medications should be promptly administered. An intravenous access should be quickly obtained, preferably in two peripheral catheters. After a venous access is obtained, a Dextrostix test should be performed, and if the patient is hypoglycemic, a 25% dextrose solution, 2–4 ml/kg, should be administered. Other blood samples should be sent for appropriate laboratory studies. Toxicology screening may be valuable in certain clinical situations. Although laboratory data are helpful in evaluating the cause of SE, it is imperative that treatment not be delayed while awaiting test results.

## Diagnostic Evaluation

A list of diagnostic tests helpful in evaluating a patient with SE is provided in Table 28.1. The physician must initiate a diagnostic evaluation seeking the cause of the SE while simultaneously stabilizing and directing therapy to control seizure activity. Laboratory tests and imaging studies should be performed based

*Table 28.1*    Diagnostic evaluation in status epilepticus

| |
| --- |
| Complete blood cell count, blood culture |
| Electrolyte, glucose levels |
| Calcium, magnesium, phosphate levels |
| Blood urea nitrogen, creatinine levels |
| Urinalysis |
| Toxicology screen |
| Ammonia levels |
| Anticonvulsant blood levels |
| Cerebrospinal fluid analysis (glucose, protein, cell count) and culture |
| Electroencephalogram |
| Computed tomographic scan |
| Magnetic resonance imaging |
| Other studies as indicated |

on the history and physical examination. Anticonvulsant levels should be drawn on all patients with a known seizure disorder. A computed tomographic (CT) scan of the head should be performed on all patients with head trauma, focal neurologic deficit, focal seizure, or evidence of increased intracranial pressure. When there is a history or physical examination compatible with neck injury, careful cervical spine evaluation should be undertaken.

A lumbar puncture is indicated for all febrile patients, because the presence or absence of meningeal signs is often difficult to ascertain after a prolonged bout of seizures or after anticonvulsant medications have been administered. Lumbar puncture is also indicated for those patients presenting with meningeal signs or first episode of SE and for immunocompromised patients. Contraindications to lumbar puncture include the presence of thrombocytopenia, marked coagulopathy, hydrocephalus, intracranial mass or midline shift on CT scan, and evidence of increased intracranial pressure. It is a good practice to obtain imaging studies of the brain before a lumbar puncture for all patients and especially for patients who have focal seizures or for whom focal neurologic signs are present. If the patient has cardiopulmonary instability or if there is an unclear neurologic picture, the lumbar puncture may be delayed; antibiotics should be administered immediately to cover for possible meningitis.

## Antiepileptic Drugs

The goal of therapy in SE is to control the seizures promptly before irreversible neuronal damage occurs. Irreversible damage begins between 20 and 60 minutes after the start of SE in experimental animals, despite adequate oxygenation and ventilation [6]. Most of the antiepileptic drugs used to stop seizures may compromise airway and breathing and, therefore, should be used with great caution. Intravenous administration is the preferred route because of its reliability and rapid action; intramuscular administration may be erratic. If intravenous access is not easily available, a rectal or intramuscular route may be used as a temporary measure.

Of the 22 drugs approved by the U.S. Food and Drug Administration to treat seizures, diazepam, lorazepam, phenytoin, and phenobarbital are all effective in the management of generalized tonic-clonic SE. However, clinical trials comparing any of these drugs are few. In refractory status epilepticus (RSE), more rapidly acting drugs like midazolam hydrochloride, pentobarbital sodium, and thiopental sodium are used.

The first-line antiepileptic drugs for SE include (1) benzodiazepines (lorazepam; diazepam; midazolam hydrochloride), (2) phenytoin, and (3) phenobarbital.

## Benzodiazepines

Benzodiazepines have been used extensively as initial antiepileptic drugs for SE. The reliable anticonvulsant activity of lorazepam (0.05–0.10 mg/kg per dose), its tendency to cause less respiratory depression, and its longer duration of action have made it the drug of first choice, and its use surpasses that of diazepam. Even though diazepam (0.1–0.3 mg/kg per dose) has a faster onset of action because of greater lipid solubility, lorazepam appears to show sustained anticonvulsant effect and may require less frequent dosing [10,11]. Occasionally, intramuscular midazolam hydrochloride (0.05–0.20 mg/kg per dose) is useful, particularly if there is difficulty achieving intravenous access [12]. The possibility of respiratory depression is always present whenever benzodiazepines are used. Therefore, one must be able to control the airway when benzodiazepines are administered and must be prepared to assist ventilation if necessary. Rectal administration of diazepam is effective in the acute therapy of convulsions in children (0.2–0.5 mg/kg per dose) and has been used outside the United States [13]. A rectal gel preparation of diazepam (Diastat; Athena Neuro) has been recently released that might encourage its wider use in the United States.

## Phenytoin

The benefit of administering phenytoin [14] is that it does not cause respiratory depression or sedation; thus, its use is ideal in a setting where one might want to preserve the ability to carry out a neurologic examination, particularly evaluation of mental status. When phenytoin is given intravenously, blood pressure should be monitored closely during its administration to avoid hypotension. Phenytoin should be infused only in normal saline. A loading dose of up to 18–20 mg/kg should maintain a therapeutic level for up to 24 hours. The duration of therapeutic level may not be as long in children; measurement of drug level 2 hours after the loading dose is given may help guide timing of the maintenance of phenytoin therapy.

Fosphenytoin sodium [15,16] is a phosphate ester prodrug of phenytoin that is highly water soluble and buffered to a pH of 8.6–9.0. It is rapidly converted to phenytoin by endogenous phosphatases once it reaches the vascular compartment. Fosphenytoin sodium has a high affinity for phenytoin albumin binding sites. Doses and infusion rates of fosphenytoin sodium are expressed as the amount of phenytoin delivered. In contrast to phenytoin, extravasation of fosphenytoin sodium from the veins into perivenous tissue does not cause tissue reaction or pain. Intravenous or intramuscular administration of fosphenytoin sodium at doses corresponding to customary phenytoin loading doses (15–20 mg/kg) rapidly and consistently produces therapeutic levels within 10 minutes of rapid intravenous infusion and within 30 minutes of intramuscular injection. Fosphenytoin sodium can also be given intramuscularly as a loading dose or maintenance dose at up to 20 mg/kg without causing muscle tissue reaction at the injection site. Although intramuscular administration of fosphenytoin sodium may be an effective method, only the intravenous route should be used in a patient in active SE if prompt venous access is available. Unlike with phenytoin, adverse cardiovascular side effects and hypotension do not appear to occur with fosphenytoin sodium, even with rapid intravenous infusion.

## Phenobarbital

Phenobarbital is widely used as the first drug to control generalized tonic-clonic seizures in infants and neonates [12,13]. The intravenous route is always the preferred way to administer phenobarbital in the management of tonic-clonic status. Peak brain concentrations occur 30–60 minutes after intravenous loading, although seizure control is achieved within 20 minutes. Loading doses of 15–20 mg/kg are required to achieve therapeutic serum levels. Further doses of phenobarbital to achieve a very high serum concentration may be used in specific situations where the seizures are difficult to control [17,18]. In such cases, the integrity of the patient's airway should be ensured with endotracheal intubation, and intravenous infusion should be performed slowly to avoid cardiovascular complications. The maintenance dose of phenobarbital (3–6 mg/kg per day) is started 8–12 hours after the loading dose. One must be cautious when phenobarbital is used in conjunction with a benzodiazepine because of the possibility of respiratory depression.

## Strategy of Drug Therapy

A number of strategies are used in the treatment of SE, but there is lack of uniformity [9,12,19]. A pragmatic approach is intended to provide rational and practical therapy in the management of SE. Anticonvulsant drug dosages and steps in the pharmacotherapy of the patient with SE are given in Table 28.2 and Table 28.3, respectively.

After venous access is obtained, lorazepam is given intravenously at a dose of 0.05–0.10 mg/kg. If seizures continue, we recommend intravenous loading with phenytoin immediately after the first dose of lorazepam is administered. The intravenous loading dose of phenytoin is 20 mg/kg at a rate no faster than 1 mg/kg per minute. Electrocardiogram results and blood pressure must be monitored during the infusion, and a close watch should be kept on the intravenous site. It takes approximately 20 minutes for phenytoin to be infused; if needed during this period, an additional three to four doses of lorazepam may be administered (maximum = 4 mg per dose). It is not unusual for a few additional doses of lorazepam to be required when phenytoin is being infused early in the treatment of SE. Diazepam is now less commonly used because of its short duration of action.

*Table 28.2*  Anticonvulsant drugs and dosages for generalized tonic-clonic status epilepticus

| Drug | Route | Loading dose | Onset of action | Maintenance dose |
|---|---|---|---|---|
| Phenobarbital | IV | 20 mg/kg, infuse at 1 mg/kg/min Max median dose: 60 mg/kg Max rate: 100 mg/min | 20–30 mins | 3–6 mg/day |
| Phenytoin | IV | 15–20 mg/kg, infuse at 1 mg/kg/min Max rate: 50 mg/min | 15–20 mins | 3–6 mg/day |
| Fosphenytoin sodium | IV/IM | 15–20 mg/kg | 20–30 mins | 3–6 mg/day |
| Lorazepam | IV | 0.05–0.10 mg/dose every 10–15 mins Max: 4 mg/dose Max total: 3–4 doses | 2–3 mins | |
| Diazepam | IV | 0.1–0.3 mg/kg/dose Max: 10 mg/dose | 1–2 mins | |
| | PR | 0.2–0.5 mg/kg/dose | | |
| Midazolam hydrochloride | IV/IM | 0.05–0.20 mg/kg/dose every 10–15 mins Max: 5 mg/kg/dose | 2–5 mins | Continuous IV infusion 0.2–0.4 mg/kg/dose |
| Paraldehyde | PR | 0.3 ml/kg | | Every 4–6 hrs Max total: 4–6 doses |
| Valproic acid | PR/NGT | 20–30 mg/kg | | 10–20 mg/kg/day |
| | IV | 15 mg/kg bolus | | 1 mg/kg/hr infusion |
| Carbamazepine | PR/NGT | 10–30 mg/kg | | 10–30 mg/kg/day |
| Pentobarbital | IV | 2–8 mg/kg bolus | | Continuous infusion 1–3 mg/kg/hr |
| Lidocaine | IV | 2–3 mg/kg | | |
| Thiopental sodium | IV | 5 mg/kg IV bolus | | Continuous infusion 5 mg/kg/hr |
| Isoflurane | Inhalation | 0.5–3.0% | | |
| Propofol | IV | 2 mg/kg | | Infusion rate 5–10 mg/kg/hr |
| Vitamin $B_6$ | IV | 100–200 mg | | |

IV = intravenous; IM = intramuscular; PR = per rectum; NGT = nasogastric tube.

If seizures continue after three or four doses of lorazepam and phenytoin loading, load the patient with 20 mg/kg of phenobarbital. The combination of benzodiazepine and phenobarbital may lead to respiratory depression requiring tracheal intubation and mechanical ventilation. The airway should be carefully secured and mechanical ventilation initiated if additional phenobarbital doses

*Table 28.3*　Management of generalized tonic-clonic status epilepticus

1. Assess neurologic, general physical, and cardiorespiratory status; elicit quick history and obtain samples of blood for laboratory studies. Insert intravenous catheter and oral airway and administer oxygen as needed.
2. Begin intravenous infusion with 5% dextrose and 0.45% saline solution. Administer a bolus of 2–4 ml/kg of 25% dextrose if no cause is obvious or patient is hypoglycemic.
3. Administer intravenous lorazepam 0.05–0.10 mg/kg. If seizures continue, infuse phenytoin 20 mg/kg over 20 mins.
4. If seizures persist, administer additional doses of lorazepam as above at least three times every 10 mins while phenytoin is being infused until seizures are controlled. Protect airway and be ready to intubate the trachea. Continuously assess airway, breathing, and circulation. If seizures still persist, give intravenous phenobarbital, 20 mg/kg over 20 mins. If seizures continue, administer another round of intravenous phenobarbital, 5–10 mg/kg and intravenous phenytoin, 5 mg/kg.
5. If seizures still continue, consider diagnosis of refractory status epilepticus. Look for a cause and for metabolic complications and review therapy. Arrange for continuous bedside electroencephalographic (EEG) monitoring. If seizures persist, administer rectal paraldehyde (0.3 ml/kg/dose) or, in selected cases, rectal or intravenous valproic acid (15–20 mg/kg loading dose). High-dose phenobarbital therapy or the use of continuous intravenous midazolam hydrochloride infusion (0.1–0.4 mg/kg/hr) may be considered. Anticipate the need for pentobarbital-sodium-induced coma or general anesthesia, consult anesthesia team, and start preparations. Review all laboratory data.
6. Undertake pentobarbital-sodium-induced coma (2–8 mg/kg loading dose followed by 1–2 mg/kg hourly) until burst suppression on EEG is established and maintained. Aim to maintain pentobarbital sodium blood levels between 25 and 30 mg/liter. Maintain cardiovascular support with vasopressors as needed. Slow the rate of infusion every 2–4 hrs to determine whether seizures have stopped.
7. If seizure control is well achieved, reverse pentobarbital-sodium-induced coma gradually, while maintaining adequate therapeutic levels of phenytoin and phenobarbital. Attempt pentobarbital sodium withdrawal 72 hrs after achieving adequate seizure control; judge its necessity every 12–24 hrs. Introduction of valproate sodium or carbamazepine via nasogastric tube to maintain seizure control may be considered.
8. At all times in refractory status epilepticus, the prevention and control of infections, nutritional support, and excellent nursing are important.

become necessary. When higher doses of phenobarbital are required, cardiovascular functions must be closely monitored and additional cardiovascular support (e.g., inotropic agents) provided if necessary.

As soon as the laboratory results become available, appropriate treatments for metabolic and electrolytic abnormalities (hypocalcemia, hypoglycemia, hyponatremia, and hypernatremia) should be administered. Furthermore, if an infectious cause of SE is suspected, antimicrobial therapy should be initiated as soon as possible. Diagnostic imaging and lumbar puncture should be performed only after the patient has been stabilized. If seizure activity continues even after treatment with benzodiazepines, phenytoin, and phenobarbital, the patient is considered to have RSE and may require pentobarbital-sodium-induced coma for further management. This treatment should always be undertaken in a pediatric intensive care unit with invasive hemodynamic monitoring and continuous EEG monitoring.

Refractory Status Epilepticus

Some of the factors that contribute to RSE include inadequate drug therapy, medical and metabolic complications, encephalitis, metabolic acidosis, intractable epilepsy, and the presence of a large cerebral lesion (tumor, hematoma). In the management of RSE, particular attention should be paid to metabolic acidosis, electrolyte imbalance, hyperpyrexia, and fluid therapy. At all times, adequate ventilation should be maintained by tracheal intubation and, if necessary, by assisted ventilation and neuromuscular blockade (e.g., with pancuronium bromide or vecuronium bromide). Several approaches appear to be effective in terminating RSE when conventional drug therapy fails. Continuous bedside EEG monitoring of RSE patients should become part of the standard care. The following steps are helpful in drug therapy.

*First-Line Drugs*

A round of previously used first-line drugs is a reasonable step. Seizure control by administration of high doses and repeated boluses of phenobarbital (15–20 mg/kg) aimed at achieving a very high therapeutic level (30–120 mg/ml) has been successfully reported [17]. Repeated doses of lorazepam may also sometimes be helpful. We do not advocate the use of a continuous intravenous diazepam infusion.

*Second-Line Drugs*

**Paraldehyde** [20].    Rectal administration of paraldehyde is frequently effective, with peak concentrations achieved in 20–30 minutes without any major complications. The drug may be repeated every 4–6 hours to a maximum of four to six doses in a 24-hour period. Neither an intravenous nor an intramuscular route of administration should be used. Administer a dose of 0.3 ml/kg diluted 2 to 1 in oil (olive or cottonseed).

**Valproic Acid** [21].    When valproic acid is given rectally or by nasogastric tube, therapeutic blood levels can be rapidly achieved to control RSE. Rectally, valproic acid at 20–25 mg/kg per loading dose is reasonably well absorbed and reaches peak levels 2–4 hours after administration. Valproate sodium syrup is diluted 1 to 1 with tap water and administered as retention enema. Doses of 10 mg/kg can be given every 6–8 hours thereafter, with a careful monitoring of blood cell count, platelet count, liver functions, and valproic acid blood levels.
    Intravenous valproate sodium (Depacon, Abbott Laboratories) [22] may be used when oral administration is not feasible or rapid elevation of valproate concentration is necessary. The pharmacokinetics of intravenous valproate sodium is similar to that of the oral forms. Experience with its use has been more extensive in Europe than in the United States. The same precautions regarding oral valproate should be applied to the intravenous form.

**Carbamazepine** [23].    Nasogastric administration of carbamazepine is often effective in rapidly achieving therapeutic blood levels. The dose administered is

10–30 mg/kg per loading dose followed by maintenance doses of 10–30 mg/kg in divided doses.

Both valproic acid and carbamazepine may be beneficial as adjuncts when major drugs have failed to control generalized tonic-clonic and complex partial status. They are particularly useful when frequent breakthrough seizures have continued despite administration of maximal doses of first-line drugs. However, one should expect delay in onset of action of these drugs compared with intravenously administered first-line drugs. Significant sedative effects, hyperammonemia, and hepatotoxicity should not be overlooked.

**Midazolam Hydrochloride.**    Reports [24–26] have indicated that continuous intravenous infusion of midazolam hydrochloride can be effective in treating RSE when other measures have failed. The drug has rapid onset of action, but its effects are of short duration (1–5 hours). The dose administered for continuous intravenous infusion is 0.05–0.10 mg/kg per loading dose and then titration as needed to 0.2–0.4 mg/kg per hour. The drug is tapered once seizures are under control, usually within 48–72 hours. Significant sedative effects due to its metabolites preclude its use for a longer duration of therapy.

**Anesthetics.**    Lidocaine, isoflurane, and thiopental sodium have been effective in controlling RSE. However, currently they are not commonly used. Intravenous administration of lidocaine can itself cause seizures. Isoflurane and thiopental sodium are both rapid-acting, and their effects wear off quickly; therefore, they do not adequately sustain seizure control. Recent reports describe the use of propofol in the management of SE [27]. Propofol is an intravenously administered alkylphenyl anesthetic agent that has two main advantages: its potency and rapid onset of action with a short duration of effects. Initial loading dose is 2 mg/kg.

**Pentobarbital Sodium** [18].    High-dose intravenous pentobarbital sodium therapy is one of the standard therapies for RSE [9,12,18,19,27,28]. This drug reduces tonic-clonic seizure activity promptly and flattens EEG seizure discharges. However, the duration of action and efficacy are somewhat limited. The benefits include the ease of administration, its ameliorating effects on intracranial pressure, the ability to monitor the dosage, and the ease of reversing treatment. Cerebral metabolism is also reduced during high-dose pentobarbital sodium therapy. Disadvantages of this drug include its short duration of action and severe cardiorespiratory depression, and the high rate of recurrence of seizures. The duration of therapy and adjustment of dosage are guided by continuous bedside EEG monitoring and clinical seizure control. Pentobarbital sodium is given as a bolus of 2–8 mg/kg for loading followed by 1–2 mg/kg per hour until a therapeutic level of 25–30 mg/liter is achieved. This level usually produces burst suppression on the EEG, but achieving a burst-suppression pattern does not ensure that seizures will not occur. Blood levels should be monitored frequently. In addition to tracheal intubation and mechanical ventilation, continuous hemodynamic monitoring is necessary. Hypotension may require the use of vasopressors. In high doses, pentobarbital sodium may cause pulmonary edema and ileus. The optimal duration of pentobarbital sodium coma is uncertain. However, transition from high-dose barbiturate withdrawal may be attempted 72 hours after satisfactory seizure control is achieved. We withdraw pentobarbital sodium slowly, reducing the dose every 12–24 hours while maintaining an adequate level of phenytoin and phenobarbital. The transition can be further aided in certain situations by introducing valproate sodium or carbamazepine delivered by nasogastric tube to maintain seizure control. The time over which this transition can be accomplished depends on the duration of SE, pre-existing brain disease, the cause of the seizures, and concurrent medical complications. For example, in some cases of encephalitis, several weeks of therapy may be required.

**Pyridoxine (Vitamin B₆)** [29].   In any young infant with a developmental disability and refractory generalized tonic-clonic SE of unknown etiology, an intravenous infusion of 100–200 mg pyridoxine (vitamin B₆) may be considered to cover the possibility of pyridoxine-dependent epilepsy. Continuous bedside EEG monitoring is essential. A successful response is characterized by prompt abolition of epileptic activity on EEG.

In summary, prompt and aggressive management of the child with SE is likely to reduce both morbidity and mortality. The strategy should include the following four goals: ensure adequate cardiorespiratory function, abolish seizure activity, maintain seizure control, and diagnose and treat the underlying cause.

## REFERENCES

1. Epilepsy Foundation of America. Treatment of convulsive status epilepticus statement: recommendation of the Epilepsy Foundation of America's working group on status epilepticus. JAMA 1993;270:854–859.
2. Ramsey RE. Treatment of Status Epilepticus. Annual Course Syllabus of Status Epilepticus. Hartford, CT: American Epilepsy Society, 1991.
3. Treiman DM. Status epilepticus: current opinion. Crit Care 1996;1:104–110.
4. Hauser WA. Status epilepticus: epidemiologic considerations. Neurology 1990;40(suppl 2):9–13.
5. Lothman E. The biochemical basis and pathophysiology of status epilepticus. Neurology 1990;40(suppl):13–23.
6. Meldrum B. Metabolic factors during prolonged seizures and their relation to nerve cell death. Adv Neurol 1983;34:261–275.
7. Maytal J, Shinnar S, Moshe SL, Alvarez LA. Low morbidity and mortality of status epilepticus in children. Pediatrics 1989;83:323–331.
8. Phillips SA, Shannahan RJ. Etiology and mortality of status epilepticus in children: a recent update. Arch Neurol 1989;46:74–76.
9. Roberts MR, Eng-Courquin J. Status epilepticus in children. Emerg Med Clin North Am 1995;13:489–507.
10. Giang DW, McBride MC. Lorazepam versus diazepam for the treatment of status epilepticus. Pediatr Neurol 1984;4:358–361.
11. Crawford TO, Mitchell WG, Snodgrass SR. Lorazepam in childhood status epilepticus and serial seizures. Neurology 1987;37:190–195.
12. Tunik MG, Young GM. Status epilepticus in children. Pediatr Clin North Am 1992;39:1007–1030.
13. Camfield CS, Camfield PR, Smith E, Dooley JM. Home use of rectal diazepam to prevent status epilepticus in children with convulsive disorders. J Child Neurol 1989;4:125–126.
14. Leppick TE, Boucher BS, Wilder BJ, et al. Pharmacokinetics and safety of phenytoin prodrug given IV or IM in patients. Neurology 1990;40:456–460.
15. Wilder BJ. The use of parenteral antiepileptic drugs and the role for fosphenytoin. Neurology 1996;46(suppl):S1–S2.
16. Morton LD, Rizkallah E, Pellock JM. New drug therapy for acute seizure management. Semin Pediatr Neurol 1997;4:51–63.

17. Crawford TO, Mitchell WG, Fishman LS, Snodgrass SR. Very high dose phenobarbital for refractory status epilepticus. Neurology 1988;38:1035–1040.
18. Mirski MA, Williams MA, Hanley DF. Prolonged pentobarbital and phenobarbital coma for refractory generalized status epilepticus. Crit Care Med 1995;23:399–404.
19. Lockman LA. Treatment of status epilepticus in children. Neurology 1990;40:43–46.
20. Curless RH, Holzman BH, Ramsey RE. Paraldehyde therapy in childhood status epilepticus. Arch Neurol 1983;40:477–480.
21. Snead OC, Miles MV. Treatment of status epilepticus in children with rectal sodium valproate. J Pediatr 1985;106:323–325.
22. Giroud M, Gras D, Escousse A, et al. Use of injectable valproic acid in status epilepticus. Drug Invest 1993;5:154–159.
23. Miles MV, et al. Rapid loading of critically ill patients with carbamazepine suspension. Pediatrics 1990;86:263–267.
24. Rivera R, Segnini M, Baltodano A, Peter V. Midazolam in the treatment of status epilepticus in children. Crit Care Med 1993;21:991–994.
25. Parent JM, Lowenstein DH. Treatment of refractory generalized status epilepticus with continuous infusion of midazolam. Neurology 1994;44:1837–1840.
26. Kumar A, Bleck TP. Intravenous midazolam for the treatment of refractory status epilepticus. Crit Care Med 1992;20:483–487.
27. Runge JW, Allen FH. Emergency treatment of status epilepticus. Neurology 1996;46(suppl):820–823.
28. Kinoshita H, Nakagawa E, Iwasaki YJ, et al. Pentobarbital therapy for status epilepticus in children. Pediatr Neurol 1995;13:164–168.
29. Neil Gordon. Pyridoxine dependency: an update [annotation]. Dev Med Child Neurol 1997;39:63–65.

# 29
# Management of Acute Intracranial Hypertension (Increased Intracranial Pressure)

Kalpathy S. Krishnamoorthy

The sustained and prolonged elevation of intracranial pressure (ICP), or intracranial hypertension, has a catastrophic effect on the respiratory and vasomotor centers, causing a failure of brain stem functions. It is important to note that an increase in intracranial pressure frequently may not be detected by clinical examination alone. When intracranial pressure rises acutely and rapidly (i.e., there is acute brain swelling), the clinical changes include bradycardia, shallow respirations, widening of the pulse and pressure, and rapid alteration in mental status. In addition, ipsilateral or bilateral motor posturing and pupillary dilation may occur. In contrast, a patient with a gradual and generalized increased ICP, such as in pseudotumor cerebri, is likely to present with headache, nausea, vomiting, and papilledema. It is important to keep in mind that papilledema is not always a consistent finding when there is an acute rise of ICP. Prompt recognition and treatment of raised ICP increases survival and may improve neurologic outcome.

## ETIOLOGY

Some of the important conditions that may be associated with intracranial hypertension in children are as follows:

1. Severe head injury
2. Hypoxic-ischemic encephalopathy
    a. Cardiorespiratory arrest
    b. Near drowning
3. Metabolic encephalopathy
    a. Hepatic failure
    b. Diabetes mellitus
    c. Inborn error of metabolism (e.g., urea-cycle disorder/hyperammonemia)
    d. Organic acid disorders (e.g., maple syrup urine disease)

4. Intracranial infections and complications
   a. Bacterial meningitis
   b. Viral meningoencephalitis
   c. Subdural empyema
   d. Cerebral abscess
5. Tumor
6. Vascular disorder
   a. Arterial occlusion
   b. Venous sinus thrombosis

Cerebral edema is usually classified into vasogenic, cytotoxic, and interstitial edema, according to its pathogenesis. Disruption of the blood-brain barrier is the foundation of vasogenic cerebral edema. The increased capillary permeability allows intravascular fluid to enter brain interstitial fluid. Vasogenic edema is typically encountered in head trauma, bacterial meningitis, brain abscess, tumor, hypertensive encephalopathy, and lead poisoning. In cytotoxic cerebral edema, intracellular water is increased, as is the potential of water in the brain intercellular compartment, in order to maintain osmotic equilibrium between intracellular fluid and the plasma.

Severe traumatic brain injury is by far the most common condition associated with intracranial hypertension aside from central nervous system infections and hypoxic-ischemic encephalopathy. Significant intracranial hypertension is not frequently encountered in the first 72 hours after a hypoxic-ischemic event, however. Even after circulation and oxygenation are restored, significant neuronal damage may continue to occur in hypoxic-ischemic encephalopathy. Increased ICP, cerebral edema, excessive accumulation of cytosolic calcium, and damage from oxygen-derived free radicals are some of the proposed mechanisms of hypoxic-ischemic neuronal injury [1].

## DIAGNOSIS

Once increased ICP is clinically suspected, computed tomographic (CT) brain scan is an important diagnostic test for diffuse and localized cerebral swelling. CT scanning remains the initial diagnostic imaging modality of choice; it allows rapid diagnosis of the majority of head injuries as well as the evaluation of other causes of intracranial hypertension. However, magnetic resonance imaging is useful in the subacute and chronic stages to assess brain stem and white matter shearing injuries. CT scans help to identify intracranial pathology and provide accurate information on surgically amenable lesions, midline position, intracranial hemorrhage, ventricular size, and cerebral edema. The presence of hypodense areas, poor gray-white differentiation, small compressed ventricles, midline shift, and compression of the basal cisterns are all typical findings seen with cerebral swelling. CT scans do not, however, provide direct information on the intracranial pressure or blood flow dynamics.

## MONITORING OF INTRACRANIAL PRESSURE

In certain clinical settings, ICP monitoring has enabled physicians to evaluate and manage ICP promptly. However, ICP monitoring is not a substitute for a careful neurologic examination. ICP monitoring offers the benefit of allowing the changes in ICP to be correlated with various therapeutic interventions in the management. ICP monitoring measures ICP gradients and serves as an index to determine cerebral perfusion; thus, it is useful in preventing cerebral herniation and ischemia. ICP monitoring can also be used to guide therapy to minimize the multiple risks that accompany the treatment modalities for intracranial hypertension.

## Indications for Intracranial Pressure Monitoring

The selection of patients for ICP monitoring should be based on both clinical and radiographic evaluation. The most common indication for ICP monitoring is unresponsiveness in any child with a closed head injury and a score of less than 8 on the Glasgow Coma Scale or less than 5 (i.e., not following commands) on the Glasgow Coma Motor Scale. In severe traumatic brain injury, the occurrence of intracranial hypertension is very high in the acute stage. Lowering of ICP in such situations has not been definitely associated with improved outcome, even though there is a wide body of evidence to support the role of ICP monitoring [2]. Those patients with severe head injury who show CT scan findings of diffuse injury and compression of cisterns with midline shift of more than 5 mm would be considered candidates for ICP monitoring. Any patient with a moderate head injury and an abnormal CT scan who is not available for close neurologic examination is a potential candidate for monitoring.

Diffuse cerebral swelling that causes elevation of ICP in selected metabolic encephalopathies (hepatic failure, hyperammonemia, diabetic coma) is an indication for the measurement of ICP. Other selective indications include certain forms of meningoencephalitis, such as herpes simplex and equine virus encephalitis. In postoperative patients, after evacuation of a hematoma, and when craniotomy closure is difficult, ICP monitoring may be indicated, especially when diffuse cerebral swelling is anticipated. Another possible indication for ICP monitoring is uncertainty of neurologic findings when a clinical examination cannot be performed because of the use of muscle relaxants or anesthetics in a patient at high risk for increased ICP. Rapid and unexplained neurologic deterioration in a patient at potential risk for elevated ICP with high airway pressure would be an important indication for prophylactic monitoring of ICP, provided a repeat CT scan is performed to rule out a new or recurrent surgical lesion. The enthusiasm for monitoring ICP in cases of global and severe hypoxic-ischemic encephalopathy has greatly diminished, because the prognosis in these patients is uniformly poor. The benefits and risks of the procedure must be taken into consideration before ICP monitoring is undertaken.

## Measurement of Intracranial Pressure

The concurrence of the attending neurosurgeon and the intensivists, along with the availability of a team of trained intensive care physicians and nursing personnel, is a prerequisite for ICP monitoring. The use of a ventricular catheter connected to an external strain gauge transducer is the most reliable method for ICP monitoring [3,4]. This method also allows therapeutic cerebrospinal fluid (CSF) drainage. Minimal CSF drainage of a few milliliters through a ventricular catheter often dramatically reduces ICP. Parenchymal catheter-tip pressure-transducer devices, subarachnoid or subdural fluid-coupled devices, and epidural ICP devices are also used. In our unit, a fiberoptic parenchymal or subdural catheter-tip device (Camino No. 110-4C) is often used rather than the ventricular catheter. Practices vary in different centers. Under the direction of a trained neurosurgeon, the pressure device is inserted in the operating room or, rarely, at the bedside in acute emergencies. The pressure device is usually left in place for 5–7 days. Pressure is transduced with the patient in a 30-degree head-up position with the transducer level with the external auditory canal. The pressure device must be kept strictly sterile. To confirm patency, the pressure wave must be apparent on the oscilloscope and must respond to venous occlusion or abdominal pressure.

Ventricular cannulation can be successfully accomplished even in patients with ventricular effacement, characterized by significantly reduced ventricular size (often referred to as *slit ventricles*) [3,4]. Complications of ICP device use include infection, hemorrhage, malfunction, obstruction, and malposition. However, none of these complications produces any long-term morbidity in patients. The incidence of malfunction or obstruction of ICP devices ranges from 6.3% to 16% [5,6]. In maintaining an optimal ICP monitoring system, it is important to calibrate, monitor for infection, and check fluid-coupled devices for obstruction. Interested readers can refer to articles describing the procedure for the placement of ventricular catheters for ICP monitoring [3,4]. Once an ICP monitor is inserted, treatment is directed toward controlling ICP; specifically, a cerebral perfusion pressure (CPP) level between 60 and 70 mm Hg is a most reasonable goal, and such perfusion should be established and maintained in the management of intracranial hypertension. This goal should be accomplished after CT imaging and any necessary surgical procedure.

## Normal and Abnormal Measurements

An ICP of less than 10 mm Hg is considered normal, while an ICP of up to 15 mm Hg is considered tolerable. An ICP greater than 15 mm Hg should be considered abnormal. Intracranial hypertension is generally defined as an ICP greater than 20 mm Hg. A spontaneous and sudden elevation of ICP to greater than 20 mm Hg for more than 3 minutes (plateau wave) is a dangerous signal heralding possible herniation and ischemia. An elevation of ICP of any magnitude associated with pupillary dilation and bradycardia should alert the physician to the need for urgent intervention with appropriate therapy. Once intracranial hypertension is documented, prompt therapy must be initiated to prevent secondary cerebral ischemia. Increases in pressure must be interpreted in the context of the clinical situation. Treatment to lower ICP is usually initiated when ICP is in the range of 15–30 mm Hg, depending on the individual situation [2]. When there is a pressure of 20–25 mm Hg lasting longer than 30 minutes, it is essential to initiate measures to lower ICP.

## GENERAL MEASURES

A team approach, in which physicians and nurses in an intensive care unit work in harmony with neurologists and neurosurgeons, is very important for treating ICP.

It is critical to maintain an adequate airway and adequate ventilation and circulation. When it is necessary to intubate the patient, the procedure should be performed under adequate anesthesia to protect the brain from secondary damage caused by acute rises in ICP that may be associated with laryngoscopy. The same applies to comatose patients as well. One of the goals of therapy is to safeguard cerebral perfusion and prevent secondary cerebral ischemia. Maintaining an adequate systemic mean arterial pressure (mBAP) at all times helps to ensure adequate cerebral perfusion. CPP is the critical variable influencing brain perfusion. CPP is the difference between mBAP and ICP (CPP = mBAP – ICP). CPP is an important clinical indicator of cerebral blood flow (CBF). Maintaining adequate CBF requires an elevated minimal CPP. The generally accepted range for CPP is about 70 mm Hg; optimally, it should be higher than 60 mm Hg. In order to maintain circulatory volume, a large majority of patients require pressors to elevate mBAP sufficiently to meet the CPP range. Positioning the head at a 30-degree elevation is important to maximize jugular venous drainage. The head should be kept in midline. Intensive care techniques should be undertaken to provide adequate ventilation to maintain $pO_2$ greater than 100 mm Hg. Nutritional requirements also should be taken into consideration, especially when the situation becomes subacute or chronic. Appropriate antibiotic coverage should be provided for infections. Electrolyte levels, osmolality, and blood chemistry should be measured frequently. In cases of severe head injury, hypoxia and hypotension should be avoided in order to prevent secondary brain injury. Techniques to monitor the status of cerebral oxygen delivery, such as photoplethysmography and continuous measurement of jugular venous oxygen saturation by fiberoptic catheters placed in the jugular bulb, may be helpful [4].

## SPECIFIC MEASURES

The specific measures discussed below are very helpful in reducing intracranial hypertension, either alone or in combination. A summary of the medical management of ICP is provided in Table 29.1. The management of increased ICP consists of a combination of treatment modalities executed by the team based on the individual clinical situation and the experience of the consultant.

## Hyperventilation

The cerebral vasculature is exquisitely sensitive to acute changes in $pCO_2$. A traditional cornerstone of the treatment of cerebral edema used to be prolonged prophylactic hyperventilation to reach $pCO_2$ levels of 25–28 mm Hg. Carbon dioxide tension is an important factor that directly influences vascular tone and ICP. Hyperventilation reduces ICP by causing arterial vasoconstriction and an overall decrease in the intracranial arterial compartment [4]. However, the vasoconstrictive effects of hyperventilation eventually diminish, usually within 48 hours, because renal compensatory mechanisms respond to the induced respiratory alkalosis. At this point, cerebral arterioles return to their normal state of vascular tone, so that increased hyperventilation is required if a similar level of vasoconstriction is desired [7]. The potential deleterious effects of severe hyperventilation should not be underestimated. Therefore, aggressive and prolonged hyperventi-

*Table 29.1*   Medical management of intracranial hypertension

| | |
|---|---|
| Positioning | Head elevation 30 degrees, at midline |
| Adequate oxygenation | Circulation, ventilation |
| Neuromuscular blockade | Pancuronium bromide, 0.1 mg/kg/dose; repeat as needed |
| | Vecuronium, 0.1 mg/kg/dose |
| Hyperventilation* | $pCO_2$ at 30–35 mm Hg |
| Fluid restriction | 1,200 ml/M² daily maintenance IV fluids ($D_5$ in 0.45% saline) |
| | Serum osmolality at 310–320 mOsm/liter |
| | Urine output 1.0 ml/kg/hr |
| | Serum sodium 140–150 mEq/liter |
| Hypertonic solutions* | Mannitol 0.25–0.50 g/kg IV boluses per dose every 2–4 hrs |
| | Discontinue mannitol when desired osmolality of 300–310 mOsm/liter is achieved and use as needed |
| Temperature control | Maintain normal or slightly decreased temperature with cooling blanket and antipyretics; rarely, hypothermia to 32°C |
| Anesthetics, narcotics, and sedatives | IV morphine, 0.1 mg/kg/hr |
| | IV midazolam hydrochloride, 0.4 mg/kg loading dose; 0.1 mg/kg/hr maintenance dose |
| | IV fentanyl, 3–10 μg/kg/hr |
| Barbiturates* | IV pentobarbital sodium, 5 mg/kg loading dose; 2–5 mg/kg/hr maintenance dose |
| Diuretics | Furosemide, 0.5–1.0 mg/kg IV bolus in selected situations |
| Corticosteroids | IV dexamethasone, 0.5 mg/kg in 4 divided doses in selected situations |
| Seizure control | IV phenytoin (Dilantin), 10–20 mg/kg loading dose; 5 mg/kg/day maintenance dose |
| | IV phenobarbital, 10–20 mg/kg loading dose; 5 mg/ kg/day maintenance dose |
| | IV diazepam, 0.2–0.4 mg/kg/dose |

*See text for specific indications.

lation of several days' duration with $pCO_2$ levels often reaching the low 20s (mm Hg) is not currently recommended as the first line of therapy for intracranial hypertension or as prophylactic therapy for severe head injury [8]. Evidence based on abnormalities in cerebral blood flow and metabolism that result from traumatic brain injury and other causes of cerebral edema suggests that prophylactic severe hyperventilation therapy might exacerbate secondary brain injury and can cause decrease in cerebral blood flow without a concomitant reduction in ICP [8]. However, this form of therapy is clearly indicated when there is acute neurologic deterioration or when intracranial hypertension is refractory to sedation, paralysis, CSF drainage, and osmotic diuretics [7,9]. In some situations, short-term use of hyperventilation is very helpful and is indicated, as when a patient with acute neurologic deterioration is awaiting an emergent CT scan procedure or is on the way to the operating room for surgery to evacuate a large intracranial mass, or when there is an impending cerebral herniation. Except in these circumstances, the $pCO_2$ should be maintained at the lower end of the normal range (i.e., 35 mm Hg).

## Fluid Restriction

Although fluid restriction has been long advocated for intracranial hypertension and cerebral edema, recently it has been suggested that this restriction has a minimal effect on cerebral edema and results in episodes of hypotension that may decrease ICP and thus affect the neurologic outcome [10]. Administration of hypo-osmolar solutions such as 5% dextrose and water reduces serum sodium and increases brain water in ICP. As a rule, even hypotonic solutions (e.g., 0.45% saline, 5% dextrose, and water) should not be given rapidly in large volumes to patients with intracranial hypertension. Excess free water should be restricted, because these solutions are likely to lower plasma osmolality and drive water across the blood-brain barrier, thereby increasing cerebral water content and ICP. Serum sodium is kept in the range of 140–150 µg/liter. Therefore, therapy in intracranial hypertension must balance the desire for adequate volume against the need to minimize exacerbation of cerebral edema and swelling. An isotonic crystalloid solution, preferably 0.9% saline, is often the first solution to be infused in hypotensive trauma patients [11]. If the initial patient evaluation suggests intracranial hypertension, administration of mannitol may also be appropriate.

It is prudent to keep the hemoglobin concentration greater than 13 g% to provide adequate oxygen delivery. Packed-red-blood-cell transfusion may be indicated for those patients with rising ICP who are not responding to other modalities of management. This treatment allows increased oxygen delivery and limits the blood volume. Routine use of diuretics is controversial in ICP management and is not recommended, but diuretics may be used in some clinical situations.

## Administration of Hypertonic Solutions

Administration of hypertonic solutions (osmotic agents) constitutes the major therapy for reduction of ICP. Mannitol has replaced other diuretics as the agent of first choice for control of ICP. Urea is rarely used now. Osmotic agents create an osmotic gradient between the blood and brain, so that fluid is drawn from the brain into the intravascular space. The risks associated with the use of osmotic agents are severe hyperosmolality and potential rebound rises in ICP. An intact blood-brain barrier is essential for mannitol to be effective. Mannitol is used in the management of intracranial hypertension before hyperventilation is initiated. However, prophylactic use of mannitol is not recommended. Bleeding diathesis is a relative contraindication.

Mannitol crosses the blood-brain barrier rapidly, along with other small molecules in the circulation. Multiple doses may become potentially harmful, however, because mannitol may accumulate in the brain, causing a reverse osmotic shift, raising brain osmolality, and thus theoretically worsening brain ICP by increasing brain swelling. However, this theoretical concern has not been conclusively shown to be valid for humans [12]. This accumulation in the brain is more likely to occur when mannitol stays in the circulation for long periods. Even though the administration of mannitol is a standard practice in the management of acute ICP, mannitol has never been subjected to controlled clinical trials against a placebo [13].

Mannitol has an immediate plasma-expanding effect that reduces the hematocrit level, reduces blood viscosity, increases CBF, and increases cerebral oxygen metabolism and CPP [14–16]. These hemorheologic effects probably explain why mannitol reduces the ICP level within a few minutes following its administration. Theoretically, it should reduce the incidence of delayed secondary ischemic damage [13]. The osmotic effect of mannitol is probably delayed for 15–20 minutes until osmotic gradients can be established between the plasma and the cells. It should be given as a bolus intravenous infusion over 10–30 minutes in doses ranging from 0.25 to 1.00 g/kg of body weight. The ICP-lowering effect of mannitol is better and safer when mannitol is administered in bolus doses than as a continuous infusion. Serum osmolality should be measured frequently after mannitol administration and should be maintained at less than 320 mOsm to avoid renal complications. Mannitol is given in an emergent situation to patients who develop a fixed dilated pupil or neurologic deterioration. The use of large volumes of 0.45% saline solution or 0.45% saline/5.0% dextrose solution over 4–6 hours has been advocated to counteract the hyperosmolar effect of mannitol [13]. The goal during mannitol therapy is still to maintain intravascular volume and to optimize mBAP and maintain high CPP levels.

## Hypothermia Induction

Moderate hypothermia has been shown to produce high levels of cerebral protection in well-established models of global ischemia in brain injury; these results have led to a recent resurgence of interest in the use of moderate systemic hypothermia as a treatment modality for intracranial hypertension, especially following brain injury [17]. The induction of moderate hypothermia (32°C) of 24–48 hours' duration with slow warming in patients with brain injury might enhance neurologic improvement, and the incidence of hypothermia complications is low; the trial testing of this mode of therapy is currently in progress [18].

## Seizure Control

Seizures are dangerous because of their effects on metabolic demands, elements of cerebral blood flow, blood volume, and ICP. Therefore, seizures should be treated aggressively with anticonvulsants. In specific situations in which continuous seizures are suspected in patients who are paralyzed (with muscle relaxants), continuous bedside electroencephalographic (EEG) monitoring should be performed to look for evidence of seizure activity, and any such activity should be treated as needed. Phenytoin is used in the standard loading dose of 10–20 mg/kg; for maintenance, 5 mg/kg is given intravenously divided in two doses. The use of phenytoin does not alter the mental status and allows the neurologic signs and symptoms to be monitored. In treating patients with moderate to severe head injury, we routinely use phenytoin for short-term seizure prophylaxis. In certain situations, benzodiazepines or phenobarbital may be also used to control seizure activity.

## Administration of Sedative and Neuromuscular Blocking Drugs

Sedative and neuromuscular blocking drugs are often used in neurologic intensive management to facilitate care of patients with intracranial hypertension. The use of sedation should be considered as one of the earliest treatment modalities for intracranial hypertension. Neuromuscular blockade is also extremely useful in treating patients whose intracranial hypertension is exacerbated by motor activity that is not adequately controlled by sedation. Although neuromuscular blocking drugs are used as an adjunctive therapy in controlling or limiting intracranial hypertension, delayed emergence of severe weakness in some patients undergoing neuromuscular blockade after prolonged sedation and reports of such effects in the intensive care unit are reasons for caution [19].

Sedatives are used to decrease anxiety and diminish awareness of noxious stimuli. The use of morphine (0.05–0.10 mg/kg per hour), midazolam hydrochloride (0.04 mg/kg loading dose followed by 0.1 mg/kg per hour maintenance dose), and fentanyl (2 µg/kg per dose) has been beneficial in some patients in preventing abrupt elevations of ICP when there are blood pressure fluctuations; during endotracheal intubation, pharyngeal and tracheal suctioning, mechanical ventilation, and bucking on the respirator; and in other situations involving physical stimulation. Neuromuscular blocking drugs (e.g., pancuronium bromide, 0.1 mg/kg per hour or vecuronium bromide, 0.1 mg/kg per dose) given alone may be inadequate; therefore, they are used in combination with opioids or benzodiazepines. Propofol has also been used in patients with severe head injuries, especially before short procedures. Rarely, general anesthesia may be necessary.

## Barbiturate Therapy

In the treatment of intracranial hypertension, high-dose barbiturate therapy has been shown to control ICP and reduce mortality in a small but definite number of patients who are refractory to conventional therapy. Barbiturates have been shown to have consistent and measurable effects on several important physiologic variables, including CBF, cerebral metabolic rate of oxygen ($CMRO_2$), brain electrical activity (EEG), and systemic hemodynamic changes [20]. Kassel and colleagues demonstrated that administration of barbiturates induced a 55% reduction in $CMRO_2$ and a 48% reduction in CBF [20]. The ICP-lowering effects of barbiturates have been attributed to several mechanisms. By metabolically reducing CBF requirements, barbiturates directly decrease the blood volume and thus directly decrease ICP. There is less convincing evidence for other mechanisms of action by barbiturates, such as reduction of ICP by increasing cerebral vascular resistance, and lipid peroxidation of neuronal cell membranes by acting as free-radical scavengers [21]. There appears to be a dose-dependent barbiturate suppression of EEG activity, and the pattern of EEG burst suppression correlates well with observed maximal metabolic depression [22]. Using electrocerebral silence as the end point with increasing barbiturate doses does not appear to further diminish $CMRO_2$ or CBF [23,24].

Various barbiturates have been advocated for controlling ICP. Pentobarbital sodium has been the most commonly used drug. A loading dose of pentobarbital sodium of 5 mg/kg administered intravenously followed by an infusion of 2–5 mg/kg per hour usually produces a serum concentration of 20–30 mg/liter. All therapeutic regimens have in common the need for both loading and maintenance dosing. No clear correlation has been established between serum pentobarbital sodium level and therapeutic efficacy. The dosage may be increased to the most commonly used end point of barbiturate therapy, which is the EEG pattern of burst suppression, although this is not necessary in the management of ICP. The potential dangers of barbiturate therapy include cardiovascular complications, hypothermia, and infections [22,25]. High-dose barbiturate therapy has no prophylactic role in the management of severe head injury, and it is initiated only to control increased ICP. Severe hypotensive episodes should be anticipated. The administration of intravenous colloids and dopamine hydrochloride may be necessary to maintain mean arterial pressure above 60 mm Hg to ensure adequate control cerebral perfusion.

Some of the other indications for high-dose barbiturate therapy include (1) persistent and sustained elevation of ICP above 20 mm Hg without stimulation, despite adequate trial of hyperventilation and osmotherapy, and (2) ICP elevation to 20 mm Hg or higher that occurs with stimulation (e.g., suctioning), does not respond to mannitol administration or hyperventilation, and does not return to normal within 3–5 minutes after stimulus removal.

## Corticosteroid Therapy

High dosages of steroids have been used to reduce ICP without good evidence of their efficacy [26]. Despite several studies with various dosage schedules, steroid administration does not appear to be effective in patients with high ICP related to head trauma or hypoxic-ischemic encephalopathy (cytotoxic edema). However, focal vasogenic edema due to brain tumors or mass lesions responds well to high dosages of steroids.

## CONTINUATION AND WITHDRAWAL OF THERAPY

ICP is considered to be stabilized successfully when there is adequate CPP without dangerous rises in ICP or deterioration of neurologic signs. All necessary therapeutic measures are usually continued for at least 72 hours and for at least 24 hours after the last significant rise in ICP. ICP monitoring is usually continued for 5–7 days. Various therapeutic measures should be reduced slowly, starting with discontinuation of hyperventilation, barbiturates, opioids, and mannitol. Withdrawal of therapy is accomplished gradually, with the most recently instituted therapy usually withdrawn first. Recurrence of ICP elevation requires resumption of therapy for another 24 hours. Frequent assessment of neurologic functions should be performed by the neurologic consultant during these critical hours of therapy discontinuance. Sporadic elevations of ICP to greater than 30 mm Hg may still occur due to the patient's responsiveness. The child withdrawing from prolonged barbiturate-induced coma or fentanyl may exhibit disturbing withdrawal symptoms, such as tremor, agitation, delirium, or visual hallucinations, and these symptoms may persist for days to weeks. Usually they do not require therapy; however, if the symptoms are severely distressing, longer acting benzodiazepines may be helpful. Once the patient shows signs of awakening, the clinical examination is more reliable, and all modalities of therapy may be withdrawn. If uncontrollable intracranial hypertension persists and adequate cerebral perfusion cannot be maintained or the clinical course suggests irreversible deterioration, then the neurologic consultant and intensivist in charge must consider the possibility of brain death using standard criteria.

To summarize, patients who are clinically suspected of brain swelling and intracranial hypertension should be treated vigorously. Mannitol should be used first. Hyperventilation is used in cases of acute deterioration as indicated by pupillary signs, posturing, or changes in vital signs. When hyperventilation is initiated, the $pCO_2$ should be maintained in the range of 30–35 mm Hg to ensure a minimal associated risk of ischemia. Excessive hyperventilation should be avoided, because a decrease in cerebral blood flow below the ischemic threshold may occur. Repetition of CT scanning should be considered at any point at which ICP control becomes difficult. High dosages of barbiturates have a distinct role in the management of refractory intracranial hypertension. The combined use of hyperventilation and mannitol administration is important in situations in which there is impending cerebral herniation as well as ventriculostomy and CSF drainage. Decompressive craniectomy as a surgical procedure has a role in rare situations. Thus, the management of ICP consists of a combination of treatment modalities that are executed based on the individual clinical situation and the experience of the team of consultants.

# REFERENCES

1. Kochanek PM, Uhl MW, Schoettle RJ. Hypoxic-Ischemic Encephalopathy: Pathophysiology and Therapy of the Postresuscitation Syndrome in Children. In BP Fuhrman, JJ Zimmerman (eds), Pediatric Critical Care. St. Louis: Mosby–Year Book, 1992;637–652.
2. Lang EW, Chesnut RM. Intracranial pressure and cerebral perfusion pressure in severe head injury. New Horiz 1995;3:400–409.
3. Ghajar J. Intracranial pressure monitoring techniques. New Horiz 1995;3:395–399.
4. Ghajar J, Hariri R. Management of pediatric head injury. Pediatr Clin North Am 1992;39:1093–1125.
5. Mayhall C, Archer N, Lamb A, et al. Ventriculostomy-related infections: a prospective epidemiologic study. N Engl J Med 1984;310:553–559.
6. North B, Reilly P. Comparison among three methods of intracranial pressure recording. Neurosurgery 1986;18:730–732.
7. Marion DW, Firlik A, McLaughlin MR. Hyperventilation therapy for severe traumatic brain injury. New Horiz 1995;3:439–447.
8. Mulzelaar JP, Marmaron A, Ward JD, et al. Adverse effects of prolonged hyperventilation in patients with severe head injury: a randomized clinical trial. J Neurosurg 1991;75:731–739.
9. Chestnut RM. Medical management of severe head injury: present and future. New Horiz 1995;3:581–593.
10. Zornow MH, Prough DS. Fluid management in patients with traumatic brain injury. New Horiz 1995;3:488–498.
11. Shapira Y, Artru AA, Qassam N, et al. Brain edema and neurologic status with rapid infusion of 0.9% saline or 5% dextrose after head trauma. J Neurosurg Anesthesiol 1995;7:17–25.

12. Kaufman AM, Cardozo E. Aggravation of vasogenic cerebral edema by multiple dose mannitol. J Neurosurg 1992;77:584–589.
13. Bullock R. Mannitol and other diuretics in severe neurotrauma. New Horiz 1995;3:448–452.
14. Mendellow AD, Teasdale GM, Russell T, et al. Effect of mannitol on cerebral blood flow and cerebral perfusion pressure in human head injury. J Neurosurg 1985;63:43–48.
15. Mulzelaar JP, Lutz HA, Becker DP. Effect of mannitol on ICP and CBF and correlation with pressure autoregulation. J Neurosurg 1984;61:700–706.
16. Mulzelaar JP, Wei EP, Kontos HA, et al. Mannitol causes compensatory cerebral vasoconstriction and vasodilation in response to blood viscosity changes. J Neurosurg 1983;59:822–828.
17. Clifton GL, Allen S, Beery J, et al. Systemic hypothermia in treatment of brain injury. J Neurotrauma 1992;9:S487–S495.
18. Clifton GL, Allen S, Barrodall P, et al. A phase II study of moderate hypothermia in severe brain injury. J Neurotrauma 1993;10:263–271.
19. Watling SM, Daston JF. Prolonged paralysis in intensive care unit patients after use of neuromuscular blocking agents: a review of the literature. Crit Care Med 1994;22:884–893.
20. Kassell NF, Hitchar PW, Gerk MK, et al. Alterations in cerebral blood flow, oxygen metabolism, and electrical activity produced by high-dose thiopental. Neurosurgery 1980;7:598–603.
21. Smith DS, Rehncrona S, Seiesro BK. Inhibitory effects of different barbiturates on lipid peroxidation in brain tissue in vitro. Anesthesiology 1980;33:186–194.
22. Wilberger JE, Cantella D. High-dose barbiturates for intracranial pressure control. New Horiz 1995;3:469–473.
23. Michenfelder J. The interdependence of cerebral functional and metabolic effects following massive doses of thiopental in the dog. Anesthesiology 1974;41:231–236.
24. Smith A. Barbiturate protection in cerebral hypoxia. Anesthesiology 1977;47:285–293.
25. Neuwelt EA, Kikuchi K, Hill SA, et al. Barbiturate inhibition of lymphocyte function. Differing effects of various barbiturates used to induce coma. J Neurosurg 1982;56:254–259.
26. Dearden NM, Gibson JS, McDowall DC, et al. Effect of high-dose dexamethasone on outcome from severe head injury. J Neurosurg 1986;64:81–88.

# 30
# Pediatric Cardiology and Cardiac Surgery

Adré J. du Plessis

Children with congenital heart disease (CHD) form one of the largest inpatient populations in major pediatric centers. Each year approximately 30,000 infants are born with some form of CHD; half of them will require surgery in the first year of life [1]. Neurologic dysfunction is one of the most common extracardiac complications of heart disease in children and may be related to the underlying heart defect or to its surgical repair. In addition, cardiac and neurologic dysfunction may both occur as complications of other inherited or acquired disorders.

While a broad spectrum of mechanisms may underlie the neurologic injury seen in pediatric heart disease, the most common final pathway is hypoxia-ischemia/reperfusion (HI/R) injury related to the exquisite demands of the brain for a constant supply of oxygen and glucose. Children with CHD are at risk for both global cerebral hypoperfusion (e.g., cardiac arrest) and focal vaso-occlusive disease (e.g., cardiogenic stroke). Both the mechanisms and clinical profile of neurologic injury in this population have undergone major changes in recent years, largely as a result of dramatic advances in infant cardiac surgery. In the past, the neurologic complications of CHD were related in large part to the effects of chronic cyanosis, polycythemia, and right-to-left shunts. Because repeated palliative surgery often preceded final repair, the exposure to such factors was often prolonged and the neurologic effects cumulative [2].

Surgical advances have facilitated definitive anatomic repair of CHD at ever younger ages, and in many centers neonatal repair has become commonplace. These developments have had several important consequences for neurologic outcome in this population. This earlier surgical repair has decreased the exposure to the chronic risk factors mentioned above; on the other hand, there has been a paradoxical increase in the prevalence of other forms of neurologic injury. Many of the previously lethal congenital heart conditions that present with shock and acidosis in the newborn period are now amenable to early correction. Increasing numbers of these infants are surviving only to manifest the long-term neurologic consequences of neonatal hemodynamic compromise. Furthermore, this surgical advance into the newborn period has been facilitated by support techniques such as deep hypothermic circulatory arrest and low-flow cardiopulmonary bypass, techniques with their own inherent risk for neurologic injury. Consequently, the striking increase in survival of infants with severe CHD has been accompanied by the emergence of a population in whom cardiac morbidity has been exchanged for chronic, often lifelong, neurodevelopmental dysfunction.

This discussion is divided into two parts and reviews (1) the perioperative complications of cardiac surgery and catheterization and (2) the nonoperative neurologic issues in children with heart disease. The latter section includes a discussion of inherited and acquired conditions with clinical profiles that combine cardiac and neurologic manifestations. Because in this era of CHD management neurologic complications appear to manifest most commonly in the perioperative period, these are discussed first.

## NEUROLOGIC COMPLICATIONS RELATED TO CARDIAC SURGERY

The perioperative period is of particular importance to the neurologist for a number of reasons. Preoperatively, the hemodynamic instability experienced by many of these infants predisposes to cerebrovascular injury. Such injury not only challenges the neurologist's diagnostic skills but also raises complex management issues. It is estimated that up to 25% of children undergoing open heart surgery develop neurologic complications in the early postoperative period [3]. In addition, the multiple factors influencing cerebral hemodynamics and metabolism during the perioperative period are complex, dynamic, and poorly understood, a situation that limits the formulation of informed management strategies. Furthermore, the widespread use of sedating and paralyzing agents in the early postoperative period makes this a particularly challenging time for neurologic bedside diagnosis. Finally, the efficacy of future neuroprotective "rescue" therapies will be critically dependent upon early and accurate diagnosis within the window of therapeutic opportunity. Early postoperative neurologic dysfunction is likely, in most cases, to be the result of intraoperative HI/R injury, presumably sustained during periods of low-flow cardiopulmonary bypass or total deep hypothermic circulatory arrest. Such periods of attenuated perfusion are required for intracardiac repair, particularly in young infants, and occur under the protective cover of techniques such as deep hypothermia that are aimed at suppressing cerebral metabolism. Despite current neuroprotective strategies, an unacceptable incidence of postoperative neurologic dysfunction persists [4–6]. The risk for brain injury extends into the early postoperative period, when disturbances in cerebral perfusion and intrinsic vasoregulation [7–9] may occur in the setting of postoperative cardiorespiratory instability.

Finally, the often-transient acute course of early postoperative neurologic complications led to the notion that these manifestations were prognostically insignificant; this notion has been challenged by more rigorous long-term follow-up studies [5]. As the long-term impact of these early complications becomes clear, neurologists are likely to be called on with increasing frequency

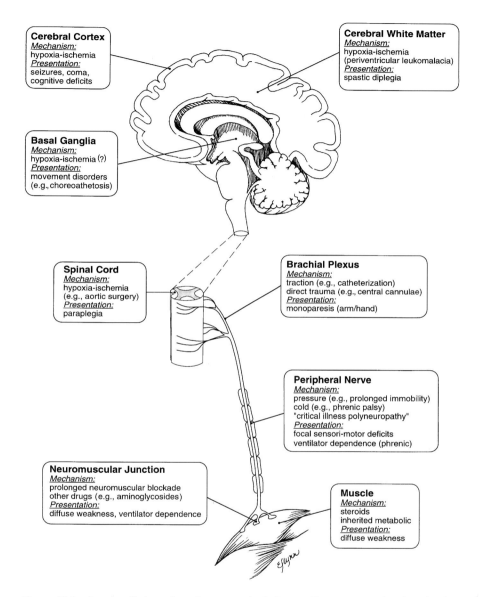

*Figure 30.1* Levels of injury along the neuroaxis during cardiac surgery and catheterization.

to evaluate and treat these often challenging conditions. Intraoperative and post-operative injury to the nervous system may be sustained at any level of the neuroaxis (Figure 30.1). A detailed discussion of the entire spectrum of neurologic manifestations is beyond the scope of this chapter. What follows is a discussion of the more common clinical issues facing the child neurologist in this setting.

### Preoperative Neurologic Complications: Cerebrovascular Disease

In the newborn population overall, cerebrovascular disease constitutes one of the principal forms of neurologic injury. The premature infant is at particular risk for intraventricular-periventricular hemorrhage (IVH-PVH), as well as ischemic injury, particularly periventricular leukomalacia (PVL). Possibly as a consequence of the associated hemodynamic instability, the risk period for cerebrovascular injury characteristic of premature infants (i.e., IVH-PVH and PVL) [10] appears to extend further into maturity in infants with CHD. For instance, cranial ultrasonography has demonstrated IVH-PVH in 24% of full-term infants with CHD [11], while autopsy studies have demonstrated an increased incidence of PVL [12,13]. Furthermore, in infants with CHD, this cerebrovascular injury appears to have an antenatal onset in many cases [11]. Certain cardiac lesions—such as the hypoplastic left heart syndrome, with its inherent hemodynamic instability [12], and coarctation of the aorta, with its associated intracranial vascular malformations and hypertension—may present particular risk for cerebrovascular injury [10,14].

The diagnosis of cerebrovascular disease in the newborn with CHD complicates surgical planning. In these infants, the use of anticoagulation, the increase in fibrinolytic activity [15], and the marked changes in cerebral perfusion pressure during cardiopulmonary bypass may predispose to extension of IVH-PVH or hemorrhagic transformation of ischemic lesions. As the advances in neonatal cardiac surgery extend the surgical procedures to smaller and less mature infants, these difficult diagnostic and management issues will increasingly challenge clinicians.

Currently these decisions are made without the benefit of prospective outcome data. However, similar dilemmas have confronted clinicians using extracorporeal membrane oxygenation (ECMO). The ECMO experience has shown that infants with minor subependymal hemorrhages are at minimal risk for extension of hemorrhage [16,17]. Most centers, however, consider IVH, and particularly intraparenchymal hemorrhage, to be contraindications to ECMO. Differences in anticoagulation and perfusion pressure changes make a direct extrapolation of the ECMO experience to neonatal cardiac surgery difficult. The timing and management of cardiac surgery in infants with IVH-PVH should attempt to balance the risks of extending the IVH-PVH during cardiac surgery against the risks of HI/R injury and further hemorrhagic extension during the persistent cardiorespiratory instability associated with uncorrected heart disease. This decision should consider the severity of the cardiac illness, the expected complexity of the surgery, and the severity of the intracranial hemorrhage. Hemorrhage confined to the subependymal region should not delay surgery. In infants with IVH, it is probably advisable to delay cardiopulmonary bypass for at least 1 week and preferably longer for those with intraparenchymal hemorrhage. The use of antifibrinolytic and proteinase-inhibiting agents [18,19] to decrease the risk of further hemorrhage during cardiopulmonary bypass (CPB) has not been investigated. The indications for cranial ultrasonography and management guidelines used in our cardiac intensive care unit for infants with IVH-PVH are summarized in Table 30.1.

*Table 30.1* Neonatal intracranial hemorrhage: diagnosis and management in newborn infants with congenital heart disease

*Indications for preoperative cranial ultrasound (CUS)*
 Birth weight under 1,500 g
 Evidence of coagulopathy
 Clinical neurologic dysfunction
 Hemodynamic instability with metabolic acidosis
 High-risk cardiac diagnosis (e.g., hypoplastic left heart syndrome; coarctation of the aorta)

*Timing of cardiopulmonary bypass in the newborn with intracranial hemorrhage*

| Intraventricular-periventricular hemorrhage | Cardiac morbidity | Surgical postponement |
|---|---|---|
| Subependymal | Any degree | No delay |
| Intraventricular | Mild or moderate | Delay for 1 wk |
| | Critical | No delay; CUS surveillance |
| Intraparenchymal | Mild or moderate | Delay for >1 wk |
| | Critical | No delay; CUS surveillance |

## Early Postoperative Neurologic Complications

### Delayed Recovery of Consciousness

Inappropriately delayed recovery of mental status following cardiac surgery, anesthesia, and postoperative sedation is a common indication for neurologic consultation. Such patients should be evaluated according to the well-established diagnostic and therapeutic guidelines for stupor and coma [20]. In most cases of postoperative mental status depression, no clear cause is established, although many of these infants ultimately demonstrate features compatible with HI/R injury. In the acute setting, a number of other specific causes should be excluded. Postoperative hepatic or renal impairment may result in the accumulation of toxic metabolites or in impaired metabolism or excretion of sedating drugs. Prolonged use of neuromuscular blocking agents may be associated with delayed recovery of motor function [21–23] (see below), which in more severe cases may mimic a state of impaired consciousness. This condition may be excluded at the bedside with a peripheral nerve stimulator or more formal nerve conduction studies. As discussed in the next section, a significant minority of infants develop postoperative seizures, which may recur serially and are often clinically silent [4]. A persistent depression of consciousness warrants consideration of occult seizures or a prolonged postictal state.

### Postoperative Seizures

Seizures are probably the most common neurologic complication of infant open heart surgery and are clinically manifest in up to 15% of cases in the early post-

operative period [4,24,25]. More recently, prospective long-term videoelec-
troencephalographic (video-EEG) monitoring has demonstrated a significantly
higher incidence of electrographic seizure activity in this early postoperative period,
frequently without typical behavioral seizure manifestations [4].

Etiologically, postoperative seizures may be divided into (1) seizures with a
readily identifiable cause, and (2) seizures of unknown cause. Although postoperative seizures may have many causes, of most concern are seizures resulting from
HI/R injury, due to either generalized cerebral hypoperfusion or focal vaso-occlusive disease. More commonly, however, these early postoperative seizures remain
cryptogenic and are often referred to as *postpump seizures*. Although these postpump seizures are often assumed to be HI/R in origin, they differ in several respects
from other forms of post-HI/R seizure. First, these seizures are typically later in
onset than, for instance, those occurring after birth asphyxia. Whereas the majority of asphyxial seizures commence within the first 12 hours after birth, the onset
of postpump seizures is most commonly during the second postoperative 24 hours.
Second, although the prognosis for postpump seizures may be less benign than previously believed [5], it is nonetheless significantly better than the prognosis for
asphyxial seizures, which leave up to 50% of infants with neurologic disability
[26–28]. The delayed onset of these postpump seizures and their more favorable
outcome may reflect a beneficial modulating effect of intraischemic hypothermia
during the cardiac operation, which may provide partial protection [29].

Postpump seizures follow a fairly typical clinical course and appear to be confined to a relatively narrow time window. After their onset, usually between 24
and 48 hours postoperatively, these seizures tend to occur serially and often
evolve to status epilepticus. The tendency toward further seizures persists for several days and then appears to decrease rapidly.

The clinical manifestations of these electrographic seizures depend on the
presence of sedating and paralyzing drugs. However, even in the absence of such
medications, clinical manifestations are often minimal, and may be confined to
paroxysmal changes in autonomic function and pupillary size. Convulsive activity, when evident, is often focal or multifocal. Bedside EEG is a useful diagnostic technique for several reasons. First, it distinguishes true epileptic phenomena
from other behavioral or autonomic changes [30,31]. Second, EEG can guide the
level of anticonvulsant drug therapy required, because it continues to detect
seizure activity even after this activity becomes clinically inapparent. Finally,
highly focal EEG abnormalities may reflect an underlying stroke and hence may
indicate the need for neuroimaging.

The following therapeutic approach is based on the typical clinical course of
postpump seizures. First, in view of the tendency toward repeated seizures and
status epilepticus, an initial goal is the rapid achievement by an intravenous
route of therapeutic levels of anticonvulsant drugs. At the same time, reversible
causes such as hypoglycemia, hypomagnesemia, and hypocalcemia should be
identified and corrected [32,33]. The vast majority of postoperative seizures are
controlled by the anticonvulsant drug strategy outlined in Figures 30.2 and
30.3. A particular concern for the infant after cardiac surgery is the potential car-
diotoxicity of several major anticonvulsant drugs. Although this issue has not
been addressed prospectively, the potential for underlying myocardial or rhythmic disturbances necessitates careful cardiorespiratory monitoring, particularly
during the induction phase of anticonvulsant drug therapy. In infants with established myocardial dysfunction, cautious administration of phenobarbital is

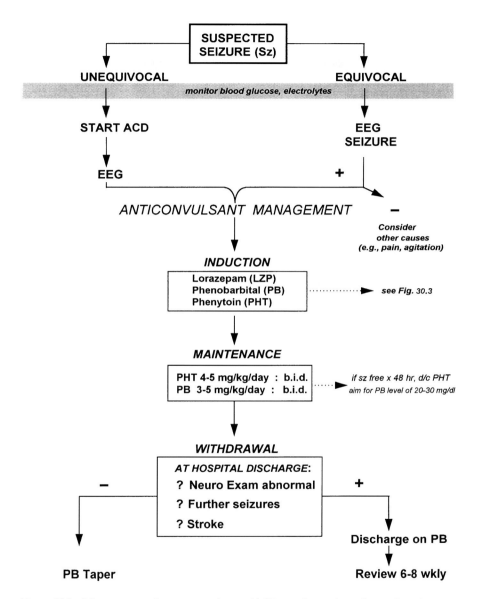

*Figure 30.2* Management of postpump seizures. (ACD = anticonvulsant drugs; d/c = decrease; EEG = electroencephalogram.)

advisable, while pre-existent conduction disturbances, particularly bra-dyarrhythmias, require careful use of phenytoin [34]. Once seizures have been successfully controlled for several days, anticonvulsant drug therapy may be reduced to monotherapy. The apparently circumscribed window of susceptibil-ity to these postpump seizures allows successful withdrawal of anticonvulsant

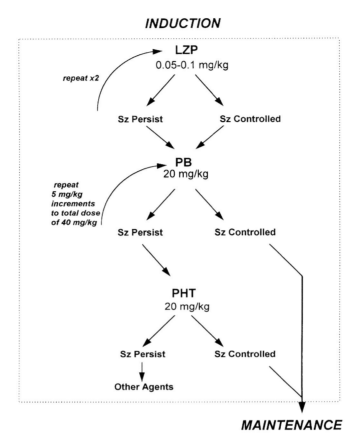

*Figure 30.3* Treatment of postpump seizures. (LZP = lorazepam; Sz = seizure; PB = phenobarbital; PHT = phenytoin.)

drugs before hospital discharge in many cases. Guidelines for anticonvulsant drug withdrawal are given in Figure 30.2.

The prognosis for postoperative seizures depends on the underlying cause. Seizures without an obvious cause (e.g., postpump seizures) were previously considered benign and of no prognostic significance. However, a recent prospective study using continuous video-EEG demonstrated a significant correlation between postoperative seizures and worse neurodevelopmental outcome at age 1 year [5]. None of these infants developed epilepsy by age 1 year (Newburger, personal communication), a finding that supports earlier reports [25]. Therefore, in most cases of cryptogenic postpump seizure, early discontinuation of anticonvulsant therapy may be considered. Rarely, after more intractable postpump seizures, West's syndrome may develop [35], and in these cases developmental delay, cerebral palsy, and epilepsy are likely.

Among those infants with an identified cause for their postoperative seizures, long-term outcome is related to etiology. For instance, cerebral dysgenesis may present with seizures in the early postoperative period, and here the long-term outcome is generally poor, with epilepsy a common sequel. Patients whose seizures have stroke as an underlying cause have a 19–28% risk for subsequent epilepsy [36,37]. Within this group, the epilepsy risk relates to age at the time of stroke and the latency to first seizure following the stroke. In the newborn, the risk for subsequent epilepsy is low [38], while longer latency to first seizure is associated with greater incidence of epilepsy [36]. These features may assist long-term anticonvulsant therapy decisions.

## Movement Disorders

Soon after the advent of deep hypothermic cardiac surgery, reports of striking movement disorders began to appear in the literature [39,40], and approximately 100 cases have been described [39,41–51]. The incidence of movement disorders in these case series has ranged from 0.5% [52] to 19.0% [48]. However, it is likely that these dyskinesias are underdiagnosed and underreported, so that a true incidence is difficult to ascertain. Despite their relative rarity, these movement disorders are often dramatic, frequently intractable, and, particularly in severe cases, associated with a substantial mortality. While choreoathetosis is the most frequent form of dyskinesia complicating cardiac surgery, other movement disorders have been described, including oculogyric crises [53] and parkinsonism [54].

These postoperative movement disorders follow a relatively typical clinical course. The involuntary movements are preceded in most cases by a latency period of 2–7 days during which there is an apparently uncomplicated neurologic recovery from surgery. The dyskinesia is usually heralded by a subacute onset of delirium, with marked irritability, insomnia, confusion, and disorientation, followed soon thereafter by the emergence of abnormal involuntary movements. These movements commence in the distal extremities and orofacial muscles and progress proximally to involve the girdle muscles and trunk; in severe cases violent ballismic thrashing may develop. The abnormal movements are present during wakefulness, peak with distress, and resolve during periods of sleep, brief as these may be. In addition, an apraxia of oculomotor and oromotor function develops, with a loss of feeding and expressive language skills. A supranuclear ophthalmoplegia becomes apparent; voluntary gaze is lost, but reflex extraocular movements are spared. This occurrence often leads to concerns of blindness, because the infants do not look at parents or caretakers and show minimal facial signs of recognition. The onset of involuntary movements is usually followed by a period of deterioration lasting about 1 week, a plateau period of 1–2 weeks during which the movements remain relatively constant, and, finally, a recovery phase, which is more variable in duration.

Diagnosis of these postoperative hyperkinetic syndromes is essentially clinical, and adjunct neurodiagnostic tests have been useful only insofar as they exclude other disorders. Neuroimaging studies, including computed tomographic (CT) scans and magnetic resonance imaging (MRI), have shown nonspecific changes, most commonly diffuse cerebral atrophy. Focal abnormalities are rare [41–44]. Single photon emission computed tomography (SPECT) functional brain-imaging studies have shown a high incidence of both cortical and subcortical perfusion defects, even in the absence of structural defects on CT scans and MRI [55]. EEG studies are most commonly normal or show diffuse slowing; ictal activity is not seen during these movements. Autopsy studies of these patients are limited and the neuropathology inconsistent [49,56]; findings range from normal to extensive degrees of neuronal loss and gliosis, particularly focused in the external globus pallidus [56]. Typical features of infarction are characteristically absent.

The mechanisms underlying these movement disorders that follow cardiac surgery have remained elusive. While HI/R injury has been implicated by many, the neuropathologic features are not characteristic of this mechanism. Recent data from an animal model of cardiopulmonary bypass has suggested that deep hypothermia may modify the topography and evolution of HI/R injury [57,58]. A relatively distinct form of selective neuronal necrosis was described, with the globus pallidus being a region of vulnerability [57,58]. Data from a rodent model suggest a transient expression of glutamate receptors in the globus pallidus during development [59].

The prognosis for these conditions depends largely on their initial severity. Mild cases tend to resolve within weeks to months, while more severe cases have an associated mortality approaching 40% and a high incidence of persistent neurodevelopmental deficits in survivors [41]. Only about 10% of survivors among the severe cases demonstrate normal neurologic outcome [41]. Common residual deficits include generalized hypotonia, developmental delay, and expressive language impairment. However, these reports are anecdotal, and detailed long-term follow-up remains lacking in these patients.

Despite the lack of a unifying mechanism for these dyskinesias, a number of risk factors have been identified. At particular risk are children with cyanotic CHD, particularly those with (1) systemic-to-pulmonary collaterals from the head and neck, (2) age at surgery older than 9 months, and (3) excessively short cooling periods before attenuation of intraoperative blood flow. Some authors have even implicated deep hypothermia itself as a cause [51]. Of note, there have been several reports of postoperative dyskinesias in the setting of prolonged use of fentanyl and midazolam hydrochloride. These drug-related dyskinesias tend to be relatively mild and to resolve over a period of weeks [60–62].

The pursuit of preventive and effective management strategies for these movement disorders has proved as frustrating as the search for an etiology. In response to the risk factors identified in the previous paragraph [41], specific changes have been made in the management of CHD at Boston Children's Hospital, including earlier corrective surgery, careful attention to systemic-to-pulmonary collaterals, gradual cooling, and decreased use of deep hypothermic circulatory arrest. Since these changes were instituted, there has been a marked decline in the incidence of postoperative dyskinesia [52].

Management of these postoperative dyskinetic syndromes remains a difficult and stressful task for parents and caretakers. The essential management goals should address the delirium, the involuntary movements, and the increased nutritional demands. The delirium is often severe, with profound irritability and insomnia. General measures should include decreasing the level of external stimuli (e.g., noise, light) and internal stimuli (e.g., pain). Sedation should be used judiciously and should aim to restore the fragmented sleep-wake cycle. Reducing the level of agitation also decreases the intensity of involuntary movements. Consistently effective pharmacologic control with agents specifically directed at the dyskinesia remains elusive. Medications effective against other forms of hyperkinetic movement disorders have proved largely ineffective against these postoperative dyskinesias. The wide spectrum of agents described highlights our current ignorance of the neurochemical disturbances underlying these conditions. Such agents have included dopamine-receptor blockers (phenothiazines and butyrophenones), dopamine-depleting agents (reserpine, tetrabenazine), dopamine agonists (L-dopa), gamma-aminobutyric-acid–stimulating agents (benzodiazepines, barbiturates, baclofen), and other agents including valproic acid, carbamazepine, phenytoin, diphenhydramine hydrochloride, and chloral hydrate. Successful movement control usually has been achieved only at the expense of excessive sedation. In general, mild dyskinesias can be managed during the acute phases by sedating agents alone, such as benzodiazepines and chloral hydrate. For severe dyskinesias, a cautious trial of more specific agents, such as haloperidol, is warranted. If a clear beneficial response is evident, the dose may be increased gradually while the patient is monitored closely for potential cardiac depressant effects of dopamine blockade. However, if sedation becomes evident without a clear decrease in involuntary movements, or if myocardial depression develops, these agents should be replaced by more specific sedating agents, such as clonazepam. The often prominent oromotor dyskinesia impairs feeding and predisposes to aspiration. Nasogastric or even gastrostomy tube feedings may be necessary to meet the high caloric demands of the constant involuntary movements.

## Spinal Cord Injury

Fortunately, spinal cord injury is relatively rare during pediatric cardiac surgery. This complication is most commonly seen after aortic coarctation repair, occurring in 0.4% [63] to 1.5% [64,65] of cases; however, it is not confined to this operation [66]. Injury to the spinal cord during aortic surgery results primarily from a watershed-type cord ischemia. The spinal circulation has end-zone or watershed regions at a transverse, lower thoracic level and at a longitudinal level between the anteromedial supply of the anterior spinal artery and the posterolateral supply of the posterior spinal arteries. Transverse cord ischemia occurs when aortic blood flow is interrupted distal to the subclavian arteries; this interruption results in persistent proximal perfusion through the anterior spinal artery but inconsistent distal cord perfusion through a highly variable collateral supply. Furthermore, the hypertension associated with aortic clamping increases cerebrospinal fluid pressure, further decreasing perfusion pressure to the lower cord. Such intraoperative cord ischemia manifests as postoperative paraplegia, with or without an abnormal thoracolumbar sensory level. While intraoperative monitoring with somatosensory evoked potentials has been advocated, it is not universally used and may be unreliable, because it tests the posterolateral columns rather than the more vulnerable anterior horn cells [67]. Watershed ischemia has been described following birth asphyxia [68] as well as CHD [69] with anterior-posterior spinal artery end-zone injury and selected anterior horn cell loss.

## Brachial Plexus and Peripheral Nerve Injury

The often sustained immobility, both intraoperatively and postoperatively, predisposes to postoperative pressure palsies and traction injuries in children undergoing cardiac procedures. Brachial plexus injury is not uncommon after cardiac catheterization [70], a procedure that requires extreme and sustained abduction of the arm. This complication usually involves the lower plexus and results from neuropraxia, which gradually improves. The upper brachial plexus may be injured by indwelling central venous catheters, particularly those through an internal jugular approach. Recovery after such injury depends on the extent of direct physical trauma to the plexus.

Pressure palsies may occur at any dependent site but are most common in the peroneal and ulnar nerves. Phrenic nerve injury with diaphragmatic palsy is another peripheral neuropathy fairly unique to hypothermic cardiac surgery; it manifests as postoperative ventilator dependence. Phrenic injury is thought to result from the ice packed around the heart or from direct intraoperative transection [71–73]. Bedside neurophysiologic confirmation of this lesion has been described [74,75]. Although most phrenic injuries are transient and presumably neuropraxic in origin, some cases are permanent and require diaphragmatic plication or, in rare instances, diaphragmatic pacing [76].

Generalized peripheral polyneuropathy has been described after prolonged nondepolarizing neuromuscular blockade, a technique widely used for more effective postoperative ventilatory management. Commonly implicated agents include vecuronium bromide, an agent with a relatively less adverse cardiovascular profile, and pancuronium bromide. A number of reports [21,23,77–84] have described a prolonged neuromuscular syndrome following the withdrawal of these agents. The concomitant use of steroids may be an added risk factor [81,82,84]. The neuropathology in these cases is highly variable but may include an axonal motor neuropathy with variable sensory involvement and, in some cases, features of a myopathy [82,83]. Precise differentiation between this condition and so-called critical-illness polyneuropathy [77] may be difficult.

## Delayed Postoperative Neurologic Complications

Many of the acute postoperative complications of cardiac surgery appear to be transient. The long-term sequelae of these acute complications are becoming more appreciated. For example, postpump seizures, for many years considered benign transient events, appear to be significant risk factors for worse neurodevelopmental outcome [5]. Overall, though, there is a glaring lack of prospectively gathered long-term outcome data in this population. This section will focus on two delayed complications of cardiac surgery: stroke and headaches. Clearly, stroke may occur at any time in the preoperative, intraoperative, and early postoperative periods. However, the majority of such events appear to occur remote from surgery and hence are discussed here.

### Cerebrovascular Accident (Stroke)

The incidence of vaso-occlusive stroke in childhood has been found to range from 2.5 [85] to 7.9 [86] per 100,000 children each year. Among the conditions associated with stroke in childhood, CHD is the most common and is present in 25–30% of cases [37,85,87]. Earlier initiation of corrective cardiac surgery has decreased previous risk factors for stroke, such as polycythemia and right-to-left

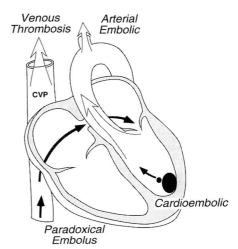

*Figure 30.4* Mechanisms of cardiogenic stroke in childhood cardiac disease. The three principal mechanisms of cerebrovascular occlusive disease associated with cardiac disease are shown: cardioembolic, from an intracardiac thrombotic source; paradoxical, from a systemic venous source with a cardiac anatomy that permits direct access to the systemic arterial system; and cerebral venous thrombotic, due to elevated central venous pressure (CVP) and polycythemia.

shunt. Autopsy reports from earlier studies demonstrated an incidence of cerebrovascular ischemic lesions in children with CHD of as high as 20% [88,89]; more recent neuropathologic studies are lacking. Stroke of cardiac origin—that is, cardiogenic stroke—has three broad mechanisms (Figure 30.4). First, arterial emboli may be generated from an intracardiac embolic source (*cardioembolic stroke*). Second, emboli may arise from a systemic venous or right heart source and bypass the pulmonary circulation through a right-to-left shunt (*paradoxical embolic stroke*). Finally, *cerebral venous thrombosis* may result from a combination of central venous hypertension, venous stasis, and polycythemia. Risk factors for cardiogenic stroke include Virchow's triad (i.e., altered vascular surface, stasis, and hypercoagulability) and paradoxical vascular pathways.

A number of intraoperative mechanisms may lead to cerebral vaso-occlusive disease. Particulate and gaseous emboli originating from the CPB apparatus or surgical field bypass the normal pulmonary filtration system during CPB and thus enter the systemic circulation directly [90–93]. Improvements in bypass circuits, particularly the switch from bubble to membrane oxygenators, have decreased the incidence of macroembolization [94]; the impact of these advances on the incidence of microvascular disease [95] has not been examined. A further potential mechanism of intraoperative vascular injury relates to the often marked inflammatory response triggered by the extensive and prolonged exposure of bypass blood to artificial surfaces [96–98]. These inflammatory processes in turn trigger complex cascades, including endothelial-leukocyte interactions [99–102].

Establishing the precise timing of stroke presenting in the early postoperative period may be complicated by the widespread use of postoperative sedating and paralyzing agents. At the same time, a number of risk factors may predispose to stroke during this early postoperative period. Vascular stasis, both intracardiac and extracardiac, may result from localized areas of low flow within the heart [103–105] or global ventricular dysfunction. Transient pressure elevations in the right heart and central veins, resulting from postoperative pulmonary hypertension, further slow flow through the right heart chambers. Vascular surfaces may be altered by both injured native tissue and the presence of prosthetic tissue, and when such altered surfaces lie within areas of low flow, the risk of thrombosis increases. A number of these risk factors converge in patients undergoing the Fontan procedure, in many centers the most common operation for CHD with a single ventricle physiology. In a retrospective review of 645 patients who underwent the Fontan procedure, we found a 2.6% incidence of stroke [103]. This stroke risk extends over 3 [103] to 15 [104] years. Stroke in the early postoperative period may present with focal motor weakness and speech and visual dysfunction. Seizures are a particularly common presentation of stroke in young infants [37,106].

Stroke therapy may be broadly considered to encompass preventive and rescue strategies. Rescue strategies include therapies aimed at limiting the extent of stroke by salvaging potentially viable brain. Such therapies may include the use of thrombolytic agents [107,108] or agents directed at biochemical cascades triggered during HI/R insults [109–111]. These rescue therapies are currently confined to adult and experimental trials and are not discussed further here. Preventive stroke management in children is based almost entirely on the experience in adults. Stroke prevention may be regarded as primary (i.e., treatment of high-risk patients to prevent a first stroke); or secondary (i.e., treatment aimed at preventing stroke recurrence) [112]. Many aspects of preventive stroke therapy in adults remain controversial. This debate intensifies in childhood stroke therapy, because both the stroke mechanisms and long-term consequences differ markedly in these two age groups. Furthermore, there have been no prospective therapeutic trials for childhood stroke. Nevertheless, there is consensus regarding certain aspects of primary stroke prophylaxis in children. Specifically, most agree on the use of prophylactic anticoagulant therapy in children with prosthetic heart valves, dilated cardiomyopathy, or intracardiac thrombus on electrocardiography (ECG). Stroke prophylaxis should be individualized and should consider risk factors such as elevated right atrial pressure, intracardiac prosthetic material, and existence of a right-to-left shunt in children requiring prolonged bed rest. As mentioned above, such a constellation of factors may converge after a patient undergoes the Fontan procedure, and low-dose aspirin is now commonly used postoperatively for several months in these patients, particularly those with a "fenestrated" anatomy.

Secondary stroke prophylaxis aims to balance the risk of recurrent embolism and that of hemorrhagic transformation of a bland infarction. In the adult post–myocardial infarction population, the recurrence rate for stroke is approximately 1% per day over the first 2 weeks [113–115]. There is no equivalent documented incidence rate in children following cardiogenic stroke. In adults, the risk for hemorrhagic transformation is particularly high in cardioembolic strokes [116], where such secondary hemorrhage may occur in 20–40% of the cases [116–120]. Although the use of anticoagulant therapy in the setting of stroke remains highly controversial [121], it has been demonstrated that significant clinical deterioration is more likely when hemorrhagic transformation occurs in the presence of anticoagulant therapy [119,120]. While the prediction of subsequent hemorrhagic transformation in individual strokes remains difficult, certain guidelines have been formulated. Seventy percent of strokes that ultimately undergo hemorrhagic transformation do so within the first 48 hours following the onset of cerebral infarction [120]. In addition, large infarcts, particularly those involving an entire cerebral lobe or more than 30% of a hemisphere, appear to be at greater risk for secondary hemorrhage [119,120,122]. Other risk factors for bleeding into stroke include uncontrolled systemic hypertension, stroke due to septic emboli, and cerebral venous thrombosis. Guidelines for anticoagulant therapy are discussed in Chapter 7. Seizures are a common complication of childhood stroke [37,38,106]. Combining anticonvulsant drugs with antithrombotic therapies may result in serious drug interactions. Phenobarbital and carbamazepine tend to decrease the anticoagulant effect of warfarin sodium (Coumadin), necessitating higher warfarin sodium dosages, while phenytoin may either increase or decrease the anticoagulant effect. Consequently, the coagulation profile should be followed closely, particularly after discontinuation of anticonvulsant drug when excessive anticoagulation may occur.

Headache

Headaches in patients with congenital heart disease may originate from a number of possible sources. First, acute severe headache should always raise the question of subarachnoid hemorrhage, particularly in patients with a history of coarctation of the aorta. Headache is the most common presenting feature [123] in the otherwise often subtle clinical presentation of brain abscess. Second, patients with severe polycythemia tend to experience more frequent headaches. Finally, raised central venous pressure such as may be seen in some situations—for example, following the Fontan procedure or the bidirectional Glenn procedure—may result in increased cerebral venous pressure, which by itself may be associated with headaches. Increased central venous pressure may also impair cerebrospinal fluid (CSF) absorption, however, resulting in communicating hydrocephalus [124] with elevated intracranial pressure and headache. Papilledema is a common clinical finding in brain abscess and may also be seen in communicating hydrocephalus. Before the direct measurement of CSF pressure, a brain abscess should be excluded by neuroimaging (MRI or CT scan with contrast), in order to exclude mass effect before a spinal tap is performed.

## NEUROLOGIC COMPLICATIONS OF CARDIAC DISEASE NOT RELATED TO CARDIAC SURGERY

Because the mechanisms and manifestations of neurologic dysfunction may depend on the underlying form of heart disease, the following discussion categorizes cardiac disease as (1) structural congenital heart disease; (2) inherited disease of the heart, brain, and muscle; and (3) acquired heart disease.

### Structural Congenital Heart Disease

The neurologic complications of structural CHD may be developmental, cerebrovascular, or infectious in etiology. Both dysgenetic and cerebrovascular disorders may present in early infancy, while infectious complications tend to occur later in infancy and childhood.

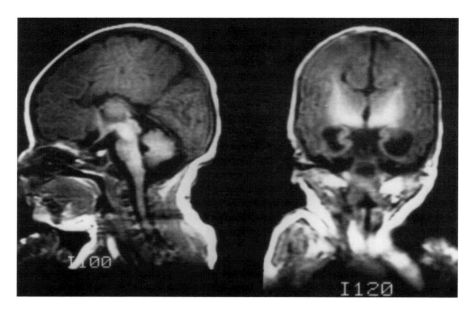

*Figure 30.5*   Brain magnetic resonance image (T1 weighted) of an infant with congenital heart disease (transposition of the great arteries) and dysgenetic brain disease (agenesis of the corpus callosum).

## Cerebral Dysgenesis

The prevalence of brain dysgenesis in children with CHD ranges from 10% to 29% in autopsy studies and may relate to the underlying cardiac lesion [89,125,126] (Figure 30.5). Infants with hypoplastic left heart syndrome may be at particular risk for associated developmental brain lesions, which range in severity from microdysgenesia to gross malformations like holoprosencephaly [125]. With the increasing availability and use of neuroimaging, the association between cardiac and brain dysgenesis is likely to become more clearly defined. Clinically, these dysgenetic lesions may present in the newborn period with seizures, alterations in level of consciousness, and abnormalities in motor tone. Conversely, the lesions may remain clinically occult until later infancy and childhood, when they present with developmental delay, epilepsy, and cerebral palsy. For these reasons, it is important to consider cerebral dysgenesis in any child with CHD and neurologic manifestations.

## Infectious Complications

Children with congenital heart disease are at increased risk for *infectious endo-carditis* (IE) and brain abscess. The neurologic manifestations of IE are protean and include meningitis, brain abscess, seizures, and, most commonly, cerebrovascular injury. Despite modern antibiotic advances, approximately one-third of children with IE develop neurologic complications, approximately half of which are embolic in origin [127]. Cerebrovascular complications are not only the most common form of neurologic injury but also carry the highest mortality, which reaches 80–90% in mycotic aneurysm hemorrhage [128]. The high risk of hemorrhagic transformation of septic infarction or the direct subarachnoid hemorrhage through mycotic aneurysms contraindicates the use of anticoagulant therapy in children with IE and cerebrovascular disease [129] (Figure 30.6).

*Brain abscess* is rare during childhood and in acyanotic forms of CHD [130]. Cyanotic CHD, on the other hand, constitutes a major predisposing factor for brain abscess, particularly in the setting of polycythemia and right-to-left shunt [131]. In earlier reports, the incidence of brain abscess in cyanotic CHD ranged from 2% to 6% [132]. CHD is present in almost one-half of childhood cases of brain abscess [133], with tetralogy of Fallot being the most common underlying CHD lesion. Arterial oxygenation is inversely correlated with the incidence, morbidity, and mortality of brain abscess in CHD [132]; infants with higher oxygen saturations are less likely to develop brain abscess and more likely to recover. Overall, the incidence of brain abscess in CHD has decreased markedly, primarily as a result of earlier corrective surgery and the decreased exposure to polycythemia and hypoxia.

In cyanotic infants with polycythemia, periods of systemic illness and dehydration may critically disturb cerebral microvascular perfusion, producing subsequent localized areas of ischemia. Organisms crossing a right-to-left shunt bypass the pulmonary filtration system and gain direct access to the brain, where they breach the disrupted blood-brain barrier and pass into necrotic areas to form focal septic cerebritis and, subsequently, frank cerebral abscess. Seventy-five percent of brain abscesses are supratentorial, predominantly in the middle cerebral artery territory. Posterior fossa abscesses, while less common, are more dangerous; cerebellar abscesses may remain clinically silent until the onset of a rapid deterioration from tonsillar herniation and brain stem compression. Cerebral abscesses are multifocal in about 20% of cases.

In children with CHD, brain abscess is rare before the age of 2 years; peak incidence is at 4–7 years of age [134]. The clinical manifestations of brain abscess result from a combination of intracranial hypertension, focal neurologic injury, and sepsis. Headache is the predominant and usual presenting symptom. The initial presentation is often subtle and the course slowly progressive. Conversely, when there are complications like seizures, the presentation may be abrupt. The most common symptoms are headache and vomiting, which are present in 50% and 72% of cases, respectively [123]. Fever is absent in up to 75% of cases, and peripheral leukocytosis may be minimal. The cerebrospinal fluid, which should be obtained only after brain imaging excludes significant mass effect, may show elevated protein but often shows only mild leukocytosis. The diagnosis of brain abscess is best confirmed by contrast-enhanced CT scan or MRI. On CT scan, brain abscess presents as an area of hypodensity with contrast ring enhancement; marked cerebral edema often surrounds the abscess. While diagnostic and therapeutic advances have reduced the mortality of brain abscess from 40% [134] to 10% [135], the 35–45% prevalence of neurologic sequelae in survivors has remained largely unchanged [133,135]. Epilepsy develops, often years later, in up to 30% of survivors [133]. This outcome pro-

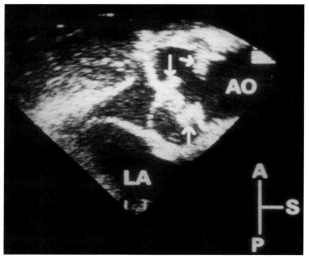

A

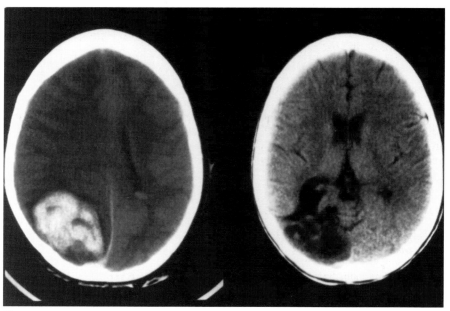

B

*Figure 30.6* (**A**) Echocardiogram showing vegetations (*arrows*) on the aortic valve and sinus of Valsalva. (AO = aorta; LA = left atrium.) (**B**) Computed tomographic brain scan of the same patient showing, on the left, a massive acute intracerebral hemorrhage in the right occipital-parietal region, presumably due to ruptured mycotic aneurysm, and on the right, the large residual cavitation after 3 months.

file has changed little over the past three decades, despite advances in surgical and medical management.

The *optimal management of brain abscess* remains controversial [135]. Surgery is still widely considered the definitive first-line treatment. Whether direct resection or aspiration of the abscess under CT guidance is the preferable surgical approach remains unclear. More recently, advances in both antibiotic therapy and neuroimaging have allowed more conservative, antibiotic management to be monitored closely by brain scans [136,137]. While still controversial, this approach may prove effective, particularly in early cases of focal cerebritis without rapid progression. Whether used in combination with surgery or not, high-dose antibiotic therapy should be maintained for at least 6 weeks. The management of brain abscess is outlined in Table 30.2. Mixed organisms, particularly streptococci (aerobic and anaerobic) and staphylococci, are the most common causative organisms [130]. While earlier initial antibiotic regimens have now been largely superseded by third-generation cephalosporins, together with anti-staphylococcal and antianaerobic agents, subsequent therapy should be guided by culture results, when available. In patients who are immunosuppressed (e.g., after cardiac transplant), other lower virulence organisms as well as fungi (e.g., *Aspergillus*) and parasites (e.g., *Toxoplasma*) should be considered.

Because the clinical presentation of brain abscess closely resembles that of aseptic stroke in up to 30% of cases [138], it has been suggested that children with cyanotic CHD and a stroke-like presentation should be managed with antibiotics until a brain abscess is excluded [138].

## Inherited Disorders of Heart, Muscle, and Nervous System

Combined cardiac and neurologic dysfunction may be seen in a number of inherited disorders of metabolism and neuromuscular degeneration. While these syndromes are generally rare, their early diagnosis is important because some are treatable, and, in some cases, antenatal diagnosis is available. In addition, the phe-

---

*Table 30.2*   Management of brain abscess

---

1. *Surgery*: Aspiration or resection may still be first-line therapy
2. *Pharmacologic therapy*
   a. Antibiotics
      First-line antibiotic regimen should include one agent each from (1), (2), and (3) below:
      (1) Ceftazidine, 50 mg/kg IV every 8 hrs or ceftriaxone sodium, 50 mg/kg IV every 12 hrs
      (2) Nafcillin or oxacillin, 50 mg/kg IV every 6 hrs or vancomycin, 10 mg/kg IV every 6 hrs
      (3) Metronidazole hydrochloride, 15 mg/kg IV loading dose, then 7.5 mg/kg every 6 hrs; once causative organism(s) is isolated, adjust antibiotic regimen on sensitivities
   b. Steroids: if significant mass effect, dexamethazone, 10–12 mg IV loading dose, then 0.25 mg/kg every 12 hrs
   c. Anticonvulsant drugs: Prophylactic treatment with anticonvulsant drugs remains controversial

notype of certain chromosomal disorders may include combined developmental abnormalities of the heart and nervous system. Only the most common of these disorders are discussed here.

## Inborn Errors of Metabolism

Cardiac dysfunction may be a prominent feature of several inherited metabolic disorders [139] and is often the cause of death. The inheritance of these conditions is usually recessive (autosomal, rarely X-linked) or mitochondrial. In general, the cardiac defects are not primarily structural and tend to reflect either myocardial infiltration or energy failure. Manifestations of hypertrophic or dilated cardiomyopathy include myocardial failure, valvular insufficiency, arrhythmias, and coronary insufficiency (in storage disorders) with myocardial ischemia. Because in most cases of infantile hypertrophic cardiomyopathy the cause remains unknown, it is important that these uncommon inherited metabolic causes be excluded by endomyocardial biopsy [140]. The neurologic presentation may be a primary manifestation of the enzyme defect or may be secondary to underlying heart disease accompanied by a global decrease in cerebral perfusion or focal cardiogenic stroke.

### Disorders of Energy Production

*Mitochondrial fatty acid oxidation defects* are a group of autosomal recessive disorders presenting with recurrent, sometimes catastrophic, episodes of hypoketotic hypoglycemia, hyperammonemia, and a Reye's syndrome–like picture, with vomiting and stupor-coma, particularly during periods of fasting and intercurrent infection. Among these conditions are several with prominent cardiac dysfunction, particularly acyl–coenzyme A (CoA) dehydrogenase deficiency and primary systemic carnitine deficiency. The latter condition is caused by a carnitine transporter defect and is the only disorder of *carnitine metabolism* with prominent cardiac dysfunction. Serum levels of carnitine are often very low, and, while L-carnitine supplementation rapidly restores these serum levels, the often severe cardiomyopathy often recovers incompletely. The *acyl-CoA dehydrogenase deficiencies* are a group of disorders in which there is impaired mitochondrial oxidation of short-, medium-, and long-chain fatty acids. Of these conditions, only long-chain acyl-CoA dehydrogenase (LCAD) deficiency is commonly associated with cardiac dysfunction, which results from myocardial fat deposition and is accompanied by cardiomyopathy (hypertrophy or dilatation) and arrhythmias. The liver fat deposition results in a typical microvesicular steatosis. Long-chain hydroxy-acyl dehydrogenase deficiency causes hypertrophic cardiomyopathy. It resembles LCAD deficiency in many respects but has the additional features of severe liver dysfunction and pigmentary retinopathy. *Multiple acyl-CoA dehydrogenase deficiency (glutaric aciduria type II)* may present as a severe, often catastrophic, illness within the first days of life. This neonatal-onset form frequently has other associated dysmorphic features and produces a "sweaty feet" odor. It usually causes death within weeks to months, often from severe cardiomyopathy. Less severe enzyme deficiency presents with episodic vomiting, hypoketonemic hypoglycemia, and lactacidosis. In this form, the characteristic urine and CSF organic acid abnormalities may be present only during periods of decompensation. In addition to cardiomyopathy, infants with this disorder develop an ataxic and dyskinetic syndrome, with caudate and putaminal atrophy on brain imaging due to neuronal loss and gliosis [141].

Management of these mitochondrial fatty acid oxidation defects includes avoidance of fasting and ingestion of frequent high-carbohydrate, low-fat meals. During acute illnesses, intravenous glucose infusions should be used. Medium-chain triglycerides (MCTs) provide a useful caloric source in LCAD deficiency, because they usually enter lipid pathways distal to the enzyme block. This is not the case in glutaric aciduria type II, and MCTs should not be used in this condition. Carnitine supplementation is critical in primary carnitine deficiency; its role in treating the other fatty acid oxidation defects discussed above is unclear.

*Disorders of oxidative phosphorylation* result from enzyme defects in pyruvate metabolism and the mitochondrial electron transport chain and display autosomal recessive, X-linked recessive, or mitochondrial patterns of inheritance. These conditions generally involve multiple systems and are clinically and biochemically heterogeneous. Their clinical presentation, which ranges in onset from the neonatal period to adulthood, most frequently reflects an encephalopathy or myopathy. In certain disorders, cardiac dysfunction is prominent, with myocardial failure or arrhythmias. The age at presentation appears to determine the cardiac features; cardiomyopathy is the primary presentation in early infancy, while cardiac dysrhythmias and conduction defects are the more common cardiac complications in older patients [142]. Furthermore, early-onset cardiomyopathy is usually rapidly progressive and fatal by 2 years of age [142]. The distention of myocytes by mitochondrial accumulation results in concentric hypertrophy of the septum and ventricular walls, especially the posterior wall, without outflow tract obstruction [142]. *Kearns-Sayre syndrome* is a later-onset disorder, usually associated with complex I or complex IV deficiency. It presents with retinal degeneration and chronic progressive external ophthalmoplegia; between late childhood and adulthood, atrioventricular heart block may develop with syncopal spells or sudden death.

Cardiac dysfunction is most commonly seen in certain respiratory chain enzyme defects, specifically complex I (NADH CoQ reductase) [140] and complex IV (cytochrome c oxidase) [143] deficiencies, which often occur in combination [144]. In addition, complex III (reduced CoQ–cytochrome c reductase) deficiency may cause an isolated cardiomyopathy. Cytochrome c oxidase deficiency may present in the newborn or young infant as a severe, rapidly fatal condition or in a benign, reversible form. Initially, the benign form may be indistinguishable from the lethal form; in fact, the lactacidemia may be more severe in the benign form [145]. Because infants with the benign form may recover fully with supportive management, an aggressive approach is warranted until the clinical distinction becomes evident.

The diagnostic evaluation of these respiratory chain defects includes measurement of blood or CSF lactate levels, muscle biopsy to look for ragged red fibers, and enzyme assays on muscle, fibroblasts, or lymphocytes.

Treatment of these disorders includes general measures such as avoidance of extremes in temperature and exercise, and aggressive treatment of infection and dehydration. The existence of Kearns-Sayre syndrome, with its risk of sudden death from cardiac conduction defects, may be an indication for prophylactic cardiac pacing. In addition, a number of more specific approaches have been directed at the likely mechanisms of cellular injury in these conditions (i.e., energy failure with membrane depolarization, calcium influx, generation of free radicals, and lactic acid accumulation) [146]. Agents used in these conditions, often in the form of "cocktails," include free-radical scavengers (vitamins C and E and coenzyme $Q_{10}$), calcium channel blockers, and low-dose steroid therapy and dichloroacetate to decrease lactic acid production. In addition, electron transfer mediators (vitamins $K_3$, C, and $B_2$ or riboflavin) that bridge specific electron transfer chain defects have been used [146,147]. Carnitine supplementation may be appropriate, because a secondary deficiency often develops in these conditions. Details of these therapies are outlined elsewhere [146,147].

## Storage Disorders of the Heart and Nervous System

*Glycogen storage diseases* take on a number of different forms, but combined cardiac-neurologic dysfunction is largely confined to the type II form, or Pompe's disease, an autosomal recessive condition resulting from acid maltase (acid alpha-glucosidase) deficiency. Glycogen is deposited in multiple tissues, including the myocardium, anterior horn cells, and skeletal muscle. Nervous system glycogen deposition is most marked in the spinal cord and brain stem; the cerebral cortical neurons are spared [148]. This disorder has a spectrum of severity that is inversely related to age. The classic severe early infantile form presents with a hypertrophic cardiomyopathy, macroglossia, and diffuse myopathy; there is striking hypotonia and rapidly progressive muscle weakness. Deep tendon reflexes may be absent as a result of the anterior horn cell involvement. Despite the profound weakness, the muscles often appear hypertrophic and firm. With the progressive cardiomyopathy, usually evolving to left ventricular outflow obstruction, and progressive respiratory weakness (due to myopathy and anterior horn cell injury), this condition usually culminates in death due to cardiorespiratory failure before the age of 1 year. Early-onset Pompe's disease may resemble infantile spinal muscular atrophy, but the prominent cardiomegaly and other storage features, such as macroglossia and hepatomegaly, help distinguish these two conditions. Later-onset forms of acid maltase deficiency are slowly progressive and resemble limb-girdle dystrophy. Patients presenting with the disease after age 2 do not have associated cardiac involvement.

The ECG typically shows a short PR interval and large-amplitude QRS complexes. Serum creatine phosphokinase may be elevated up to tenfold. Hypoglycemia is uncommon in Pompe's disease. Diagnosis is supported by the presence of myotonic bursts on electromyography (EMG) and glycogen deposits on muscle biopsy and is confirmed by enzyme assays. Treatment is supportive.

The *lysosomal storage diseases* are autosomal recessive or X-linked diseases that are slowly progressive and may be complicated by hypertrophic or dilated cardiomyopathy. A review of these disorders is beyond the scope of this chapter. Generally, however, the phenotype—which usually includes coarse facial features, hepatomegaly, and corneal clouding—as well as the neurodegenerative process are evident well before the emergence of cardiac failure and arrhythmias. In the mucopolysaccharidoses, myocardial thickening, valvular dysfunction, coronary insufficiency, and pulmonary hypertension may develop. The diagnosis is clinical and is confirmed by enzyme assay. The treatment is supportive.

*Refsum's disease* is an autosomal recessive peroxisomal disorder with abnormal storage of phytanic acid due to a phytanic acid oxidase deficiency. While an infantile form exists and is associated with mental retardation and dysmorphic features, the cardiac complications are seen in the later-onset form and include atrioventricular conduction defects and bundle branch block, progressive cardiac failure, and sudden death. The onset of these cardiac complications is usually some time after the typical development of retinitis pigmentosa, peripheral polyneuropathy, cerebellar ataxia, sensorineural deafness, and elevated CSF protein. The diagnosis is made on the basis of elevated serum phytanic acid levels and fibroblast enzyme diagnosis. Because the stored phytanic acid in these patients is of exogenous origin, dietary exclusion effectively reduces the storage load. During periods of acute deterioration, plasmapheresis may be required.

## Inherited Disorders of Muscle and Nerve with Cardiac Complications

The *X-linked muscular dystrophies* include the *"dystrophinopathies"* of *Duchenne* (DMD) and *Becker* (BMD) (Xp21 locus) as well as *Emery-Dreifuss muscular dystrophy* (Xq28 locus). Both DMD and BMD may be complicated by a dilated cardiomyopathy. The skeletal muscle involvement in these conditions is usually well established years before the cardiac presentation. Patients with more severe, early-onset, and rapidly progressive DMD may develop papillary muscle dysfunction with subsequent valvular (particularly mitral) incompetence, cardiac (mainly atrial) arrhythmias, and myocardial fibrosis. Diagnosis is clinical, electromyographic, and cytogenetic. Genetic analyses have eliminated the need for muscle biopsy in most typical cases. Currently, treatment remains supportive. Although BMD is milder, later in onset, and has slowly progressive skeletal muscle involvement, the cardiac involvement in BMD may be severe and rapidly progressive. Emery-Dreifuss muscular dystrophy presents with slowly progressive muscle weakness and wasting in a humeral-peroneal distribution; there are prominent, early contractures of the heel cords, elbow flexors, and neck extensors. The cardiac involvement in this condition is that of atrial flutter, fibrillation, and permanent atrial paralysis (standstill) in which the entire atrial wall becomes inexcitable. These patients often require pacemakers, which may be lifesaving. Cardiac dysfunction is frequently the cause of death. Two other X-linked forms of dilated cardiomyopathy are of interest because of their relationship to conditions discussed previously. First, a rapidly progressive cardiomyopathy has been described in previously well adolescents; this condition has a gene locus in the same Xp21 region as the dystrophin gene involved in DMD and BMD. Second, an X-linked cardioskeletal myopathy (Barth syndrome) with congenital dilated cardiomyopathy (often with endocardial fibroelastosis), a mitochondrial myopathy, and growth retardation has been described; interestingly, the gene locus is in the same region as that in Emery-Dreifuss muscular dystrophy.

*Myotonic dystrophy* is an autosomal dominant condition with multisystem involvement of skeletal, smooth, and cardiac muscle, as well as cataracts, testicular atrophy, and mental deterioration. The skeletal muscle disease shows prominent neck flexor weakness and wasting, together with grip and percussion myotonia. Although myocardial dystrophic features develop, these are usually mild, and the more important cardiac manifestations involve the conduction system with the development of arrhythmias and heart block. The diagnosis is based on the clinical features and the typical EMG findings of myotonia.

*Friedreich's ataxia* is an autosomal recessive condition that forms part of a wide spectrum of spinocerebellar degenerations. Unlike the muscular disorders discussed above, this condition combines neuropathic and cardiomyopathic processes. The neurologic presentation occurs in childhood and includes gait disturbance, limb and trunk ataxia, areflexia, loss of position sense, and pes cavus. The neurologic disturbances are established well before the onset of cardiac dysfunction, which usually occurs during adolescence or early adulthood. There appear to be two distinct forms of cardiac involvement in this condition: a more common hypertrophic cardiomyopathy and a less common but more serious dilated (dystrophic) cardiomyopathy, in which fatal arrhythmias and heart failure may develop. Ultimately, up to 90% of patients with Friedreich's ataxia develop cardiac involvement, which is often the cause of death.

## Chromosomal Disorders Involving the Heart and Brain

A number of chromosomal disorders may have prominent cardiac and neurologic manifestations. The *trisomies*, particularly those of chromosomes 21, 11, and 18, may have combined cerebral and cardiac malformations as part of their often grossly abnormal dysmorphic phenotypes. About 40% of children with trisomy 21 have associated CHD, most commonly in the form of endocardial cushion defects. The most common neurologic manifestation in these children is cognitive dysfunction; 5% of cases develop epilepsy. Trisomy 13 is associated with ventricular septal defects and patent ductus arteriosus; the associated cerebral dysgenesis in this syndrome is often severe, the most common lesions being holoprosencephaly and agenesis of the corpus callosum. The most common cardiac lesions in infants with trisomy 18 are ventricular septal defects and patent ductus arteriosus, while the cerebral lesions are usually in the form of neuronal migration defects.

Interest has focused on *chromosome 22* because of the association between specific deletions, particularly in the 22q11 region [149], and a variety of cardiac malformation syndromes [150–153]. The acronym CATCH 22 (*c*ardiac defect, *a*bnormal facies, *t*hymic hypoplasia, *c*left palate, *h*ypocalcemia, chromosome *22*q11 deletions) has been used to designate this group of apparently related syndromes. These deletions appear to be of maternal origin in many cases [151], and the resultant syndromes include the DiGeorge syndrome and velocardiofacial (Shprintzen's) syndrome. Both these latter conditions have neurologic or cognitive disturbances [154] in association with structural cardiac defects. The DiGeorge syndrome results from a developmental defect of the third and fourth pharyngeal pouches, with hypoplasia of the thymus and parathyroids, and conotruncal cardiac malformations (interrupted aortic arch type B, truncus arteriosus, and tetralogy of Fallot). The neurologic presentation of these infants often takes the form of hypocalcemic seizures due to hypoparathyroidism. The velocardiofacial syndrome may also present with neonatal hypocalcemia and cardiac malformations, most commonly ventricular septal defects or tetralogy of

Fallot. In addition, these patients have cleft palate or velopharyngeal insufficiency and a typical facial appearance that includes a broad, prominent nose and retrognathia. These children usually present to neurologists with developmental and learning disabilities, and are often hearing and speech impaired. The mean IQ in this syndrome is around 70 [154], and there is often a marked discrepancy between verbal and performance IQs. As children, these patients may demonstrate a peculiar and inappropriately blunt affect [155]; during adolescence and adulthood, there is an increased risk for psychotic illness [156,157]. Structural brain abnormalities, including a small posterior fossa and vermis and small cystic lesions adjacent to the frontal horns of the lateral ventricle, have been described on neuroimaging studies.

Williams syndrome is a relatively rare condition related in most cases to a deletion of the elastin gene on chromosome 7. These patients present with CHD lesions, typical facial features, and social, cognitive, and learning disabilities, as well as gross motor, fine motor, and oromotor dysfunction. The average IQ in this syndrome is about 55. The most frequent cardiac lesions in Williams syndrome are supravalvular aortic stenosis, peripheral pulmonary stenosis, or ventricular/atrial septal defects. These patients also have particular visuospatial and constructional difficulties [158]. Reports have also indicated an increased risk of stroke with associated intracranial arteriopathy [159–161].

## Acquired Heart Disease: Rheumatic Heart Disease

Sydenham's chorea is the major neurologic complication of acute rheumatic fever (ARF) [162] and in earlier years was the most common form of acquired chorea in childhood [163]. There had been a steady decline in the incidence of Sydenham's chorea. This trend was associated not only with a worldwide, decades-long decline in the incidence of ARF but also with a relative decrease in the occurrence of chorea as a complication of ARF [163]. While the reason for this trend is unknown, it possibly relates to an alteration in the virulence or epitopes of rheumatogenic streptococci and a decrease in antigen cross-reactivity with the basal ganglia. Outbreaks of ARF in both the United States [164] and developing countries [165] have once again raised the awareness of this debilitating condition.

Chorea presents during the acute phase of ARF in only 25% of cases [163]. The latency from the onset of ARF to the emergence of chorea ranges from 1 week to 8 months; once established, the chorea persists for 1–6 months [163]. Sydenham's chorea is rare under the age of 3 years and occurs more commonly in girls than in boys. In some cases, chorea may be the only clinical manifestation of ARF.

The onset of this disorder is often subtle, and the abnormal movements tend to be preceded by psychoemotional symptoms such as anxiety, emotional lability, distractibility, the emergence or exacerbation of attention-deficit hyperactivity disorder, obsessive-compulsive symptoms, and sleep disturbances [166]. On occasion, both the psychoemotional prodrome and the dyskinesia may be explosive in onset. The motor activity, which at first is described as "fidgety," soon becomes frankly choreiform, evolving from initial brief, myoclonic-like proximal muscle jerks to more complex, writhing distal movements. The chorea may be asymmetric, and in some cases pure hemichorea develops. Muscle hypotonia and mild to moderate weakness are often present. Speech and oral motor activity are often affected. An explosive dysarthria develops that in severe cases may evolve into complete mutism. Other features include difficulty initiating spontaneous motor activity, an inconsistently sustained grip ("milkmaid's grip"), and motor impersistence. These symptoms usually begin to subside after about 6 months but may recur in the setting of subsequent illnesses, particularly streptococcal infections, pregnancy (chorea gravidarum), or oral contraceptive use.

The diagnosis of this condition is clinical and is based on specific criteria (Jones' criteria) [162]. Additional laboratory findings, such as an elevated antistreptolysin O titer, positive throat cultures for group A beta-hemolytic streptococci, an elevated C-reactive protein, and specific ECG features, may be helpful. Despite the causal relationship with streptococcal infection, the onset of chorea is often delayed; consequently, serologic evidence of streptococcal disease is absent in 25% of cases. Rheumatogenic strains of group A streptococci contain particular (M-type) proteins that share antigenic determinants with neurons in the basal ganglia, particularly in the caudate and subthalamic nuclei. Autoantibodies against these neurons (antineuronal antibodies) have been detected in up to 90% of cases in some studies [166].

The neuropathology of Sydenham's chorea is limited, because the condition is seldom fatal. Neuronal loss with vascular and perivascular inflammatory changes have been demonstrated in the caudate and putamen, as well as the frontoparietal cortex. The topography of these earlier neuropathologic findings has been supported by MRI [167,168] and SPECT [167] scans. These techniques have also demonstrated disturbances in the blood-brain barrier with localized edema, presumably resulting from vasculitis [167].

Management of the dyskinesia is usually accomplished with dopamine-blocking agents, such as haloperidol, 0.5–1.0 mg twice a day, which is maintained for 2–6 months and then gradually withdrawn. Other agents used include carbamazepine and valproic acid [166,169]. While the intensity of the chorea may be diminished by these agents, the effect is often incomplete. In severe cases, prednisone has been used, usually with limited success. Prophylaxis against group A streptococcal infections with penicillin V potassium or monthly intramuscular injections of penicillin G benzathine is recommended, because even asymptomatic future infections may precipitate a recurrence of chorea. Studies have found a high incidence of antineuronal [166] and, more recently, anticardiolipin antibodies [170] in these patients; these findings have led to trials of plasmapheresis and intravenous immunoglobulin therapy.

## REFERENCES

1. Benson D. Changing profile of congenital heart disease. Pediatrics 1989;83:790–791.
2. Newburger J, Silbert A, Buckley L, Fyler D. Cognitive function and age at repair of transposition of the great arteries in children. N Engl J Med 1984;310:1495–1499.
3. Ferry P. Neurologic sequelae of cardiac surgery in children. Am J Dis Child 1987;141:309–312.
4. Newburger J, Jonas R, Wernovsky G, et al. A comparison of the perioperative neurologic effects of hypothermic circulatory arrest versus low-flow cardiopulmonary bypass in infant heart surgery. Am J Dis Child 1993;329:1057–1064.

5. Bellinger D, Jonas R, Rappaport L, et al. Developmental and neurologic status of children after heart surgery with hypothermic circulatory arrest or low-flow cardiopulmonary bypass. N Engl J Med 1995;332:549–555.

6. Ferry P. Neurologic sequelae of open-heart surgery in children: an irritating question. Am J Dis Child 1990;144:369–373.

7. du Plessis A, Newburger J, Jonas R, et al. Cerebral $CO_2$ vasoreactivity is impaired in the early postoperative period following hypothermic infant cardiac surgery. Eur J Neurol 1995;2(suppl 2):68A.

8. Rodriguez R, Austin E, Audenaert S. Postbypass effects of delayed rewarming on cerebral blood flow velocities in infants after total circulatory arrest. J Thorac Cardiovasc Surg 1995;110:1686–1691.

9. Ohare B, Bissonnette B, Bohn D, et al. Persistent low cerebral blood flow velocity following profound hypothermic circulatory arrest in infants. Can J Anaesth 1995;42:964–971.

10. Volpe JJ. Intracranial Hemorrhage. In JJ Volpe (ed), Neurology of the Newborn (3rd ed). Philadelphia: Saunders, 1994;373–463.

11. van Houten J, Rothman A, Bejar R. Echoencephalographic (ECHO) findings in infants with congenital heart disease (CHD). Pediatr Res 1993;33:376A.

12. Glauser T, Rorke L, Weinberg P, Clancy R. Acquired neuropathologic lesions associated with the hypoplastic left heart syndrome. Pediatrics 1990;85:991–1000.

13. Leviton A, Gilles F. Astrocytosis without globules in infant cerebral white matter: an epidemiologic study. J Neurol Sci 1974;22:329–340.

14. Young R, Liberthson R, Zalneraitis E. Cerebral hemorrhage in neonates with coarctation of the aorta. Stroke 1982;13(4):491–494.

15. Giuliani R, Szwarcer E, Aquino E, Palumbo G. Fibrin-dependent fibrinolytic activity during extracorporeal circulation. Thromb Res 1991;61:369–373.

16. Rudack D, Baumgart S, Gross G. Subependymal (grade 1) intracranial hemorrhage in neonates on extracorporeal membrane oxygenation. Clin Pediatr 1994;33:583–587.

17. von Allmen D, Babcock D, Matsumoto J, et al. The predictive value of head ultrasound in the ECMO candidate. J Pediatr Surg 1992;27:36–39.

18. Wilson J, Bower L, Fackler J, et al. Aminocaproic acid decreases the incidence of intracranial hemorrhage and other hemorrhagic complications of ECMO. J Pediatr Surg 1993;28:536–541.

19. Brunet F, Mira J, Belghith M, et al. Effects of aprotinin on hemorrhagic complications in ARDS patients during prolonged extracorporeal $CO_2$ removal. Intensive Care Med 1992;18:364–367.

20. Plum F, Posner J. Multifocal, Diffuse, and Metabolic Brain Diseases Causing Stupor or Coma. In F Plum, J Posner (eds), The Diagnosis of Stupor and Coma (3rd ed). Philadelphia: Davis, 1985; 177–303.

21. Gooch J, Suchyta M, Balbierz J, et al. Prolonged paralysis after treatment with neuromuscular junction blocking agents. Crit Care Med 1991;19:1125–1131.

22. Partridge B, Abrams J, Bazemore C, et al. Prolonged neuromuscular blockade after long-term infusion of vecuronium bromide in the intensive care unit. Crit Care Med 1990;18:1577–1582.

23. Waitling S, Dasta J. Prolonged paralysis in intensive care unit patients after use of neuromuscular blocking agents: a review of the literature. Crit Care Med 1994;22:884–891.

24. Miller G, Eggli K, Contant C, et al. Postoperative neurologic complications after open heart surgery on young infants. Arch Pediatr Adolesc Med 1995;149:764–768.

25. Ehyai A, Fenichel G, Bender H. Incidence and prognosis of seizures in infants after cardiac surgery with profound hypothermia and circulatory arrest. JAMA 1984;252:3165–3167.

26. Volpe JJ. Neonatal Seizures. In JJ Volpe (ed), Neurology of the Newborn (3rd ed). Philadelphia: Saunders, 1994;172–207.

27. Andre M, Matisse N, Vert P. Prognosis of Neonatal Seizures. In C Wasterlain, P Vert (eds), Neonatal Seizures. New York: Raven Press, 1990;61–67.

28. Bergman I, Painter M, Hirsch R, et al. Outcome in neonates with convulsions treated in an intensive care unit. Ann Neurol 1983;14:642–647.

29. Dietrich W, Busto R, Alonso O, et al. Intraischemic but not postischemic brain hypothermia protects chronically following global forebrain ischemia in rats. J Cereb Blood Flow Metab 1993;13:541–549.

30. Scher M, Painter M. Electroencephalographic Diagnosis of Neonatal Seizures: Issues of Diagnostic Accuracy, Clinical Correlation, and Survival. In C Wasterlain, P Vert (eds), Neonatal Seizures. New York: Raven Press, 1990;15–25.

31. Mizrahi E. Neonatal seizures: problems in diagnosis and classification. Epilepsia 1987;28(suppl 1): S46–S55

32. Satur C, Jennings A, Walker D. Hypomagnesemia and fits complicating pediatric cardiac surgery. Ann Clin Biochem 1993;30:315–317.

33. Lynch B, Rust R. Natural history and outcome of neonatal hypocalcemic and hypomagnesemic seizures. Pediatr Neurol 194;11:23–27.
34. Cranford R, Leppik I, Patrick B, at al. Intravenous phenytoin: clinical and pharmacological aspects. Neurology 1978;28:874–880.
35. du Plessis A, Kramer U, Jonas R, et al. West syndrome following deep hypothermic cardiac surgery. Pediatr Neurol 1994;11:246–251.
36. Yang J, Park Y, Hartlage P. Seizures associated with stroke in childhood. Pediatr Neurol 1995;12:136–138.
37. Lanska M, Lanska D, Horwitz S, Aram D. Presentation, clinical course and outcome of childhood stroke. Pediatr Neurol 1991;7:333–341.
38. Levy S, Abroms I, Marshall P, et al. Seizures and cerebral infarction in the full-term newborn. Ann Neurol 1985;17:366–370.
39. Bergouignan M, Fontan F, Trarieux M. Syndromes choreiformes de l'enfant au de cours d'interventions cardio-chirurgicales sous hypothermic profounde. Rev Neurol 1961;105:48–59.
40. Bjork V, Hultquist G. Contraindications to profound hypothermia in open-heart surgery. J Thorac Cardiovasc Surg 1962;44:1–13.
41. Wong P, Barlow C, Hickey P, et al. Factors associated with choreoathetosis after cardiopulmonary bypass in children with congenital heart disease. Circulation 1992;85(suppl II):II 118–II 126.
42. Robinson R, Samuels M, Pohl K. Choreic syndrome after cardiac surgery. Arch Dis Child 1988; 63:1466–1469.
43. Medlock M, Cruse R, Winek S, et al. A 10-year experience with postpump chorea. Ann Neurol 1993;34:820–826.
44. Huntley D, Al-Mateen M, Menkes J. Unusual dyskinesia complicating cardiopulmonary bypass surgery. Dev Med Child Neurol 1993;35:631–641.
45. Donaldson D, Fullerton D, Gollub R, et al. Choreoathetosis in children after cardiac surgery [abstract]. Neurology 1990;40(suppl 1):337.
46. Wical B, Tomasi L. A distinctive neurologic syndrome after profound hypothermia. Pediatr Neurol 1990;6:202–205.
47. Barrat-Boyes B. Choreoathetosis as a complication of cardiopulmonary bypass. Ann Thorac Surg 1990;50:693–694.
48. Brunberg J, Doty D, Reilly E. Choreoathetosis in infants following cardiac surgery with deep hypothermia and circulatory arrest. J Pediatr 1974;84:232–235.
49. Chaves E, Scaltes-Persson I. Severe choreoathetosis (CA) following congenital heart disease (CHD) surgery [abstract]. Neurology 1988;38(suppl):284.
50. Curless R, Katz D, Perryman R, et al. Choreoathetosis after surgery for congenital heart disease. J Pediatr 1994;124:737–739.
51. DeLeon S, Ilbawi M, Arcilla R, et al. Choreoathetosis after deep hypothermia without circulatory arrest. Ann Thorac Surg 1990;50:714–719.
52. Wessel D, du Plessis A. Choreoathetosis. In R Jonas, J Newburger, JJ Volpe (eds), Brain Injury and Pediatric Cardiac Surgery. Boston: Butterworth–Heinemann, 1995;353–362.
53. du Plessis A. Pediatric cardiovascular intensive care: neurologic problems. Prog Pediatr Cardiol 1995;4:135–141.
54. Straussberg R, Shahar E, Gat R, Brand N. Delayed parkinsonism associated with hypotension in a child undergoing open-heart surgery. Devel Med Child Neurol 1993;35:1007–1014.
55. du Plessis A, Treves S, Hickey P, et al. Regional cerebral perfusion abnormalities after cardiac operations. J Thorac Cardiovasc Surg 1994;107:1036–1043.
56. Kupsky W, Drozd M, Barlow C. Selective injury of the globus pallidus in children with post-cardiac surgery choreic syndrome. Dev Med Child Neurol 1995;37:135–144.
57. Redmond J, Gillinov A, Zehr K, et al. Glutamate excitotoxicity: a mechanism of neurologic injury associated with hypothermic circulatory arrest. J Thorac Cardiovasc Surg 1994;107:776–786.
58. Johnston M, Redmond J, Gillinov A, et al. Neuroprotective Strategies in a Model of Selective Neuronal Necrosis from Hypothermic Circulatory Arrest. In M Moskowitz, L Caplan (eds), Cerebrovascular Disease. Boston: Butterworth–Heinemann, 1995;165–174.
59. Greenamyre T, Penney J, Young A, et al. Evidence for transient perinatal glutamatergic innervation of globus pallidus. J Neurosci 1987;7:1022–1030.
60. Bergman I, Steeves M, Burckart G, et al. Reversible neurologic abnormalities associated with prolonged intravenous midazolam and fentanyl administration. J Pediatr 1991;119:644–649.
61. Lane J, Tennison M, Lawless S, et al. Movement disorder after withdrawal of fentanyl infusion. J Pediatr 1991;119:649–651.
62. Petzinger G, Mayer SA, Przedborski S. Fentanyl-induced dyskinesias. Mov Disord 1995;10:679–680.

63. Brewer L, Fosberg R, Mulder G, Verska J. Spinal cord complications following surgery for coarctation of the aorta. J Thorac Cardiovasc Surg 1972;64:368–379.
64. Pennington D, Liberthson R, Jacobs M, et al. Critical review of experience with surgical repair of coarctation of the aorta. J Thorac Cardiovasc Surg 1979;77:217–229.
65. Lerberg D, Hardesty R, Siewers R, et al. Coarctation of the aorta in infants and children: 25 years of experience. Ann Thorac Surg 1982;33:159–170.
66. Puntis J, Green S. Ischemic spinal cord injury after cardiac surgery. Arch Dis Child 1985;60:517–520.
67. Laschinger J, Owen J, Rosenbloom M, Kouchoukos N. Direct noninvasive monitoring of the spinal cord motor function during thoracic aorta occlusion: use of motor evoked potentials. J Vasc Surg 1988;7:161–171.
68. Sladky JT, Rorke LB. Perinatal Hypoxic/Ischemic Spinal Cord Injury. In JT Sladky, LB Rorke (eds), Pediatric Pathology. New York: Hemisphere Publishing Corp, 1986;87–101.
69. Rousseau S, Metral S, Lacroix C, et al. Anterior spinal artery syndrome mimicking infantile spinal muscular atrophy. Am J Perinatol 1993;10:316–318.
70. Lederman R, Breuer A, Hanson M, et al. Peripheral nervous system complications of coronary artery bypass graft surgery. Ann Neurol 1982;12:297–301.
71. Watanabe T, Trusler T, Williams W, et al. Phrenic nerve paralysis after pediatric cardiac surgery. J Thorac Cardiovasc Surg 1987;94:383–388.
72. Mok Q, Ross-Russell R, Mulvey D, et al. Phrenic nerve injury in infants and children undergoing cardiac surgery. Br Heart J 1991;65:287–292.
73. Dunne J, Reutens D, Newman M, et al. Phrenic nerve injury in open heart surgery [abstract]. Muscle Nerve 1991;14:883.
74. Bolton C. Clinical neurophysiology of the respiratory system. Muscle Nerve 1993;16:809–818.
75. Swenson M, Rubenstein R. Phrenic nerve conduction studies. Muscle Nerve 1992;15:597–603.
76. Weese-Mayer D, Hunt C, Brouillett R, et al. Diaphragm pacing in infants and children. J Pediatr 1992;120:1–8.
77. Sheth R, Pryse-Phillips W, Riggs J, Bodensteiner J. Critical illness neuromuscular disease in children manifested as ventilatory dependence. J Pediatr 1995;126:259–261.
78. Heckmatt J, Pitt M, Kirkham F. Peripheral neuropathy and neuromuscular blockage presenting as prolonged respiratory paralysis following critical illness. Neuropediatrics 1993;24:123–125.
79. Kuper Y, Namba T, Kaldawi E, Tessler S. Prolonged weakness after long-term infusion of vecuronium bromide. Ann Intern Med 1992;117:484–486.
80. Segredo V, Caldwell J, Matthay M, et al. Persistent paralysis in critically ill patients after long-term administration of vecuronium. N Engl J Med 1992;20:524–528.
81. Bird S, Mackin G, Schotland D, Raps E. Acute myopathic quadriplegia: a unique syndrome associated with vecuronium and steroid treatment [abstract]. Muscle Nerve 1992;15:1208.
82. Subramony S, Carpenter D, Seshadri R, et al. Myopathy and prolonged neuromuscular blockage after lung transplant. Crit Care Med 1991;19:1580–1582.
83. Danon M, Carpenter S. Myopathy with thick filament (myosin) loss following prolonged paralysis with vecuronium during steroid treatment. Muscle Nerve 1991;14:1131–1139.
84. Benzing G, Iannacone S, Bove K, et al. Prolonged myasthenic syndrome after one week of muscle relaxants. Pediatr Neurol 1990;6:190–196.
85. Schoenberg B, Mellinger J, Schoenberg D. Cerebrovascular disease in infants and children: a study of incidence, clinical features, and survival. Neurology 1978;28:763–768.
86. Giroud M, Lemesle M, Gouyon J-B, et al. Cerebrovascular disease in children under 16 years of age in the city of Dijon, France: a study of incidence and clinical features from 1985 to 1993. J Clin Epidemiol 1995;48:1343–1348.
87. Riela A, Roach E. Etiology of stroke in children. J Child Neurol 1993;8:201–220.
88. Berthrong M, Sabiston D. Cerebral lesions in congenital heart disease. Bull Johns Hopkins Hosp 1951;89:384.
89. Terplan K. Brain changes in newborns, infants and children with congenital heart disease in association with cardiac surgery: additional observations. J Neurol 1976;212:225–236.
90. Moody D, Bell M, Challa V, et al. Brain microemboli during cardiac surgery or aortography. Ann Neurol 1990;28:477–486.
91. Solis R, Kennedy P, Beall A, et al. Cardiopulmonary bypass: microembolization and platelet aggregation. Circulation 1975;52:103–108.
92. Boyajian R, Sobel D, DeLaria G, et al. Embolic stroke as a sequela of cardiopulmonary bypass. J Neuroimag 1993;3:1–5.

93. Padayachee T, Parsons S, Theobold R, et al. The detection of microemboli in the middle cerebral artery during cardiopulmonary bypass: a transcranial Doppler ultrasound investigation using membrane and bubble oxygenators. Ann Thorac Surg 1987;44:298–302.
94. Nussmeier N, McDermott J. Macroembolization: Prevention and Outcome Modification. In M Hilberman (ed), Brain Injury and Protection during Heart Surgery. Boston: Martinus Nijhoff Publishing, 1988;85–108.
95. Fish K. Microembolization: Etiology and Prevention. In M Hiberman (ed), Brain Injury and Protection during Cardiac Surgery. Boston: Martinus Nijhoff Publishing, 1988;67–84.
96. Kirklin J, Westaby S, Blackstone E, et al. Complement and the damaging effects of cardiopulmonary bypass. J Thorac Cardiovasc Surg 1983;86:845–857.
97. Millar A, Armstrong L, van der Linden J, et al. Cytokine production and hemodilution in children undergoing cardiopulmonary bypass. Ann Thorac Surg 1993;56:1499–1502.
98. Steinberg J, Kapelanski D, Olson J, et al. Cytokine and complement levels in patients undergoing cardiopulmonary bypass. J Thorac Cardiovasc Surg 1993;106:1008–1016.
99. Lucchesi B. Complement activation, neutrophils, and oxygen radicals in reperfusion injury. Stroke 1993;24(12, suppl 1):I41–I47.
100. del Zoppo G. Microvascular changes during cerebral ischemia and reperfusion. Cerebrovasc Brain Metab Rev 1994;6:47–96.
101. Elliot M, Finn A. Interaction between neutrophils and endothelium. Ann Thorac Surg 1993;56: 1503–1508.
102. Feuerstein G, Liu T, Barone F. Cytokines, inflammation, and brain injury: role of tumor necrosis factor-a. Cerebrovasc Brain Metab Rev 1994;6:341–360.
103. du Plessis A, Chang A, Wessel D, et al. Cerebrovascular accidents following the Fontan procedure. Pediatr Neurol 1995;12:230–236.
104. Rosenthal D, Friedman A, Kleinman C, et al. Thromboembolic complications after Fontan operations. Circulation 1995;92(suppl II):287–293.
105. Rosenthal D, Bulbul Z, Friedman A, et al. Thrombosis of the pulmonary artery stump after distal ligation. J Thorac Cardiovasc Surg 1995;110:1563–1565.
106. Clancy R, Malin S, Laraque D, et al. Focal motor seizures heralding stroke in full-term infants. Am J Dis Child 1985;139:601–606.
107. del Zoppo G, Ferbert A, Otis S, et al. Local intra-arterial fibrinolytic therapy in acute carotid territory stroke: a pilot study. Stroke 1988;19:307–313.
108. Mori E, Tabuchi M, Yoshida T, Yamadori A. Intracarotid urokinase with thromboembolic occlusion of the middle cerebral artery. Stroke 1988;19:802–812.
109. Gerlach M, Riederer P, Youdim M. Neuroprotective therapeutic strategies: comparison of experimental and clinical results. Biochem Pharmacol 1995;50:1–16.
110. Lees K. Therapeutic interventions in acute stroke. Br J Clin Pharmacol 1992;34:486–493.
111. Vannucci R. Current and potentially new management strategies for perinatal hypoxic-ischemic encephalopathy. Pediatrics 1990;85:961–968.
112. Anderson D. Cardioembolic stroke: primary and secondary prevention. Postgrad Med 1991;90(8):67–77.
113. Cerebral Embolism Study Group. Immediate anticoagulation of embolic stroke: brain hemorrhage and management options. Stroke 1984;15:779–789.
114. Cerebral Embolism Study Group. Cardioembolic stroke, immediate anticoagulation, and brain hemorrhage. Arch Intern Med 1987;147:636–640.
115. Cerebral Embolism Task Force. Cardiogenic brain embolism. The second report of the Cerebral Embolism Task Force. Arch Neurol 1989;46:727–743.
116. Hart R, Easton J. Hemorrhagic infarcts. Stroke 1986;17:586–589.
117. Furlan A, Cavalier S, Hobbs R, et al. Hemorrhage and anticoagulation after nonseptic brain infarction. Neurology 1982;32:280–282.
118. Horning C, Dorndorf W, Agnoli A. Hemorrhagic cerebral infarction—a prospective study. Stroke 1986;17:179–185.
119. Okada Y, Yamaguchi T, Minematsu K, et al. Hemorrhagic transformation in cerebral embolism. Stroke 1989;20:598–603.
120. Sherman D, Dyken M, Fisher M, et al. Antithrombotic therapy for cerebrovascular disorders. Chest 1992;102:529S–537S.
121. Pessin M, Estol C, Lafranchise F, Caplan L. Safety of anticoagulation after hemorrhagic infarction. Neurology 1993;43:1298–1303.
122. Yatsu F, Hart R, Mohr J, Grotta J. Anticoagulation of embolic strokes of cardiac origin: an update. Neurology 1988;38:314–316.

123. Aicardi J. Diseases of the Nervous System in Childhood. In Clinics in Developmental Medicine (vol 115/118). London: Mac Keith Press, 1992;590–696.
124. Rosman P, Shands K. Hydrocephalus caused by increased intracranial venous pressure: a clinico-pathological study. Ann Neurol 1978;3:445–450.
125. Glauser T, Rorke K, Weinberg P, Clancy R. Congenital brain anomalies associated with the hypoplastic left heart syndrome. Pediatrics 1990;85:984–990.
126. Jones M. Anomalies of the brain and congenital heart disease: a study of 52 necropsy cases. Pediatr Pathol 1991;11:721–736.
127. Saiman L, Prince A, Gersony W. Pediatric infective endocarditis. Brain 1993;122:847–853.
128. Jones H, Sieker R. Neurologic manifestations of infective endocarditis. Brain 1989;122:1295–1315.
129. Pruitt A, Rubin R, Karchmer A, et al. Neurologic complications of bacterial endocarditis. Medicine 1978;57:329–343.
130. Ghosh S, Chandy M, Abraham J. Brain abscess and congenital heart disease. J Indian Med Assoc 1988;88:312–314.
131. Tyler R, Clark D. Cerebrovascular accidents in patients with congenital heart disease. Arch Neurol Psychiatry 1957;77:483–489.
132. Shu-yuan Y. Brain abscess associated with congenital heart disease. Surg Neurol 1989;31:129–132.
133. Aebi C, Kaufman F, Schaad U. Brain abscess in congenital heart disease. J Neurosurg 1991;150:282–286.
134. Kagawa M, Takeshita M, Yato S, Kitamura K. Brain abscess in congenital heart disease. J Neurosurg 1983;58:913–917.
135. Dodge P, Pomeroy S. Parameningeal Infections (Including Brain Abscess, Epidural Abscess, Subdural Empyema). In R Feigin, J Cherry (eds), Textbook of Pediatric Infectious Diseases (3rd ed) (vol II). Philadelphia: Saunders, 1992;455–459.
136. Berg B, Franklin G, Cuneo R, et al. Nonsurgical cure of brain abscess: early diagnosis and follow-up with computerized tomography. Ann Neurol 178;3:474–478.
137. Rosenblum M, Hoff J, Norman D, et al. Nonoperative treatment of brain abscess in selected high-risk patients. J Neurosurg 1980;52:217–225.
138. Kurlan R, Griggs R. Cyanotic congenital heart disease with suspected stroke. Should all patients receive antibiotics? Arch Neurol 1983;40:209–212.
139. Lyon G, Adams R, Kolodny E (eds). Neurology of Inherited Metabolic Diseases of Children. New York: McGraw-Hill, 1996;327–339.
140. Rustin P, Lebidois J, Chretien D, et al. Endomyocardial biopsies for early detection of mitochondrial disorders in hypertrophic cardiomyopathies. J Pediatr 1994;124:224–228.
141. Chow C, Frerman F, Goodman S, et al. Striatal degeneration in glutaric aciduria type II. Acta Neuropathol 1989;77:554–556.
142. Guenthard J, Wyler F, Fowler B, Baumgartner R. Cardiomyopathy in respiratory chain disorders. Arch Dis Child 1995;72:223–226.
143. Zeviani M, Van Dyke D. Myopathy and fatal cardiopathy due to cytochrome c oxidase deficiency. Arch Neurol 1986;43:1198–1202.
144. Nagai T, Tuchiya Y, Taguchi Y, et al. Fatal infantile mitochondrial encephalomyelopathy with complex I and IV deficiencies. Pediatr Neurol 1993;9:151–154.
145. DiMauro S, Lombes A, Nakase H, et al. Cytochrome c oxidase deficiency. Pediatr Res 1990;28: 536–541.
146. Peterson PL. The treatment of mitochondrial myopathies and encephalomyopathies. Biochem Biophys Acta 1995;1271:275–280.
147. Przyrembel H. Therapy of mitochondrial disorders. J Inherited Metab Dis 1987;10:129–146.
148. Martin JJ, De Barsy T, De Schrijver T, et al. Acid maltase deficiency (type II glycogenosis): morphological and biochemical study of a childhood phenotype. J Neurol Sci 1976;30:155–166.
149. Morrow B, Goldberg R, Carlson C, et al. Molecular definition of the 22q11 deletions in velo-cardio-facial syndrome. Am J Hum Genet 1995;56:1391–1403.
150. Driscoll D. Genetic basis of DiGeorge and velocardiofacial syndromes. Curr Opin Pediatr 1994;6: 702–706.
151. Demczuk S, Levy A, Aubry M, et al. Excess of deletions of maternal origin in the DiGeorge/velo-cardio-facial syndromes. A study of 22 new patients and review of the literature. Hum Genet 1995; 96:9–13.
152. Shprintzen R, Goldberg R, Young D, Wolford L. The velo-cardiofacial syndrome: a clinical and genetic analysis. Pediatrics 1981;67:167–172.
153. Lindsay E, Goldberg R, Jurecic V, et al. Velo-cardio-facial syndrome: frequency and extent of 22q11 deletions. Am J Med Genet 1995;57:514–522.

154. Moss E, Wang P, McDonald-McGinn D, et al. Characteristic cognitive profile in patients with a 22q11.2 deletion: verbal IQ exceeds nonverbal IQ. Am J Hum Genet 1995;57:A20.
155. Golding-Kushner K, Weller G, Shprintzen R. Velo-cardio-facial syndrome: language and psychological profiles. J Craniofac Genet 1995;5:259–266.
156. Shprintzen R, Golding R, Golding-Kushner K, Marion R. Late-onset psychosis in the velo-cardio-facial syndrome. Am J Med Genet 1992;42:141–142.
157. Pulver A, Nestadt G, Goldberg R, et al. Psychotic illness in patient diagnosed with velo-cardio-facial syndrome and their relatives. J Nerv Ment Dis 1994;182:476–478.
158. Chapman C, du Plessis A, Pober B. Neurologic findings in children and adults with Williams syndrome. J Child Neurol 1995;10:63–65.
159. Ardinger R, Goertz K, Matteolli L. Cerebrovascular stenosis with cerebral infarction in a child with Williams syndrome. Am J Med Genet 1994;51:200–202.
160. Soper R, Chaloupka JC, Fayad PB, et al. Ischemic stroke and intracranial multifocal cerebral arteriopathy in Williams syndrome. J Pediatr 1995;126:945–948.
161. Kaplan P, Levinson M, Kaplan B. Cerebral artery stenoses in Williams syndrome cause strokes in childhood. J Pediatr 1995;126:943–945.
162. Special Writing Group of the Committee on Rheumatic Fever, Endocarditis, and Kawasaki Disease of the Council on Cardiovascular Disease in the Young of the American Heart Association. Guidelines for the diagnosis of rheumatic fever: Jones' criteria, updated 1992. JAMA 1992;268:2069–2073.
163. Eschel G, Lahat E, Azizi E, et al. Chorea as a manifestation of rheumatic fever: a 30 year survey (1960–1990). Eur J Pediatr 1993;152:645–646.
164. Ayoub E. Resurgence of rheumatic fever in the United States. Postgrad Med 1992;92:133–142.
165. Karademir S, Demirceken F, Atalay S, et al. Acute rheumatic fever in children in the Ankara area in 1990–1992 and comparison with a previous study in 1980–1989. Acta Paediatr 1994;83:862–865.
166. Swedo S, Leonard H, Schapiro M, et al. Sydenham's chorea: physical and psychological symptoms of St. Vitus dance. Pediatrics 1993;91:706–713.
167. Heye N, Jergas M, Hotzinger H, et al. Sydenham chorea: clinical, EEG, MRI, and SPECT findings in the early stages of the disease. J Neurol 1993;240:121–123.
168. Giedd J, Rapoport J, Kruesi M, et al. Sydenham's chorea: magnetic resonance imaging of the basal ganglia. Neurology 1995;45:2199–2202.
169. Aicardi J. Para-Infectious and Other Inflammatory Disorders of Immunologic Origin. In Diseases of the Nervous System in Childhood (vol 115/118). London: Mac Keith Press, 1992;698–699.
170. Figueroa F, Berrios X, Gutierrez M, et al. Anticardiolipin antibodies in acute rheumatic fever. J Rheumatol 1992;19:1175–1180.

# Index

Note: Page numbers followed by *f* indicate figures; page numbers followed by *t* indicate tables.

Hypertensive crisis, acute, headache due to, 11
Hypertensive encephalopathy, 377–379, 511–512, 512f
 causes of, 378
 clinical presentation of, 377–378
 headache due to, 11
 laboratory diagnosis of, 378
 treatment of, 378–379
Hypertonic solutions, for increased intracranial pressure, 681–682
Hyperventilation, for increased intracranial pressure, 679–681
Hyperventilation syndrome, behavioral disturbances and, 69
Hyperviscosity, headache due to, 7
Hyperviscosity syndromes, 280
 headache due to, 10
Hypocalcemia, 165–166
Hypoglycemia, coma and, management of, 38
Hypokalemia, 164–165
Hypomagnesemia, 167–168
Hypomania, differential diagnosis of, 623t
Hyponatremia, 159–163
 duration of, 159–160
 headache due to, 9
 myelinolysis following correction of, 160–162
 onset of, rapidity of, 159–160
 prognosis of, 160
 treatment of, 162–163
Hypophosphatemia, 169
Hypophyseal-pituitary axis, tumors of, headache due to, 14
Hypoprothrombinemia, 277–278
Hypothermia, for increased intracranial pressure, 682
Hypoxia, coma and, management of, 38–39
Hysteria
 behavioral disturbances and, 70–78
 conversion reaction and, 71–72
 defined, 70–71
 globus hystericus, 72
 hallmarks of, 71
 hemisensory loss with, 72–73
 hysterical deafness, 76
 hysterical gait, 74–75
 hysterical hemiparesis, 74
 hysterical hemiplegia, 73
 hysterical pain, 76–78
 hysterical rigidity, 75
 paralysis of extraocular muscles in, 73

 secondary gain in, 71
 visual hysterical symptoms, 75–76

Idiopathic vasculitides, 332–338
Iliohypogastric nerve, orthopedic surgery for, 583
Ilioinguinal nerve
 entrapment neuropathies of, 572–573
 orthopedic surgery for, 583
Immunosuppressant(s), following organ transplantation, neurologic complications of, 447–451
Inborn errors of metabolism, in children, 706–709
Incomitance, defined, 478
Incontinence, urinary, 597–603. *See also* Urinary incontinence
Industrial toxins, 127, 131, 131t
Infarcts of unknown cause, 154
Infection(s)
 drug abuse and, 113–114, 114t
 paraproteinemias and, 281
 structural congenital heart disease and, 702–705, 704f
 vasculitis due to, 338–339
Infectious diseases, headaches in patients with, 18–20. *See also specific disease, e.g.,* Meningitis
 diagnostic measure–related, 20
 neurologic, urologic problems associated with, 606–608
 treatment-related, 20
Infective endocarditis, neurologic complications of, 322–324, 323t, 324t
Infective enteritides, headache due to, 14
Inflammation
 ocular, 486–487
 orbital, 486–487
Inflammatory bowel diseases, headache due to, 14
Inflammatory demyelinating polyneuropathy, in HIV-positive patients, 197, 199
Inflammatory disease, stroke due to, 362–364, 362t
Inflammatory myopathy, in pregnancy, 527
Informed consent, ethical issues related to, 213–215
 absence of coercion in, 214–215
 adequate information in, 214
 competence in, 213–214
Infratentorial lesion, coma due to, management of, 38
Inhalant(s), 112, 112t